The Guide to the Clinical Application of Electrothermal Acupuncture Therapy

汉英对照

电热针临床应用指南

夏玉清 著　邱玺文 译

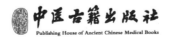

中医古籍出版社
Publishing House of Ancient Chinese Medical Books

图书在版编目（CIP）数据

电热针临床应用指南：汉英对照 / 夏玉清著；邱玺文译 . —北京：中医古籍出版社，2020.5

ISBN 978-7-5152-1839-7

Ⅰ . ①电… Ⅱ . ①夏… ②邱… Ⅲ . ①电热式—针刺疗法—指南—汉、英 Ⅳ . ① R245.31-62

中国版本图书馆 CIP 数据核字（2019）第 001819 号

电热针临床应用指南

夏玉清　著　邱玺文　译

责任编辑	张　磊　张凤霞
封面设计	韩博玥
出版发行	中医古籍出版社
社　　址	北京东直门内南小街 16 号（100700）
电　　话	010-64089446（总编室）010-64002949（发行部）
网　　址	www.zhongyiguji.com.cn
印　　刷	北京市泰锐印刷有限责任公司
开　　本	787mm×1092mm　1/16
印　　张	52
字　　数	1148 千字
版　　次	2020 年 5 月第 1 版　2020 年 5 月第 1 次印刷
书　　号	ISBN 978-7-5152-1839-7
定　　价	248.00 元

凡 例

General Principles

一、本书分上篇、下篇两部分，上篇阐述经络腧穴的概论、针灸处方的原则、针灸手法的体会；下篇论述100余种疾病以电热针为主的针灸治疗方法，是作者的临床治法以及典型病例。

二、疾病的命名与分型参照《希氏内科学》《辞海·医学卫生分册》等权威医学书籍。少数疾病无相应西医病名，针灸治疗确有良好效果者，亦酌情取录。

三、多数疾病分为诊断及辨证要点、治疗方法、注意事项、典型病例四项，少数疾病增设现代临床治疗。

四、诊断及辨证要点论述疾病的诊断、证候分类及临床表现，难以分证的病证略去此项。

五、注意事项介绍针灸处方、操作中的注意要点、针灸

1. The book is divided into two parts: Part I and Part II. Part I consists of an introduction of meridian and acupoints, the principles of acupuncture and its techniques. Part II describes more than 100 types of diseases mainly rely on electrothermal acupuncture therapy, including the author's clinical approaches and typical cases.

2. The nomenclature and classifications of diseases are based on authoritative medical textbooks, such as *Goldman's Cecil Medicine* or *Cihai: Medicine and Health*. For the few diseases that are very responsive to acupuncture but lack corresponding western names, they may also be included as appropriate.

3. Most diseases are presented from four categories, including guidelines for diagnosis and its dialectic, treatment, precautions and typical cases.

4. Guidelines for diagnosis and its dialectic consist of the actual diagnosis of the disease and classification of its manifestations as well as clinical phenomena, but those manifestations difficult to classify should be excluded.

5. Notes indicate acupuncture approaches, precautions during application, indications and treatment regi-

疗法的适应范围、疾病的调护方法等。

六、典型病例即从作者多年临床治疗本病效果确切有效者，选出典型病例，否则删去此项。

七、现代临床治疗择录了国内外针灸操作简便的临床资料，亦包括个人研究资料。部分疾病临床报道较少者，则删去此项。

八、穴位图解便于读者能准确选取穴位，尤其对自我治疗者，更有助于了解穴位的位置。

九、处方取穴遵循传统取穴原则，无论是对症取穴，还是循经取穴、局部取穴等，均以实用有效并利于国际针灸交流为基点。

十、十四经穴和部分经外奇穴，均标明英文经穴名称缩写字母及编号。穴位编号标准依据1990年国家技术监督局颁布的中华人民共和国国家标准（GB 12346-90）《经穴部位》而命名。尚未标准化的腧穴英文缩写名称，原则上不注明编号。

mens.

6. Typical cases refer to those diseases that respond positively to standard care. If no such cases are found, this item will not be included.

7. Modern clinical therapy not only quotes international and national clinical data concerning acupuncture approaches, but also includes personal research results. Those diseases with less frequent clinical reports should be ignored.

8. Anatomical illustrations of acupuncture points help readers locate acupoints accurately, particularly for self-operations.

9. The selection of acupoints relies either on disease symptoms or on meridian channels and specific locations, all of which are based on traditional principles of operational practices which led to positive results and may further facilitate research exchanges at international level.

10. Standard locations of 14 meridian points and the extraordinary meridians are all labeled with English names and abbreviations as well as codes. The principles for meridian point codes are based on the *National Standard of the People's Republic of China* (GB 12346-90), namely "Locations of Points" enacted by the State Bureau of Technical Supervision in 1990. For those English acupoint abbreviations whose standardization is still pending, in principle no coding specification is required.

前言

电热针是以中医学的经络学说和针灸"焠刺"(火针)的理论为基础,结合现代科学技术而改进的一种针刺方法,对经络学说的探讨、针麻原理的研究、针刺手法的改进、临床疗效的提高、扩大针灸的治疗病种都有一定的价值。

电热针针具的诞生,是1973年由内蒙古中蒙医研究所唐学正主任最初试制成功的(一台简易的交流电热针治疗机),之后经过不断地研究改进,最后研制成多针位晶体管直流电热针机。这种电热针机设有稳压、滤波、正流等装置,灵敏度高,温度恒定可调,适合临床应用和科学实验研究。

1974年,电热针已在门诊及巡回医疗中应用,如对风湿痹痛、脾胃病、妇科病、肾虚遗精、腱鞘囊肿等有较好的

Preface

electrothermal acupuncture therapy is an improved method based on the theory of Traditional Chinese Medicine (TCM) and acupuncture meridians appropriate to *cui ci* (the fire needle) combined with modern science and technology. It also has certain influence on the discussion of meridian theory, research of acupuncture and anesthesia principles, improved acupuncture techniques, increased clinical efficiency as well as the expanding range of diseases treatable through acupuncture.

The electrothermal needle (a simple AC electrothermal acupuncture equipment) was originally invented by Dr. TANG Xuezheng in 1973, the chairman of Graduate Institute of Traditional Chinese and Mongolian Medicine, Inner Mongolia Autonomous Region. After continuous testing and improvement, a multi-needle transistorized DC electrothermal acupuncture equipment was eventually developed. The equipment composes a stabilizer, a filter and a rectifier, with a highly-sensitive thermostat and is applicable to clinical practice as well as scientific research.

In 1974, electrothermal acupuncture therapy was used in outpatient clinics and mobile health care. Because of its better efficacy for rheumatic pain, digestive diseases, gynecological diseases, insufficient kidney

疗效，深受患者的欢迎。1979年，电热针开始用于治疗肿瘤的动物实验研究，运用电热针对3种小鼠可移植性癌有抑制作用，治疗长径为0.7～1cm的肿瘤时宜用140～195卡，治疗时间为40分钟。治疗时，肿瘤中心的温度（56℃）高于肿瘤周围的温度（44～47℃）。经1次治疗后，对荷前胃鳞癌小鼠的治愈率为60%，肿瘤完全消退率为78%～83.3%，肿瘤生长抑制率为84.8%～90.6%；对荷乳腺癌小鼠的治愈率为50%～68%，肿瘤完全消退率为76%～83.3%，肿瘤生长抑制率为84.8%～90.6%；对荷肝癌小鼠的治愈率为70%～88%，肿瘤完全消退率为88.2%～90%，肿瘤生长抑制率为84.2%～94.4%；对肝癌小鼠进行重复实验时，治疗组的转移率为0/17，对照组的转移率为7/17，说明电热针并不增加小鼠肝癌的转移率。经过3年多的努力，完成了电热针对小鼠可移植性癌抑制作用的实验研究。1983年通过了阶段性的成果鉴定，肯定了电热针对3种小鼠可移植性癌（肝癌、乳腺癌、前胃鳞癌）的抑

output as well as ganglion cysts, electrothermal acupuncture therapy was well received by patients. In 1979, electrothermal acupuncture therapy started to be used for tumor treatment in animal research. The application of electrothermal acupuncture therapy has shown inhibitory effects on three transplantable mice cancer models. For example, when treating a diameter of 0.7～1cm tumor, the therapeutic dose should be approximately 140～195 calories for 40 minutes, and the central temperature of the tumor shall reach up to 56 ℃, which is higher than the surrounding temperature (44～47℃). After a session of treatment, the cure rate of squamous carcinoma of gastric cardia in mice was about 60%, the tumor complete regression rate was between 78%～83.3%, and the tumor growth inhibition rate was between 84.8%～90.6%. For breast adenocarcinoma in mice, the cure rate was between 50%～68%, the tumor complete regression rate was between 76%～83.3%, and the tumor growth inhibition rate was between 84.8%～90.6%. For liver cancer in mice, the cure rate was between 70%～88%, the tumor complete regression rate was between 88.2%～90%, and the tumor growth inhibition rate was between 84.2%～94.4%. When conducting repeated experiments in mice with liver cancer, the cancer metastatic rate of therapeutic group was 0/17 while that of control group was 7/17, suggesting that the electrothermal acupuncture therapy did not increase the metastatic rate of liver cancer in mice models. Over more than 3 years of efforts, the experimental study investigating inhibitory effects of electrothermal acupuncture therapy on three transplantable mice cancer models has been completed. According

制作用,为开展电热针治癌临床应用提供了科学依据。

1983年6月9日,中蒙医研究所接受首例患者。包某,女性,74岁,确诊为左颜面部鳞状上皮癌Ⅰ级,经电热针治疗5次,瘤体结痂,21天后痂皮自然脱落,经组织学检查,未发现癌细胞。复经1年5个月的随访,患者健康状态良好,并无复发。1983年11月2日,我院(中国中医科学院针灸研究所)接受2例患者,一例为神经细胞癌,经8次电热针治疗后痊愈,1年后随访未见复发。一例为晚期乳腺癌手术后复发,已不能接受放、化疗,并有播散性转移,经电热针治疗后,局部病灶明显缩小,转移灶消失,半年后患者返回原籍。1年后随访,该患者复发灶尚存,但生活尚可自理。

to the preliminary results in 1983, the inhibitory effects of electrothermal acupuncture therapy on three transplantable mice cancer models (i.e. liver cancer, breast adenocarcinoma and squamous carcinoma of gastric cardia) was confirmed, which also provided scientific evidence for its clinical applications.

Therefore, the Graduate Institute of Traditional Chinese and Mongolian Medicine received the first patient for electrothermal acupuncture therapy on June 9th, 1983. The patient (BAO) was a 74-year-old female with a definite diagnosis of Class I squamous cell carcinoma (SCC) on her left face. After 5 electrothermal acupuncture therapy treatments, the tumor started to form scars, and the crust fell off 21 days after treatment. The histology results then showed freedom from cancer cells during the 1 year and 5 months' follow-ups, the patient remained healthy without any cancer recurrence. On November 2nd, 1983, the Institute of Acupuncture and Moxibustion, China Academy of Chinese Medical Sciences admitted 2 cases, and one of the patients had neural cell carcinoma. The patient was cured after receiving 8 electrothermal acupuncture treatments, and showed no recurrence during the 1-year follow-up. Another case was a breast cancer patient at an advanced stage with post-operative recurrence and metastasis, who was not indicated for radio- or chemotherapy. After receiving electrothermal acupuncture therapy, the size of the local lesion was significantly reduced, and the metastatic lesions also disappeared. Six months later, the patient was discharged and returned home. During the 1-year follow-up, the patient still had recurrent lesions, but was able to function inde-

截至1985年末,我院相继用电热针治疗各种浅表肿瘤130例。其中,皮肤鳞状上皮癌38例,原位癌37例,乳腺癌8例,直肠癌5例,宫颈癌4例,纤维肉瘤4例,神经细胞瘤5例,黑色素瘤4例,腭扁桃体瘤2例,溶骨性成骨肉瘤4例,乳腺癌淋巴转移3例,其他肿瘤16例。

1985年7月,课题组接受卫生部课题《电热针治疗皮肤癌的临床疗效及机理研究》,1986年接受国家中医药管理局课题《电热针治疗女阴白色病变的临床疗效与机理研究》,1987年接受中国中医科学院课题《电热针治疗萎缩性胃炎的临床疗效及机理研究》,上述课题的研究目的是预防肿瘤的发生。经过研究发现,电热针能够使食道黏膜、胃黏膜以及外阴黏膜的非典型增生部位的组织细胞转化为正常组织细胞,这是预防癌症发生的可喜苗头。同时,开展治疗免疫系统疾病(如类风湿性关节炎、系统红斑狼疮)、内分泌系统疾病(如2型糖尿病)等25种疾病,并逐步扩大了电热针在临

pendently for daily living.

Until the end of 1985, we used the electrothermal acupuncture therapy to treat a total of 130 cases with various superficial tumors. Among them, there were 38 skin squamous cell carcinoma, 37 in carcinoma, 8 breast cancer, 5 colorectal cancer, 4 cervical cancer, 4 fibrosarcoma, 5 neural cell carninoma, 4 melanoma, 2 palatine and tonsil cancer, 4 osteolytic osteosarcoma, 3 breast cancer with lymphatic metastasis, and 16 other tumor types.

In July 1985, the research team was delegated by the Ministry of Health of PRC with a research topic entitled "The Clinical Efficacy and Mechanism of Prescription of electrothermal Acupuncture Therapy for Patients with Melanoma". In 1986, the State Administration of Traditional Chinese Medicine of PRC delegated a topic entitled "The Clinical Efficacy and Mechanism of Prescription of electrothermal Acupuncture Therapy for Patients with Leukoplakia Vulvae" to us. In 1987, we received an assignment from China Academy of Chinese Medical Sciences regarding "The Clinical Efficacy and Mechanism of Prescription of electrothermal Acupuncture Treatment for Patients with Atrophic Gastritis". All of the above topics focus on the prevention of tumors. After a series of research, the results showed that electrothermal acupuncture therapy could revert atypical mucosal hyperplasia in esophagus, stomach and vulvae to normal cells/tissues, which was a positive sign for cancer preventions. At the same time, electrothermal acupuncture therapy was also found effective on treatment for

床上的应用及适应证。

电热针在临床上取得较好的疗效，深受患者的欢迎。为了使更多的患者能够有机会接受电热针治疗，首先应积极向基层医疗单位培训人才，推广应用，为广大患者造福；其次，电热针具现已有厂家研制，针的质量、电热针机的功能越来越精细，越来越实用，再也不必为电热针具供不应求而担心和焦急。

2009年12月，我编写的《电热针临床应用指南》（中文版）出版，由此夙愿得偿，此书受到了广大热心读者、行业专家的欢迎和肯定。自此至2019己亥之年，十年期间，电热针在文化传承和技术发展、治疗应用方面又有长足进步：一是中医针灸凭借国家"一带一路"的倡议走出去的势头更猛，随着国家的崛起和软实力的提升，针灸等中国文化更加被全球认可和接受；二是电热针在美容等领域有新的应用。

25 types of illnesses such as immune dysfunctions (e.g. rheumatoid arthritis, systemic lupus erythematosus) and endocrine system diseases (e.g. type II diabetes). In other words, the clinical applications and indications of electrothermal acupuncture therapy were at a broader scale.

Given its visible effects, electrothermal acupuncture therapy has become a popular approach nowadays. To enable more patients to gain access to such therapy and to benefit the mass public, the priority is to promote professional training and clinical applications at local medical institutes. electrothermal acupuncture equipment has become available now through R&D by manufacturers. Not only has the quality of the needles has improved, the functioning of the equipment has also become more accurate, allowing more practical applications. Therefore, the problem of supplying and obtaining electrothermal acupuncture equipments and tools is no longer an issue.

In December 2009, as I published the "The Guide to the Clinical Application of Electrothermal Acupuncture Therapy" (Chinese version), my hope has been realized. This book has been welcomed and affirmed by enthusiastic readers and industry experts. 2019, in this Chinese year of the pig, for a decade, the electrothermal acupuncture therapy has made great progress in its cultural inheritance, technology development and therapeutic application. First, acupuncture of Traditional Chinese Medicine has borrowed the stronger momentum of "Belt and Road" Initiative, along with the country's improvement in status and soft power. Acupuncture and Chinese culture have then been recognized and accepted across the world. Second, electrothermal acupuncture has had new

面对新情况、新发展、新需求,我深感需要对电热针临床及教学、科研经验再次进行总结和研究,编著出版《电热针临床应用指南》(中英文),以助电热针疗法能够在国内、国际上更好地推广和应用。本书在各方支持下如期出版,在此,衷心感谢清华大学,和参与出版的我的学生们、其他人士所做之贡献,也感谢卢兰兰女士为本书出版的协调。一并致谢如下(以下排名不分先后):

合作机构:清华大学教育基金会 清华大学公共健康研究中心

英文翻译:邱玺文

英文校对:卢兰兰 符晓东 曹代勇

英文审定:林 巍

(杭州师范大学 外国语学院 翻译研究所 特聘教授)

项目组:陈 晨 邓娅男 綦菁菁

由于时间有限,书中错误

applications in the fields of beauty and so on. In the face of new situations, developments and demands, I deeply feel the need to re-synthesize and research the clinical and teaching experience of electrothermal acupuncture, and thus publish the "The Guide to the Clinical Application of electrothermal Accupuncture Therapy" (in both Chinese and English) to help electrothermal acupuncture therapies, in order to better promote and apply it both nationally and internationally. The book was published as scheduled with the support of all parties. Here, I would like to express my sincere gratitude to Tsinghua University, to the contributions of my students and other people who participated in the publication, and to Mrs. LU Lanlan for the coordination of the publication of this book. Acknowledgments are as follows (the following rankings are in no particular order):

Partners: Tsinghua University Education Foundation, Tsinghua University Research Center for Public Health

English translation: Simon CHIU

English Proofreading: LU Lanlan, FU Xiaodong, CAO Daiyong

English certification: LIN Wei

(Special Professor, Institute of Translation Studies, School of Foreign Languages, Hangzhou Normal University)

Project Group: CHEN Chen, DENG Yanan, QI Jingjing

Due to the limited time, the mistakes in the book

之处在所难免，望广大读者提出宝贵的意见和建议。

夏玉清

2019 年 8 月于北京

are inevitable, and the readers are expected to provide valuable comments and suggestions.

XIA Yuqing

August 2019, Beijing

目 录

凡例	i
前言	iii

上篇 理论溯源

电热针概论   **1**

概述	1
特点	4
实验与临床	6
防治肿瘤	9
电热针量化问题	18

电热针应用   **21**

传统针具概述	21
电热针结构名称、保养和消毒	21
针刺练习法	23
针刺前准备	26
进针	28
针感	33
行针	34

Table of Contents

General Principles	i
Preface	iii

Part I Theories and History

Introductions of electrothermal acupuncture therapy   **1**

Overview	1
Features	4
Experiments and clinical applications	6
Cancer prevention	9
Quantitative issues	18

The application of electrothermal acupuncture therapy   **21**

Overview of traditional needles	21
The components of the electrothermal needle, the maintenance and aseptic measures	21
Needling practice	23
Preparations before needling	26
Needle insertion	28
Needling sensation	33
Needle manipulation	34

留针	36	Needle retention	36
出针	36	Needle withdrawal	36
针次与间隔	37	Needling frequency and intervals	37
异常现象及处理	37	Abnormalities and the handlings	37

经络总论 44

General principles of meridians 44

经络系统的内容与分类	44	The contents and categories of the meridian system	44
十二经脉命名、分布及循行规律	46	The nomenclature, distribution and running rules of twelve regular meridians	46
经络的作用	48	The functions of meridians	48

腧穴 51

Acupoints 51

概述	51	Overview	51
取穴方法	52	Methods of locating acupoints	52
十四经穴选要	56	Acupoint guidelines for fourteen meridians	56

电热针的治疗原则 117

Therapeutic principles of the electrothermal acupuncture therapy 117

辨证论治	117	Treatment for syndrome differentiation	117

下篇 临床论治

Part II: Clinical Treatment

内科疾病	**127**	**Medical illness**	**127**
慢性支气管炎	127	Chronic Bronchitis	127
支气管哮喘	136	Asthma	136
支气管扩张症	145	Bronchiectasis	145
原发性高血压	153	High Blood Pressure	153
低血压	163	Low Blood Pressure	163
冠状动脉粥样硬化性心脏病	166	Coronary Atherosclerotic Heart Diseases	166
风湿性心脏病	175	Rheumatic Heart Diseases	175

病毒性心肌炎	181	Viral Myocarditis	181
心律失常	184	Arrhythmia	184
心脏神经官能症	187	Cardiac Neurosis	187
慢性胃炎	194	Chronic Gastritis	194
胃下垂	207	Gastroptosis	207
幽门梗阻	212	Pylorochesis	212
胆道疾病及结石症	219	Biliary Tract Diseases and Lithiasis	219
腹痛	223	Abdominal Pain	223
肠麻痹	232	Enteroparalysis	232
慢性腹泻（肠炎）	234	Chronic Diarrhea (Enteritis)	234
慢性结肠炎	239	Chronic Colitis	239
营养障碍性水肿	249	Trophopathic Edema	249
慢性肾小球肾炎	256	Chronic Glomerulonephritis	256
肾盂肾炎	263	Pyelonephritis	263
尿失禁	269	Urinary Incontinence	269
尿道炎	272	Urethritis	272
膀胱炎	275	Urocystitis	275
老年痴呆症	279	Alzheimer's Disease	279
脑卒中	287	Cerebrovascular Diseases	287
共济失调	304	Ataxia	304
大脑发育不全	310	Cerebral Agenesis	310
多发性神经炎	316	Multiple Neuritis	316
坐骨神经痛	324	Sciatica	324
臀上皮神经麻痹	330	Superior Gluteal Cutaneous Nerve Paralysis	330
脊髓炎	332	Myelitis	332
强直性脊柱炎	338	Ankylosing Spondylitis	338
进行性肌营养不良	342	Progressive Muscular Dystrophy（Type DMD）	**342**
多发性硬化	355	Multiple Sclerosis	355
脊髓空洞症	367	Syringomyelia	367
重症肌无力	376	Myasthenia Gravis	376
脑外伤后神经症	382	Neurosis After Traumatic Brain Injury	382

风湿性关节炎	386	Rheumatoid Arthritis	386
类风湿性关节炎	392	Rheumatoid Arthritis	392
雷诺病	398	Raynaud Disease	398
多发性大动脉炎（无脉症）	401	Takayasu's Arteritis (Pulseless Disease)	401
高脂血症	404	Hyperlipidemia	404
糖尿病	409	Diabetes	409
甲状腺腺瘤	422	Thyroid Adenoma	422
多汗症	426	Hyperhidrosis	426
食道癌	430	Esophagus Cancer	430
肺癌	447	Lung Cancer	447
胃癌	462	Stomach Cancer	462
肝癌	477	Liver Cancer	477
大肠癌	495	Colorectal Cancer	495
晚期癌肿	509	Advanced Cancer	509
肿瘤放疗与化疗之副反应	512	Side Effects of Tumor Radiotherapy and Chemotherapy 512	

妇科疾病	**516**	**Gynecological diseases**	**516**
月经不调	516	Menoxenia	516
痛经	529	Dysmenorrhea	529
闭经	538	Amenorrhea	538
白带增多症	546	Leukorrhagia	546
盆腔炎	556	Pelvic Inflammatory Disease	556
外阴瘙痒	563	Pruritus Vulvae	563
女阴白色病变	567	Vulva White Lesion	567
功能性子宫出血	573	Functional Uterine Hemorrhage	573
子宫脱垂	579	Uterine Prolapse	579
不孕症	583	Infertilitas Feminis	583
更年期综合征	594	Menopausal Syndrome	594
子宫肌瘤	607	Hysteromyoma	607
乳房纤维腺瘤	609	Breast Fibroadenoma	609

中文	页码	English	Page
乳腺癌	612	Breast Cancer	612
宫颈癌	622	Cervical Cancer	622
男科疾病	**627**	**Men's diseases**	**627**
阳痿	627	Asynodia	627
早泄	636	Premature Ejaculation	636
遗精	644	Spermatorrhea	644
不射精症	652	Anejaculation	652
无精子症	659	Azoospermia	659
精液异常	662	Semen Abnormalities	662
前列腺炎	670	Prostatitis	670
皮外骨伤科疾病	**682**	**Diseases of dermasurgery and orthopedics**	**682**
皮肤鳞状细胞癌	682	Squamous Cell Carcinoma of Skin	682
指间关节扭伤	689	Sprain of Interphalangeal Joint	689
腕关节扭伤	691	Sprain of Waist Joint	691
菱形肌劳损	693	Strain of Rhomboid Muscle	693
胸壁挫伤	695	Contusion of Thoracic Wall	695
肩关节周围炎	697	Scapulohumeral Periarthritis	697
肱二头肌短头肌腱损伤	700	Tendon Injuries of Short Head of Biceps Brachii	700
三角纤维软骨盘损伤	702	Injuries of Triangular Fibrous Cartilage Plate	702
腰肌扭伤	704	Sprain of Psoas	704
梨状肌损伤综合征	706	Syndrome of Piriformis Injuries	706
踝关节扭伤	708	Sprain of Ankle Joint	708
足跟腱扭伤	710	Achilles Tendon Sprain	710
足跟外侧皮神经损伤	712	Heel Lateral Cutaneous Nerve Injuries	712
腓肠肌损伤	714	Gastrocnemius Injuries	714
颈椎病	716	Cervical Spondylosis	716
腰椎间盘突出症	724	Protrusion of Lumbar Intervertebral Disc	724
增生性骨性关节病	729	Proliferative Osteoarthritis	729

五官科疾病	735	ENT diseases	735
眼睑跳动症	735	Eyelid Subsultus	735
虹膜睫状体炎	739	Iridocyclitis	739
视网膜色素变性	745	Retinal Pigment Degeneration	745
视神经萎缩	750	Optic Atrophy	750
夜盲	753	Nyctalopia	753
保健与美容	**758**	**Health and beauty**	**758**
预防慢性支气管炎和支气管哮喘	758	Prevention of Chronic Bronchitis	758
预防胃肠病	764	Prevention of Gastro-intestinal Diseases	764
预防高血压	767	Prevention of High Blood Pressure	767
预防冠心病	774	Prevention of Coronary Heart Disease	774
预防中风	778	Stroke Prevention	778
预防感冒	785	Cold Prevention	785
预防流行性腮腺炎	789	Mumps Prevention	789
防治痢疾	791	Dysentery Prevention	791
减肥	794	Antiobesity	794
美容	804	Cosmetology	804

上篇　理论溯源　Part I Theories and History

电热针概论

Introductions of electrothermal acupuncture therapy

概述

"焠刺"（即火针）是针灸中重要的针刺方法。《灵枢·官针》载："凡刺有九，以应九变……九曰焠刺，焠刺者，刺燔针则取痹者也。"在《灵枢·经筋》中，凡属十二经筋的疾病，都有"治在燔针劫刺，以知为数，以痛为输"的论述。从《内经》的记载中看出，"焠刺"对于"诸痹"和"经筋"的疾病是一种有效的针刺方法，历代医家都积累了丰富的实践经验，在民间也广为流传。

Overview

Cui Ci (namely the "fire needle") is one of the important approaches in acupuncture therapy. In the book *Lingshu Jing* (a theoretical book regarding Traditional Chinese Medicine), section "Guan Zhen (concerning recognized acupuncture tools and approaches)": "For 9 different types of diseases, there should be 9 types of acupuncture approaches."; "The 9th approach is the fire needle; that is, using a fire needle to treat paralysis." As to the treatment for diseases associated with the musculature of the 12 meridians, the same book, section "Jing Jin (musculature)": "Find the trigger point as the target acupoint, apply a fire needle into the acupoint with quick insertion and withdrawal. The patient should feel warmth at the insertion site." The book *Neijing* (the oldest medical theoretical book) indicated that *Cui Ci* (the fire needle)" was an effective approach for diseases such as

前人的成就和实践经验，给予我们很大的启示，电热针是根据经络学说及《内经》"燔针""焠刺"的理论，并结合现代科学技术研发的一种新型针具，它是对传统火针的继承与改进，具有针刺与温灸之共性，类似火针，但又优于火针。传统的火针一般在刺入机体后，针体自然冷却，温度随之降低，因而很难在体内维持恒定的温度；并且火针只能疾刺疾出，不能留针，刺入"太深恐伤经络，太浅不能去病"。电热针利用电能转换为热能，在针刺得气后的留针时间内，使针体保持恒定的温热效应，可根据患者的机体状态，较准确地调整针体的温度。根据《素问·缪刺论》"寒则热之"和《灵枢·经脉》"虚则补之"的理论，改善、调节气血在经络中的运行状态，通过扶正祛邪，调整阴阳，达到防病治病的目的。这样可使古典的"焠刺"与现代技术结合起来而得到改进。

"paralysis" or concerning "aponeurotic systems". From this, previous physicians (practitioners) clearly had accumulated experience in clinical practice, and the approach was widely disseminated.

These ancestors' achievements and clinical experience have provided great inspiration to modern approaches. electrothermal acupuncture therapy is an advanced approach/equipment based on meridian theories and the "fire needle" concept described in *Neijing*, and in combination with modern technology. It is not only an improvement which inherited the core idea of traditional fire needles, but also has the common features of acupuncture and thermal therapy. In other words, it is an approach similar to fire needles but with superior functions. One of the drawbacks of traditional fire needles was their rapid drop in temperature. In other words, the acupuncture needle cooled down automatically once needle insertion was performed. In this case, the control of needle temperature at a constant level is very challenging. In addition, fire needles only allow quick insertion and withdrawal, needle retention being prohibited. More importantly, the depth of needle insertion is also strictly regulated since "too deep may injure the meridian while too shallow is not curative". The electrothermal acupuncture therapy transforms electricity into heat. After needle insertion, the needle remains at constant temperature during retention. Moreover, the practitioner is allowed to control the temperature of the needle more accurately based on the status of the patient. Based on the principles "treating cold syndromes with hot-natured drugs" (described in the book *Neijing*, "Suwen" part, Section "Miu

电热针针温范围为30～700℃（暗红色），温度集中在针尖部位，临床应用并无皮肤损伤。动物测温实验中可见体外针温在350℃以内，与体内针温相差3倍，无组织坏死，临床针温监测基本相同。针温超过350℃，随着温度的升高，可引起组织炎性反应，700℃可引起针体周围的组织坏死甚至炭化。根据电热针针温调节的控制范围，其具有针刺、温针、火针的共同作用。当输入电流后，温热感可透入机体深部并可传导扩散，随着电流的增大，温度的增高，其作用同于火针，且温度恒定可调，它是目前将热辐射引入机体深部而使中心散热的较为理想的送热工具。

Ci (one of the acupuncture approaches)"); and "treating a deficiency syndrome with enhancing methods" (in the Book *Lingshu Jing*, Section "Jing Mai(channel)"), electrothermal acupuncture therapy can improve and modulate Qi and blood circulation, strengthen vital Qi and eliminate pathogenic factors, and balance Yin-Yang in order to achieve disease prevention and treatment. So electrothermal acupuncture therapy is a refined method combining traditional "fire needle" concepts and modern technologies.

The temperature control of the electrothermal acupuncture equipment ranges from 30~700℃ (dark red), and the heat mainly accumulates on the tip of the needle. Therefore, no skin lesion has been observed during clinical practice. In animal studies, if the temperature of the needle in vitro were within 350℃, which is 3 times differences relative to in vivo temperature, no tissue necrosis is observed. Based on the same principles of clinical monitoring over needle temperature, if the temperature of the needle was above 350 ℃ or even higher, tissue inflammatory issue reactions started to appear. For example, needle temperature up to 700 ℃ could cause tissue necrosis or even charring of the surrounding areas. According to the temperature control of the electrothermal acupuncture equipment, the needle can function as acupuncture, warm needle or fire needle. After turning on the power, the heat will be generated inside the equipment and transmitted to the needle through heat dissemination. The stronger the power, the higher the temperature. The function of electrothermal acupuncture therapy is similar to fire needles, but the temperature of the former is stable and controllable. It is an ideal heat generation and transmission technology by disseminating heat into precise depth while at the same time maintaining the temperature at the core.

特点

一、电热针对针刺感应稳定可调

近年来，科研人员对经络实质的探讨及针麻原理的研究做了大量的科学研究工作，尽管学说各异、结论不同，但在研究方法上都是从针刺的感应入手。电热针的针刺感应稳定可调，在留针时间内，电热针传导感应的强弱和温度的变化与输入电流成正比，电流截断后，感应立即消失，接通电源后，电热感应立即再现。感应的痕迹作用，可继续保留数小时或1～2天。由于在留针时间内始终保持针感且稳定可调，这样就便于固定经络传导放散的部位，对经络实质的探讨提供了有利的条件。

Features

I. The needling sensation of the electrothermal acupuncture therapy is stable and adjustable.

In recent years, research scientists have conducted massive scientific studies on substantial meridians and acupuncture principles. Although the theories and conclusions were diversified, all studies investigated the needling sensation as the starting point. The needling sensation of the electrothermal acupuncture therapy is stable and adjustable. During needle retention, the intensity of the needling sensation as well as the changes in temperature of electrothermal acupuncture therapy are proportional to the input current. If the power is switched off, the needling sensation disappears immediately; however, the sensation resumes promptly once the power is switched back again. The needling sensation may remain for a few hours to 1-2 days. Because the needling sensation of the electrothermal acupuncture therapy remains stable and adjustable during needle retention, it provides stability to target meridian channels, and therefore provides a useful condition to explore the essence of meridians.

二、电热针与电针的针感差异

电热针利用电能转化为热能的原理作用于机体而产生针感,它不同于针麻仪或电针直流脉冲的作用,电热针针体绝缘,刺入机体不发生电干扰现象。电热针与普通电针产生的针感不同,前者利用电热刺激产生感应,后者利用电脉冲刺激产生针感。

三、电热针具有针刺、火针、灸疗的共同作用

电热针刺入机体后,在未输入电流前同于一般针刺,输入电流后具有火针与灸疗的作用。温热感可透入机体的深部并传导扩散,且不会烫伤皮肤。随着电流的加大,温度增高,则具有"焠刺"(火针)的作用,并且温度恒定持久。

II. The differences in the needling sensation between the electrothermal acupuncture and electrical acupuncture therapy.

The generation of needling sensation is based on the principle of converting electrical energy into heat. Unlike the direct current impulses generated by the acupuncture anesthesia apparatus or the electrical acupuncture therapy, the needle body of the electrothermal acupuncture therapy is an insulator, which does not cause electrical interference when the needle is inserted into human bodies. The needling sensation generated by the electrothermal acupuncture therapy is therefore different from that of regular electrical needles. The former uses electrothermal stimulation to develop the needling sensation while the latter uses electrical pulses to create this sensation.

III. electrothermal acupuncture therapy combines the effects derived from needle insertion, fire needles and acupuncture therapy.

Electrothermal acupuncture therapy combines the effects derived from needle insertion, fire needles and acupuncture therapy. Before switching on the power, the effects of the electrothermal acupuncture therapy are similar to regular needle insertion into human bodies. It works like fire acupuncture needles once the power of the equipment has been switched on. The warm-to-hot sensation penetrates into human bodies to the required depth and is transmitted to surrounding tissues without burning the skin. The temperature of the needle increases with the strength of the current, and the thermostatic effects remain for a long time, are both the common features of *Cui Ci* (fire needle)

实验与临床

电热针研制工作始于 1973 年初，经过几十年的科学实验和临床观察，认为电热针对经络实质的探讨、针灸理论的研究、临床疗效的提高都有一定的价值。

一、经络感传的定向、定位

经络是人体客观存在的独立生理系统，在针刺条件下能更明显地观察到经络的感传和隐现。由于电热针对机体内部的感应器官具有持续性温热刺激且稳定可调的独特效应，因此，给经络感传的定向、定位提供了客观的观察手段。通过几十年的临床观察，凡接受电热针治疗的患者，不分年龄、性别、病种、穴位，在针刺后的留针时间内，均保留有经络感传的方向、部位、范围，并可重复再现。这样就改善了在"得气"停施手法后，经络感传瞬间消失的现象，同时也可以减少患者对感传现象的暗示

Experiments and clinical applications

The establishment of electrothermal acupuncture therapy started at the beginning of 1973. After decades of scientific research and clinical observations, electrothermal acupuncture therapy was regarded as beneficial from substantial research exploration into meridian research on the theory of acupuncture and improving its clinical efficacy.

I. The orientation and location of meridian routes

Meridians are an independent and objective physiological system which exists in human bodies. The conductance and appearance of meridian sensation is more obvious during needle insertion. Because electrothermal acupuncture therapy specifically provides constant thermal stimulation at a steady and adjustable level in human bodies, the orientation and localization of meridian therapy supplies an objective measure for clinical observations. Based on decades of clinical observations, patients in all ages and genders or with different illnesses and acupoints who received electrothermal acupuncture therapy, usually retain their sensation of meridian directions, locations and range during needle retention. And the sensation is repeatable when receiving the same meridian therapy. Such features improve the "arrival of Qi", compensates the sudden disappearance of meridian conduction, and reduce the impact for transmission on

因素。

二、针刺手法的强化和模拟

针刺手法是唤起经络感传和调节气血运行的重要手段。电热针可以强化针刺手法的持续作用,通过对家兔心电 Rvr、Svr 振幅影响的观察发现,在家兔心电 Rvr、Svr 振幅降低时,如果针刺后可见升高,加用电热针后随着温度的升高则出现继续升高的现象。在家兔心电 Rvr、Svr 振幅升高时,如果针刺后可见降低,加用电热针后随着温度的升高则出现继续降低的现象。

电热针针刺后产生的温热效应,从一定意义上可看作是传统手法"烧山火"的模拟。《针灸大成·三衢杨氏补泻》载:"烧山火之能除寒,一退三飞病自安。"临床上运用"烧山火"手法,一方面是因人而异、因病而异、因穴而异,另一方面是因术而异。有些患者出现针下热感,有些患者只出现胀、酸、麻等感觉,这与电热针出现的温热与酸、胀相兼的针感基本上是相符的。

patients after the therapy is discontinued.

II. The reinforcement and simulation of needle insertion techniques

Needle insertion is an important approach to awake meridian conduction and to regulate Qi-blood circulation. The electrothermal acupuncture therapy reinforces the tolerance of needle insertion. Echocardiograms on rabbits showed that when needle insertion increased the amplitude of rapid/slow ventricular response (RVR/SVR), the amplitude was proportional to the increase in temperature of the electrothermal acupuncture therapy. On the contrary, if needle insertion decreased the amplitude of rapid/slow ventricular response (RVR/SVR), the amplitude was inversely proportional to the increase of temperature of the electrothermal acupuncture therapy.

From a certain point of view, the thermal effects generated by electrothermal acupuncture therapy are similar to the traditional approach of "pyrogenic needling". "Yang's Three Qu Acupoints Reinforcement and Reduction" of the Book "Compendium of Acupuncture and Moxibustion" states "Pyrogenic needling with one deep insertion and three withdrawals dispels cold and heals the disease automatically." In clinical practice, the approach of "pyrogenic needling" varies depending on the practitioner, the disease, the acupoint and the technique. Some patients demonstrate thermal sensation at the insertion site; some only display swelling, soreness or numbness. All the above sensations (e.g. thermal, soreness and swelling effects) are identical to those of

三、对"调气"的探讨

动物实验中，对家兔心率变化的观察发现，心率慢的家兔（200次/分）加电热针后趋于正常心率（260次/分），心率快的家兔（300次/分）加电热针后也趋于正常心率（260次/分）。不论心率慢或快，接受电热针治疗后均是趋向正常值的，即向中的。

临床实验中，通过对肢体血流描记的观察发现，由于患者机体功能状态的差异（阴虚或阳虚），在同一条件、同一刺激量的情况下，会产生两种血管容积变化（扩张或收缩）的不同反应。说明针刺有调节气血、改善机体功能活动的双相效应。"随变而调气"中"调气"实质上是以手法唤起机体自我调节功能，针刺手法则是一种信息的输入，通过反馈过程使气血运行恢复有序状态。

四、提高针刺效果

"焠刺"可以治疗"诸痹""经筋病"等疾病已经被历代医家在长期实践中证实。电热针将温热效应引入

III. The discussion about "Qi regulation"

A study on rabbit heart-beating rates showed that the rate returned to normal (260bpm) after applying electrothermal acupuncture therapy on rabbits with bradycardia (200bpm), but the heart rates of rabbits with tachycardia (300bpm) also returned to normal (260 bpm) after receiving such therapy. Whether bradycardial or tachycardial, abnormal heart rates can be rectified by electrothermal acupuncture therapy.

In clinical settings, the results of body blood flow using plethysmography demonstrated that under the same condition and stimulation but different physical status (deficiency of Yang or Yin), changes in vascular volume may respond differently (vessel dilation or constriction). This indicated that needle insertion had improved both Qi-blood modulation and physical functions improvement. The ancients said, "Acupuncture therapy is flexible depending on the circumstances through regulating Qi." "Qi modulation" itself is basically an approach to awake self-regulatory function, and needle insertion is a means for signal input to make smooth Qi-blood circulation through the circular flow process.

IV. Enhance the efficacy of needle insertion

The efficacy of *Cui Ci* on "paralysis" or "musculoskeletal disorders" has been proven for a long time in earlier medical practice. The temperature of the electrothermal acupuncture needle inside human body can range

机体内部，它的温度范围是30～700℃，因而适应的病种也比较广泛，特别对于风寒湿痹、虚寒诸症有较好的效果。电热针可以温通经络、疏风散寒，改善气血运行，近几十年来，凡接受电热针治疗的患者，一般反映镇痛效果较好。我们认为，电热针疗法是一种能使热辐射导入机体深部，直达病所，使热效应集中，最大限度地不使热量散失的热疗手段。

防治肿瘤

中医药及针灸在治疗肿瘤方面已取得了较好的临床疗效，并引起国内外医学界的高度关注。电热针具有调节气血、疏通经络、软坚散结、解凝化瘀的作用，并能集中热量于一定的区域，可在病灶中心散热，且有温度可调的特点，填补了目前国内外高温治肿瘤送热方法的不足。

根据中医学和历代医家对肿瘤的相关论述可知，任何邪毒蕴积、寒结痰凝、滞留不去都可致瘤。我们参阅国内外

from 30 to 700 ℃; therefore, it can treat wider range of diseases. For those with arthralgia caused by wind-cold-damp pathogens or deficient cold, the effects are particularly positive. electrothermal acupuncture therapy is known to warm up and dredge meridians, dispel cold and improve Qi-blood circulation. In recent decades, patients receiving electrothermal acupuncture therapy often reflected better analgesic effects. We believe that electrothermal acupuncture therapy is a thermal therapy, which transmits heat radiation directly in-depth into human bodies and accumulates thermal effects with minimum heat dispersion.

Cancer prevention

Traditional Chinese Medicine and acupuncture therapy have achieved great clinical efficiency, and therefore gained national and international recognition. electrothermal acupuncture therapy may regulate Qi-blood circulation, dredge the meridians, soften and resolve hard masses, invigorate blood circulation, eliminate stasis and accumulate heat within a specific geometric area in order to disseminate heat from the center of the lesion. Moreover, its function of adjustable temperature compensates for the insufficiency of heat transmission in current hyperthermia cancer treatment in the country.

According to the descriptions and discussions about neoplasm in Traditional Chinese Medical publications and ancient works, it was believed that the pathogenic factors of neoplasm consisted pathogenic toxin accu-

高温治瘤的有关文献，运用中医辨证施治，结合针灸固有穴位的特异作用，经过3年多的努力，完成了电热针对小鼠可移植性癌抑制作用的实验研究，通过了阶段性成果鉴定，肯定了电热针对3种小鼠可移植性癌（肝癌、乳腺癌、前胃鳞癌）的抑制作用，为电热针治疗肿瘤的临床应用提供了科学依据。实验结果显示，经一次性治疗对荷前胃鳞癌小鼠治愈率为60%，肿瘤完全消退率为78%～83.3%，肿瘤生长抑制率为84.8%～90.6%；对荷肝癌小鼠治愈率为70%～88%，肿瘤完全消退率为88.2%～90%，肿瘤生长抑制率为82.4%～94.4%（《中国针灸》1984年第1期）。

通过动物实验发现，荷肝癌小鼠治愈后再接种同种瘤株70日无一例死亡，而对照组全部死亡。这一现象表明，电热

mulation/retention, cold-induced constipation as well as yang-insufficiency-induced sputum accumulation. By reviewing domestic and international literatures on hyperthermia cancer treatments, applying Traditional Chinese Medicine to syndrome differentiation and treatment and combining the specific mechanisms of prescription of acupuncture therapy, we have completed the experiments concerning the inhibitory effects of electrothermal acupuncture therapy on cancer transplantable mice models with more than three years of efforts. The interim results proved that electrothermal acupuncture therapy was effective on the inhibition of three cancers (i.e. liver cancer, breast adenocarcinoma, and squamous cell carcinoma of gastric cardia) in transplantable mice models. Such results provided scientific evidences for the application of electrothermal acupuncture therapy in clinical practice. The study results showed that in mice model with squamous cell carcinoma of gastric cardia, the effects of one-time treatment on mice cure rate was 60%, the tumor complete regression rate was 78%-83.3%, and the tumor growth inhibition rate was 84.8%-90.6%. In mice model with liver cancer, the effects of one-time treatment on mice cure rate was 70%-88%, the tumor complete regression rate was 88.2%-90%, and the tumor growth inhibition rate was 82.4%-94.4%. ("Chinese of Acupuncture & Moxibustion"; 1984, volume:1)

A study revealed that mice cured of previous liver cancer were found zero death in 70 days after receiving the same cancer cell line implantation. While none of the mice survived in the other sample group. The results

针治愈的荷肝癌小鼠对再接种同种肿瘤有明显的抑制作用，该结果是否可考虑电热针治疗能使小鼠获得较强的免疫力。电热针治肿瘤不仅是热物理效应，对热生物学、非热效应及免疫功能方面的研究也是一项值得探讨的课题。

一、临床观察

1983年6月9日治疗首例患者，包某，女，74岁，蒙古族，确诊为左颜面部鳞状上皮癌1级。经电热针治疗5次，瘤体结痂，21天痂皮自然脱落，经组织学检查，未发现癌细胞，复经1年5个月的随访，患者健康状态良好，并无复发。

截至1985年末，我院相继用电热针接受并治疗各种浅表肿瘤患者120例（表1）。

indicated that electrothermal acupuncture therapy had significant inhibitory effects on mice with recurrent liver cancer. This outcome may make researcher to consider if electrothermal acupuncture therapy boost up the immune system of the mice. In other words, electrothermal acupuncture therapy may not only possess a thermophysical effect, but its effects on enhancing immune system is also worth of further scientific research.

I. Clinical observation

On June 9th, 1983, we first used electrothermal acupuncture therapy to treat a 74-year-old female patient (Bao) with 1st-degree squamous cell carcinoma (SCC) on her left face. After five treatments of electrothermal acupuncture therapy, the tumor started to encrust and the crust fell naturally 21 days later. The histology results demonstrated completely cancer-free tissues. At the follow-up visit one year and 5 months later, the patient remained healthy without recurrence.

Until the end of 1985, we applied electrothermal acupuncture therapy on total of 120 patients with varieties of superficial tumors (Table 1).

表 1 电热针对 120 例浅表肿瘤疗效统计
Table 1. The statistics of the efficacy of electrothermal acupuncture therapy on 120 superficial tumors

病种 Tumor types		例数 Case number	疗效判定 Efficacy					备注 Remarks
			痊愈 Cured	肿瘤消退 Tumors efficacy	显效 Subsidence	有效 Effective	无效 Non-effective	
皮肤癌 Melanoma	鳞状细胞癌 Squamous cell carcinoma	38	5	8	6	6	13	
	原位癌（包文氏癌） In squamous cell carcinoma (Bowen's diseases)	37	2	6	7	7	14	
乳腺癌 Breast adenocarcinoma		8			4		4	
直肠癌 Colorectal cancer		5		2	2		1	
宫颈癌 Cervical cancer		4		2		2		
纤维肉瘤 Fibrosarcoma		4	1		3			
神经细胞癌 Neuroblastoma		5	1	2			2	
黑色素瘤 Melanoma		4		1	2	1		
其他肿瘤 Others tumors	腭扁桃体癌 Palatine tonsil cancer	2	1	1				
	外瘤 External tumor	6	2	1	2	1		
	溶骨性成骨肉瘤 Osteolytic osteosarcoma	4			2	1	2	
	乳腺癌淋巴结转移 Breast cancer combined with lymph node involvement	3		1	2			
合计 Total		120	12	24	30	18	26	120
百分比 Percentages			0%	20%	25%	15%	30%	100%

二、典型病历介绍

病例1：

尚某，女，59岁，患外阴肿物3月余，肿瘤大小为2cm×2cm×1cm，呈菜花状，表面合并溃疡，经病理检查诊断为"外阴鳞状细胞癌"。1983年7月20日开始接受电热针治疗，治疗10次后，瘤体已脱落，但局部仍有溃疡，经取活组织病检，示"未见癌细胞，有大量炎性细胞浸润"。继续在溃疡处用电热针治疗4次，溃疡面完全愈合，随访2年，肿瘤未见复发。

病例2：

范某，男，60岁。患者于1981年6月左踝部长一肿物，1983年6月手术切除，术后1个月肿瘤复发，瘤体大小为3.5cm×2cm，局部皮肤粗、硬，经病理检查诊断为"皮肤原位癌"。1983年7月开始用电热针治疗。治疗2次后，肿瘤坏死脱落。因针刺较深，局部形成溃疡，使跟腱暴露，经外敷中药"珍珠生肌散"后，疮面2个月愈合，病理检查示"未见癌细胞"。半年后左足功

II. Several Typical Cases

Case 1:

Shang, a 59-year-old female. She suffered from a cauliflower-shaped vulval lump with superficial ulcer over three months, and the size of the tumor was 2cm×2cm×1cm. After biopsy, the lesion was confirmed to be "vulval squamous cell carcinoma". She started to receive electrothermal acupuncture therapy on July 20th, 1983. After 10 times' treatments, the tumor become encrusted and fell naturally, but a localized ulcer was still noted. The biopsy results indicated "cancer-free tissues with massive inflammatory cells infiltration". We continued applying electrothermal acupuncture therapy over the lesion site for additional 4 times till the ulcer was completely healed. The patient had no cancer recurrence in the following two years.

Case 2:

Fan, a 60-year-old male. Patient found a tumor over his left ankle in June, 1981. He received surgical removal in June, 1983, but the cancer recurred a month later with a size of 3.5cm×2cm coarse and stiff tumor as well as a localized texture. The biopsy results indicated as a "carcinoma in situ of skin". The patient started to receive electrothermal acupuncture therapy in July, 1983. The tumor became encrusted and necrotic, and fell naturally after twice treatments. Because of deeper needle insertion, there was a localized ulcer along with tendon exposure at the needle insertion site. After 2 months of external application with Chinese herb "Zhenzhu Shengji San", the wound healed completely. The biopsy results showed

能完全恢复，随访 2 年，肿瘤未见复发。

1983 年 11 月，中国中医研究院针灸研究所治疗 2 例患者，1 例为神经细胞癌，经 8 次电热针治疗后痊愈，1 年后随访未见复发；1 例为晚期乳腺癌手术后复发，已不能接受放、化疗，并有播散性转移，经电热针治疗后，局部病灶明显缩小，转移灶消失，半年后患者返回原籍。1 年后随访，该患者复发灶尚未愈合，生活尚可自理。

三、体会

目前，加温治疗肿瘤法引起了国内外学者的极大兴趣，大量科学实验证明，加温可以选择性地抑制肿瘤细胞的生长，促进肿瘤细胞的凋亡。由于现在的热治疗技术（如微波、射频、超声波、水浴等方法）具有一定的局限性，国内外学者多致力于探索新的热疗手段，特别是力图寻找一种使热辐射能集中对准瘤体或体内

"cancer-free tissues". Six months later, the patient regained his left foot functions fully and had no cancer recurrence in the following 2 years.

In November, 1983, the Institute of Acupuncture and Moxibustion, China Academy of Chinese Medical Sciences cured 2 patients. One of them was a patient with Neuroblastoma, who was cured after 8 treatments of electrothermal acupuncture therapy. The patient showed no recurrence during the following year. Another one was a breast cancer patient at advanced stage with post-operative recurrence and metastasis, who was not suited for radio- or chemotherapy anymore. After receiving electrothermal acupuncture therapy, not only the size of the local lesion significantly reduced, but the metastatic lesions disappeared. Six months later, the patient was discharged and returned home. During 1-year of follow-up, the patient still had recurrent lesions, but was able to function independently for daily living.

III. Experiences

Currently the anti-cancer effects of thermal therapy become of great interest to national and international scientists. A large number of scientific studies have proven that thermal therapy may selectively inhibit the growth of cancer cells and therefore accelerate cancer cell apoptosis. Because of the limitations of current thermal therapies (e.g. microwave, radio frequency, ultrasound, water bath, etc.), most international and national scientists focus on exploring advanced thermal approaches, especially the kind aiming at radiation heat directly and centrally on the tumor or a specific area. Such therapy

的一定几何区域，使深部瘤体中心受热的方法，提高加温治肿瘤的疗效。但是，现有的其他方法送热途径均由外向内，从表皮到深部组织，瘤体深部吸收热能较少，不够集中，散热不均匀。

电热针治肿瘤是中医针灸治肿瘤的一个组成部分，在理论、方法、临床上充分体现了中医传统针灸"燔针""焠刺"的特色，是一种新的治疗手段。电热针治肿瘤的特点是把热效应直接引入瘤体中心，热辐射途径由内向外，由组织深部到体表，从根本上改变了高温治肿瘤的送热途径，同时可以根据瘤体的不同部位和不同大小，从不同方向进行多点针刺，因此，瘤体内散热比较均匀且不损伤正常组织。

根据现有加温治肿瘤的临床报道，均须配合放疗、化疗方能取得较为显著的疗效。电热针治肿瘤则仅用电热针单一方法，无须配合放疗、化疗而取效。尤其是电热针治肿瘤可根据中医理论辨证施治，除在瘤体针刺外，亦可配合循经

may increase anti-cancer effects of hyperthermia therapy through transmitting heat directly and deeply to the center of the tumor. Unfortunately, contemporary thermal therapies are transmitting heat internally (deeper tissues) from external environment (cutaneous epidermis), of which the amount of heat accumulated in the core of the tumor is insufficient and uneven due to heat dispersion.

Electrothermal acupuncture therapy is one of the Chinese acupuncture approaches used for anti-cancer treatment. The principles and clinical techniques of electrothermal acupuncture therapy is practically consistent with the traditional Chinese acupuncture therapies such as *Fan Zhen* and *Cui Ci*, and thus has been considered as an advanced therapeutic measure. The feature of electrothermal acupuncture therapy includes transmitting heat directly into the center of the tumor, that is, a paradigm shift of heat transmission from internal source (deep tissue) to external environment (body surface). In this case, based on the location and the size of the tumor, the practitioner may apply multiple needle insertions at different sites in various directions. electrothermal acupuncture therapy will create a more even and focused thermal effect on tumor itself without damaging healthy tissues.

According to available clinical reports, present thermal therapies are required to be combined with radiotherapy or chemotherapy to achieve more significant anticancer effects. However, electrothermal acupuncture therapy itself is working effectively without the requirement of other combination therapies such as radiotherapy or chemotherapy. The anti-cancer effects of electrothermal acupuncture therapy are based on the

取穴施治，增强机体的抗病能力。我们临床治疗的全部患者均未配合其他放、化疗，经观察未发现转移及恶化现象。值得探讨的是，内蒙古医院接受一位晚期乳腺癌患者，瘤体大小为 9.8cm×8.8cm×3cm，经 2 个疗程治疗后，瘤体缩小为 3.5cm×5.5cm×1.5cm，而后进行局部手术切除，手术发现瘤体中心坏死，腋窝转移灶也转化为阴性，瘤体周围出现环行被膜，包绕瘤体，这种情况在既往手术中尚属少见。另有，内蒙古医学院附属医院治疗 1 例左股内侧纤维肉瘤 2 次手术后复发的患者，瘤体大小为 10cm×12cm×10cm，由于瘤体与股动脉粘连，无法进行手术剥离。经电热针治疗 2 个疗程后，瘤体缩小 1/2，从体表可触及瘤体与股动脉分离，经手术局部切除，效果满意。随访 1 年半，身体健康，未见复发，现已恢复工作。

肿瘤防治研究工作是国家科学技术委员会重点攻关项目，电热针治肿瘤引起了国内

traditional Chinese medical theory "syndrome differentiation", hence in addition to direct needle insertion on tumor, acupuncture therapy on meridian channels as well as acupoints are also needed to reinforce the human body's resistance against disease. All of our patients did not receive additive radiotherapy or chemotherapy, but no cancer metastasis or progression was observed, either. It is worth noting that a hospital in Inner Mongolia admitted a patient with advanced breast adenocarcinoma with a tumor size of 9.8cm×8.8cm×3cm. After two treatment sessions, the tumor size was reduced partially to 3.5cm×5.5cm×1.5cm, followed by a local surgical resection. During the surgery, a membrane-encapsulated tumor plus a necrotic lesion at the center along with axillary metastasis (-) was noted, and such condition was very rare in previous surgical history. The affiliated hospital of Inner Mongolia Medical University admitted a patient with recurrent fibrosarcoma on the left inner thigh after twice surgeries, whose tumor size was of 10cm×12cm×10cm. The tumor was unresectable due to its adherence to the femoral artery. After receiving two sessions of electrothermal acupuncture therapy, the tumor size was reduced to half and separable from the femoral artery through surface palpation. Therefore, the patient subsequently received surgical resection and the effect was quite satisfactory. During the 1.5 year-follow-up visit, no disease recurrence was found at all, so the patient returned to work successfully.

Cancer prevention is one of the essential scientific projects of the State Scientific and Technological Commission. Since electrothermal acupuncture therapy has

外学者的重视，并被寄予希望。电热针治肿瘤临床观察见到了初步成效，预测其将在创建具有中医特色的肿瘤防治研究工作中占有一定的位置。

电热针治肿瘤与近代加温治疗的比较（见表 2）。

drawn great attention to the national and international scientists, we are looking forward to applying such advanced therapy in greater extent of clinical practice. The clinical observation of electrothermal acupuncture therapy has finally shown favorable effects. It will play an important role as an innovative Traditional Chinese Medicine-based cancer prevention/treatment.

Please refer to Table 2 for the comparison between electrothermal acupuncture therapy and modern thermal therapies.

表 2　电热针、微波、超声波热疗治癌比较
Table 2. A comparison between electrothermal acupuncture therapy, ultra-short wave and ultrasonic hyperthermia therapy on anti-cancer effects

项目 Method / 热疗方法 Thermal therapy	微波、超声波 ultra-shortwave, ultrasounds	电热针 electrothermal acupuncture therapy
意义 Significance	国外称之为"一种全新治疗方法"，可有效控制肿瘤，是医学界的新发现 A so-called "brand new therapy" to effectively control tumor, which is also a new discovery in medical field	中医针灸治肿瘤的重要组成部分，体现中医传统"燔针""焠刺"的特色，且为国内独创 It is an important part of Chinese acupuncture therapy for anti-cancer treatment, which is a unique innovation reflecting the features of Traditional Chinese Medicine (e.g. *Fan Zhen* or *Cui Ci*)
温度范围 Temperature range	45℃聚焦，尚待研究 45℃ focused heat, remained to be studied	30～700℃，稳定可调 30-700℃, stable and controllable
送热途径 Heat transmission pathways	从表皮到深部组织，扇形辐射，从外向内，表面温度高于深部 The heat was transmitted from epidermis (outside) to deep tissues (inside) through a fan-shaped radiation pattern, so the temperature at surface is much higher than the deep tissues	从深部组织到表层，病灶中心散热，从内向外，深部温度高于表面 The heat was transmitted from deep tissues (inside) to epidermis (outside); that is, heat dispersion from the center of the lesion, so the temperature in deep tissues is much higher than at the surface
临床温度 Clinical temperature	深部 42.5～45℃，表面须加冷风设备降温 42.5-45℃ in deep tissues, a surface cold air equipment is required to cool down the temperature	从深部组织到表层，病灶中心散热，从内向外，深部温度高于表面 The heat was transmitted from deep tissues (inside) to epidermis (outside); that is, heat dispersion from the center of the lesion, so the temperature in deep tissues is much higher than at the surface

续表

项目 Method 热疗方法 Thermal therapy	微波、超声波 ultra-shortwave, ultrasounds	电热针 electrothermal acupuncture therapy
热辐射 Radiation heat	受机器性能限制,从上向下辐射,穿透力不等 From up to down radiation, uneven penetration due to limited equipment performance	不受机器限制,可在病灶中心散热,根据临床需要可用斜刺、平刺或直接刺入瘤体基底部 The heat can be transmitted from the center of the lesion through needle insertions (e.g. diagonal, horizontal or direct insertion into the tumor) based on clinical requirements without being limited by the equipment
测温 Temperature measurement	微波场下由于电磁波场干扰产生误差 Errors may occur due to the electromagnetic interference under ultra-shortwave	无电磁干扰,误差小 No electromagnetic interference, fewer errors
仪器使用 Instructions of equipment use	仪器较复杂,操作过程须有屏蔽设备 Complicated operation and require a shielding device during operation	操作简单,不须屏蔽,易携带,可在家庭、病床应用 Easy operation, no shielding is required, portable, and applicable to both home-based or ward-based practice
临床应用 Clinical applications	配合放疗、化疗同时应用,有降低白细胞之弊 Should be combined with radiotherapy or chemotherapy, may cause leukocytopenia	不用配合其他放、化疗,根据中医辨证施治配合中药治疗,提高机体抗病能力 No other radiotherapy or chemotherapy is required, it can be applied along with Chinese herb therapy based on the principles of Traditional Chinese Medicine "syndrome differentiation", so as to increase human body's resistance against diseases
预测与展望 Expectations and perspectives	热疗技术尚不成熟,肿瘤深部受热不均匀,专用辐射器研究不足 Immature thermal therapy, uneven heat transmission in deep tumor tissue and insufficient studies on specific heat radiators	临床观察有重复性,是一项突出中医特色,有较好前景的科研课题,预测在防治肿瘤工作中占有一定的位置 It is a prominent feature of TCM to provide repeatable clinical results, and focus on prospective scientific topics, as well as pay attention to cancer prevention

电热针量化问题

Quantitative issues

随着现代医学的发展,越来越突显针灸学在医学领域中

As modern medical development progresses, the treatment of acupuncture has become more important in

所占有的重要地位。当前，现代科学技术正向定量科学深化，如何使针灸学逐步成为定量科学，是针灸学发展面临的一个重要问题，也是针灸学发展的必然趋势。

几千年来，针灸发展过程中缺乏量化的指标。即使进入现代，对针灸也还没有能够做出可靠的量化规定，因而阻碍了针灸学向定量科学方面发展的进程。实践证明，针灸学只有建立在定量化的基础上，才能够准确地提供可靠的科学研究的定量数据，以便充实和丰富针灸学的理论体系，指导临床实践，阐明针灸学的内在规律。也只有定量化才能更有力地说明针灸学的学术价值，为针灸学的发展创造条件。

工具改革是推动定量化的手段，任何工具改革都将加速其科学的发展，针灸仪器的研制、工具的改革是针灸学科学发展的一个重要途径。把现代科学技术引进针灸学的领域，促进针灸工具的改革有着怡人的前景，但这方面目前还是我国针灸研究工作的薄弱环节。当然，工具改革和科学定量化并不意味着抛弃传统精华，任

medical fields. So far, the trend of modern science and technology is focusing on quantitative science. Therefore, how to make the science of acupuncture a quantifiable science has become an important issue and an inevitable trend.

Over thousands of years of acupuncture therapy development, quantitative indices were missing. Even in modern society, the regulations for reliable measurements on acupuncture therapy are still missing, which impedes the development of quantitative nature of acupuncture treatment. Clinical observations have proven that the science of acupuncture is only accurate on the basis of quantitative data as well as reliable scientific studies in order to enrich the principles and theories of acupuncture therapy, guide clinical practice, and elaborate internal rules/requirements. In addition, the academic value of acupuncture therapy only becomes more significant through quantitative measurement.

Tool reform is a means to promote quantitative science, and it will accelerate the development of acupuncture therapy. Research and development of acupuncture equipments and tool reform are both important measures to promote the advancement of acupuncture therapy. The tool reform by introducing modern science and technology into acupuncture therapy is very promising, but it is still its weakness which requires improvement together with the accumulation of clinical practice. Of course, tool reform and quantitative science do not mean abandon traditions. Any metaphysical "reforms" that deviates

何形而上学的观点偏离针灸传统特色的"改革"都是不值得提倡的。

通过几十年的实验和临床研究，我们发现电热针不但是针刺工具的改进，而且打破了传统针灸定量不明的弊端，对针灸理论的研究也提出了一些新的问题。我们以后将着重对电热针进行临床和理论研究，特别要运用中医辨证施治的原则，结合针灸固有穴位的特异作用，提高治疗效果，扩大病种。这将是一项有意义的研究工作。笔者殷切地希望得到各位学者、专家及相关单位的支援，以期为继承和发扬针灸学做出更大的贡献。

from traditional acupuncture features/concepts are worth of attention and to be alerted.

Through decades of experiments and clinical studies, we have found that electrothermal acupuncture therapy not only reformed needling tools, but also overcame the previous hurdle of "non measurable" of traditional acupuncture and brought a new perspective into acupuncture theories. In the future, we will focus on the research, theories and clinical practice of electrothermal acupuncture therapy based on the principles of syndrome differentiation in Traditional Chinese Medicine. Through utilization of the specific mechanisms of acupoints, we will try to further enhance the efficiency of acupuncture and apply it to wider range of illnesses. This can be a significant research work. The authors sincerely hope for the support and contribution by scholars, experts and related medical institutions and wish that this book will pass on the essence of Traditional Chinese Medicine and further elaborate the effectiveness of the scientific nature of acupuncture.

上篇 理论溯源　Part I Theories and History

电热针应用

The application of electrothermal acupuncture therapy

传统针具概述

针灸针的质料随着社会发展、医疗工具的改进而逐渐演变，古代有石、骨、竹、铜、铁的针质；近代有金、银、铜等合金针。目前，以不锈钢针的针质为佳，被临床广泛应用。

古有"九针"，即镵针、圆针、锟针、锋针（三棱针）、铍针、圆利针、毫针、长针、大针（火针、燔针、焠针）。其中，毫针、圆利针、三棱针、火针等经历代改进，沿用至今，当代新发展的尚有皮内针、皮肤针、电热针等。

电热针结构名称、保养和消毒

电热针针具内部结构精细，外部结构由金属制成，其尖锋利，针体细，然较普通

Overview of traditional needles

The materials for acupuncture needles have evolved with social development and medical device improvement. In ancient times, acupuncture needles were made of stones, bones, bamboos, copper or iron, but now they are made of gold, silver or copper-nickel alloy. At present, the stainless acupuncture needle is the best quality and therefore has become very popular and applied extensively.

There were nine classical needles, namely shear needle, round needle, spoon needle, lance needle (triangular needle), stiletto needle, round sharp needle, filiform needle, long needle, and big needle (fire needle or warm needle). Among them, the filiform needle, round sharp needle, triangular needle and fire needle have been reformed from time to time and are still applicable up to now. New developed needles include the intradermal needle, cutaneous needle and electrothermal needle.

The components of the electrothermal needle, the maintenance and aseptic measures

The internal structure of the electrothermal needle is very delicate. The outer structure is made of metal. The needle tip is sharp and the needle is thin. However, it is

· 21 ·

毫针略粗。外表结构形态及各部名称分别为：针尖、针身（针体）、针根、针柄、针尾（图1）。

still thicker than the filiform needle. The outer structure and component of the needle are as the following: tip, body, base, handle and tail. (Figure 1)

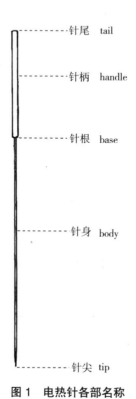

图 1 电热针各部名称
Figure 1. The components of the electrothermal needle

一般所说的电热针的长度，是指针身而言，计算以市尺5分为基本单位，其中5分～1.5寸较为常用。电热针的粗细以针体横截面计算，以毫米为单位，临床常用的电热针型号有1～5号（表3），一般临床习惯以"短而细，长而粗"的类型应用购置。

Generally speaking, the length of the electrothermal needle refers to the length of the body. If used "chi (=1/3m)" as the unit, the length of 5 "fen (= 1/3cm)" ~ 1.5 "cun (=1/3dm)" is more popular. The thickness of the electrothermal needle is based on the cross-section area using "mm" as unit. In clinical practice, popular needle number ranges from 1~5 (Table 3). Usually the procurement of needles is based on the types of "short and thin" or "long and thick".

表 3 电热针直径

Table 3. The diameters of electrothermal acupuncture needles

号数 Number	1	2	3	4	5
直径（毫米） Diameters (mm)	0.40	0.45	0.50	0.55	0.60

电热针使用前应先检查，原则上以通电正常、发热良好、针尖尖锐、针身直、针柄不松脱为佳，以免术中给患者造成不应有的痛苦或发生事故。针身弯曲者可用干纱布或棉片裹住针身，用指捋法捋直。使用多次后，针尖过钝或针柄松脱者应立即换用新针。

电热针使用后，应妥善放置，注意针尖勿挫钝或曲钩，针身勿压弯。一般收在藏针具中保存，如金属、电木、塑料质地的藏针管、针盒、皮夹、布包等。

电热针使用前，要根据具体条件进行消毒，一般采用干热高温消毒。

针刺练习法

针刺练习法，主要是锻炼术者持针的指力和运针手法。由于电热针质地细软，如果施术者没有一定的持针指力，很

Before application, careful checkup of its quality is required. In principle, an optimal needle consists of several properties including smooth thermal conductivity, sharp tip, straight body and well-connected handle in order to prevent from pain or accidents during the practice. For those bent needles, the practitioner may cover the needle body with gauze or cotton pads and use the fingers to twist and straighten the needle. If the tip became dull or the handle became loosening after multiple uses, a replacement of a new needle is required immediately.

The electrothermal needle should be stored properly after application. The tip of the needle should not be dull or hooked. Do not press or curve the body of the needle. Usually the needles are stored in a barrel, box, which is made of metal, Bakelite or plastic materials, or in a leather wallet or cloth-bag.

Before using the electrothermal needles, sterilization under specific conditions is required. Normally dry-heat is adopted for sterilization.

Needling practice

The purpose of needling practice is to train finger strength and needling approaches of the practitioner. Modern electrothermal needles are usually thin and soft, if the practitioner did not have certain finger strength,

难顺利进针，所以指力练习是学习针法的基础，是进针迅速、减少患者痛感、针下得气、提高疗效的根本保障。因而，在进入临床施针之前，必须经常练习指力。由于电热针价格相对昂贵，为避免针身损坏，练习时可用普通毫针代之，本着循序渐进的原则，应先练粗而短，后练细而长的毫针。只有达到一定的指力和熟练程度，方可将电热针应用于临床。针刺练习的内容有：进针、捻转、提插等。具体练习方法如下：

一、纸块练习方法

用细软的纸片，裁成 5cm×8cm 长方形，叠作 2cm 厚的纸块，用线扎成"井"字并勒紧。练习时，以左手平执纸块，右手持针，在纸块上反复进行捻进、捻出的练习。先慢后快，熟能生巧，待指力已有增进，可将纸块逐渐加厚（图 2）。

needle insertion will be very difficult. Therefore, finger strength training is essential to needling practice. In addition, fast needle insertion with Qi arrival not only reduces pain, but improves therapeutic effects. In this case, finger strength training is required before clinical practice. Because electrothermal needles are relatively expensive, trainers may practice with regular filiform needles. Needling practice should be step by step, that is, from "thick and short" to "thin and long". The trainers may start to practice electrothermal acupuncture therapy only when they become skillful and their finger strength is sufficient. Needling practice consists of needle insertion, twisting, lifting and thrusting. The specific practicing methods are as follows:

Ⅰ. Paper stack practicing

Use thin and soft paper (in 5cm×8cm rectangle) to pile a 2cm-thick paper stack, and then use a rope to tie into the shape of the character "井". During the practice, use the left hand to hold the paper stack, use the right hand to hold the needle, and then practice needle insertion and withdrawal repeatedly on the paper stack. From slow to fast, from easy to difficult, practice makes perfect. After the finger strength has been improved, the thickness of the paper stack can be increased accordingly (Figure 2).

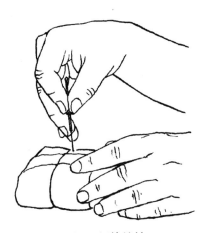

图 2 纸块练针
Figure 2. Paper stack practicing

二、棉球练习法

用脱脂棉做成一个直径5～6cm的球体,外用纱布包裹扎紧。练习时,左手持棉球,右手持针,在球上练习左右捻转、上下提插,并按各种针刺姿势和手法等要求练习,以熟练针刺的基本动作(图3)。

II. Cotton ball practicing

Use absorbent cotton to make cotton ball with 5~6cm diameter, and then cover the cotton ball tightly with gauze. During practice, use the left hand to hold the cotton ball, use the right hand to hold the needle, and then practice left-and-right twisting and twirling or up-and-down thrusting and lifting. At the same time, practice essential needling approaches in accordance with all kinds of postures and techniques (Figure 3).

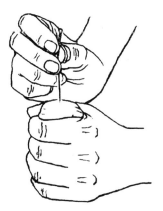

图 3 棉团练针
Figure 3. Cotton ball practicing

三、自身试针

通过以上两种方法的练习，达到了一定程度的进针指力及掌握了基本手法后，即可将电热针施于人体，但不能先用于患者，应该先自身试针。亲自体会进针手法、皮肤韧性、针感情况、匀称用力、减痛方法等，然后再在同学、同事之间相互针刺练习，更有利于临床实践。

针刺前准备

一、检查诊断

针刺前，术者首先对患者通过中医四诊（望、闻、问、切）采证，运用八纲（阴阳、表里、寒热、虚实）辨证，结合西医临床检查，以确诊并开具选穴处方。

二、选择体位

按选穴处方嘱咐患者选择适当的体位，以使患者平稳持久、舒适安全，便于针刺操作，利于取穴为原则。如体位不当，勉强支撑，患者易引起

III. Self-needling

Following the above two practicing methods, the practitioners have achieved certain finger strength and basic skills, and therefore are ready to apply electron-thermal needle into human bodies. But before applying to patients, they must practice on themselves first. Self-needling helps the practitioner exercise needling approaches, experience skin texture and needling sensation, feel needling strength and symmetry, and discover pain-free fashion. Afterward, the practice may be extended to classmates and colleagues to prepare for clinical practice.

Preparations before needling

I. Examination and Diagnosis

Before starting acupuncture therapy, the practitioner is required to examine the patient using four Chinese diagnostic methods (observation, listening, inquiry and palpation) to collection evidence, differentiate symptoms using eight principles (Yin-Yang, surface-interior, cold-hot and false-true), and then make a definitive diagnosis based on Western medicine and laboratory data in order to select appropriate acupoints for proper therapies.

II. Selection of body position

According to the accessibility of the selected acupoints, the patient should be instructed in a stable, rest, comfortable and safe position for acupuncture therapy. If patient's position were inappropriate and it makes patient restless, it may result in fatigue and therefore com-

疲劳，影响疗效。若体位移动，可能造成弯针或折针等事故。患者体位基本分为坐、卧2种，应妥善取位。

三、消毒

为防止感染，按选穴处方对患者皮肤用酒精棉球进行消毒，待酒精挥发干净后方可针刺。未进针前，术者的手亦必须用消毒水和肥皂水进行清洁消毒，以免污染针具和腧穴部位。

四、选针与检查

根据患者体质、穴位所在解剖的部位，选择相应型号的电热针。并认真检查针尖、针身、针根、针柄等各部，看是否合乎施术要求。

五、术者态度和体位

进针前，术者态度一定要庄重、和蔼、亲切，做好电热针常识的宣传和解释工作，以免初针患者精神紧张。术者同时需要选择便于针刺操作且平稳舒适持久之体位。

promise the efficiency. If a patient was moved during needling, it may result in bending or breaking the needle. There are two basic patient's positions: sitting and/or lying, which should be selected properly.

III. Sterilization

To prevent any infection, it is required to use an alcohol swab to clean the skin over acupoints. Acupuncture therapy can be performed after the alcohol gets dry. Before needle insertion, both hands of the practitioner should be disinfected and sterilized using disinfectant and soap water in order to prevent from needle and acupoints contamination.

IV. Needle selection and inspection

Select corresponding electrothermal needles based on the patient's physical condition and anatomical locations of the acupoints. Carefully inspect the tip, body, base and handle of the needle to see if all safe practice requirements have been met.

V. The attitude and position of the practitioner

Before needle insertion, the practitioner must provide common and explanatory information about electrothermal therapy with careful, thoughtful and kind attitude in order to calm the patient (especially for those first-time clinic visitors). Practitioners should also choose a stable and comfortable body position for the ease of needle insertion.

进针 / Needle insertion

一、持针式 / I. Needle holding styles

持针方式：①拇食式；②拇中式；③拇食中或执笔式。最后一种方法为临床习用。持针者必须全神贯注、精力集中在指端及针尖上（图4）。

Needle holding styles include: ① Thumb-index finger; ② Thumb-middle finger; ③ Thumb-index-middle finger or pen-holding styles. The last method is for clinical practice. The needle holders must fully concentrate on their finger tips and needle tips (Figure 4).

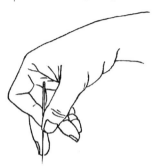

图 4 持针姿势
Figure 4. Needle holding position

二、进针方向 / II. Direction for needle insertion

进针的方向是指针身和皮肤应保持的角度。一般分为直刺、斜刺、平刺（图5）。

The direction for needle insertion refers to the angle between the needle body and the skin. Generally it can be divided into direct, diagonal and horizontal insertions (Figure 5).

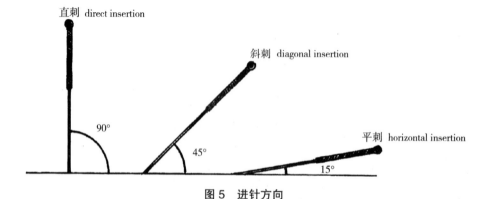

图 5 进针方向
Figure 5. Direction of needle insertion

其中，电热针直刺法最为常用，适用于全身大多数腧穴，尤其是肌肉丰厚部位的腧穴，如四肢及腹部腧穴。斜刺一般用于不能深刺的解剖部位，适用于肌肉较浅薄处或内有重要脏器的部位，或避开血管及瘢痕等特殊情况，如胸部和背部的腧穴。平刺的范围较大，适用于皮薄肉少部位的腧穴，如面部的腧穴。

三、进针法

进针法是将电热针刺入皮下的操作过程。为减轻患者疼痛，要求术者针刺速度要快、动作敏捷轻巧。主要手法如下：

1. 单手进针法

以右手拇、食指持针柄，中指辅助针身并触及皮肤，向下挫力，快速将针刺入皮肤。然后再按需要的针刺方向将针刺入一定深度。适用于1寸以下之电热针（图6）。

Among them, the direct insertion of electrothermal needle is the most popular approach applicable to most of the acupoints in human bodies, especially the acupoints with thick muscles, including acupoints in four extremities or abdomen. Diagonal insertion usually is indicated for deep anatomical locations, including acupoints with fewer muscular layers or acupoints over important organs. In some special situations, the approach is also indicated for acupoints to avoid certain vessels or scars, including acupoints in the chest or back. Since horizontal insertion involves greater area, it is indicated for acupoints with thin skin or muscle layers such as facial "Yu" acupoints.

III. Needle insertion approaches

Needle insertion approach is the process of inserting the electrothermal needle into the skin. To reduce pain, the practitioner is required to perform quick needle insertion with light and fast movement. The primary approaches are as follows:

1. Single-handed needle insertion:

Hold the needle handle with needle-holding thumb and index finger, use the middle finger to stabilize the needle body, touch the skin with the needle tip, and thrust the needle quickly into the skin. Continue inserting the needle into certain depth at required angle. The approach is applicable to electrothermal needles under 1" (one cun, equals to 1/3 decimeter) length (Figure 6).

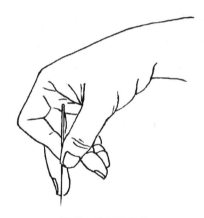

图 6 单手进针法
Figure 6. Single-handed needle insertion

2. 双手进针法

一般情况下，进针需双手协作，多以右手持针施术，称为"刺手"；左手固定穴位或扶助针身，加强进针力度，推避血管，减轻疼痛等，称为"佐手"。电热针多用之。

（1）指（爪）切进针法：以佐手拇指甲切于穴位上（古称"爪切"），或以拇、食、中指按压穴旁；刺手持针靠紧佐手拇指甲面，一捻一插快速刺入。适用于短针的进针（图 7）。

2. Double-handed needle insertion

Normally needle insertion requires the coordination of both hands. The practitioner may use right hand, namely "needle-holding hand" to hold the needle while practicing, and use the left hand, namely "supporting hand" to stabilize the acupoint or to support the needle in order to increase insertion intensity, avoid vasculatures and reduce pain. Most of the electrothermal needles apply such method.

(1) Finger pressure needle insertion: Use the needle-supporting thumb fingernail mark the acupoint or use the thumb/index finger/middle finger pressing the tissues next to the acupoint, hold the needle in the needle-holding hand and place the needle tip next to the needle-supporting thumb fingernail, and then perform a quick twist and insertion. It is an approach applicable to short needles (Figure 7).

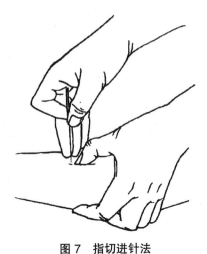

图 7 指切进针法
Figure 7. Finger pressure needle insertion

（2）夹持进针法：佐手拇、食指用消毒棉片或棉球裹住针身，露出针尖2～3分，刺手持针柄。当针尖接近穴位皮肤时，佐手将针快速刺入皮内，刺手同时随之轻加压刺力量，两手协同动作，刺手捻转针柄，佐手夹持针柄配合随捻随压刺入深处。此法适用于1.5寸以上之电热针（图8）。

（3）舒指进针法：以佐手拇、食或食、中两指向穴位两侧撑开，使皮肤紧张，便于刺手进针。此法适用于皮肤松弛的腹部及夹缝皱瘪处（图9）。

(2) Fingers-squeeze needle insertion: Use the needle-supporting thumb and index finger to pinch an alcohol swab or alcohol cotton ball along with the needle body, expose 2~3' (one fen=1/3cm) of the needle tip, and use the needle-holding hand to hold the needle handle. When the needle tip is approaching the acupoint skin, use the needle-supporting hand to thrust the needle into the skin quickly. At the same time, use the needle-holding hand to slightly increase needle insertion force. Coordinate both hands' motions, use the needle-holding hand to swirl the handle while use the needle-supporting hand to pinch the handle and apply pressure for deep needle insertion. The approach is applicable to electrothermal needles above 1.5" length (Figure 8).

(3) Skin-stretching needle insertion: Use the needle-supporting hand thumb and index finger or index finger and middle finger to stretch the acupoint skin in order to allow the needle-holding hand to insert the needle. This method is applicable to slack or wrinkled skin (such as abdomen) (Figure 9).

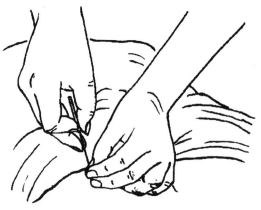

图 8 夹持进针法
Figure 8. Fingers-squeeze needle insertion

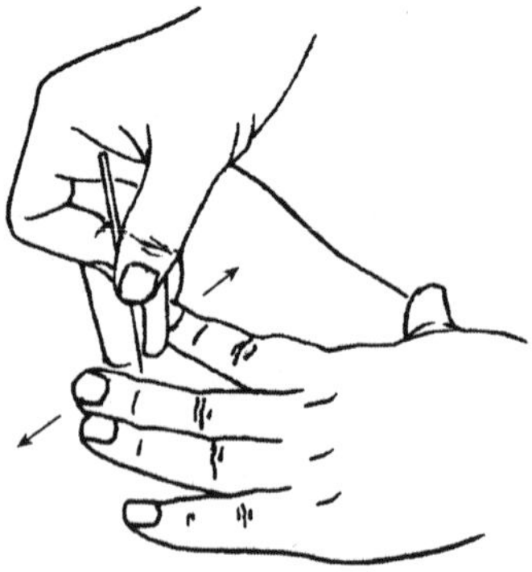

图 9 舒指进针法
Figure 9. Skin-stretching needle insertion

（4）捏起进针法：以佐手拇、食指将穴位所在的皮肤捏起，然后刺手所持之针从旁刺入。此法多用于面部需沿皮平刺的腧穴，如印堂、地仓等（图10）。

(4) Skin-pinching up needle insertion: Pinch the skin on top of the acupoint using the needle-supporting thumb and index finger, and then use the needle-holding hand to hold the needle and insert the needle through the skin. This method is often applicable to facial acupoints requiring horizontal subcutaneous insertion, including Yintang (EX-HN3) and Dicang (ST4) (Figure 10).

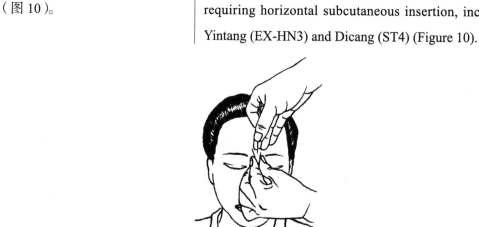

图 10 捏起进针法
Figure 10. Skin-pinching up needle insertion

四、进针的次序

古法是先上而后下，先

IV. The order of needle insertion

Ancient approach followed up-to-down and chest-

胸而后背。如今临床多先手而后足，先背而后胸；先主穴而后配穴，先病变部位而后远隔部位。这只是通常规律，根据术者习惯可灵活运用，不必拘泥。

五、进针后的深度

针刺深度应参照患者的年龄、性别、体质以及腧穴所在局部的解剖特征而"因地制宜"，关键以"得气"为度。正常成年人一般规律如下：

（1）头、指（趾）：1～3分。

（2）四肢：远体端5分～1寸；近体端1～3寸。

（3）胸背：4～6分

（4）腰腹：5～8分。

针感

当进针到一定深度时，术者在指下有"沉、涩、紧"之感；通电加温后，患者对针刺有酸、麻、胀、木、温热等感觉，统称"针感"，这一现象古典针籍称"得气"。不同的针感取决于患者的个体差异、不同腧穴以及同一腧穴的深度和方向；而术者取穴的准确性、手

to-back orders. On the contrary, modern approach follows hand-to-foot, back-to-chest, primary acupoint-to-accessory acupoint, and lesion site-to-distal part orders. These are only routine orders. The practitioner may apply the rules with flexibility instead of following the orders strictly.

V. The depth of needle insertion

The depth of needle insertion may vary based on the age, sex, physical conditions of the patient and the anatomical features of the acupoint. The key is the "arrival of Qi". Usually the depth of needle insertion for healthy adults may follow the rules as follows:

(1) For acupoints on the head or finger (toes): 1'~3' (fen).

(2) For acupoints on four limbs: Distal limbs 5'(fen)~1"(cun), proximal limbs 1"~3" (cun).

(3) For acupoints on the chest or back: 4'~6' (fen).

(4) For acupoints on lumbar or abdomen area: 5'~8' (fen).

Needling sensation

Once the needle inserts into certain depth of the skin, the practitioner may feel "deep, astringent and tense" under one's finger. At the same time, the patient may feel soreness, numbness, swelling and warmth after the power of the electrothermal acupuncture equipment is switched on and the needle is warmed. All of the above are called "needling sensations", which were described as "arrival of Qi" in ancient acupuncture books. Patients may have different needling sensations based on different

法熟练技巧尤为重要。针感和疗效关系尤为密切。一般针感出现迅速，放散传导较远，如能"气达病所"，疗效较好，反之则差，针刺的关键在于"得气"。因此，我们必须对技术精益求精，不断提高针刺疗效，保证医疗质量。

若无针感，应在腧穴周围循按，或加针，或加温，以激发针感。如初诊患者不出现针感，待针灸数次后也可出现针感。

遇有不适针感者，如针后感到疼痛、过热、不舒服等，应退针或减低温度，改变针刺方向，停止留针，以减轻刺激，或用循按法以缓解不适针感。

行针

当进针达到一定深度后，采用多种不同针刺手法，用以激发针感而提高疗效，称为

physical conditions, acupoints or depths and directions over the same acupoint. The accuracy and proficiency of the practitioner's acupuncture skill is particularly crucial to the needling sensation. Needling sensation is closely related to therapeutic efficacy. Usually the needling sensation appears promptly and may be transmitted to distal parts. In this case, needling sensation that "reaches to lesion site" achieves better efficiency; otherwise, the effects may be poor, namely, the key to needle insertion is about the "arrival of Qi". Therefore, we must practice repeatedly to pursue the best skills in order to improve acupuncture efficiency and ensure the quality of medical service.

If the lack of needling sensation occurred, massage or pressure areas next to acupoints or add more needle insertions or thermal therapy may stimulate the needling sensation. If the first-time clinic visitor did not show any needling sensations, the sensation still may appear after several acupuncture treatments.

For those have uncomfortable needling sensations (pain after acupuncture therapy, hyperthermia or discomfort), immediate needle withdrawal, reduce thermal effect, change directions for needle insertion, discontinue needle retention or apply massage or pressure over acupoints and related meridian channels may all be helpful to relieve acupuncture stimulation and discomfort.

Needle manipulation

When applying an acupuncture needle to certain depth, the practitioner may combine several different needle manipulation approaches to stimulate needling

"行针"手法。常用的有如下两种。

一、提插法

为进（插）、退（提）两种单式手法的概称。以刺手持住针柄，将针上下小幅度提插。穴位下如有重要内脏和大血管区应加以注意或尽量少用，以防刺伤。

二、捻转法

为搓（单向捻转）、拈（双向捻转）两种单式手法的综合概括，以刺手持住针柄往复地小范围内来回转动。使用该手法时，应避免针下出现组织纤维缠绕针体而产生疼痛或滞针的感觉。

当进针达到一定深度而未"得气"时，以上两种方法可用来寻找针感，在"得气"后可用来加强针感。但是，由于电热针针身较粗，做上述两种手法时不要过于勉强，以免给患者造成巨大的痛苦。

sensation in order to improve the efficiency of the therapy. This is called "needle manipulation". Two common needle manipulation approaches are as follows.

Ⅰ. Lifting and thrusting

It is an overall term for the combination of two single-handed manipulations: thrust (insertion) and lift (withdrawal). Use the needle-holding hand to hold the handle, and apply slightly up-and-down lifting and thrusting. This approach should be limited or exercised with caution at acupoints cover important organs or large vessels to prevent from stabbing incidents.

Ⅱ. Rotating

It is an overall term for the combination of two single-handed manipulations: knead (single-directional rotation) and swirl (bi-directional rotation). Use the needle-holding hand to rotate back-and-forth within a small range repeatedly. When applying such manipulation, it is required to avoid tissues/fibers kinking at the needle tip to prevent from pain or sticking needle sensation.

If the needle inserted to certain depth but still did not feel the "arrival of Qi", the practitioner may use the above two manipulations to gain needling sensation. For those who have felt the "arrival of Qi", the above two manipulations may be helpful in reinforcing needling sensation. However, due to thicker diameter of the electrothermal acupuncture needle, the application of the above manipulations should not be forced, or it may cause patients great agony.

留针

进针"得气"后留置不动，通电加温，使其延长刺激时间，以提高疗效，或缓解不适感觉和机体变化。

留针时间一般以 30～40 分钟为宜。

以镇痛、消炎、解痉为目的，常需留针。

出针

一、出针

出针时须先关闭电源，断开电热针与主机的连接，浅者用轻捷（不捻）平稳抽出法一次出针，但不宜过快。深者可分段缓慢出针。

二、出针后护理

出针前，术者必须持消毒干棉球，出针后注意观察穴孔，不出血者可不必处置；遇有出血者，随即用消毒干棉球轻压以止血。尽可能不用酒精棉球，以免刺激患者皮肤导致疼痛、过敏或发赤肿痛。

Needle retention

After the "arrival of Qi", retain the needle and switch on the power of the equipment to increase thermal effects in order to prolong stimulation and improve efficiency, or to relieve discomfort or accommodate physical changes.

Normally needle retention is recommended for 30~40 min.

The goals are to relieve pain, anti-inflammation and relieve spasm; therefore it often requires needle retention.

Needle withdrawal

Ⅰ. Needle withdrawal

Before needle withdrawal, turn off the power and disconnect the electrothermal needle from the equipment. For those with superficial needle insertion, a stable and light but not too fast needle withdrawal (without rotation) is applicable. Slow needle withdrawal is required for those with deep needle insertion.

Ⅱ. Care after needle withdrawal

Before needle withdrawal, the practitioner should carefully observe the acupoint and prepare dry sterilized cotton balls in order to stop bleeding (in certain cases). No further procedure is required for needle withdrwal. Try not to use alcohol cotton balls if possible to prevent from stimulation and skin pain, skin allergy or inflammatory reactions (e.g. redness/swelling/heat/pain).

针次与间隔

电热针针刺生效时间,多从数分钟始至 2 小时止,而针效持续时间常在 6～12 小时。如已生效而认为非 1 次可愈者,可每日 1 次或 2 次,间隔 6 小时后,便可第 2 次进针施术。若选穴处方有效,注意同一穴位连用不可超过 4 次,再次针刺须经过一段时间的休息。在连续针刺时,切忌从原针孔进针。

急性首发疾病每日可施术 1～2 次,慢性久病最好每日 1 次或隔日 1 次,体弱者隔 2 日 1 次为佳。

异常现象及处理

医务人员如能严肃认真地从事电热针医疗工作,可以减少或避免针刺时异常现象的发生。电热针临床一般所见的异常现象有如下几种:

一、晕针

现象:头晕、恶心、目眩、心悸、脉微弱、出冷汗、面色苍白、四肢厥冷,欲大小便等。

Needling frequency and intervals

The immediate efficiency of most electrothermal needling lasts between several minutes to 2 hours. But the efficiency of the therapy usually lasts for 6~12 hours. If the patient were responsive but one-time acupuncture therapy were insufficient, once or twice daily acupuncture therapy is acceptable. However, the 2nd application should be performed at minimal 6 hours interval. If the acupoint were responsive, please note that the same acupoint shouldn't be applied for more than 4 consecutive times; a period of interval is required. For continuous needling, do not apply on the same injection site.

For acute illness, the needling frequency should be 1~2 times daily. For chronic illness, the needling frequency should be once daily or once every other day. For fragile patients, the needling frequency should be once every two days.

Abnormalities and the handling

Medical/nursing staff should take caution took electrothermal acupuncture therapy more seriously in order to reduce the incidence of abnormalities or acupuncture accidents. Clinical abnormalities related to electrothermal acupuncture therapy are listed as follows:

I. Fainting during acupuncture

Manifestation: Dizziness, nausea, vertigo, palpitation, weak pulse, cold-sweating, pale face, cold extremities or incontinence.

原因：精神紧张、饥饿、疲劳、体弱或过敏、选择体位不当、取用敏感之穴或手法重、针温刺激强。

预防：做好初诊前的准备工作，以消除患者的顾虑，尽量选择卧位，饥饿、疲劳时稍事休息后再针，避免强刺激，"行针"时随时注意患者的神色和表情。

处理：调整体位，坐位改为卧位，卧时头部放低，足部垫高，并饮以热茶。

附：毫针针刺补救法

通则：针上晕则取下，针下晕则取上。

方法：出针法、补针法。

通治穴：足三里、人中、合谷、百会、少商。

误刺、深刺分别处理方法（补针法）如下：

Cause: First time receiving acupuncture therapy, fear for needles, anxiety, hunger, fatigue, weak physical condition or hypersensitivity, poor body position, sensitive acupoints or over-stimulation, or needle overheating.

Prevention: Properly prepare the patient and answer all questions about acupuncture at the first clinic visit, choose to have the patient be in a lying position if possible, take a break before next treatment session if it were caused by hunger or fatigue, avoid strong stimulation, closely observe the patient's facial expression and physical condition when applying "needle insertion".

Treatment: Adjust body positions, change sitting position to lying position, lower head position while lying and elevate feet, and drink hot tea.

Note: Remedial measures for filiform needling

General principles: Fainting during needle insertion, withdraw needle; fainting after needle withdrawal, supply with a needle.

Methods: Needle withdrawal or needle supplementation.

Tongzhi acupoints: Zusanli (ST36), Renzhong (GV26), Hegu (HI4), Baihui (GV20), Shaoshang (LU11).

Remedial measures for wrong prodding or deep needling (needle supplementation)

误刺 Wrong prodding:
- 神道——取长强补 / Acupuncture at Shendao (GV11) – Supply with Changqiang (GV1)
- 承灵——取肾俞补 / Acupuncture at Chengling (GB18) – Supply with Shenshu (BL23)
- 囟会——取风门补 / Acupuncture at Xinhui (GV22) – Supply with Fengmen (BL12)
- 膻中——取天突补 / Acupuncture at Danzhong (CV17) – Supply with Tiantu (CV22)
- 鸠尾——取中脘补 / Acupuncture at Jiuwei (CV15) – Supply with Zhongwan (CV12)
- 神门——取脊中补 / Acupuncture at Shenmen (HT7) – Supply with Jizhong (GV6)
- 手三里——取阳溪补 / Acupuncture at Shousanli (LI10) – Supply with Yangxi (LI5)

深刺 Deep needling:
- 血海——取足三里补 / Deep acupuncture at Xuehai (SP10) – Supply with Zusanli (ST36)
- 肩井——取足三里补 / Deep acupuncture at Jianjing (GB21) – Supply with Zusanli (ST36)

二、滞针

现象：针体在人体腧穴内一时性提插或捻转涩滞、困难，甚至不能提插捻转和出针者。

原因：患者精神紧张而引起肌肉痉挛；单向捻转幅度过大，组织纤维缠绕针体；留针过久。

处理：解除患者顾虑，以缓解其精神紧张，使肌肉松

II. Needle stagnation

Manifestation: Temporal needle lifting/thrusting in human acupoints, encounter stringent, sticking or difficult needle rotation, or even unable to perform needle lifting/thrusting/rotation and withdrawal.

Cause: Muscle spasm caused by anxiety, the needle was kinked with tissues or fibers due to excessive single-directional needle rotation, or prolonged needle retention.

Treatment: Answer patients' all questions concerned to soothe or calm anxiety, relax the acupoints by mas-

弛，按摩穴位四周，即可出针或留针待缓；轻弹针柄、加补一针，以解除痉挛；若组织纤维缠绕针体，可试用反方向捻针，待松动后即可出针。

三、弯针

现象：针体在腧穴内发生弯曲，针柄和原来方向偏离，手法受阻，患者疼痛，出针困难者。

原因：在手法上指力不均，刺激过猛而引起肌肉突然强烈收缩，留针期间体位变动，或受物体外力碰撞、压迫等。

预防：熟练指力，避免强刺激，嘱患者留针期间体位不要变动，防止外物碰压。

处理：若系体位变动者，应先矫正姿势，恢复进针时体位，然后视针弯曲的程度进行处理。一处折弯者，可沿着针柄偏斜的方向，顺势出针；数处折弯者，须放手观察，顺势分段，顺应方向出针。切忌强力抽拔或捻转，以免折针。

saging surrounding muscles, or to lightly flicking on the needle handle plus one additional needle insertion to relieve muscle spasm. If the needle were kinked with tissues or fibers, a reverse rotation may be helpful to loosen the kinked tissues or fibers, and therefore allow needle withdrawal.

III. Bent Needle

Manifestation: The needle is bent inside the acupoint (i.e. the needle-holder is deviated from the original direction), and the application has been limited along with pain at the injection site, so needle withdrawal becomes difficult.

Cause: Sudden muscle tetanic contraction caused by uneven finger strength, excessive stimulation, changes in body position during needle retention or external collision/compression.

Prevention: Strengthen finger power, avoid strong stimulation, remain steady and unchanged position during needle retention, and prevent from foreign object collision/compression.

Treatment: If needle bending were caused by changes in body position, correct the position and return to the original position, and then process the bent needle based on the severity of the situation. For those with one bent needle, the practitioner may withdraw the needle following the deviated direction. However, for those with several bent needles, the practitioner should evaluate and observe the entire situation, and withdraw the needle one by one following the deviated directions. Forceful needle withdrawal or twisting is prohibited to avoid bending needles.

四、折针

现象：在针刺过程中或做行针手法时，针体突然折断，针柄在术者手中，断端留于患者体内。

原因：针具质量不佳，保养不当，针体特别是针根部氧化生锈，有损伤剥蚀；患者体位移动较大；提插或捻转用力太猛，刺激过强，肌肉强力收缩；弯针时用力强拔。

预防：术前认真选择针具，行针运针手法防止用力过猛、过强刺激；进针时，根部留于体外1/3（至少约留2分），不可全部刺入；留针时，嘱患者不要移动体位。

处理：术者遇到折针时，首先要镇静，并嘱患者不要移动体位，以免断针继续深陷。如有残针露于体外，可用镊子钳出；残端与皮肤相平，可用手指轻轻压低周围组织，使残端外出，然后用镊子钳出；残端完全陷没皮内者，根据部位可用硬物顶过对侧取出；运动范围小、留于体内氧化者，由外科手术取出最安全。

IV. Broken Needle

Manifestation: Sudden needle break during application or approach; i.e. the needle-holder is still in the practitioner's hand, but the tip retains inside the patient's body.

Cause: Poor quality of the needle, poor maintenance, the needle especially the root is rusted due to oxidation, or the needle is damaged or with erosions; excessive movement of the patient during application; a profound lifting, thrusting or twisting of the needle; tetanic contraction of the muscle due to excessive stimulation; a forceful withdrawal when the needle is bent.

Prevention: Choose proper needles carefully before application, avoid forceful or excessive stimulation when applying; retain about 1/3 of the needle outside of the patient's body (at least 2cm); do not insert the needle completely; remind the patient not to move during the treatment.

Treatment: If the needle breaks, the practitioner should remain calm, and then remind the patient not to move to avoid further insertion of the broken needle. If any parts of the broken needle were visible, use the forceps to remove the retaining part. If the broken needle were at the same level of the skin, use fingers to press down the surrounding tissues in order to expose the retaining part, and then use the forcep to remove the retaining part. If the broken needle were completely submerged under the skin, use a hard object to push the needle where applicable, so the needle will penetrate through the opposite site and be removed easily. For those tiny or rusted broken needles retaining in the patient's body, it is safer to be removed by surgical approaches.

V. Bleeding and Hematoma

Manifestation: Bleeding at the injection site after needle withdrawal, or swelling or pain, followed by local bruises.

Cause: The needle tip is bent or hooked; a profound lifting or thrusting of the needle; or a penetration through subcutaneous vessels due to enriched capillaries under the acupoints.

Prevention: Examine the needles carefully; avoid vessel penetration when applying acupuncture, do not use lifting and thrusting approach at vessel-enriched areas, and use a sterile cotton ball to pressurize the injection site once the needle has been withdrawn.

Treatment: For those with bleeding at the injection site, it should be stopped by using a sterile cotton ball to pressurize the injection site for a moment. If local bruises appeared due to mild subcutaneous bleeding, normally it does not require any treatment because the bruises will naturally disappear. However, for those with severe local bruises, swelling or pain, or those with limited mobility, a local ice packing to stop bleeding should be applied, followed by hot packing or local gentle massage to improve bruises absorption.

VI. Pneumothorax

Manifestation: Those with mild conditions present chest pain, chest tightness and uncomfortable breathing while those with severe conditions show shock-like

绀、汗出、血压下降、虚脱等休克现象。

原因：术者对解剖部位不熟悉，针刺胸、背、腋、肋及缺盆等处腧穴时，因针刺角度和深度不当而使空气进入胸膜腔，造成创伤性气胸。

预防：针刺胸、背、腋、肋及缺盆等处腧穴时，要严格掌握针刺的角度和深度，不宜直刺过深和大幅度提插。

处理：轻者可给予消炎、镇痛药物，密切观察，休息3~5天，气体可自行吸收。严重者应立即采取急救措施，如胸腔抽气减压、输氧、抗休克等。

symptoms such as dyspnea, tachycardia, cyanosis on lips/nails, cold sweating, low blood pressure and fainting.

Cause: A traumatic pneumothorax is caused by inappropriate acupuncture angle and depth due to unfamiliar with anatomical structures. In other words, the air enters the pleural cavity resulting from needle penetration through acupoints on the chest, back, axillary ribs or quepen (ST12) point.

Prevention: When applying acupuncture over acupoints on the chest, back, ribs, or quepen (ST12) and jiangjing (GB21) acupoints, the angle and depth of application is strictly regulated. Excessive perpendicular insertion or profound lifting and thrusting of the needle are prohibited.

Treatment: Anti-inflammatory agents or analgesics along with close monitoring shall be provided to those with mild conditions. The air shall be automatically absorbed after 3~5 days of rest. Resuscitation procedures including chest decompression, oxygenation or anti-shock procedures shall be provided to those with severe conditions.

经络总论

经络是人体运行气血，联络脏腑，沟通内外，贯穿上下的通道。"直行者为经"，是主干，多循行于深部，纵行于固定的轨道；"支而横者为络"，是旁支，它是由经脉分出的大小分支，横行如网络一般。脉行络连，故通称"经络"。经络贯穿人体，形成纵横交错的罗网，就像自然界的河流渠道一样。气血就是通过经络昼夜运行，周流不息，使人体各部的功能活动保持共济和协调，故经络系统起着内连脏腑，外络肢节，兼理阴阳的作用。

经络系统的内容与分类

经络系统是由十二经脉、奇经八脉、十二经别、十二经筋、十二皮部和络脉紧密联系而成的。

经脉都有一定的循行路线，十五络脉也有一定的

General principles of meridians

Meridians are the channel to circulate up-to-bottom Qi and blood, connect visceral organs, and communicate internal and external signals. "The straight channel is Jing mai", which is the principal network located longitudinally at fixed channels and mostly circulates in deep tissues. "The horizontal channel is Luo mai", which is the collateral branches derived from Jing mai and runs across human body like a network. Pulse line connects to each other, and therefore is normally called "meridian". The meridians run through the human body and form a cross-linked network like natural river channels. The Qi and blood circulate through these meridian channels nonstop so as to coordinate the functions and activities of individual parts of the human body. Therefore, the meridian system not only communicates internal organs and activates extremities, but regulates Yin and Yang.

The contents and categories of the meridian system

The meridian system contains a closely connected network composed of the 12 principal meridians, the 8 extraordinary vessels, the 12 divergent meridians, the 12 cutaneous regions as well as the collaterals.

All of the Jing mai have fixed flow patterns, so do the 15 Luo mai. As to the smaller "tertiary collaterals" or

循行路线，而更细小的"孙络""浮络"则无一定的循行路线。

奇经八脉不同于十二经，既无脏腑属络关系，又无表里相合关系，其主要功能是对十二经气血流注盛衰起着联系、统率、调节溢蓄的作用。奇经八脉中，除了任、督二脉有本经所属的腧穴外，其余六脉均无本经腧穴，而是依附于与十二经脉相交的腧穴。

十五络脉，是从十二正经、督脉、任脉各自分出的一支络脉，再加上脾之大络，共为十五络。其主要功能是沟通表里两经，渗灌局部气血，加强经脉的循环传注作用。在正虚邪乘的情况下，络脉是病邪传注的途径。按络脉所主病证，针灸临床常采用原络配穴法而奏效。从十五络脉分出的小络脉称为"浮络"和"孙络"，即《灵枢·脉度》所说："经脉为里，支而横者为络，络之别者为孙。"络脉遍布全身，作用主要是"溢奇邪""通

"superficial collaterals", no fixed flow pattern is required.

The 8 extraordinary vessels are different from the 12 principal meridians; i.e. the 8 extraordinary vessels neither connect to visceral organs nor match the internal vessels with superficial collaterals. The primary functions of the 8 extraordinary vessels are to coordinate, dominate and regulate the outflow/inflow as well as the excitation/inhibition of the 12 principal meridians and Qi. Among the 8 extraordinary vessels, except the conception (Ren channel) and governor (Du channel) vessels, the rest 6 vessels do not consist of any acupoints mentioned in the *Shennong's Classic of Materia Medica*. On the contrary, the 6 vessels only contain acupoints which cross-over the 12 principal meridians.

Fifteen Luo mai refer to the collateral Luo mai exit from the 12 principal meridians, Du channel and Ren channel plus a major spleen Luo mai, total of 15 Luo mai. The primary functions of Luo mai are to communicate the superficial and internal Jing mai, increase local Qi-blood perfusion, and improve the circulation of the meridian. Under the circumstances of deficient vital Qi leading to lingering of pathogen, the Luo mai becomes the pathogen transmission pathway. Therefore, the acupuncture therapy in combination with the "Yuan-primary point and Luo-connecting point combination" is effective in the treatment for Luo mai-based syndromes. The small Luo mai branches derived from the 15 Luo mai are called "tertiary collaterals" or "superficial collaterals", which also mentioned in the Book "Lingshu Jing (a theoretical

营卫"。

任脉总督一身的阴经,称为"阴脉之海",因其调节十二经气血,故又称"十二经脉之海";督脉总督一身的阳经,称为"阳脉之海"。

十二经脉命名、分布及循行规律

一、十二经脉的命名原则

1. 根据中医阴阳理论及经脉中阴阳盛衰不同

阴经分为太阴、少阴、厥阴;阳经则分为阳明、太阳、少阳。

2. 根据藏象学说

手足之三阴和手足之三阳分别和脏腑相配,阴经配脏,阳经配腑。

book regarding Traditional Chinese Medicine)", Section "Mai Du (meridian measurement)": "The longitudinal channel is called *jing mai* while the horizontal channel is called luo mai. The collateral channel of Luo mai is called tertiary collateral." The Luo points cover the entire human body, whose primary function is to "defense against extraordinary pathogens" and "regulate Ying and Wei-Qi".

The conception (Ren) channel governs the overall Yin meridians and the Qi-blood of the 12 principal meridians, and thus is called "the sea of the Yin meridians" or "the sea of the 12 principal meridians". The governor (Du) channel controls the overall Yang meridians, and therefore is called "the sea of the *yang* meridians".

The nomenclature, distribution and running rules of twelve regular meridians

I. The nomenclature of twelve regular meridians

1. The Yin-Yang theory of Traditional Chinese Medicine is different from the aspect of Yin (inhibition, degeneration)/Yang (excitation, growth) in Meridian.

Yin meridian consists of Tai Yin, Shao Yin and Jue Yin meridians while yang meridian consists of Yang-Ming, Tai-Yang and Shao-Yang meridians.

2. According to the theory of visceral manifestations

The three Yin meridians of Hand/Foot and the three Yang meridians of Hand/Foot match with Zang and Fu organs respectively; i.e. the Yin meridian dominates Zang (Yin organs including heart, liver, spleen, lung and kidneys) while the Yang meridian controls Fu (Yang organs including small/large intestines, stomach, gallbladder, urinary bladder and three Jiaos).

II. The distribution of twelve meridians

十二经脉的分布情况见表4、表5。

Please refer to Table 4 and 5 for the distribution of twelve meridians.

表 4 十二经脉在四肢的分布规律及脏腑络属关系
Table 4. The distribution pattern and associate Zang-Fu pathways of twelve meridians at four extremities

十二经脉 Twelve meridians	阴经（属脏络腑，行于四肢内侧）Yin meridian (Zang-to-Fu pathway, runs along the inner side of four extremities)	手三阴（上肢）three Yin meridians of Hand(Tai-Yin, Shao-Yin, Jue-Yin) meridians for upper extremity 足三阴（下肢）three Yin meridians of Foot (Tai-Yin, Shao-Yin, Jue-Yin) for lower extremity	太阴在前
			厥阴在中
			少阴在后
	阳经（属腑络脏，行于四肢外侧）Yang meridian (Fu-to-Zang pathway, runs along the external side of four extremities)	手三阳（上肢）three Yang meridians of Hand (Yang-Ming, Tai-Yang, Shao-Yang) for upper extremity 足三阳（下肢）three Yang meridians of Foot (Yang-Ming, Tai-Yang, Shao-Yang) for lower extremity	阳明在前
			少阳在中
			太阳在后

注：足太阴脾经在内踝上8寸以下行于足厥阴肝经之后。
Note: Tai-Yin Spleen Meridian of Foot is located 8" above the inner ankle, so it can run downward and behind the Jue-Yin Liver Meridian of Foot.

表 5 十二经脉在头面躯干的分布规律
Table 5. The distribution of twelve meridians over the head, face and trunk

部位 Arrangement \ 经脉 Meridian \ 分布 Distribution	头面部 Craniofacial	躯干部 trunk
前 Front	手足阳明 Yang-Ming Meridians of Hand/Foot	手足三阴、足阳明 Tai-Yin, Shao-Yin, Jue-Yin Meridians of Hand/Foot;Yang-Ming Meridian of Foot
侧 Lateral	手足少阳、手太阳、足阳明 Shou-Yang Meridians of Hand/Foot; Tai-Yang Meridian of Hand; Yang-Ming Meridian of Foot	足少阳、手足厥阴 Shao-Yang Meridian of Foot; Jue-Yin Meridians of Hand
后 Back	足太阳、足少阳 Tai-Yang, Shao-Yang Meridian of Foot	足太阳 Tai-Yang Meridian of Foot

三、十二经脉的走向规律

手之三阴，从胸走手；手之三阳，从手走头；足之三阳，从头走足；足之三阴，从足走腹。

四、十二经脉的循行顺序规律

始于手太阴肺经→手阳明大肠经→足阳明胃经→足太阴脾经→手少阴心经→手太阳小肠经→足太阳膀胱经→足少阴肾经→手厥阴心包经→手少阳三焦经→足少阳胆经→足厥阴肝经→手太阴肺经。

经络的作用

一、生理方面

经脉以其运行的全身气血，对机体五脏六腑、四肢九窍起着营养调节作用。通过经络将体表与内脏等组织器官联成一个统一的整体，得以进行正常的生命活动。

III. The patterns of twelve meridian flows

The three Yin meridians of hand flow from the chest to hands; the three Yang meridians of hand flow from hands to the head; the three Yang meridians of foot run from the head to feet; and the three Yin meridians of foot run from feet to the abdomen.

IV. The running rules of twelve meridian flows

From Tai-Yin Lung Meridian of Hand→Yang-Ming Large Intestine Meridian of Hand→Yang-Ming Stomach Meridian of Foot→Tai-Yin Spleen Meridian of Foot→Shao-Yin Heart Meridian of Hand→Tai-Yang Small Intestine Meridian of Hand→Tai-Yang Bladder Meridian of Foot→Shao-Yin Kidney Meridian of Foot→Jue-Yin Pericardium Meridian of Hand→Shao-Yang Three-Jiao Meridian of Hand→Shao-Yang Gallbladder Meridian of Foot→Jue-Yin Liver Meridian of Foot→to Tai-Yin Lung Meridian of Hand

The functions of meridians

I. Physiology

The systemic blood running in the meridians coordinates nutritional regulation of the body's internal organs, and limbs Jiuqiao. Through the meridians of the body and visceral tissues and organs together into a unified whole, can be carried out normal life activities. The meridian systems regulate the nutritional status of the internal organs (Five-Zang and Six-Fu) and the four limbs as well as the nine orifices in human bodies through running the entire circulation Qi and blood. The meridian system links the superficial channels to the internal organs and therefore forms a unified entity to perform normal living activities.

二、病理方面

外邪侵袭人体通过经络传入脏腑，而内脏功能失调也可以通过经络反映到其经脉所属的体表，这便给临床提供了辨证与施治的参考依据。

Ⅱ. Pathology

External pathogens may invade internal organs in human bodies through the meridian system. At the same time, the organ dysfunctions may also be reflected through meridian system to the surface Jing mai zones, which provides the evidence base for syndrome differentiation and treatment.

三、诊断方面

发展地运用了经络传导刺激和反映证候的临床特征来查知脏腑经络的病变，主要根据经络所属的体表部位出现的过敏点或压痛点及异常现象。常用的方法有：望诊、切脉、经络按诊法及"经络探测仪"测量等。

Ⅲ. Diagnosis

The conduction and stimulation of the meridian systems have been developed to reflect the clinical manifestations of the syndromes, and to verify the pathological changes of the internal organs as well as the meridians. The hypersensitive points or tender points and abnormalities occurred on the surface of body parts basically are all linked to the meridian channels. Common methods consist of observation, palpation, meridian pressation and modern "meridian detector" measurements.

四、治疗方面

中医的内治法和外治法皆以经络为指导，特别是对针灸尤其重要。针灸是通过给予经穴、压痛点或过敏点一定的理

Ⅳ. Treatment

The internal treatment and external treatment of Traditional Chinese Medicine are both based on the guidance of the meridians, which thereby are particularly important to the acupuncture therapy. The acupuncture ther-

化刺激，产生针感，激发经络的传导扩散作用，从而调整气血阴阳，使人体脏腑功能恢复正常。

apy is a physicochemical stimulation with fixed intensity applied through the meridian acupoints, tender points or hypersensitive points to generate needling sensations. The conductance and transmission of activated meridians may regulate the Qi, blood, Yin and Yang, and thus affects the functions of the internal organs, consequently recover human body functions.

腧穴

Acupoints

概述

Overview

腧穴是人体脏腑经络气血输注于体表的特殊部位，亦称"气穴""穴位""孔穴""穴道"，它通过经络与脏腑器官发生联系。针灸或其他外治法在体表所选的腧穴，通过经络调整气血阴阳，从而达到防治疾病的目的。腧穴的发展，经历了无定名、无定位（即以痛为输）到定名、定位、分部、分经等不断提高、完善的漫长过程，历代医家对其进行过多次整理，归纳起来可将腧穴分为经穴、经外奇穴、阿是穴三类。

Acupoints: The special body parts that the Qi and blood from internal organs are transported to the body surface though the meridian system in human bodies, so they are also called "Qi points", "acupuncture points", "acupuncture holes" or "acupuncture channels". Acupoints connect to the internal organs through the meridian channels. The acupuncture therapy or other external treatment-selected acupoints on body surface may regulate Qi-blood and Yin-Yang through the meridian system and then achieve the goal of disease prevention. The evolvement of acupoints, from no name, no location (i.e. painful site equals to an acupoint); to the definition of name, location, division and meridian. The long-term categorization process has been sophisticated and completed. After multiple summarizations by previous physicians, the acupoints now can be divided into three major types, including meridian points, extraordinary points and Ashi points.

一、经穴

I. Meridian points

指归属于十二经脉与任、督二脉的腧穴，称为十四经穴，简称"经穴"。经穴共361个。

It refers to acupoints linking to twelve regular Jing mai and the Ren channel as well as the Du channel, which are called "acupoints of fourteen meridians" or "meridian points" in brief. There are total of 361 meridi-

二、经外奇穴

指没有归属于十四经，但有穴名、定位、主治的一类腧穴。

三、阿是穴

这类穴位既无定名，又无定位，以病痛局部或与病痛有关的压痛点或反应点作为腧穴。

腧穴的作用主要为输注气血、反应病证、协助诊断和防治疾病。

取穴方法

寻找腧穴的位置，称为取穴。取穴准确与否可直接影响治疗效果，因而标定其位置必须参阅有关的取穴法。临床上常用的腧穴取穴法可分为以下3类：

一、骨度分寸折量取穴法

本法是指以体表骨节为主要标志折量全身各部的长度和宽度，定出分寸，用于经穴定位的方法，其主要用于头、胸、腹、上肢和下肢等穴位间距离的量度。由于此法不受人

an points.

II. Extraordinary points

It refers to the acupoints that do not belong to 14 meridians, but with certain acupoint names, locations and specific indications.

III. Ashi Acupoints

Such acupoints do not have specific names or locations, only relate to tender points or responsive points that are relevant to local painful or lesion sites.

The primary functions of acupoints are to infuse Qi and blood, reflect symptoms, assist diagnoses and disease prevention.

Methods of locating acupoints

The method to search for locations of acupoints is called acupoint locating. The accuracy of acupoint locating may directly influence the therapeutic effects. Therefore, the locating of acupoints must refer to relevant methods. There are three common methods of acupoint locating used in clinical practice:

I. Locating acupoints by bone-length proportional measurement

This method uses body surface bony landmarks to proportionally measure the length and width of all body parts, and thereby determines scales that can be used to locate acupoints. The method is primarily based on the measurements between acupoints located on the head, chest, abdomen, upper and lower extremities. Because

体高矮胖瘦的影响，成人、小孩均可准确定位，在临床上较为常用。现将临床常用定位总结如下（表6、图11）。

body features (e.g. height and weight) do not have impacts on the accuracy of acupoint locating, and the method is applicable to both adults and children, it is therefore becoming a common strategy applied in clinical practice. Now, we have summarized common methods of acupoint locating used in clinical practice as follows (Table 6, Figure 11).

表6 常用骨度分寸表
Table 6. Table of common bone-length proportional measurement

部位 Parts	起止点 Starting and ending points	折量寸 Proportional length (1" =1 cun=1/3dm)	说明 Notes
头部 Head	前发际至后发际 Front hairline to back hairline	12	如发际不明显者，可自眉间（印堂）至第7颈椎棘突折作18寸 For those who do not have clear hairlines, the length between inter-eyebrow space (ophryon, Yintang) and the spinous process of C7 is 18"
	前发际至眉心 Front hairline to the midpoint between eyebrows	3	
	后发际至第7颈椎棘突 Back hairline to the spinous process of C7	3	
	两前额角之间 The length between angulus frontalis	9	两乳突最高点间亦作9寸 The length between the highest points of two mastoid process is 9"
胸腹部 Chest and Abdomen	两乳头之间 The length between two nipples	8	胸部直寸一般以肋骨隙为取穴依据，每一肋骨大约折作1.6寸 The measurement of acupoints located on the chest is usually based on the length of intercostal space; i.e. each intercostal space roughly equals to 1.6"
	胸骨体下缘至脐中 The lower border of sternum body to the navel	8	
	脐中至耻骨联合上缘 The navel to the upper boarder of symphysis pubis	5	
	腋窝横纹至第11肋 Armpit stripes to the 11th rib	12	
背腰 Back and waist	肩胛骨内缘至背正中线 The inner boarder of the scapula to the midline of the back	3	背部直寸以椎序、棘突间隙取 The locations of the acupoints on the back depend on the measurements between the vertebral level and the spinous process.
上肢 Upper extremities	腋前横纹至肘横纹 Armpit stripes to the elbow stripes	9	上肢内、外侧同用 Applicable to both inner and outer sides of the upper and lower extremities
	肘横纹至腕横纹 Elbow stripes to the wrist stripes	12	

续表

部位 Parts	起止点 Starting and ending points	折量寸 Proportional length (1" =1 cun=1/3dm)	说明 Notes
下肢 Lower extremities	股骨大粗隆（大转子）至膝中 (Femoral) greater trochanter to the middle of the knee	9	同用于下肢前、外、后侧 Applicable to both anterior, external and lateral sides of the lower extremities
	膝中至外踝尖 The middle of the knee to external ankle apex	16	
	耻骨联合上缘至股骨内上髁上缘 The upper boarder of symphysis pubis to the upper boarder of the femoral medial condyle	8	同用于下肢内侧 Applicable to inner sides of the lower extremities
	胫骨内侧髁下缘至内踝尖 The lower boarder of the tibial medial condyle to the inner ankle apex	13	

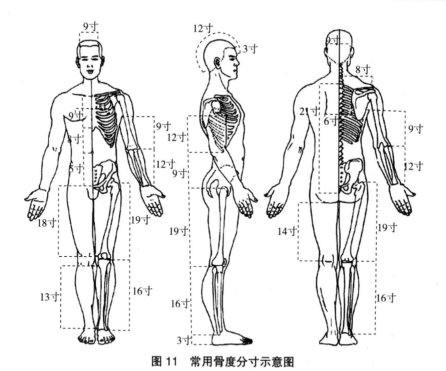

图 11 常用骨度分寸示意图

Figure 11. The schematic diagram of common bone-length measurement used for acupoint locating(in cun)

二、指寸取穴法

本法是指依据患者本人手指的某些部位折作一定分寸用

II. Locating acupoints by fingers

This method uses the patient's fingers as units to measure the location of acupoints. There three approach-

以比量腧穴位置的方法，分为中指同身寸、拇指同身寸、横指同身寸三种。

1. 中指同身寸

《太平圣惠方》曰："手中指第二节内度两横纹相去为一寸。"《针灸大全》指出："大指与中指相屈如环，取中指中节横纹，上下相去，长短为 1 寸。"（图 12）

2. 拇指同身寸

《备急千金要方》曰："取手大拇指第一节横度为一寸。"（图 13）

3. 横指同身寸（一夫法）

《备急千金要方》曰："凡量一夫之法，覆手并舒四指，对度四指上中节上横过为一夫。""四指"分别指食指、中指、无名指、小指，宽度相当于 3 寸。本法多用于四肢、下腹部的直寸和背部的横寸定穴（图 14）。

es including proportional unit of middle finger, proportional unit of the thumb and four-finger-breadth measurement.

1. Proportional unit of the middle finger

The Book *Taiping Shenghui Fang* mentioned that "The distance between the proximal and the distal phalange of the middle finger equals to 1"." The Book *Compendium of Acupuncture and Moxibustion* pointed out that "When circle the middle finger with the thumb (thumb opposition), the distance between the proximal and the distal phalange of the middle finger equals to 1"." (Figure 12)

2. Proportional unit f the thumb

Essential Recipes for Emergent Use Worth a Thousand Gold mentioned that "The diameter of the thumb around the phalange equals to 1"." (Figure 13)

3. Four-finger-breadth measurement (four-finger-width measurement)

Essential Recipes for Emergent Use Worth a Thousand Gold mentioned that "It refers to the width across four proximal phalanges (index, middle, ring and little fingers) when using four-finger-breadth measurement by approximating all fingers while relaxing the phalanges." The width equals to 3". This method is mostly used to locate acupoints on the extremities, the vertical meridians on the lower abdomen and the horizontal meridian on the back (Figure 14).

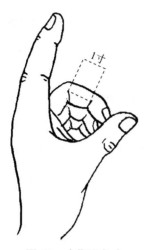

图 12 中指同身寸

Figure 12. Proportional unit of the middle finger

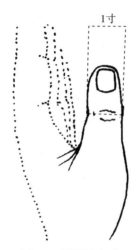

图 13 拇指同身寸

Figure 13. Proportional unit of the thumb

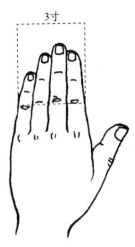

图 14 横指同身寸

Figure 14. Four-finger-breadth measurement

三、体表解剖标志取穴法

本法是指以体表解剖学的各种体表标志为依据来确定经穴位置的方法。

III. Locating acupoints by using the method of anatomical landmarks

This method uses various body surface anatomical landmarks to confirm and locate the acupoints.

十四经穴选要

Acupoint guidelines for fourteen meridians

一、手太阴肺经（左右各11穴，共22穴）

I. Tai-Yin Lung Meridian of Hand (11 acupoints on each arm, total of 22 acupoints)

（一）循行路线

手太阴肺经起于上腹部中焦，下络大肠，回绕过来沿着胃的上口，穿过横膈，入属于肺，从肺系（肺与喉咙相联系的部位）横行出来（中府），向下沿上臂内侧，行于手少阴经

(I) Meridian pathway

The Tai-Yin Lung Meridian of Hand originates in the upper abdomen (Middle Jiao), and runs downwards connecting with the large intestine. It then turns along with the upper boarder of the stomach, and passes through the diaphragm to connect with the lungs. This meridian branch out horizontally from the lung meridian

和手厥阴经的前面，下行到肘窝中，沿着前臂内侧前缘，入寸口，经过大鱼际，沿着大鱼际的边缘，出拇指桡侧末端（少商）。

分支：从腕后（列缺）分出，一直走向食指桡侧端（商阳），与手阳明大肠经相接。

（二）联系脏腑器官

肺经属肺，络大肠，与中焦（胃）、肺系（气管）、喉咙有联系。

（三）主治

主治肺、胸、咽喉等病及本经脉循行部位的病症。

（四）经穴

中府（LU1）、云门（LU2）、天府（LU3）、侠白（LU4）、尺泽（LU5）、孔最（LU6）、列缺（LU7）、经渠（LU8）、太渊（LU9）、鱼际（LU10）、少商（LU11）。

(the joint connection between the lung and the throat) (Zhongfu, LU1), runs down the medial aspect of the upper arm where it crosses the front of Shao-Yin of Hand and Jue-Yin of Hand meridians, then runs down to the axilla (armpit) together with the medial aspect of the forearm, and enter into the medial aspect of the radial artery (Cunkou). It continues until it passes the thenar muscle (Yuji, LU10) and emerges at the tip of the thumb (radial side, Shao-shang, LU11).

Another branch emerges from the back of the wrist (Lieque, LU7) and ends at the radial side of the tip of the index finger (Shangyang, LI1) to connect with the Yang-Ming Large Intestine Meridian of Hand.

(II) Relevant Zang, Fu and organs

Lung meridian governs the lung, the large intestine collateral, and connects with the Middle-Jiao (stomach), pulmonary system (bronchus) and throat.

(III) Main indications

Acupuncture points in the Lung Meridian are indicated for throat, chest and lung ailments and for other symptoms that are presented along the meridian's pathway.

(IV) Meridian points

Zhongfu (LU1), Yunmen (LU2), Tianfu (LU3), Xiabai (LU4), Chize (LU5), Kongzui (LU6), Lieque (LU7), Jingqu (LU8), Taiyuan (LU9), Yuji (LU10), Shaoshang (LU11).

（五）要穴简介（图15）　　（Ⅴ）Introductions of key acupoints (Figure 15)

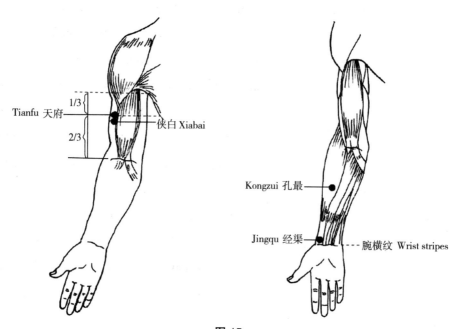

图 15
Figure 15

1. 天府（LU3）

定位：在臂内侧面，肱二头肌桡侧缘，腋前纹头下3寸。

主治：气喘，鼻衄，肺出血，风湿，瘿气，上臂内侧痛。

2. 侠白（LU4）

定位：在臂内侧面，肱二头肌桡侧缘，腋前纹头下4寸。

主治：咳嗽，气喘，烦满，肋间神经痛，上臂内侧痛。

1. Tianfu (LU3)

Location: The medial aspect of the arm, the lateral boarder of the biceps brachii, 3" below the anterior axillary line.

Main indications: Asthma, epistaxis, pulmonary hemorrhage, rheumatism, simple goiter, and pain in the medial side of the upper arm.

2. Xiabai (LU4)

Location: The medial aspect of the arm, the lateral boarder of the biceps brachii, 4" below the anterior axillary line.

Main indications: Cough, asthma, dysphoria, intercostal neuralgia, and pain in the medial side of the upper arm.

3. 孔最（LU6）（郄穴）

定位：在前臂掌面桡侧，尺泽与太渊连线上，腕横纹上7寸。

主治：咯血，咳嗽，气喘，咽喉肿痛，痔疾，肘臂挛痛。

4. 经渠（LU8）（经穴）

定位：在前臂掌面桡侧，桡骨茎突与桡动脉之间的凹陷处，腕横纹上1寸。

主治：咳嗽，气喘，咽喉肿痛，小儿急性支气管炎，胸痛，腕部疼痛。

二、手阳明大肠经（左右各20穴，共40穴）

（一）循行路线

手阳明大肠经起于食指桡侧端（商阳），沿食指桡侧上行，经过合谷穴，行于上肢外侧前缘，上至肩关节前上缘，过肩后，到项后第7颈椎棘突下（大椎），再向前下行入锁骨上窝（缺盆），进入胸腔络肺，向下通过膈肌下行，属大肠。

3. Kongzui (LU6)(Xi acupoint, also called xi-cleft point)

Location: Radial palmer side of the forearm, connects with Chize (LU5) and Taiyuan (LU9), 7" above the wrist.

Main indications: Hemoptysis, cough, asthma, sore throat, hemorrhoids, and elbow/arm spasm and pain.

4. Jingqu (LU8)(meridian point)

Location: Radial palmer side of the forearm, the concavity between radial stolid process and radial artery, 1" above the wrist.

Main indications: Cough, asthma, sore throat, pediatric acute bronchitis, chest pain, and wrist pain.

II. Yang-Ming Large Intestine Meridian of Hand(20 acupoints on each arm, total of 40 acupoints)

(Ⅰ) Meridian pathway

The Yang-Ming Large Intestine Meridian of Hand starts from the radial side tip of the index finger (Shangyang, LI1) and runs up between the thumb and the index finger and passes Hegu (LI4) point. It then proceeds along the lateral side of the forearm and the anterior side of the upper arm, until it reaches the anterior upper boarder of the shoulder. After passing the shoulder, it goes around the neck and runs down to the spinous process of C7 (Dazhui, DU14), then goes anterior and down to the supraclavicular fossa (Quepen, ST12), enters into chest meridian system, and runs down through the diaphragm to govern the large intestine.

上行的支脉：从锁骨上窝（缺盆）上行，经颈部至面颊，过大迎，入下齿中，复返出挟口角两旁，过地仓，绕至上唇与鼻下的中央（人中），左右交叉于人中（右脉左行，左脉右行），分别至对侧鼻翼旁（迎香），交于足阳明胃经。

（二）联系脏腑器官

大肠经属大肠，络肺，与口、下齿、鼻有联系。

（三）主治

主治头面、口鼻、唇齿、胃肠、神志、皮肤、发热等病及本经脉循行部位的病症。

（四）经穴

商阳（LI1）、二间（LI2）、三间（LI3）、合谷（LI4）、阳溪（LI5）、偏历（LI6）、温溜（LI7）、下廉（LI8）、上廉（LI9）、手三里（LI10）、曲池（LI11）、肘髎（LI12）、手五里（LI13）、臂臑（LI14）、肩髃（LI15）、巨

The other travels externally upwards from the supraclavicular fossa (Quepen, ST12), where it passes the neck, cheek and Daying (ST5), and enters the lower teeth and gums. It then curves around the corner of the mouth, passes Dicang (ST4), goes around to the upper lip and the center under the nose (the philtrum), and crosses at the philtrum (right meridian goes to left and left meridian goes to right), and crosses to the opposite side of the nose (Yingxiang, LI20) as well as the Yang-Ming Stomach Meridian of Foot.

(Ⅱ) Relevant Zang, Fu and organs

The large intestine meridian governs the large intestine, lung collateral, and connects with the mouth, lower teeth and nose.

(Ⅲ) Main indications

Acupuncture points in this meridian are indicated for diseases affecting the head, face, mouth, nose, lips and teeth, stomach and intestines, consciousness, skin, febrile conditions and other symptoms along the meridian pathway.

(Ⅳ) Meridian points

Shanyang (LI1), Erjian (LI2), Sanjian (LI3), Hegu (LI4), Yangxi (LI5), Pianli (LI6), Wenliu (LI7), Xialian (LI8), Shanglian (LI9), Shousanli (LI10), Quchi (LI11), Zhouliao (LI12), Shouwuli (LI13), Binao (LI14), Jianyu (LI15), Jugu (LI16), Tianding (LI17), Futu (LI18), Heliao (LI19), Yingxiang (LI20).

骨（LI16）、天鼎（LI17）、扶突（LI18）、禾髎（LI19）、迎香（LI20）。

（五）要穴简介（图 16）

1. 合谷（LI4）（原穴）

定位：手背第1、2掌骨间第2掌骨桡侧中点处。

(V) Introductions of key acupoints (Figure 16)

1. Hegu (LI4) (Yuan acupoint, or yuan-primary point)

Location: On the dorsal side of the hand; between the 1st, and 2nd metacarpal bone; at the mid-point, radial side of the 2nd metacarpal bone.

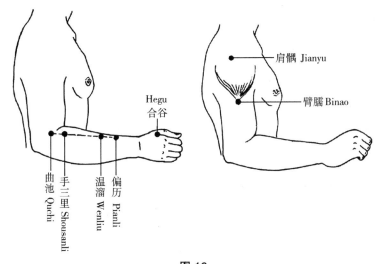

图 16
Figure 16

主治：头痛，咽喉肿痛，牙痛，面神经麻痹，口眼㖞斜，三叉神经痛，胃痛，月经不调，半身不遂。

2. 偏历（LI6）（络穴）

定位：曲肘，前臂背面桡侧，阳溪与曲池连线上，腕横纹上3寸。

Main indications: Headache, sore throat, toothache, facial palsy, deviation of the eye, trigeminal neuralgia, stomachache, menoxenia, paralysis.

2. Pianli (LI6) (collateral point)

Location: Flex the elbow, dorsal side of the forearm, radial side, connects with Yangxi (LI5) and Quchi (LI11), 3" above the wrist.

主治：耳鸣耳聋，目赤，齿痛，喉痛，手臂疼痛，水肿。

3. 温溜（LI7）（郄穴）

定位：曲肘，前臂背面桡侧，阳溪与曲池连线上，腕横纹上5寸。

主治：头痛，面肿，咽喉肿痛，口舌肿痛，手臂痛。

4. 手三里（LI10）

定位：前臂背面桡侧，阳溪与曲池连线上，肘横纹下2寸。

主治：齿痛颊肿，上肢不遂，肩臂疼痛，腹痛腹泻。

5. 曲池（LI11）（合穴）

定位：屈肘，肘横纹桡侧端凹陷中。

主治：热病，咽喉肿痛，齿痛，目赤肿痛，半身不遂，手臂肿痛，癫狂，头晕，瘰疬，瘾疹，腹痛吐泻，高血压。

6. 臂臑（LI14）

定位：臂外侧三角肌止点处，曲池与肩髃连线上，曲池上7寸。

主治：肩臂痛，颈项痉挛，目疾，瘰疬。

7. 肩髃（LI15）（手阳明经、阳跷脉交会穴）

定位：肩峰与肱骨大结节

Main indications: Tinnitus, deaf, red eye, toothache, sore throat, pain on the arms, swelling.

3. Wenliu (LI7) (Xi acupoint)

Location: Flex the elbow, dorsal side of the forearm, radial side, connects with Yangxi (LI5) and Quchi (LI11), 5" above the wrist.

Main indications: Headache, face swelling, sore throat, mouth and tongue swelling and pain, pain on the arms.

4. Shousanli (LI10)

Location: Dorsal side of the forearm, radial side, connects with Yangxi (LI5) and Quchi (LI11), 2" below the elbow.

Main indications: Toothache, cheeks swelling, upper extremity paralysis, shoulder/upper arm pain, abdominal pain, diarrhea.

5. Quchi (LI11) (He acupoint, also called he-sea point)

Location: Flex elbow, the concavity at the radial side of the elbow

Main indications: Fever, sore throat, toothache, red eye, eye swelling and pain, paralysis, arm swelling and pain, manic-depressive psychosis, dizziness, scrofula, urticaria, abdominal pain, vomiting, diarrhea, high blood pressure.

6. Binao (LI14)

Location: At the terminal end of the deltoid on the lateral side of the upper arm, connects with Quchi (LI11) and Jianyu (LI15), 7" above the Quchi (LI11).

Main indications: Shoulder and upper arm pain, neck spasm, eye problem, scrofula.

7. Jianyu (LI15) (the cross over point of the Yang-Ming Meridian of Hand and the Yangqiao Meridian)

Location: The concavity between the acromion and

之间的凹陷中。

主治：肩臂疼痛，手臂挛急，风热瘾疹，瘰疬，半身不遂。

三、足阳明胃经（左右各 45 穴，共 90 穴）

（一）循行路线

足阳明胃经起于鼻翼两侧（迎香），挟鼻上行至鼻根部，旁行入目内眦（睛明），与足太阳经相交，向下沿鼻柱外侧，过承泣、巨髎，进入上齿龈内，还出，挟口两旁，环绕嘴唇，左右相交于颏唇沟（承浆），再向后沿下颌骨后下缘到大迎处，上行过耳前，经上关，沿着前发际到达额前（头维）。

分支：由下颌分出，沿喉咙入锁骨上窝，下膈，属胃络脾。其支脉起于胃口，循腹里，与锁骨上窝直行脉会合于腹股沟。

其直行的支脉，从锁骨上窝下行，经乳头，沿腹正中线旁开 2 寸到腹股沟，循下肢外侧前缘，行走至次趾末端

the greater tubercle of the humerus.

Main indications: Shoulder and upper arm pain, acute arm spasm, wind-heat, urticaria, scrofula, paralysis.

III. Yang-Ming Stomach Meridian of Foot (45 acupoints on each leg, total of 90 acupoints)

(I) Meridian pathway

The Yang-Ming Stomach Meridian of Foot starts from the side of the nose (Yingxiang, LI20), cross with Tai-Yang Meridian of Foot, goes down along with the lateral side of the nose, passes Chengqi (ST1), Juliao (ST3), enters into upper gum and then goes out and curves around the lips and lower jaw. The right and left collateral crosses over the mentolabial furrow (Chengjiang, CV24), and runs backward along with the lower mandible posterolateral boarder to the Daying (ST5). It then turns upwards, passing in front of the ear, passes through Shangguan (GB3) until it reaches the corner of the forehead (Touwei, ST8).

One branch emerges from the lower jaw, running from the throat to the supraclavicular fossa and then downwards through diaphragm until it reaches its pertaining organ, the stomach and the spleen. The collateral meridian starts from the stomach, runs down along with the abdomen rectus and merges with the supraclavicular fossa vertical collateral at the groin.

The vertical collateral goes downward from the supraclavicular fossa, through the nipples, and runs 2" aside with the linea mediana ventralis to the groin, and then it goes further downward along the front of the

（厉兑）。

分支：从膝下3寸（足三里）而别，下行到第3趾外侧端。

别络：从足背（冲阳）分出，前行进入足大趾内侧端（隐白），交于足太阴脾经。

（二）联系脏腑器官

胃经属胃，络脾，与鼻、眼、口、上齿、喉咙、乳房相联系。

（三）主治

主治头面、口鼻、口齿、胃肠、神志疾患及本经脉循行部位的病症。

（四）经穴

承泣（ST1）、四白（ST2）、巨髎（ST3）、地仓（ST4）、大迎（ST5）、颊车（ST6）、下关（ST7）、头维（ST8）、人迎（ST9）、水突（ST10）、气舍（ST11）、缺盆（ST12）、气户（ST13）、库房（ST14）、屋翳（ST15）、膺窗（ST16）、乳中（ST17）、乳根（ST18）、

thigh and the lower leg, until it reaches the top of the 2nd toe (Lidui, ST45).

Other collateral branches from 3" below the knee (Zusanli, ST36) and runs down to the lateral side of the 3rd toe.

The collateral branch out from the dorsal foot (Chongyang, ST42), enters anteriorly into the inner side of the big toe (Yinbai, SP1), and crosses over with the Tai-Yin Spleen Meridian of Foot.

(II) Relevant Zang, Fu and organs

The stomach meridian governs stomach, collaterals with spleen, and connects to the nose, eyes, mouth, upper teeth, throat and the breasts.

(III) Main indications

Acupuncture points in this meridian are indicated for head, face, mouth and nose, mouth and teeth, gastro-enteric diseases, mental illnesses and other symptoms along the meridian pathway.

(IV) Meridian points

Chengqi (ST1), Sibai (ST2), Juliao (ST3), Dicang (ST4), Daying (ST5), Jiache (ST6), Xiaguan (ST7), Touwei (ST8), Renying (ST9), Shuitu (ST10), Qishe (ST11), Quepen (ST12), Qihu (ST13), Kufang (ST14), Wuyi (ST15), Yingchuang (ST16), Ruzhong (ST17), Rugen (ST18), Burong (ST19), Chengman (ST20), Liangmen (ST21), Guanmen (ST22), Taiyi (ST23), Huaroumen (ST24), Tianshu (ST25), Wailing (ST26), Daju (ST27), Shuidao (ST28), Guilai (ST29), Qichong (ST30), Biguan

不容（ST19）、承满（ST20）、梁门（ST21）、关门（ST22）、太乙（ST23）、滑肉门（ST24）、天枢（ST25）、外陵（ST26）、大巨（ST27）、水道（ST28）、归来（ST29）、气冲（ST30）、髀关（ST31）、伏兔（ST32）、阴市（ST33）、梁丘（ST34）、犊鼻（ST35）、足三里（ST36）、上巨虚（ST37）、条口（ST38）、下巨虚（ST39）、丰隆（ST40）、解溪（ST41）、冲阳（ST42）、陷谷（ST43）、内庭（ST44）、厉兑（ST45）。

(ST31), Futu (ST32), Yinshi (ST33), Liangqiu (ST34), Dubi (ST35), Zusanli (ST36), Shangjuxu (ST37), Tiaokou (ST38), Xiajuxu (ST39), Fenglong (ST40), Jiexi (ST41), Chongyang (ST42), Xiangu (ST43), Neiting (ST44), Lidui (ST45).

（五）要穴简介（图17、图18）

（Ⅴ）Introductions of key acupoints (Figure 17, 18)

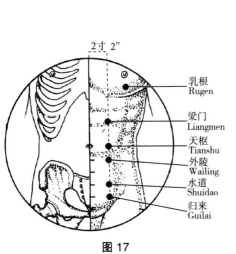

图 17
Figure 17

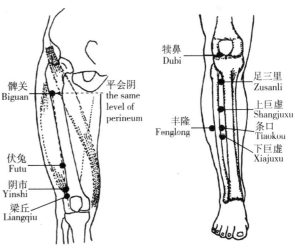

图 17
Figure 17

1. 乳根（ST18）

定位：胸部，乳头直下，

1. Rugen (ST18)

Location: Breast, nipple directly down to the base

· 65 ·

乳房根部，第5肋间隙，距前正中线4寸。

主治：咳喘，胸闷胸痛，乳痈，乳汁少。

2. 梁门（ST21）

定位：上腹部，脐中上4寸，距前正中线2寸。

主治：胃痛，呕吐，腹胀，腹泻，食欲不振。

3. 天枢（ST25）（大肠募穴）

定位：腹中部，距脐中2寸。

主治：腹胀肠鸣，绕脐腹痛，泄泻，便秘，痢疾，肠痈，月经不调，痛经。

4. 外陵（ST26）

定位：下腹部，脐中下1寸，距前正中线2寸。

主治：腹痛，疝气，痛经。

5. 水道（ST28）

定位：下腹部，脐中下3寸，距前正中线2寸。

主治：小便不利，小腹胀满，痛经，疝气。

6. 归来（ST29）

定位：下腹部，脐中下4寸，距前正中线2寸。

主治：小腹疼痛，疝气，

of the breast, the 5th intercostal space, 4" away from the anterior median line.

Main indications: Cough, short of breath, chest tightness, chest pain, acute mastitis, oligogalactia.

2. Liangmen (ST21)

Location: Upper abdomen. 4" above the navel, 2" away from the anterior median line.

Main indications: Stomachache, vomiting, abdominal distention, diarrhea, poor appetite.

3. Tianshu (ST25) (Mu acupoint, or front-mu point of Large Intestine)

Location: Middle of abdomen, 2" away from the navel.

Main indications: Abdomen distention, borborygmus, cord entanglement, abdominal pain, diarrhea, constipation, malaria, acute appendicitis, menoxenia, dysmenorrhea.

4. Wailing (ST26)

Location: Lower abdomen, 1" below the navel, 2" away from the anterior median line.

Main indications: Abdominal pain, hernia, dysmenorrhea.

5. Shuidao (ST28)

Location: Lower abdomen, 3" below the navel, 2" away from the anterior median line.

Main indications: Dysuria, lower abdomen distention, dysmenorrhea, hernia.

6. Guilai (ST29)

Location: Lower abdomen, 4" below the navel, 2" away from the anterior median line.

Main indications: Lower abdomen pain, hernia,

月经不调，闭经，白带，阴挺，前阴痛。

7. 髀关（ST31）

定位：大腿前面，髂前上棘与髌底外侧端连线上，平臀横纹处。

主治：髀股痿痹，腰腿疼痛，足麻木不仁，筋骨屈伸不利。

8. 伏兔（ST32）

定位：大腿前面，髂前上棘与髌底外侧端连线上，髌底上6寸。

主治：腰痛膝冷，下肢麻痹，疝气，脚气。

9. 阴市（ST33）

定位：大腿前面，髂前上棘与髌底外侧端连线上，髌底上3寸。

主治：腿膝麻痹酸痛，屈伸不利，疝气。

10. 梁丘（ST34）（郄穴）

定位：大腿前面，髂前上棘与髌底外侧端连线上，髌底上2寸。

主治：胃痛，膝部肿痛，下肢不遂，乳痈。

11. 足三里（ST36）（合穴、胃下合穴）

定位：小腿外侧，犊鼻下3寸，距胫骨前缘1横指。

dysmenorrhea, amenorrhea, leucorrhea, uterine prolapse, anterior vaginal pain.

7. Biguan (ST31)

Location: Anterior thigh, connects with anterior superior iliac spine and the lateral side of patellar base, the same level as buttocks line.

Main indications: Femur atrophy, low back and leg pain, feet numbness, musculoskeletal stiffness and hard to extend.

8. Futu (ST32)

Location: Anterior thigh, connects with anterior superior iliac spine and the lateral side of patellar base, 6" above patellar base.

Main indications: Low back pain, chill knees, lower extremities numbness, hernia, weak feet.

9. Yinshi (ST33)

Location: Anterior thigh, connects with anterior superior iliac spine and the lateral side of patellar base, 3" above patellar base.

Main indications: Leg and knees numbness, sore and pain, stiffness and hard to extend, hernia.

10. Liangqiu (ST34) (Xi acupoint)

Location: Anterior thigh, connects with anterior superior iliac spine and the lateral side of patellar base, 2" above patellar base.

Main indications: Stomachache, knee swelling and pain, lower extremities paralysis, acute mastitis.

11. Zusanli (ST36) (He acupoint, He acupoint under the stomach)

Location: Lateral side of the leg, 3" below Dubi (ST35), one-finger width away from the anterior side of

主治：胃痛，腹胀，泄泻，呕吐，便秘，心悸，气短，癫狂，脚气，中风。

12. 上巨虚（ST37）（大肠下合穴）

定位：小腿前外侧，犊鼻下6寸，距胫骨前缘一横指。

主治：腹痛，肠鸣，泄泻，痢疾，便秘，肠痈，下肢痿痹。

13. 条口（ST38）

定位：小腿外侧，犊鼻下8寸，距胫骨前缘一横指。

主治：小腿冷痛，麻痹，转筋，肩臂痛。

14. 下巨虚（ST39）（小肠下合穴）

定位：小腿前外侧，犊鼻下9寸，距胫骨前缘一横指。

主治：小腹痛，腰脊痛引睾丸，泄泻，痢疾，下肢痿痹。

15. 丰隆（ST40）（络穴）

定位：小腿前外侧，外踝尖上8寸，条口外，距胫骨前缘2横指。

主治：痰多，咳嗽，哮

the tibia.

Main indications: Stomachache, abdomen distention, diarrhea, vomiting, constipation, palpitation, short of breath, manic-depressive psychosis, weak feet, stroke.

12. Shangjuxu (ST37) (He acupoint below the large intestine)

Location: Anterior lateral side of the leg, 6" below Dubi (ST35), one-finger width away from the anterior side of the tibia.

Main indications: Abdominal pain, borborygmus, diarrhea, malaria, constipation, acute appendicitis, lower extremities atrophy.

13. Tiaokou (ST38)

Location: Lateral side of the leg, 8" below Dubi (ST35), one-finger width away from the anterior side of the tibia.

Main indications: Cold and painful leg, numbness, spasm, shoulder and upper arm pain.

14. Xiajuxu (ST39) (He acupoint below the small intestine)

Location: Lateral side of the leg, 9" below Dubi (ST35), one-finger width away from the anterior side of the tibia.

Main indications: Lower abdominal pain, lower back and spine pain and spread to the testicles, diarrhea, malaria, lower extremity atrophy.

15. Fenglong (ST40) (collateral point)

Location: Lateral side of the leg, 8" above the lateral ankle apex, outside of the Tiaokou (ST38), two-finger width away from the anterior side of the tibia.

Main indications: Phlegm, cough, asthma, dizzi-

喘，头晕，呕吐，水肿，癫狂痫，下肢不遂，便秘，筋骨屈伸不利。

四、足太阴脾经（左右各共 21 穴，共 42 穴）

（一）循行路线

足太阴脾经起于足大趾内侧端（隐白），沿足背内侧赤白肉际，上行经过内踝缘（商丘），沿小腿内侧正中线上行，在内踝上 8 寸处交叉，行于足厥阴肝经之前，上行沿大腿内侧前缘至冲门，进入腹部，属脾，络胃。再向上穿过膈肌，沿食道两旁上行，挟咽两旁，连于舌根，散于舌下。

分支：从胃分出，上行通过膈肌，注入心中，交于手少阴心经。

（二）联系脏腑器官

脾经属脾，络胃，与心脏、舌、咽有联系。

（三）主治

主治胃肠、前阴、妇科等病以及经脉循行部位的病症。

ness, vomiting, swelling, manic-depressive psychosis, epilepsy, lower extremities paralysis, constipation, musculoskeletal stiffness and hard to extend.

IV. Tai-Yin Spleen Meridian of Foot (21 acupoints on each leg, total of 42 acupoints)

(I) Meridian pathway

The Tai-Yin Spleen Meridian of Foot begins at the medial side of the big toe (Yinbai, SP1) and runs along the inside of the foot, the border between red and white muscles, crossing the inner ankle (Shanqiu, SP5). It then travels up along the inner side of the median lower leg, cross over at 8" above the inner ankle. It runs in front of the Jue-Yin Liver Meridian of Foot, goes up along the inner anterior thigh to Chongmen (SP12), and enters into abdomen, pertaining to spleen and collaterals stomach. It then goes up through the diaphragm, along with the bilateral sides of the esophagus, to the throat, connects to the root of the tongue, and spreads under the tongue.

It branches from the stomach, goes up through the diaphragm, enters into the heart, and crosses over with the Shao-Yin Heart Meridian of Hand.

(II) Relevant Zang, Fu and organs

Spleen meridian governs to spleen, collaterals with stomach, and connects to the heart, tongue and throat.

(III) Main indications

Acupuncture points in this meridian are indicated for gastroenterol, genital and gynecological diseases and

(四)经穴

隐白(SP1)、大都(SP2)、太白(SP3)、公孙(SP4)、商丘(SP5)、三阴交(SP6)、漏谷(SP7)、地机(SP8)、阴陵泉(SP9)、血海(SP10)、箕门(SP11)、冲门(SP12)、府舍(SP13)、腹结(SP14)、大横(SP15)、腹哀(SP16)、食窦(SP17)、天溪(SP18)、胸乡(SP19)、周荣(SP20)、大包(SP21)。

(五)要穴简介(图19)

other symptoms along the meridian pathway.

(IV) Meridian points

Yinbai (SP1), Dadu (SP2), Taibai (SP3), Gongsun (SP4), Shangqiu (SP5), Sanyinjiao (SP6), Lougu (SP7), Diji (SP8), Yinlingquan (SP9), Xuehai (SP10), Jimen (SP11), Chongmen (SP12), Fushe (SP13), Fujie (SP14), Daheng (SP15), Fuai (SP16), Shidou (SP17), Tianxi (SP18), Xiongxiang (SP19), Zhourong (SP20), Dabao (SP21).

(V) Introductions of key acupoints (Figure 19)

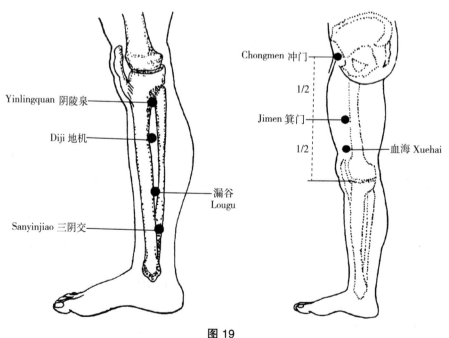

图 19

Figure 19

1. 三阴交（SP6）（足三阴经交会穴）

定位：小腿内侧，足内踝尖上3寸，胫骨内侧缘后方。

主治：脾胃虚弱，腹胀，腹泻，月经不调，痛经，白带过多，子宫出血，失眠，高血压，脏躁，神经衰弱，遗尿，尿路感染，阴部肿痛，下肢瘫痪。

2. 漏谷（SP7）

定位：小腿内侧，内踝尖与阴陵泉的连线上，内踝尖上6寸，胫骨内侧缘后方。

主治：腹胀，肠鸣，小便不利，下肢麻木。

3. 地机（SP8）（郄穴）

定位：小腿内侧，内踝尖与阴陵泉的连线上，阴陵泉下3寸。

主治：腹胀，泄泻，食欲不振，月经不调，痛经，小便不利，遗精。

4. 阴陵泉（SP9）（合穴）

定位：小腿内侧，胫骨内侧髁下方凹陷处。

主治：腹胀，泄泻，痢疾，水肿，小便不利，黄疸，膝痛。

5. 血海（SP10）

定位：大腿内侧，髌底内侧上2寸，股四头肌内侧头的

1. Sanyinjiao (SP6) (Zusanyin meridian cross over point)

Location: Medial side of the leg, 3" above the inner ankle apex, medial and posterior tibia.

Main indications: Deficiency of the spleen and stomach, abdomen distention, diarrhea, menoxenia, dysmenorrhea, leucorrhea, uterine bleeding, insomnia, high blood pressure, hysteria, neurasthenia, enuresis, urinary tract infection, genital swelling and pain, and lower extremity paralysis.

2. Lougu (SP7)

Location: Medial side of the leg, the connection between inner ankle apex and Yinlingquan (SP9), 6" above the inner ankle apex, medial and posterior tibia.

Main indications: Abdomen distention, borborygmus, dysuria, and lower extremities numbness.

3. Diji (SP8) (Xi acupoint)

Location: Medial side of the leg, the connection between inner ankle apex and Yinlingquan (SP9), 3" below the Yinlingquan (SP9).

Main indications: Abdomen distention, diarrhea, poor appetite, menoxenia, dysmenorrhea, dysuria, and spermatorrhea.

4. Yinlingquan (SP9) (He acupoint point)

Location: Medial side of the leg, the concavity below the tibial medial condyle.

Main indications: Abdomen distention, diarrhea, malaria, swelling, dysuria, jaundice, and knee pain.

5. Xuehai (SP10)

Location: Medial side of the leg, 2" above the patellar base, the bulge of the inner head of quadriceps.

隆起处。

主治：月经不调，闭经，崩漏，痛经，湿疹，瘾疹，皮肤瘙痒，丹毒，股内侧痛。

6. 箕门（SP11）

定位：小腿内侧，血海与冲门的连线上，血海上6寸。

主治：小便不利，遗尿，腹股沟肿痛。

7. 冲门（SP12）（足太阴经、足厥阴经交会穴）

定位：腹股沟外侧，距耻骨联合上缘中点3.5寸，髂外动脉搏动处的外侧。

主治：腹痛，疝气，带下，小便不利。

五、手少阴心经（左右各9穴，共18穴）

（一）循行路线

手少阴心经起于心中，出行后属心系，向下穿过膈肌，络小肠。

分支：从心系分出，挟食道上行，经颈、颜面深部连目系。

直行分支：从心系分出，经过肺，再浅出腋下（极泉），沿上肢内侧后缘，经肘过腕，进入掌后锐骨端，自掌后内侧

Main indications: Menoxenia, amenorrhea, uterine bleeding, dysmenorrhea, eczema, urticaria, skin rash, erysipelas, and inner thigh pain.

6. Jimen (SP11)

Location: Inner leg, the connection between Xuehai (SP10) and Chongmen (SP12), 6" above Xuehai (SP10).

Main indications: Dysuria, enuresis, groin swelling and pain.

7. Chongmen (SP12) (cross over with Tai-Yin Meridian of Foot and Jue-Yin Meridian of Foot)

Location: Outside of the groin, 3.5" above the midpoint of pubic symphysis, the lateral side of the external iliac artery pulse.

Main indications: Abdominal pain, hernia, leukorrhea, and dysuria.

V. Shao-Yin Heart Meridian of Hand (9 acupoints at each arm, total of 18 acupoints)

(Ⅰ) Meridian pathway

The Shao-Yin Heart Meridian of Hand starts from the heart, and pertaining to heart, goes downward through the diaphragm and collaterals towards the small intestine.

It branches from the heart, goes up alongside with the esophagus, passes through the neck and deep facial parts and then connects with the eyes.

The straight collateral branches from the heart, through the lung, emerges under the armpit (Jiquan (HT1)), and runs along the inner side of the forearm, elbow and upper arm. It then crosses the inner side of the

直至小指桡侧端（少冲），交于手太阳小肠经。

wrist and palm and ends at the radial side tip of the little finger, where it connects with the Tai-Yang Small Intestine Meridian of Hand.

（二）联系脏腑器官

心经属心，络小肠，与肺脏、心系、咽（食管）、目系有联系。

(Ⅱ) Relevant Zang, Fu and organs

Heart meridian governs to heart, collaterals with the small intestine, and connects with the lung, heart, throat (esophagus) and eyes.

（三）主治

主治心、胸、神志等病及本经脉循行部位的病症。

(Ⅲ) Main indications

Acupuncture points in this meridian are indicated for heart, chest and mental problems and other symptoms along the meridian pathway.

（四）经穴

极泉（HT1）、青灵（HT2）、少海（HT3）、灵道（HT4）、通里（HT5）、阴郄（HT6）、神门（HT7）、少府（HT8）、少冲（HT9）。

(Ⅳ) Meridian points

Jiquan (HT1), Qingling (HT2), Shaohai (HT3), Lingdao (HT4), Tongli (HT5), Yinxi (HT6), Shenmen (HT7), Shaofu (HT8), Shaochong (HT9).

（五）要穴简介（图 20）

(Ⅴ) Introductions of key acupoints (Figure 20)

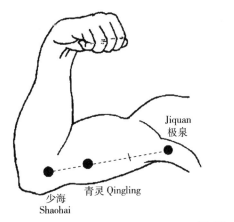
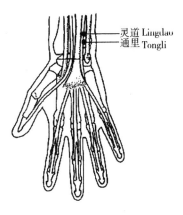

图 20
Figure 20

1. 极泉（HT1）

定位：腋窝中点，腋动脉搏动处。

主治：心痛，心悸，咽干，胸闷，瘰疬，肩臂疼痛。

2. 青灵（HT2）

定位：臂内侧，极泉与少海的连线上，肘横纹上3寸，肱二头肌的内侧沟中。

主治：肘臂疼痛，头痛，胁痛，目黄。

3. 少海（HT3）（合穴）

定位：屈肘，肘横纹内侧端与肱骨内上髁连线的中点处。

主治：心痛，肘臂疼痛、麻木，胁腋痛，头项痛，瘰疬。

4. 灵道（HT4）（经穴）

定位：前臂掌侧，尺侧腕屈肌腱的桡侧缘，腕横纹上1.5寸。

主治：心痛，心悸，舌强不语，暴喑，肘臂疼痛。

5. 通里（HT5）（络穴）

定位：前臂掌侧，尺侧腕屈肌腱的桡侧缘，腕横纹上1寸。

主治：心悸，怔忡，舌强不语，暴喑，头痛目眩，腕臂痛。

1. Jiquan (HT1)

Location: Midpoint of the armpit, the pulse of axillary artery.

Main indications: Angina, palpitation, dry throat, chest tightness, scrofula, shoulder and arm pain.

2. Qingling (HT2)

Location: Inner arm, the connection between Jiquan (HT1) and Shaohai (HT3), 3" above the elbow, the inner groove of the biceps brachii.

Main indications: Elbow and arm pain, headache, rib pain, and yellow eyes (jaundice).

3. Shaohai (HT3) (He acupoint)

Location: Flex elbow, the midpoint between the medial elbow and the medial condyle of the humerus.

Main indications: Angina, elbow and arm pain, numbness, flank and armpit pain, headache and neck pain, and scrofula.

4. Lingdao (HT4) (meridian point)

Location: Palmer side of the forearm, the radial side of the ulnar wrist flexor, 1.5" above the wrist.

Main indications: Angina, palpitation, stiff tongue and speechless, sudden aphonia, elbow and arm pain.

5. Tongli (HT5) (collateral point)

Location: Palmer side of the forearm, the radial side of the ulnar wrist flexor, 1" above the wrist.

Main indications: Palpitation, severe palpitation, stiff tongue and speechless, sudden aphonia, headache, dizziness, elbow and arm pain.

六、手太阳小肠经（左右各19穴，共38穴）

（一）循行路线

手太阳小肠经起于小指尺侧端（少泽），直上过腕部外侧（阳谷），沿上肢外侧后缘上行，过肘部，出于肩关节后面（肩贞），绕行于肩胛部（肩中俞），交会于大椎，向前经缺盆，深入胸腔，下行络心，再沿食道，穿过膈肌，到达胃部，下行属小肠。

分支：从缺盆出，沿颈部上行到面颊部，至目外眦后，折入耳中。

分支：从面颊分出，斜向目眶下缘直达鼻根部，至目内眦（睛明），交于足太阳膀胱经。

（二）联系脏腑器官

小肠经属小肠，络心，与胃、咽（食管）、眼、耳、鼻有联系。

VI. Tai-Yang Small Intestine Meridian of Hand (19 acupoints on each arm, total of 38 acupoints)

(I) Meridian pathway

The Shou Tai Yang Small Intestine Meridian starts from the ulnar side tip of the little finger (Shaoze, SI1) and crosses the lateral side of the wrist (Yanggu, SI5). It runs upwards along the lateral and posterior side of the forearm, passes through the elbow until it reaches the back of shoulder (Jianzhen, SI9) where goes around the scapula (Jianzhongshu, SI15), crosses over at Dazhui (DU14). It then goes forward through Quepen (ST12), enters deeply in the chest, and goes down to collateral the heart, then along with the esophagus, through the diaphragm and reaches toward the stomach. Finally it runs down toward the small intestine.

It branches from the Quepen (ST12), runs up along the neck to the cheeks and outer canthus, and then goes back to enter the ears.

It also branches from the cheeks, diagonally around the lower boarder of the orbit and runs downwardly to the root of the nose and the inner canthus (Jingming, BI1), crosses over with the Tai-Yang Bladder Meridian of Foot.

(II) Relevant Zang, Fu and organs

Small intestine meridian governs to small intestine, collaterals with the heart, and connects with the stomach, throat (esophagus), eyes, ears, and the nose.

（三）主治

主治后头、耳、肩胛、神志等病及本经脉循行部位的病症。

（四）经穴

少泽（SI1）、前谷（SI2）、后溪（SI3）、腕骨（SI4）、阳谷（SI5）、养老（SI6）、支正（SI7）、小海（SI8）、肩贞（SI9）、臑俞（SI10）、天宗（SI11）、秉风（SI12）、曲垣（SI13）、肩外俞（SI14）、肩中俞（SI15）、天窗（SI16）、天容（SI17）、颧髎（SI18）、听宫（SI19）。

（五）要穴简介（图 21）

(Ⅲ) Main indications

Acupuncture points in this meridian are indicated for diseases of the head, ear, shoulder, scapulas and mental illnesses, and other symptoms along the meridian pathway.

(Ⅳ) Meridian points

Shaoze (SI1), Qiangu (SI2), Houxi (SI3), Wangu (SI4), Yanggu (SI5), Yanglao (SI6), Zhizheng (SI7), Xiaohai (SI8), Jianzhen (SI9), Naoshu (SI10), Tianzong (SI11), Bingfeng (SI12), Quyuan (SI13), Jianwaishu (SI14), Jianzhongshu (SI15), Tianchuang (SI16), Tianrong (SI17), Quanliao (SI18), Tinggong (SI19).

(Ⅴ) Introductions of key acupoints (Figure 21)

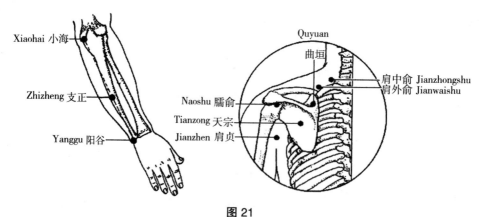

图 21
Figure 21

1. 支正（SI7）（络穴）

定位：前臂背面尺侧，阳

1. Zhizheng (SI7) (collateral point)

Location: Dorsal and ulnar side of the forearm, the

谷与小海的连线上，腕背横纹上 5 寸。

主治：项强，肘挛，手指痛，头痛，目眩，热病，癫狂。

2. 小海（SI8）（合穴）

定位：肘内侧，尺骨鹰嘴与肱骨内上髁之间的凹陷处。

主治：肘臂挛痛，颌肿，癫狂痫。

3. 肩贞（SI9）

定位：肩关节后下方，臂内收时，腋后纹头上 1 寸。

主治：肩臂疼痛，瘰疬，耳鸣。

4. 臑俞（SI10）（手足太阳经、阳维脉、阳跷脉交会穴）

定位：肩部，腋后纹头直上，肩胛冈下缘凹陷中。

主治：肩臂酸痛无力，瘰疬。

5. 天宗（SI11）

定位：肩胛部，冈下窝中央凹陷处。

主治：落枕，肩胛疼痛，肩臂外后侧痛，气喘，乳痈。

connection between Yanggu (SI5) and Xiaohai (SI8), 5" above the dorsal side of the wrist.

Main indications: Stiff neck, elbow spasm, finger pain, headache, dizziness, fever, and manic-depressive psychosis.

2. Xiaohai (SI8) (He acupoint)

Location: Inner elbow, the concavity between the olecranon process of the ulna and the supracondyle of the humerus.

Main indications: Elbow and arm spasm and pain, jaw swelling, manic-depressive psychosis, and epilepsy.

3. Jianzhen (SI9)

Location: The posterolateral side of the shoulder joint, 1" above the posterior line of the axillary when arm abduction.

Main indications: Elbow and arm spasm and pain, scrofula, and tinnitus.

4. Naoshu (SI10) (confluent acupoint between the Tai-Yang Meridians of Hand/Foot, Yang-Wei Channel, Yang Heel Channel)

Location: Shoulder, posterior line of the axillary upward toward the head, the concavity of the lower border of the scapula.

Main indications: Shoulder and arm soreness, pain and weakness, and scrofula.

5. Tianzong (SI11)

Location: Scapula, the central concavity of the infraspinous fossa.

Main indications: Acute fibrositis, shoulder and scapula region pain, posterolateral shoulder pain, asthma, and acute mastitis.

6. 曲垣（SI13）

定位：肩胛部，冈上窝内侧端，臑俞与第2胸椎棘突连线的中点处。

主治：肩胛痉挛疼痛。

7. 肩外俞（SI14）

定位：背部，第1胸椎棘突下，旁开3寸。

主治：肩背酸痛，颈项强直，上肢冷痛。

8. 肩中俞（SI15）

定位：背部，第7颈椎棘突下，旁开2寸。

主治：咳嗽，气喘，肩背疼痛，目视不明。

七、足太阳膀胱经（左右各67穴，共134穴）

（一）循行路线

足太阳膀胱经起于内眼角（睛明），上额交于头顶，经头顶与督脉交会，后分出，至耳上角部。

直行者：从头顶部分出，向后下行至枕骨处，进入颅腔，络脑，重返出来，下行到项部（天柱），再交会于大椎，然后分左右沿肩胛内侧、脊柱两旁（距后正中线1.5寸）下

6. Quyuan (SI13)

Location: Shoulder and scapula, inner side of the infraspinous fossa, the midpoint between the Naoshu (SI10) and the 2nd spinous process of T2.

Main indications: Shoulder and scapula region spasm and pain.

7. Jianwaishu (SI14)

Location: Back, infraspinous process of the T1, 3" aside.

Main indications: Shoulder and back soreness and pain, stiff neck, upper extremities cold and pain.

8. Jianzhongshu (SI15)

Location: Back, infraspinous process of the C7, 2" aside.

Main indications: Cough, asthma, shoulder and back pain, and blurred vision.

VII. Tai-Yang Bladder Meridian of Foot(67 acupoints on each leg, total of 134 acupoints)

(I) Meridian pathway

The Tai-Yang Bladder Meridian of Foot starts at the inner side of the eye (Jingming, BL1) and goes across the forehead at the Du channel to reach the top of the head where it branches into the upper corner of the ear.

One branches straight from the top of the head, directly downward to the occipital area, enters into the cranial cavity, collaterals the brain, and then comes out again and goes down to the neck (Tianzhu, BL10). It then crosses over with Dazhui (DU14), branches to bilateral sides of the interscapular space. Afterwards, it runs

行，到达腰部（肾俞），进入脊柱两旁的肌肉（膂），深入腹腔，络肾，属膀胱。

分支：从腰部继续沿脊柱两旁下行，穿过臀部，从大腿后侧外缘下行至腘窝中（委中）。

分支：从项部分出下行，经肩胛内侧，从附分穴挟脊，沿后正中线旁开3寸下行，经过股骨大转子，沿大腿后侧至腘窝中与前一支脉会合，然后下行穿过腓肠肌，出走于足外踝后的昆仑穴，在足跟部折向前，经足背外侧缘至足小趾外侧端（至阴），交于足少阴肾经。

（二）联系脏腑器官

膀胱经属膀胱，络肾，与脑、眼、鼻有联系。

（三）主治

主治眼、鼻、后头、背腰、内脏、神志等病及本经脉循行部位的病症。

down along with the spine (1.5" away from the posteromedial line) and reaches to the waist (Shenshu, BL23). It then enters into the paraspinal muscles (backbone), goes deeply into the abdominal cavity, collaterals kidney and governs the bladder.

Once branches downward from the waist along with paraspinal muscles, passes through the bottom, and goes from posterolateral thigh down to the popliteal fossa (Weizhong, BL40).

One branches downward from the neck, passes through the interscapular space, along with the Fufen (BL41), the backbone and 3" away from the posterior median line down to the greater trochanter of the femur, runs down through the posterior thigh to the popliteal fossa and merges with the previous branch. It then passes through the gastrocnemius muscle, goes out at the posterolateral ankle apex (Kunlun, BL60), turns forward at the heel, runs along with the dorsolateral feet to the lateral side of the little toe (Zhiyin, BL67), and crosses over with the Shao-Yin Kidney Meridian of Foot.

(II) Relevant Zang, Fu and Organs

Bladder meridian governs to bladder, collaterals with the kidney, and connects with the brain, eyes and nose.

(III) Main indications

Acupuncture points in this meridian are indicated for diseases in the eyes, nose, posterior head, back, waist, internal organs and mental illnesses, and other symptoms along the meridian pathway.

(四) 经穴

睛明（BL1）、攒竹（BL2）、眉冲（BL3）、曲差（BL4）、五处（BL5）、承光（BL6）、通天（BL7）、络却（BL8）、玉枕（BL9）、天柱（BL10）、大杼（BL11）、风门（BL12）、肺俞（BL13）、厥阴俞（BL14）、心俞（BL15）、督俞（BL16）、膈俞（BL17）、肝俞（BL18）、胆俞（BL19）、脾俞（BL20）、胃俞（BL21）、三焦俞（BL22）、肾俞（BL23）、气海俞（BL24）、大肠俞（BL25）、关元俞（BL26）、小肠俞（BL27）、膀胱俞（BL28）、中膂俞（BL29）、白环俞（BL30）、上髎（BL31）、次髎（BL32）、中髎（BL33）、下髎（BL34）、会阳（BL35）、承扶（BL36）、殷门（BL37）、浮郄（BL38）、委阳（BL39）、委中（BL40）、附分（BL41）、魄户（BL42）、膏肓（BL43）、神堂（BL44）、譩譆（BL45）、膈关（BL46）、魂门（BL47）、阳纲（BL48）、意舍（BL49）、胃仓（BL50）、肓门（BL51）、志室（BL52）、胞肓（BL53）、秩边（BL54）、合阳（BL55）、承筋（BL56）、承山（BL57）、飞扬（BL58）、

(Ⅳ) Meridian points

Jingming (BL1), Cuanzhu (BL2), Meichong (BL3), Qucha (BL4), Wuchu (BL5), Chengguang (BL6), Tongtian (BL7), Luoque (BL8), Yuzhen (BL9), Tianzhu (BL10), Dazhu (BL11), Fengmen (BL12), Feishu (BL13), Jueyinshu (BL14), Xinshu (BL15), Dushu (BL16), Geshu (BL17), Ganshu (BL18), Danshu (BL19), Pishu (BL20), Weishu (BL21), Sanjiaoshu (BL22), Shenshu (BL23), Qihaishu (BL24), Dachangshu (BL25), Guanyuanshu (BL26), Xiaochangshu (BL27), Pangguangshu (BL28), Zhonglüshu (BL29), Baihuanshu (BL30), Shangliao (BL31), Ciliao (BL32), Zhongliao (BL33), Xialiao (BL34), Huiyang (BL35), Chengfu (BL36), Yinmen (BL37), Fuxi (BL38), Weiyang (BL39), Weizhong (BL40), Fufen (BL41), Pohu (BL42), Gaohuang (BL43), Shentang (BL44), Yixi (BL45), Geguan (BL46), Hunmen (BL47), Yanggang (BL48), Yishe (BL49), Weicang (BL50), Huangmen (BL51), Zhishi (BL52), Baohuang (BL53), Zhibian (BL54), Heyang (BL55), Chengjin (BL56), Chengshan (BL57), Feiyang (BL58), Fuyang (BL59), Kunlun (BL60), Pucan (BL61), Shenmai (BL62), Jinmen (BL63), Jinggu (BL64), Shugu (BL65), Zutonggu (BL66), Zhiyin (BL67).

跗阳（BL59）、昆仑（BL60）、仆参（BL61）、申脉（BL62）、金门（BL63）、京骨（BL64）、束骨（BL65）、足通骨（BL66）、至阴（BL67）。

（五）要穴简介（图 22、图 23）

(V) Introductions of key acupoints (Figure 22, 23)

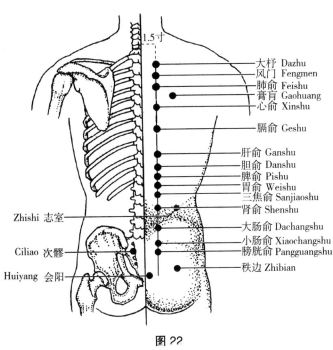

图 22

Figure 22

1. 大杼（BL11）（八会穴、骨会、手足太阳经交会穴）

1. Dazhu (BL11) (confluent acupoint between the eight influential point, bone influential point and the Tai-Yang Meridian of Hand)

定位：背部，第 1 胸椎棘突下旁开 1.5 寸。

主治：肩背痛，头项强痛，咳嗽，发热，鼻塞。

Location: Back, 1.5" aside from the infraspinous process of the T1.

Main indications: Shoulder and back pain, head and neck stiffness and pain, cough, fever, and snuffle.

2. 风门（BL12）（足太阳经、督脉交会穴）

定位：背部，第 2 胸椎棘突下旁开 1.5 寸。

主治：伤风，肩背痛，头项强痛，咳嗽发热，鼻塞。

2. Fengmen (BL12) (confluent acupoint between the Tai-Yang Meridian of Foot and the Du channel)

Location: Back, 1.5" aside from the infraspinous process of the T2.

Main indications: Cold, shoulder and back pain, head and neck stiffness and pain, cough, fever, and snuffle.

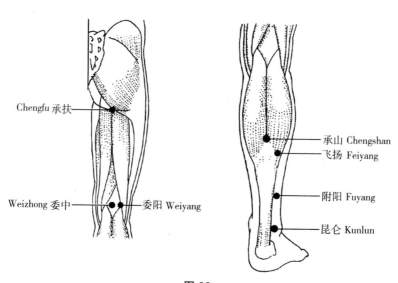

图 23
Figure 23

3. 肺俞（BL13）（背俞穴）

定位：背部，第 3 胸椎棘突下旁开 1.5 寸。

主治：咳嗽气喘，胸满，骨蒸潮热，盗汗，咯血，鼻塞。

4. 心俞（BL15）（背俞穴）

定位：背部，第 5 胸椎棘突下旁开 1.5 寸。

主治：心痛，心悸，失眠，健忘，癫狂痫，咳嗽，吐血，盗汗，梦遗。

3. Feishu (BL13) (Back-Shu acupoint)

Location: Back, 1.5" aside from the infraspinous process of the T3.

Main indications: Cough, asthma, fullness sensation in chest, hectic fever, hot flashes, sweat, hemoptysis, and snuffle.

4. Xinshu (BL15) (Back-Shu acupoint)

Location: Back, 1.5" aside from the infraspinous process of the T5.

Main indications: Angina, palpitation, insomnia, amnesia, manic-depressive psychosis, epilepsy, cough, hemoptysis, sweat, and nocturnal emission.

5. 膈俞（BL17）（八会穴）

定位：背部，第 7 胸椎棘突下旁开 1.5 寸。

主治：呕吐，呃逆，胃脘胀痛，饮食不下，咳嗽，气喘，吐血，潮热盗汗。

6. 肝俞（BL18）（背俞穴）

定位：背部，第 9 胸椎棘突下旁开 1.5 寸。

主治：黄疸，胁痛，眩晕，目赤，吐血，衄血，夜盲，癫狂痫，脊背痛。

7. 胆俞（BL19）（背俞穴）

定位：背部，第 10 胸椎棘突下旁开 1.5 寸。

主治：黄疸，胁痛，呕吐，口苦，肺痨，潮热。

8. 脾俞（BL20）（背俞穴）

定位：背部，第 11 胸椎棘突下旁开 1.5 寸。

主治：腹胀，呕吐，泄泻，痢疾，便血，黄疸，胁痛，水肿。

9. 胃俞（BL21）（背俞穴）

定位：背部，第 12 胸椎棘突下旁开 1.5 寸。

主治：胃脘痛，胸胁痛，腹胀，呕吐，肠鸣，完谷不化。

5. Geshu (BL17) (He acupoint)

Location: Back, 1.5" aside from the infraspinous process of the T7.

Main indications: Vomiting, hiccups, epigastric distention and pain, anorexia, cough, asthma, hemoptysis, hot flashes, and sweat.

6. Ganshu (BL18) (Back-Shu acupoint)

Location: Back, 1.5" aside from the infraspinous process of the T9.

Main indications: Jaundice, flank pain, dizziness, red eyes, hemoptysis, epistaxis, nyctalopia, manic-depressive psychosis, epilepsy, and spine pain.

7. Danshu (BL19) (Back-Shu acupoint)

Location: Back, 1.5" aside from the infraspinous process of the T10.

Main indications: Jaundice, flank pain, vomiting, bitter taste, tuberculosis, and hot flashes.

8. Pishu (BL20) (Back-Shu acupoint)

Location: Back, 1.5" aside from the infraspinous process of the T11.

Main indications: Abdomen distention, vomiting, diarrhea, malaria, hematochezia, jaundice, flank pain, and swelling.

9. Weishu (BL21) (Back-Shu acupoint)

Location: Back, 1.5" aside from the infraspinous process of the T12.

Main indications: Epigastric pain, chest and flank pain, abdomen distention, vomiting, borborygmus, and diarrhea with undigested food.

10. 三焦俞（BL22）

定位：腰部，第 1 腰椎棘突下旁开 1.5 寸。

主治：腹胀，呕吐，肠鸣，泄泻，痢疾，呕吐，水肿，小便不利，腰脊强痛。

11. 肾俞（BL23）（背俞穴）

定位：腰部，第 2 腰椎棘突下旁开 1.5 寸。

主治：腰膝酸软，遗精，阳痿，小便频数，月经不调，带下，水肿，目昏，耳鸣，耳聋，喘咳少气。

12. 大肠俞（BL25）（背俞穴）

定位：腰部，第 4 腰椎棘突下旁开 1.5 寸。

主治：腰痛，腹痛腹胀，肠鸣，泄泻，痢疾，遗精。

13. 小肠俞（BL27）

定位：骶部，骶正中脊旁开 1.5 寸，平第 1 骶后孔。

主治：小腹胀痛，泄泻，痢疾，遗精，遗尿，带下，腰痛。

14. 膀胱俞（BL28）（背俞穴）

定位：骶部，骶正中脊旁开 1.5 寸，平第 2 骶后孔。

10. Sanjiaoshu (BL22)

Location: Lumbar area, 1.5" aside from the infraspinous process of the L1.

Main indications: Abdomen distention, vomiting, borborygmus, diarrhea, malaria, vomiting, swelling, dysuria, and lumbar vertebra stiffness and pain.

11. Shenshu (BL23) (Back-Shu acupoint)

Location: Lumbar area, 1.5" aside from the infraspinous process of the L2.

Main indications: Sore and weak waist and knees, spermatorrhea, impotence, micturition, menoxenia, leukorrhea, swelling, dizziness, tinnitus, deaf, short of breath, cough, and hypoxemia.

12. Dachangshu (BL25) (Back-Shu acupoint)

Location: Lumbar area, 1.5" aside from the infraspinous process of the L4.

Main indications: Lower back pain, abdominal pain, abdomen distention, borborygmus, diarrhea, malaria, and spermatorrhea.

13. Xiaochangshu (BL27)

Location: At the sacrum, 1.5" aside from the sacral median ridge, the same level as the 1st posterior sacral foramen.

Main indications: Lower abdomen distention and pain, diarrhea, malaria, spermatorrhea, enuresis, leukorrhea, and lower back pain.

14. Pangguangshu (BL28) (Back-Shu acupoint)

Location: At the sacrum, 1.5" aside from the sacral median ridge, the same level as the 2nd posterior sacral

主治：小便赤涩，尿闭，遗精，遗尿，便秘，腰脊强痛，泄泻。

15. 次髎（BL32）

定位：骶部，髂后上棘内下方，第2骶后孔处。

主治：腰骶痛，月经不调，赤白带下，痛经，疝气，小便不利，遗精，下肢痿痹。

16. 会阳（BL35）

定位：骶部，尾骨端旁开0.5寸。

主治：便秘，痔疮，泄泻，阳痿，带下。

17. 承扶（BL36）

定位：大腿后面，臀横纹中点。

主治：腰、骶、臀、股部疼痛，痔疾。

18. 委阳（BL39）（三焦下合穴）

定位：腘横纹外侧端，股二头肌腱内侧。

主治：小腹胀满，小便不利，腰脊强痛，腿足挛痛。

19. 委中（BL40）（合穴、膀胱下合穴）

定位：腘横纹中点，股二头肌腱与半腱肌腱的中间。

foramen.

Main indications: Hot urination, anuria, spermatorrhea, enuresis, constipation, lumbar vertebra stiffness and pain, and diarrhea.

15. Ciliao (BL32)

Location: At the sacrum, posteromedial supraspinous sacrum, the 2nd posterior sacral foramen.

Main indications: Lumbosacral pain, menoxenia, red and white leukorrhea, dysmenorrhea, herniation, dysuria, spermatorrhea, and lower extremities atrophy.

16. Huiyang (BL35)

Location: Sacrum, 0.5" aside from the tip of coccyx.

Main indications: Constipation, hemorrhoids, diarrhea, impotence, and leukorrhea.

17. Chengfu (BL36)

Location: Posterior thigh, the midpoint of the bottom line.

Main indications: Lumbus, sacrum, bottom and femur pain, and hemorrhoids.

18. Weiyang (BL39) (He acupoint below the Sanjiao (CO17))

Location: The lateral popliteal line, the inner biceps femoris.

Main indications: Lower abdomen distention, dysuria, lumbar vertebra stiffness and pain, leg and feet spasm and pain.

19. Weizhong (BL40) (He acupoint, He acupoint below the bladder points)

Location: Midpoint of the popliteal line, the midpoint between the biceps femoris and the musculi semi-

主治：腰、背、腿、腰部疼痛，下肢不遂，腹痛吐泻，小便不利，中暑，丹毒，痈疮。

20. 膏肓（BL43）

定位：背部，第4胸椎棘突下旁开3寸。

主治：肺痨，咳嗽气喘，健忘，遗精，盗汗，脾胃虚弱。

21. 志室（BL52）

定位：腰部，第2腰椎棘突下旁开3寸。

主治：遗精，阳痿，小便不利，水肿，腰脊强痛。

22. 秩边（BL54）

定位：臀部，平第4骶后孔，骶正中嵴旁开3寸。

主治：小便不利，大便困难，腰骶痛，痔疾，下肢痿痹。

23. 承山（BL57）

定位：小腿后面正中，委中与昆仑之间，伸直小腿时，腓肠肌腹下的尖角凹陷处。

主治：痔疾，脚气，腰痛，腿痛转筋，便秘，脱肛。

24. 飞扬（BL58）（络穴）

定位：小腿后面，外踝后，昆仑直上7寸，承山外下

tendinosus.

Main indications: Lower back, back, leg and waist pain, lower extremities paralysis, abdominal pain, vomiting, dysuria, hyperthermia, erysipelas, and sore and ulcer.

20. Gaohuang (BL43)

Location: Back, 3" aside from the infraspinous process of the T4.

Main indications: Tuberculosis, cough, asthma, amnesia, spermatorrhea, sweat, deficiency of spleen and stomach.

21. Zhishi (BL52)

Location: Lumbar area, 3" aside from the infraspinous process of the L2.

Main indications: Spermatorrhea, impotence, dysuria, swelling, lumbar vertebra stiffness and pain.

22. Zhibian (BL54)

Location: At the bottom, the same level as the 4th posterior sacral foramen, 3" aside from the sacral median ridge.

Main indications: Dysuria, dyschesia, lumbosacral pain, hemorrhoids, and lower extremities atrophy.

23. Chengshan (BL57)

Location: Midline of the posterior leg, between Weizhong (BL40) and Kunlun (BL60); the concavity apex below the muscle belly of the gastrocnemius.

Main indications: Hemorrhoid, weak feet, lower back pain, leg pain and spasm, constipation, and anus prolapse.

24. Feiyang (BL58) (collateral point)

Location: Posterior leg, posterolateral ankle, 7" directly above the Kunlun (BL60), 1" obliquely below

方 1 寸。

主治：头痛，目眩，腰背疼痛，下肢痿痹。

25. 跗阳（BL59）（阳跷郄穴）

定位：小腿后面，外踝后，昆仑直上 3 寸。

主治：头重，头痛，腰骶痛，下肢痿痹。

26. 昆仑（BL60）（经穴）

定位：足外踝后方，外踝尖与跟腱之间的凹陷处。

主治：头痛，项强，目眩，鼻衄，肩背拘急，腰骶疼痛，足跟痛，小儿痫证，难产，胞衣不下。

八、足少阴肾经（左右各 27 穴，共 54 穴）

（一）循行路线

足少阴肾经起于足小趾端下，斜行于足心（涌泉），出于舟骨粗隆之下的然谷穴，沿内踝后，分出进入足跟，向上沿小腿内侧后缘，至腘内侧，直上股内侧后缘，至尾骨部（长强），贯穿脊柱，入属肾，络膀胱。

Chengshan (BL57).

Main indications: Headache, dizziness, waist and lower back pain, and lower extremity atrophy.

25. Fuyang (BL59) (Yangqiaoxi point)

Location: Posterior leg, posterolateral ankle, 3" above the Kunlun (BL60).

Main indications: Heavy head, headache, lumbosacral pain, and lower extremities atrophy.

26. Kunlun (BL60) (meridian point)

Location: Posterolateral ankle, the concavity between the outer ankle apex and the Achilles' tendon.

Main indications: Headache, stiff neck, dizziness, epistaxis, spasm in nape and back, lumbosacral pain, heel pain, pediatric epilepsy, obstructed labor, and retention of placenta.

Ⅷ. Shao-Yin Kidney Meridian of Foot (27 acupoints on each legs, total of 54 acupoints)

(Ⅰ) Meridian pathway

The Shao-Yin Kidney Meridian of Foot starts from the inferior side of the small toe. Crossing the middle of the sole (Yongquan, KI1) and the arch of the foot, goes out from the inferior tuberosity of the foot navicular bone (Rangu, KI2), circles behind the inner ankle and branches into the heel. It then travels along the posteromedial side of the lower leg to the medial popliteal fossa, and then goes straight up to the posteromedial thigh, until it enters the body near the base of the coccyx (Changqiang, GV1). It then travels through the spine, pertaining to the

直行者：从肾上行，穿过肝和膈肌，进入肺中，沿喉咙上达舌根两旁。

分支：从左右股内侧后缘大腿根部分出，向前挟阴部两侧，至下腹部，沿腹部中线两侧（距正中线 0.5 寸）上行，挟脐，抵胸部前，直到锁骨下（俞府）。

分支：从肺中分出，络于心，注于胸中（膻中），交于手厥阴心包经。

（二）联系脏腑器官

肾经属肾，络膀胱，与肝、肺、心、舌、喉咙、脊髓有联系。

（三）主治

主治肾、肺、咽喉、前阴、妇科等病及本经脉循行部位的病症。

（四）经穴

涌泉（KI1）、然谷（KI2）、太溪（KI3）、大钟（KI4）、水泉（KI5）、照海（KI6）、复溜（KI7）、交信（KI8）、筑宾（KI9）、阴谷（KI10）、

kidney, and collaterals the bladder.

The straight line branches out from the kidney, passes through the liver and the diaphragm, enters into the lung, and along with the throat up to the bilateral sides of the base of the tongue.

It branches bilaterally from the groin and the base of the posteromedial thigh, runs forward along with the genital area to the lower abdomen. It then goes up from the bilateral sides of the median abdominal line (0.5" away from the median line), along with the navel, reaches to the front chest and the infraclavicular border (Shufu, KI27).

It branches out from the lung, collaterals the heart, and enters the chest (Danzhong, CV17), and crosses over with the Jue-Yin Pericardium Meridian of Hand.

(Ⅱ) Relevant Zang, Fu and organs

Kidney meridian governs to kidney, collaterals with the bladder, and connects with the liver, lungs, heart, tongue, throat and spine.

(Ⅲ) Main indications

Acupuncture points in this meridian are used for kidney, lungs, throat, genital and gynecological diseases, and other symptoms along the meridian pathway.

(Ⅳ) Meridian points

Yongquan (KI1), Rangu (KI2), Taixi (KI3), Dazhong (KI4), Shuiquan (KI5), Zhaohai (KI6), Fuliu (KI7), Jiaoxin (KI8), Zhubin (KI9), Yingu (KI10), Henggu (KI11), Dahe (KI12), Qixue (KI13), Siman (KI14), Zhongzhu (KI15), Huangshu (KI16), Shangqu (KI17),

横骨（KI11）、大赫（KI12）、气穴（KI13）、四满（KI14）、中注（KI15）、肓俞（KI16）、商曲（KI17）、石关（KI18）、阴都（KI19）、腹通谷（KI20）、幽门（KI21）、步廊（KI22）、神封（KI23）、灵墟（KI24）、神藏（KI25）、彧中（KI26）、俞府（KI27）。

（五）要穴简介（图24、图25）

1. 然谷（KI2）（荥穴）

定位：足舟骨粗隆前下缘的凹陷中。

主治：遗精，消渴，黄疸，月经不调，阴痒，阴挺，足跗痛。

Shiguan (KI18), Yindu (KI19), Futonggu (KI20), Youmen (KI21), Bulang (KI22), Shenfeng (KI23), Lingxu (KI24), Shencang (KI25), Yuzhong (KI26), Shufu (KI27).

(V) Introductions of key acupoints (Figure 24, 25)

1. Rangu (KI2) (Xing acupoint also called Xing-spring point)

Location: The concavity at the anteroinferior tuberosity of the foot navicular bone.

Main indications: Spermatorrhea, wasting thirst, jaundice, menoxenia, itch in the vulva, uterine prolapse, and foot navicular bone pain.

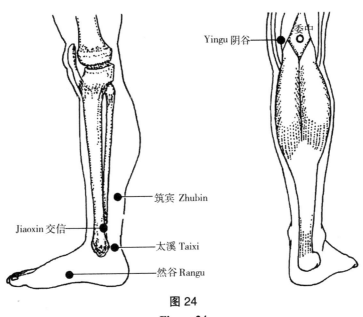

图24
Figure 24

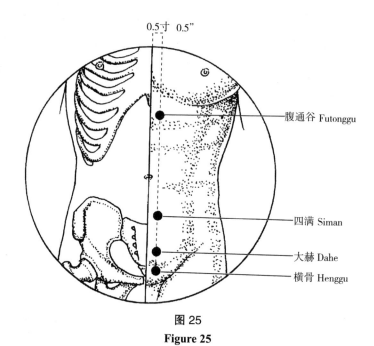

图 25
Figure 25

2. 太溪（KI3）（输穴、原穴）

定位：内踝尖与跟腱之间的凹陷中。

主治：阳痿，遗精，小便频数，消渴，月经不调，头痛，眩晕，失眠，耳聋，气喘，咽喉肿痛，腰痛，牙痛，足踝肿痛。

3. 交信（KI8）（阴跷脉郄穴）

定位：太溪穴直上2寸，复溜穴前0.5寸，胫骨内侧面后缘。

主治：月经不调，崩漏，阴挺，泄泻，疝气，股膝胫内侧痛。

2. Taixi (KI3) (shu-stream point, Yuan acupoint)

Location: The concavity between the inner ankle apex and the Achilles tendon.

Main indications: Impotence, spermatorrhea, micturition, wasting thirst, menoxenia, headache, dizziness, insomnia, deaf, asthma, throat swelling, low back pain, toothache, ankle swelling and pain.

3. Jiaoxin (KI8) (Yinqiao meridian xi-cleft acupoint)

Location: 2" directly above the Taixi (KI3), 0.5" in front of the Fuliu (KI7), posteromedial tibia.

Main indications: Menoxenia, uterine bleeding, uterine prolapse, diarrhea, herniation, and medial femur-knee-tibia pain.

4. 筑宾（KI9）（阴维脉郄穴）

定位：太溪穴与阴谷穴连线上，太溪穴直上 5 寸，腓肠肌腹下方。

主治：狂，呕吐，痫证，疝气，小腿疼痛。

5. 阴谷（KI10）（合穴）

定位：腘窝横纹内侧端，半腱肌腱与半膜肌腱之间。

主治：阳痿，遗精，月经不调，崩漏，小便不利，膝股疼痛。

6. 横骨（KI11）

定位：下腹部，脐中下 5 寸，前正中线旁开 0.5 寸。

主治：少腹痛，阳痿，遗精，小便不利，遗尿，疝气。

7. 大赫（KI12）

定位：脐中下 4 寸，距前正中线 0.5 寸。

主治：阳痿，遗精，月经不调，带下，阴部痛，阴挺，泄泻。

8. 四满（KI14）

定位：脐中下 2 寸，距前正中线 0.5 寸。

主治：腹痛，泄泻，水肿，疝气，月经不调，带下，遗精，遗尿。

4. Zhubin (KI9) (xi-cleft acupoint Yin-wei meridian)

Location: The connection between the Taixi (KI3) and the Yingu (KI10), 5" directly above the Taixi (KI3), below the muscle belly of the gastrocnemius muscle.

Main indications: Madness, vomiting, epilepsy, herniation, and leg pain.

5. Yingu (KI10) (He acupoint)

Location: medial popliteal fossa, between the tendons of the semitendinosus and the semimembranous muscle.

Main indications: Impotence, spermatorrhea, menoxenia, uterine bleeding, dysuria, knee and femur pain.

6. Henggu (KI11)

Location: Lower abdomen, 5" below the navel, 0.5" aside from the anteromedial line.

Main indications: Hypogastric pain, impotence, spermatorrhea, dysuria, enuresis, and herniation.

7. Dahe (KI12)

Location: 4" below the navel, 0.5" aside from the anteromedial line.

Main indications: Impotence, spermatorrhea, menoxenia, leukorrhea, genital pain, uterine prolapse, and diarrhea.

8. Siman (KI14)

Location: 2" below the navel, 0.5" aside from the anteromedial line.

Main indications: Abdominal pain, diarrhea, swelling, herniation, menoxenia, leukorrhea, spermatorrhea, and enuresis.

9. 腹通谷（KI20）

定位：脐中上 5 寸，距前正中线 0.5 寸。

主治：胸胁胀痛，呕吐，泄泻，咳嗽气喘。

九、手厥阴心包经（左右各 9 穴，共 18 穴）

（一）循行路线

手厥阴心包经起于胸中，出属心包络，下行，穿过膈肌，依次络于上、中、下三焦。

分支：从胸中分出，浅出胁部，当腋下 3 寸处（天池），向上至腋窝下，沿上肢内侧中线入肘，经腕后内关穴，过腕入掌中（劳宫），沿中指桡侧，出中指桡侧端（中冲）。

分支：从掌中（劳宫）分出，沿无名指尺侧，直至其指端的关冲穴，交于手少阳三焦经。

（二）联系脏腑器官

心包经属心包，络三焦。

9. Futonggu (KI20)

Location: 5" below the navel, 0.5" aside from the anteromedial line.

Main indications: Chest and flank swelling and pain, vomiting, diarrhea, cough, asthma.

IX. Jue-Yin Pericardium Meridian of Hand (9 acupoints on each arm, total of 18 acupoints)

(I) Meridian pathway

The Jue-Yin Pericardium Meridian of Hand starts from the chest, leaves the pericardium organ and runs downwards through the diaphragm to connect with three Jiaos (triple burners: upper, middle and lower burner).

A branch rising from the chest, surface out through flank, emerges from the lower chest region (3" below the axillary, Tianchi, PC1) and travels upwards to the axilla (armpit). From the medial aspect of the upper arm, it makes its way down to the elbow and the Neiguan (PC6) below the wrist, and enters into the palm (Laogong, PC8). It then runs along with and toward the radial side of the middle finger (Zhongchong, PC9).

It branches out from the palm (Zhongchong, PC9), along with the ulnar side of the ring finger toward the Guanchong (TE1) at the tip. It also crosses over with the Shao-Yang Three-Jiao Meridian of Hand.

(II) Relevant Zang, Fu and organs

Pericardium meridian governs to pericardium, collaterals with three Jiaos.

（三）主治

主治心、胸、胃、神志等病及本经脉循行部位的病症。

（四）经穴

天池（PC1）、天泉（PC2）、曲泽（PC3）、郄门（PC4）、间使（PC5）、内关（PC6）、大陵（PC7）、劳宫（PC8）、中冲（PC9）。

（五）要穴简介（图26、图27）

(Ⅲ) Main indications

Acupuncture points in this meridian are used for heart, chest, stomach as well as mental illness, and other symptoms along the meridian pathway.

(Ⅳ) Meridian points

Tianchi (PC1), Tianquan (PC2), Quze (PC3), Ximen (PC4), Jianshi (PC5), Neiguan (PC6), Daling (PC7), Laogong (PC8), Zhongchong (PC9).

(Ⅴ) Introductions of key acupoints (Figure 26, 27)

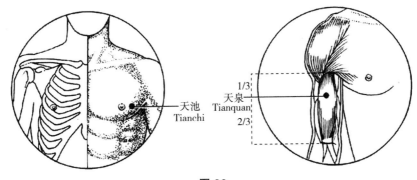

图 26
Figure 26

1. 天池（PC1）

定位：第4肋间，乳头外1寸，距前正中线5寸。

主治：胸闷，胸痛，心烦，腋肿，咳嗽气喘，瘰疬。

2. 天泉（PC2）

定位：上臂内侧，腋前纹头下2寸，肱二头肌长、短头

1. Tianchi (PC1)

Location: The 4th intercostal space, 1" outside of the nipple, 5" away from the anteromedial line.

Main indications: Chest tightness, chest pain, dysphoria, axillary swelling, cough, asthma, and scrofula.

2. Tianquan (PC2)

Location: Inner upper arm, 2" below the anterior axillary line, between the long head and short head of bi-

之间。

主治：心悸，胸胁胀痛，肘臂痛，咳嗽。

ceps brachii.

Main indications: Palpitation, chest and flank swelling and pain, elbow and arm pain, and cough.

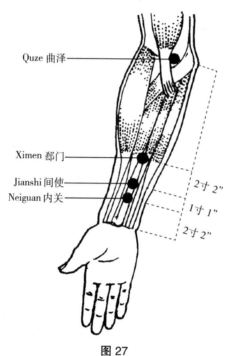

图 27
Figure 27

3. 曲泽（PC3）（合穴）

定位：肘横纹上，肱二头肌腱的尺侧缘。

主治：心悸，咳嗽，胃痛，心烦，肘臂疼痛，热病，呕吐。

4. 郄门（PC4）（郄穴）

定位：曲泽与大陵的连线上，腕横纹上 5 寸，掌上肌腱与桡侧腕屈肌腱之间。

主治：心悸，胃痛，心烦，癫痫，衄血。

3. Quze (PC3) (He acupoint)

Location: On the elbow, the ulnar side of the biceps brachii.

Main indications: Palpitation, cough, stomachache, dysphoria, elbow and arm pain, fever, and vomiting.

4. Ximen (PC4) (Xi acupoint)

Location: The connection between Quze (PC3) and Daling (PC7), 5" above the wrist, between palm tendons and radial side of the wrist flexor tendon.

Main indications: Palpitation, stomachache, dysphoria, epilepsy, and epistaxis.

5. 间使（PC5）（经穴）

定位：曲泽与大陵的连线上，腕横纹上3寸，掌长肌腱与桡侧腕屈肌腱之间。

主治：心悸，胃痛，癫痫，胸肋痛，胃痛，呕吐。

6. 内关（PC6）（络穴、八脉交会穴）

定位：曲泽与大陵的连线上，腕横纹上2寸，掌长肌腱与桡侧腕屈肌腱之间。

主治：心悸，胸痛，癫痫，失眠，肘臂痛，胃痛，呕吐。

十、手少阳三焦经（左右各23穴，共46穴）

（一）循行路线

手少阳三焦经起于无名指尺侧端（关冲），向上沿无名指尺侧至手腕背面外侧（阳池），上行于上肢外侧尺骨和桡骨之间，通过肘尖，沿上臂外侧上行至肩部（肩髎），向前行入缺盆，布于膻中，散络心包，向下穿过膈肌，依次属上、中、下三焦。

分支：从膻中分出，向上

5. Jianshi (PC5) (meridian point)

Location: The connection between Quze (PC3) and Daling (PC7), 3" above the wrist, between palm tendons and radial side of the wrist flexor tendon.

Main indications: Palpitation, stomachache, epilepsy, cheat and rib pain, stomachache, and vomiting.

6. Neiguan (PC6) (cross over with the collaterals and eight confluence points)

Location: The connection between Quze (PC3) and Daling (PC7), 2" above the wrist, between palm tendons and radial side of the wrist flexor tendon.

Main indications: Palpitation, chest pain, epilepsy, insomnia, elbow and arm pain, stomachache, and vomiting.

X. Shao-Yang Three-Jiao Meridian of Hand (23 acupoints on each arm, total of 46 acupoints)

(Ⅰ) Meridian pathway

The Shao-Yang Three-Jiao Meridian of Hand begins at the ulnar tip of the ring finger (Guangchong, SJ1) and goes along the back and ulnar side of the hand (Yangchi, SJ4), up to the lateral side of the upper extremities between the ulna and the radius). Until it passes through the elbow, reaches up to the shoulder region (Jianliao, SJ14) along with the lateral side of the upper arm, and moves forward to Quepen (ST12), distributes into Danzhong (CV17), collaterals at pericardium, and then travels downward through the diaphragm, and governs to the Upper, Middle and Lower Jiaos.

One branches from the Danzhong (CV17), goes up

出缺盆，至肩部项后，左右交会于大椎穴，上行至项，沿耳后（翳风），直上于耳上角，然后屈曲向下经面颊部，至目眶下。

分支：从耳后翳风穴分出，进入耳中，出走耳前，经上关穴前，在面颊部与前一分支相交，至目外眦（瞳子髎），交于足少阳胆经。

（二）联系脏腑器官

三焦经属三焦，络心包，与耳、眼有联系。

（三）主治

主治侧头、耳、目、咽喉、胁肋、发热等病及本经脉循行部位的病症。

（四）经穴

关冲（SJ1）、液门（SJ2）、中渚（SJ3）、阳池（SJ4）、外关（SJ5）、支沟（SJ6）、会宗（SJ7）、三阳络（SJ8）、四渎（SJ9）、天井（SJ10）、清泠渊（SJ11）、消泺（SJ12）、臑会（SJ13）、肩髎（SJ14）、天髎（SJ15）、天牖（SJ16）、

and exits Quepen (ST12) to the shoulder and posterior neck, merges bilateral routes over Dazhui (DU14), and goes up toward the upper corner of the ear along with the back of the ear (Yifeng, SJ17). It then curves back downward to the suborbital area through the face.

One branch runs from behind the ear (Yifeng, SJ17), enters into the ear, exits the ear, and passes through Shangguan (GB3). It then crosses over with the previous branch at face till outer canthus (Tongziliao, GB1), and also crosses over with the Shao-Yang Gallbladder Meridian of Foot.

(Ⅱ) Relevant Zang, Fu and organs

Three-Jiao Meridian governs three Jiaos, collaterals with the pericardium, and connects with the ears and eyes.

(Ⅲ) Main indications

Acupuncture points in this channel are used for lateral head ears, eyes, throat, flank and rubs as well as fever, and other symptoms along the meridian pathway.

(Ⅳ) Meridian points

Guanchong (SJ1), Yemen (SJ2), Zhongzhu (SJ3), Yangchi (SJ4), Waiguan (SJ5), Zhigou (SJ6), Huizong (SJ7), Sanyangluo (SJ8), Sidu (SJ9), Tianjing (SJ10), Qinglingyuan (SJ11), Xiaoluo (SJ12), Naohui (SJ13), Jianliao (SJ14), Tianliao (SJ15), Tianyou (SJ16), Yifeng (SJ17), Chimai (SJ18), Luxi (SJ19), Jiaosun (SJ20), Ermen (SJ21), Erheliao (SJ22), Sizhukong (SJ23).

翳风（SJ17）、瘈脉（SJ18）、颅息（SJ19）、角孙（SJ20）、耳门（SJ21）、耳和髎（SJ22）、丝竹空（SJ23）。

（五）要穴简介（图 28、图 29）

(V) Introductions of key acupoints (Figure 28, 29)

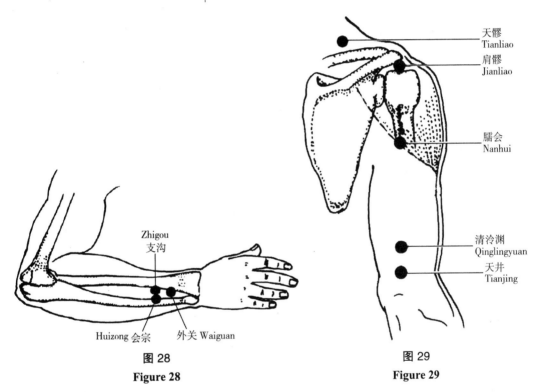

图 28
Figure 28

图 29
Figure 29

1. 外关（SJ5）（络穴、八脉交会穴）

定位：阳池与肘尖的连线上，腕背横纹上 2 寸，尺、桡骨之间。

主治：偏头痛，耳鸣、耳聋，目赤肿痛，胁痛，肩背痛，热病，瘰疬，鼻炎。

1. Waiguan (SJ5) (cross over with the collaterals and eight confluence points)

Location: The connection between Yangchi (TE4) and Zhoujian (EX-UE1), 2" above the dorsal wrist, between the ulna and the radius.

Main indications: Migraine, tinnitus, deaf, red eyes, swelling and pain, flank pain, shoulder and back pain, fever, scrofula, and rhinitis.

2. 支沟（SJ6）（经穴）

定位：阳池与肘尖的连线上，腕背横纹上3寸，尺、桡骨之间。

主治：耳鸣、耳聋，胁痛，肘臂痛，落枕，热病，便秘。

3. 会宗（SJ7）（郄穴）

定位：腕背横纹上3寸，支沟穴尺侧，尺骨桡侧缘。

主治：耳鸣、耳聋，臂痛，癫痫。

4. 天井（SJ10）（合穴）

定位：屈肘，尺骨鹰嘴上1寸的凹陷处。

主治：耳鸣、耳聋，偏头痛，胁肋痛，项肩臂痛，风疹。

5. 清泠渊（SJ11）

定位：屈肘，尺骨鹰嘴上2寸。

主治：头痛，目痛，胁痛，黄疸，肩臂疼痛、不能上举。

6. 臑会（SJ13）

定位：尺骨鹰嘴与肩髎的连线上，肩髎下3寸，三角肌后缘。

主治：肩臂痛，瘿气，瘰疬。

2. Zhigou (SJ6) (meridian point)

Location: The connection between Yangchi (TE4) and Zhoujian (EX-UE1), 3" above the dorsal wrist, between the ulna and the radius.

Main indications: Tinnitus, deafness, flank pain, elbow and arm pain, acute fibrositis, fever, and constipation.

3. Huizong (SJ7) (Xi acupoint)

Location: 3" above the dorsal wrist, the ulnar side of Zhigou, the radial aside of the ulna.

Main indications: Tinnitus, deaf, arm pain, epilepsy.

4. Tianjing (SJ10) (He acupoint)

Location: The concavity 1" above the olecranon of the ulna when flexing.

Main indications: Tinnitus, deafness, migraine, flank and rib pain, neck, shoulder and arm pain, and rubella.

5. Qinglingyuan (SJ11)

Location: 2" above the olecranon of the ulna when flexing.

Main indications: Headache, eye pain, flank pain, jaundice, shoulder and arm pain, and inability to hold arm upward.

6. Naohui (SJ13)

Location: The connection between the olecranon of the ulna and Jianliao (SJ14), 3" below the Jianliao (SJ14), posterior border of the deltoid.

Main indications: Shoulder and arm pain, Qi goiter, and scrofula.

7. 肩髎（SJ14）

定位：肩峰后下方，当上臂外展平举时，肩髃后寸许之凹陷处。

主治：肩臂痛及上举困难。

8. 天髎（SJ15）

定位：肩井与曲垣连线的中点，肩胛骨上角。

主治：肩臂痛，项背强痛，胸中烦满。

十一、足少阳胆经（左右各44穴，共88穴）

（一）循行路线

足少阳胆经起于目外眦（瞳子髎），向上至头角（颔厌），再向下到耳后（完骨），再折向上行至额部达眉上（阳白），然后向后折至耳后（风池），再沿颈部侧面下行到达肩部（肩髎），于项后左右交会于大椎，然后前行入缺盆。

分支：从耳后（完骨）分出，经翳风进入耳中，再出走于耳前，过听宫穴至目外眦后方。

7. Jianliao (SJ14)

Location: Space posterior and below the acromion process of the clavicle, and the concavity 1" behind the Jianyu (LI15) when adduction of the upper arm to the horizontal level.

Main indications: Shoulder and arm pain and cannot hold arm upward.

8. Tianliao (SJ15)

Location: The midpoint between the Jianjing (GB21) and Quyuan (SI13), the upper corner of the scapula.

Main indications: Shoulder and arm pain, neck and back severe pain, and full irritation over the chest.

XI. Shao-Yang Gallbladder Meridian of Foot (44 acupoints on each leg, total of 88 acupoints)

(I) Meridian pathway

The Shao-Yang Gall Bladder Meridian of Foot starts from the outer canthus (Tongziliao, GB1), travels up to the head corner (Hanyan, GB4), turns back down to the back of the ear (Wangu, GB12), turns up again to the forehead and above the eyebrows (Yangbai, GB14), and then goes back to the back of the ear again (Fengchi, GB20). It then runs down along with the lateral side of the neck to the shoulder (Jianliao, TE14), crosses over with Dazhui (DU14) at the back of the neck, and then goes forward to Quepen (ST12).

It branches from the back of the ear (Wangu, GB12), enters into the ear through Yifeng (TE17), comes out in front of the ear, and then travels through Tinggong (BI19) to the back of the outer canthus.

分支：从目外眦分出，下行至下颌部的大迎处，同手少阳经分布于面颊部的支脉相合，复行至目眶下，再向下经过下颌角部（颊车），下行到颈部，经颈前（人迎），与前脉会合于缺盆后，下入胸腔，穿过膈肌，络肝，属胆。沿胁里浅出气街，绕毛际，横向至髋关节（环跳）处。

直行者：从缺盆分出，下行至腋，过渊腋，沿胸侧部（日月），经过季肋，下行至环跳穴与前脉会合，再向下沿大腿外侧、膝关节外缘，行于腓骨前面，直下至腓骨下端，出外踝之前，沿足背行至足第4趾外侧端（足窍阴）。

分支：从足背（足临泣）分出，前行出足大趾外侧端，折回穿过爪甲，分布于足大趾爪甲后丛毛处，交于足厥阴肝经。

（二）联系脏腑器官

胆经属胆，络肝，与眼、

It branches out from the outer canthus, down to Daying (ST5) in the lower jaw, and then merges with the collateral branches from the Shao-Yang Meridian of Hand distributed on the face. It then travels back to the suborbital area, goes down to the neck through the lower mandibular angle (Jiache, ST6), passes through the front neck (Renying, ST9), merges the previous collateral at Quepen (ST12). It then goes down toward the thoracic cavity through the diaphragm, collaterals the liver, and governs to the gallbladder. It exist the superficial Qi passage along with the flank and goes around with the hair lines, crosses over horizontally to the hip joint (Huantiao, GB30).

One branch starts from the Quepen (ST12) straight down to the axillary, through Yuanye (GB22), passes through the hypochondriac region along with the lateral chest (Riyue, GB24), and merges with the previous collateral at lower Huantiao (GB30). It then travels down to the lateral side of the knee joint along with lateral thigh and in front of the fibula and straight downward to the inferior tip of the fibula. Before exits to the external ankle apex, it runs on the dorsal side of the foot to the lateral side of the 4th toe (Zuqiaoyin, GB44).

It branches out from the dorsal side of the foot (Zulinqi, GB41), travels forward through the lateral side of the big toe, turns backward over the onyx, distributes at the hair growth area after the big toe onyx, and finally crosses over with the Jue-Yin Liver Meridian of Foot.

(Ⅱ) Relevant Zang, Fu and organs

Gallbladder meridian governs to gallbladder, collat-

耳有联系。

（三）主治

主治头侧、耳目、咽喉、胁肋、发热、神志及本经脉循行部位的病症。

（四）经穴

瞳子髎（GB1）、听会（GB2）、上关（GB3）、颔厌（GB4）、悬颅（GB5）、悬厘（GB6）、曲鬓（GB7）、率谷（GB8）、天冲（GB9）、浮白（GB10）、头窍阴（GB11）、完骨（GB12）、本神（GB13）、阳白（GB14）、头临泣（GB15）、目窗（GB16）、正营（GB17）、承灵（GB18）、脑空（GB19）、风池（GB20）、肩井（GB21）、渊腋（GB22）、辄筋（GB23）、日月（GB24）、京门（GB25）、带脉（GB26）、五枢（GB27）、维道（GB28）、居髎（GB29）、环跳（GB30）、风市（GB31）、中渎（GB32）、膝阳关（GB33）、阳陵泉（GB34）、阳交（GB35）、外丘（GB36）、光明（GB37）、阳辅（GB38）、悬钟（GB39）、丘墟（GB40）、足临泣（GB41）、地五会（GB42）、侠溪（GB43）、足窍阴（GB44）。

erals with the liver, and connects with the eyes and ears.

(Ⅲ) Main indications

Acupuncture points in this channel are used for the lateral head, ears and eyes, flank and ribs, fever and mental illness, and other symptoms along the meridian pathway.

(Ⅳ) Meridian points

Tongziliao(GB1), Tinghui(GB2), Shangguan(GB3), Hanyan (GB4), Xuanlu(GB5), Xuanli (GB6), Qubin(GB7), Shuaigu(GB8), Tianchong (GB9), Fubai (GB10), Touqiaoyin (GB11), Wangu (GB12), Benshen (GB13), Yangbai (GB14), Toulinqi (GB15), Muchuang (GB16), Zhengying (GB17), Chengling (B18), Naokong (GB19), Fengchi (GB20), Jianjing(GB21), Yuanye(GB22), Zhejin(GB23), Riyue(GB24), Jingmen(GB25), Daimai(GB26), Wushu(GB27), Weidao(GB28), Juliao (GB29), Huantiao (GB30), Fengshi (GB31), Zhongdu (GB32), Xiyangguan (GB33), Yanglingquan (GB34), Yangjiao (GB35), Waiqiu (GB36), Guangming(GB37), Yangfu(GB38), Xuanzhong(GB39), Qiuxu(GB40), Zulinqi(GB41), Diwuhui(GB42), Xiaxi(GB43), Zuqiaoyin (GD44).

（五）要穴简介（图30、图31、图32）

1. 肩井（GB21）

定位：肩上，大椎与肩峰连线的中点。

主治：项背强痛，肩臂强痛不能举，乳痛，乳汁少，瘰疬，中风。

(V) Introductions of key acupoints (Figure 30, 31, 32)

1. Jianjing (GB21)

Location: On the shoulder, the midpoint between Dazhui (DU14) and the acromion process of the clavicle.

Main indications: Neck and back severe pain, shoulder and arm severe pain, and cannot hold upward, breast pain, oligogalactia, scrofula, and stroke.

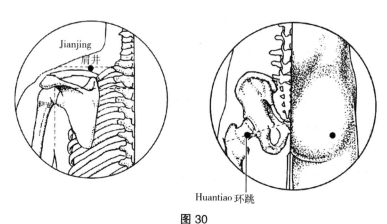

Figure 30

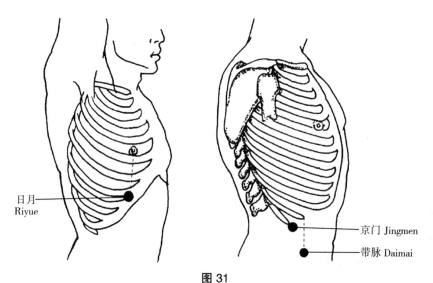

Figure 31

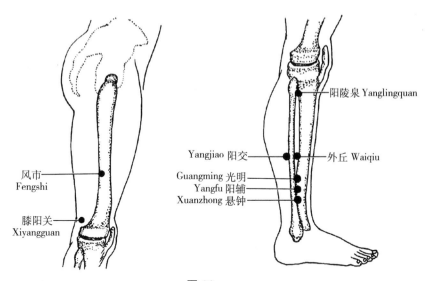

图 32
Figure 32

2. 日月（GB24）（胆募穴）

定位：乳头直下，第 7 肋间，距前正中线 4 寸。

主治：黄疸，呕吐，腹胀，胁肋胀痛。

3. 京门（GB25）（肾募穴）

定位：第 12 肋骨游离端下方。

主治：腹胀，肠鸣，腰肋痛，小便不利。

4. 带脉（GB26）

定位：第 11 肋端（章门）直下，与脐相平处。

主治：月经不调，带下，疝气，少腹痛。

5. 环跳（GB30）

定位：股骨大转子最高点与骶管裂孔连线的外 1/3 与内

2. Riyue (GB24) (Mu acupoint of Gallbladder)

Location: Directly below the nipple, the 7th intercostal space, 4" away from the anteromedial line.

Main indications: Jaundice, vomiting, abdomen distention, flank and rib swelling and pain.

3. Jingmen (GB25) (Mu acupoint of Kidney)

Location: Below the 12th rib free end.

Main indications: Abdomen distention, borborygmus, low back and rib pain, and dysuria.

4. Daimai (GB26)

Location: Directly below the 11th rib edge (Zhangmen, LR13), the same level as the navel.

Main indications: Menoxenia, leukorrhea, herniation, and lower abdominal pain.

5. Huantiao (GB30)

Location: The cross over point of the external 1/3 and the internal 2/3 of the connection between the high-

2/3 的交点处。

主治：下肢痿痹，腰胯痛，痹证。

6. 风市（GB31）

定位：大腿外侧正中，腘横纹上 7 寸处。

主治：下肢痿痹、不遂，全身痛痒，脚气。

7. 膝阳关（GB33）

定位：阳陵泉上 3 寸，股骨外上髁的凹陷处。

主治：膝部疼痛，腘窝部挛急疼痛，下肢痹痛，脚气。

8. 阳陵泉（GB34）（合穴、胆下合穴、八会穴）

定位：腓骨头前下方的凹陷处。

主治：黄疸，口苦，呕吐，胸胁痛，下肢痿痹，半身不遂，膝部疼痛。

9. 阳交（GB35）（阳维脉郄穴）

定位：外踝尖上 7 寸，腓骨后缘。

主治：胸胁胀痛，下肢痿痹，癫痫，喉痹。

est point of the greater trochanter of the femur and the sacral canal.

Main indications: Lower extremities atrophy and numbness, waist and groin pain, and arthralgia-syndrome.

6. Fengshi (GB31)

Location: Midpoint of the lateral side of the thigh, 7" above the popliteal fossa.

Main indications: Lower extremities atrophy, numbness and paralysis, systemic pain and itch, and weak feet.

7. Xiyangguan (GB33)

Location: 3" above the Yanglingquan (GB34), the concavity above the supracondyle of the femur.

Main indications: Knee pain, popliteal fossa acute spasm and pain, lower extremities numbness and pain, and weak feet.

8. Yanglingquan (GB34) (He acupoint, gallbladder lower He acupoint, eight influential point)

Location: The cavity located anterior and below the fibula head.

Main indications: Jaundice, bitter taste, vomiting, chest and flank pain, lower extremities atrophy, paralysis, and knee pain.

9. Yangjiao (GB35) (xi-cleft acupoint of Yang-wei meridian)

Location: 7" above the external ankle apex, posterior fibula.

Main indications: Chest and flank swelling and pain, lower extremities atrophy, epilepsy, and throat paralysis.

10. 外丘（GB36）（郄穴）

定位：外踝尖上 7 寸，腓骨前缘。

主治：胸胁胀痛，脚气，颈项强痛，下肢痿痹，癫痫。

11. 光明（GB37）（络穴）

定位：外踝尖上 5 寸，腓骨前缘。

主治：目痛，视物模糊，夜盲，乳胀痛，产后回乳，下肢痿痹，膝痛。

12. 阳辅（GB38）（经穴）

定位：外踝尖直上 4 寸，腓骨前缘稍前处。

主治：胸胁痛，腋肿，目痛，偏头痛，下肢痿痹。

13. 悬钟（GB39）（八会穴）

定位：外踝尖上 3 寸，腓骨前缘。

主治：胸、胁、腹部胀痛，脚气，下肢痿痹、不遂。

十二、足厥阴肝经（左右各 14 穴，共 28 穴）

（一）循行路线

足厥阴肝经起于足大趾爪甲后丛毛处，下至足大趾外侧端（大敦），沿足背向上，至内

10. Waiqiu (GB36) (Xi acupoint)

Location: 7" above the external ankle apex, anterior fibula.

Main indications: Chest and flank swelling and pain, weak feet, neck severe pain, lower extremities atrophy, and epilepsy.

11. Guangming (GB37)(collateral point)

Location: 5" above the external ankle apex, anterior fibula.

Main indications: Eye pain, blurred vision, nyctalopia, breast swelling and pain, postpartum termination lactation, lower extremities atrophy, and knee pain.

12. Yangfu (GB38) (meridian point)

Location: 4" above the external ankle apex, slightly anterior to the anterior fibula.

Main indications: Chest and flank pain, axillary swelling, eye pain, migraine, and lower extremities atrophy.

13. Xuanzhong (GB39) (eight influential point)

Location: 3" above the external ankle apex, anterior fibula.

Main indications: Chest, flank and abdominal pain, weak feet, lower extremities atrophy and paralysis.

XII. Jue-Yin Liver Meridian of Foot (14 acupoints on each leg, total of 28 acupoints)

(I) Meridian pathway

The Jue-Yin Liver Meridian of Foot goes from the big toe onyx hair lines, down to the lateral side of the big toe (Dadun, LR1), along with the dorsal side of the

踝前 1 寸处（中封），向上沿胫骨内侧前缘，在内踝上 8 寸处交出足太阴脾经之后，上行过膝内侧，沿大腿内侧中线进入阴毛中，绕阴器，抵少腹，上行至章门，循行至期门入腹，挟胃两旁，属肝，络胆。向上穿过膈肌，分布于胁肋部，沿喉咙之后，向上进入鼻咽部，上行连于目系，出于额，直达头顶部，与督脉交会于巅顶（百会）。

分支：从目系分出，下行于颊里，环绕在口唇内。

分支：从肝分出，穿过膈肌，向上注入肺中，交于手太阴肺经。

（二）联系脏腑器官

肝经属肝，络胆，与胃、肺、生殖器、喉咙、目、口唇有联系。

（三）主治

主治肝、前阴、妇科病及本经脉循行部位的病症。

foot to 1" in front of the inner ankle (Zhongfeng, LR4). It then travels up along with the anteromedial tibia to the place 8" above the inner ankle, crosses over with the Tai-Yin Spleen Meridian of Foot, and goes up along with the medial knee. It then enters into the pubic hair along with the groin, surrounds the genitals, and reaches to the lower abdomen. It then further travels up to Zhangmen (LR13), follows the line to Qimen (LR14), enters into the abdomen bypasses the stomach. It governs the liver and collaterals the gallbladder. It goes up through the diaphragm, distributes at the flank and ribs, travels further up into the nasopharyngeal space along with the posterior throat, and links to the eye connector. It then exits the forehead, straight to the top of the head, and crosses over with the Du channel at parietal lobe (Baihui, DU20).

It branches out from the eye connector, goes down to Jiali, and circulates within the mouth and lips.

It branches from the liver, through the diaphragm, goes up and enters into the lungs, crosses over with the Tai-Yin Lung Meridian of Hand.

(II) Relevant Zang, Fu and organs

Liver meridian governs to liver, collaterals with the gallbladder, and connects with the stomach, lung, genitals, throat, eyes, mouth and lips.

(III) Main indications

Acupuncture points in this meridian are indicated for liver, genital and gynecological diseases, and other symptoms along the meridian pathway.

(四) 经穴

大敦 (LR1)、行间 (LR2)、太冲 (LR3)、中封 (LR4)、蠡沟 (LR5)、中都 (LR6)、膝关 (LR7)、曲泉 (LR8)、阴包 (LR9)、足五里 (LR10)、阴廉 (LR11)、急脉 (LR12)、章门 (LR13)、期门 (LR14)。

(Ⅳ) Meridian points

Dadun (LR1), Xingjian (LR2), Taichong (LR3), Zhongfeng (LR4), Ligou (LR5), Zhongdu (LR6), Xiguan (LR7), Ququan (LR8), Yinbao (LR9), Zuwuli (LR10), Yinlian (LR11), Jimai (LR12), Zhangmen (LR13), Qimen (LR14).

(五) 要穴简介 (图 33、图 34)

(Ⅴ) Introductions of key acupoints (Figure 33, 34)

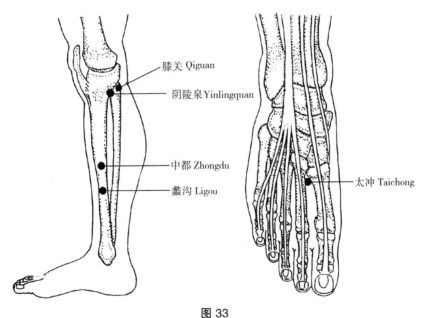

图 33
Figure 33

1. 太冲 (LR3)(输穴、原穴)

定位：足背第 1、2 跖骨结合部前的凹陷中。

主治：头痛，眩晕，呃

1. Taichong (LR3) (Shu acupoint or shu-stream point, Yuan acupoint)

Location: The concavity between the 1st and the 2nd metatarsal joint on the dorsal side of the foot.

Main indications: Headache, dizziness, hiccups,

逆，疝气，月经不调，黄疸，目赤肿痛，癫痫，小儿惊风，胸胁痛，下肢痿痹。

herniation, menoxenia, jaundice, red eyes and swelling, and pain, epilepsy, acute infantile convulsion, chest and flank pain, lower extremities atrophy.

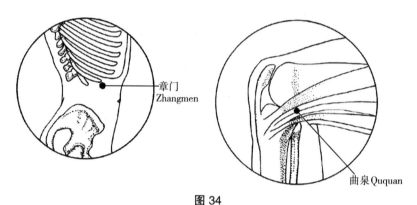

图 34
Figure 34

2. 蠡沟（LR5）（络穴）

定位：内踝上 5 寸，胫骨内侧面中央处。

主治：月经不调，带下，疝气，阴痒，小便不利，胫部疼痛。

3. 中都（LR6）（郄穴）

定位：内踝尖上 7 寸，胫骨内侧面正中央。

主治：泄泻，腹胀，疝气，胁痛，崩漏。

4. 膝关（LR7）

定位：胫骨内侧髁后下方，阴陵泉后 1 寸。

主治：咽喉肿痛，下肢痿痹，膝部肿痛。

5. 曲泉（LR8）（合穴）

定位：屈膝，膝内侧髁纹

2. Ligou (LR5) (collateral point)

Location: 5" above the inner ankle, the midpoint of the medial tibia.

Main indications: Menoxenia, leukorrhea, herniation, pruritus vulvae, dysuria, and tibia pain.

3. Zhongdu (LR6) (Xi acupoint)

Location: 7" above the inner ankle apex, midpoint of the medial-lateral tibia.

Main indications: Diarrhea, abdomen distention, herniation, flank pain, and uterine bleeding.

4. Xiguan (LR7)

Location: posterolateral condyle of the tibia, 1" posterior to the Yinlingquan (SP9).

Main indications: Throat swelling and sore throat, lower extremity atrophy, and knee swelling.

5. Ququan (LR8) (He acupoint)

Location: The concavity above the medial condyle

头上方的凹陷中。

主治：小便不利，月经不调，痛经，带下，阴挺，膝部痛。

6. 章门（LR13）（脾募穴、八会穴）

定位：第 11 肋游离端的下方。

主治：腹胀，肠鸣，泄泻，黄疸，呕吐，痞块，胸胁痛。

十三、任脉（共 24 穴）

（一）循行路线

任脉起于小腹内，下出会阴部，向上行于前阴部。沿着腹内，向上经关元到达咽部，再上行环绕口唇，经过面部，进入目眶下。

（二）联系脏腑器官

任脉与胞宫、咽喉、口唇、目有联系。

（三）主治

主治咽喉、妇科、神志等病及相应脏腑病症。

of the knee when flexing.

Main indications: Dysuria, menoxenia, dysmenorrhea, leukorrhea, uterine prolapse, and knee pain.

6. Zhangmen (LR13) (Mu acupoint of Spleen eight influential point)

Location: Below the 11th rib free end.

Main indications: Abdomen distention, borborygmus, diarrhea, jaundice, vomiting, lumps, chest and flank pain.

XIII. Ren channel (total of 24 acupoints)

(I) Meridian pathway

Ren channel starts from the lower abdomen, down to the perineum, and then goes up to the front genitals. It then travels inside the abdomen, up through Guanyuan (RN4) to the throat, and goes up further to surround the mouth and lips, passes through th face, and enters into the suborbital area.

(II) Relevant Zang, Fu and organs

Ren channel connects with the uterus, throat, mouth, lips and eyes.

(III) Main indications

Acupuncture points in this channel are used for throat, gynecological and mental illnesses, and other symptoms along the meridian pathway.

（四）经穴

会阴（RN1）、曲骨（RN2）、中极（RN3）、关元（RN4）、石门（RN5）、气海（RN6）、阴交（RN7）、神阙（RN8）、水分（RN9）、下脘（RN10）、建里（RN11）、中脘（RN12）、上脘（RN13）、巨阙（RN14）、鸠尾（RN15）、中庭（RN16）、膻中（RN17）、玉堂（RN18）、紫宫（RN19）、华盖（RN20）、璇玑（RN21）、天突（RN22）、廉泉（RN23）、承浆（RN24）。

（五）要穴简介（图35）

1. 中极（RN3）（膀胱募穴、任脉与足三阴经的交会穴）

定位：腹正中线上，脐中下4寸。

主治：小便不利，遗尿，遗精，水肿，阳痿，疝气，月经不调，阴挺。

2. 关元（RN4）（小肠募穴、任脉与足三阴经的交会穴）

定位：腹正中线上，脐中下3寸。

主治：少腹痛，吐泻，尿频，阳痿，遗尿，遗精，小便

(Ⅳ) Meridian points

Huiyin (RN1), Qugu (RN2), Zhongji (RN3), Guanyuan (RN4), Shimen (RN5), Qihai (RN6), Yinjiao (RN7), Shenque (RN8), Shuifen (RN9), Xiawan (RN10), Jianli (RN11), Zhongwan (RN12), Shangwan (RN13), Juque (RN14), Jiuwei (RN15), Zhongting (RN16), Danzhong (RN17), Yutang (RN18), Zigong (RN19), Huagai (RN20), Xuanji (RN21), Tiantu (RN22), Lianquan (RN23), Chengjiang (RN24).

(Ⅴ) Introductions of key acupoints (Figure 35)

1. Zhongji (RN3) (Mu acupoint of Bladder, and the confluent point of Ren channel and the three Yin Meridians of Foot)

Location: The midline of the abdomen, 4" below the navel.

Main indications: Dysuria, enuresis, spermatorrhea, swelling, impotence, herniation, menoxenia, and uterine prolapse.

2. Guanyuan (RN4) (Mu acupoint of Small Intestine, and the confluent point of Ren channel and the three Yin Meridians of Foot)

Location: The midline of the abdomen, 3" below the navel.

Main indications: Lower abdominal pain, vomiting, diarrhea, micturition, impotence, enuresis, spermator-

不利，月经不调，带下，阴挺，中风脱证。

rhea, dysuria, menoxenia, leukorrhea, uterine prolapse, and apoplectic collapse.

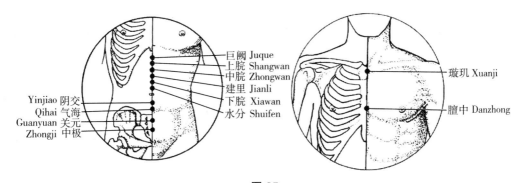

图 35
Figure 35

3. 气海（RN6）（肓之原穴）

定位：腹正中线上，脐中下 1.5 寸。

主治：小腹痛，腹胀，遗尿，小便不利，泄泻，阳痿，遗精，疝气，阴挺，中风脱证，虚劳体弱。

4. 阴交（RN7）

定位：腹正中线上，脐中下 1 寸。

主治：绕脐冷痛，腹胀，小便不利，水肿，泄泻，经闭，带下。

5. 水分（RN9）

定位：腹正中线上，脐中上 1 寸。

主治：水肿，小便不利，腹痛，腹胀，泄泻，反胃，呕吐。

3. Qihai (RN6) (Huang-primary point)

Location: The midline of the abdomen, 1.5" below the navel.

Main indications: Lower abdominal pain, abdomen distention, enuresis, dysuria, diarrhea, impotence, spermatorrhea, herniation, uterine prolapse, apoplectic collapse, consumptive disease, and weak.

4. Yinjiao (RN7)

Location: The midline of the abdomen, 1" below the navel.

Main indications: Cold pain around the umbilical region, abdomen distention, dysuria, swelling, diarrhea, amenorrhea, and leukorrhea.

5. Shuifen (RN9)

Location: The midline of the abdomen, 1" above the navel.

Main indications: Swelling, dysuria, abdominal pain, abdomen distention, diarrhea, nausea, vomiting.

6. 下脘（RN10）

定位：腹正中线上，脐中上 2 寸。

主治：胃脘痛，腹胀，泄泻，呃逆，反胃，呕吐，完谷不化。

7. 建里（RN11）

定位：腹正中线上，脐中上 3 寸。

主治：腹痛，胃胀，泄泻，呕吐，水肿。

8. 中脘（RN12）（胃募穴、八会穴）

定位：腹正中线上，脐中上 4 寸。

主治：胃脘痛，腹胀，呕吐，泄泻，完谷不化，呃逆，黄疸，脾胃虚弱。

9. 上脘（RN13）

定位：腹正中线上，脐中上 5 寸。

主治：胃脘痛，腹胀，呕吐，泄泻，癫痫。

10. 巨阙（RN14）（心募穴）

定位：腹正中线上，脐中上 6 寸。

主治：心悸，心痛，癫痫，胸痛，胃痛，呕吐。

6. Xiawan (RN10)

Location: The midline of the abdomen, 2" above the navel.

Main indications: Stomachache, abdomen distention, diarrhea, hiccups, nausea, vomiting, and diarrhea with indigestive food.

7. Jianli (RN11)

Location: The midline of the abdomen, 3" above the navel.

Main indications: Abdomen distention, stomach distention, diarrhea, vomiting, and swelling.

8. Zhongwan (RN12) (Mu acupoint of Stomach, eight influential point)

Location: The midline of the abdomen, 4" above the navel.

Main indications: Stomachache, abdomen distention, vomiting, diarrhea, diarrhea with indigestive food, hiccups, jaundice, and deficiency of the spleen and stomach.

9. Shangwan (RN13)

Location: The midline of the abdomen, 5" above the navel.

Main indications: Stomachache, abdomen distention, vomiting, diarrhea, and epilepsy.

10. Juque (RN14) (Mu acupoint of Heart)

Location: The midline of the abdomen, 6" above the navel.

Main indications: Palpitation, angina, epilepsy, chest pain, stomachache, and vomiting.

11. 膻中（RN17）（心包募穴、八会穴）

定位：胸骨正中线上，平第 4 肋间隙，两乳头连线的中点。

主治：心悸，胸痛，咳嗽，气喘，乳汁少。

12. 璇玑（RN21）

定位：胸骨正中线上，胸骨上窝中央下 1 寸。

主治：咳嗽，气喘，咽喉肿痛。

十四、督脉（共 28 穴）

（一）循行路线

督脉起于小腹内，下出于会阴，向后行于脊柱，上项行巅顶，沿前额下经鼻柱至上唇内。

（二）联系脏腑器官

督脉与胞宫、肾、脊髓、脑、鼻、眼、口唇有联系。

（三）主治

主治肛肠、腰骶、头项、妇科、发热、神志等病及相应脏腑病症。

11. Danzhong (RN17) (Mu acupoint of Pericardium, eight influential point)

Location: Midline of the sternum, the same level as the 4th intercostal space, the midpoint between the two nipples.

Main indications: Palpitation, chest pain, cough, asthma, and oligogalactia.

12. Xuanji (RN21)

Location: Midline of the sternum, 1" below the mid-suprasternal fossa.

Main indications: Cough, asthma, throat sore and swelling.

14. Du channel (total of 28 acupoints)

(Ⅰ) Meridian pathway

The Du channel arises from the lower abdomen, downward to the perineum, backward to the spine, and upward to the parietal lobe through the neck. It also runs along with the forehead down to the body of the nose and ends to the upper lip.

(Ⅱ) Relevant Zang, Fu and organs

Du channel connects with the uterus, kidney, spinal cord, brain, nose, eyes, mouth and lips.

(Ⅲ) Main indications

Acupuncture points in this channel are used for anus, intestines, sacroiliac, head and neck, gynecological, hyperthermia and mental illness, and other symptoms along the meridian pathway.

（四）经穴

长强（DU1）、腰俞（DU2）、腰阳关（DU3）、命门（DU4）、悬枢（DU5）、脊中（DU6）、中枢（DU7）、筋缩（DU8）、至阳（DU9）、灵台（DU10）、神道（DU11）、身柱（DU12）、陶道（DU13）、大椎（DU14）、哑门（DU15）、风府（DU16）、脑户（DU17）、强间（DU18）、后顶（DU19）、百会（DU20）、前顶（DU21）、囟会（DU22）、上星（DU23）、神庭（DU24）、素髎（DU25）、人中（DU26）、兑端（DU27）、龈交（DU28）。

（五）要穴简介（图36）

1. 腰俞（DU2）

定位：后正中线上，正对骶管裂孔处。

主治：腰脊强痛，癫痫，痔疮，月经不调，下肢痿痹。

2. 腰阳关（DU3）

定位：第4腰椎棘突下的凹陷中，约平髂嵴。

主治：阳痿，遗尿，遗精，月经不调，腰骶痛，下肢痿痹。

(Ⅳ) Meridian points

Changqiang (DU1), Yaoshu (DU2), Yaoyangguan (DU3), Mingmen (DU4), Xuanshu (DU5), Jizhong (DU6), Zhongshu (DU7), Jinsuo (DU8), Zhiyang(DU9), Lingtai(DU10), Shendao(DU11), Shenzhu(DU12), Taodao(DU13), Dazhui(DU14), Yamen(DU15), Fengfu(DU16), Naohu(DU17), Qiangjian(DU18), Houding (DU19), Baihui(DU20), Qianding(DU21), Xinhui(DU22), Shangxing(DU23), Shenting (DU24), Suliao(DU25), Renzhong(DU26), Duiduan(DU27), Yinjiao (DU28).

(Ⅴ) Introductions of key acupoints (Figure 36)

1. Yaoshu (DU2)

Location: On the posteromedial line, around the same level as the sacral canal foramen.

Main indications: Lumbar vertebra stiffness and pain, epilepsy, hemorrhoids, menoxenia, and lower extremities atrophy.

2. Yaoyangguan (DU3)

Location: The concavity in the infraspinous process of the L4, around the same level as iliac crest.

Main indications: Impotence, enuresis, spermatorrhea, menoxenia, lumbosacral pain, lower extremities atrophy.

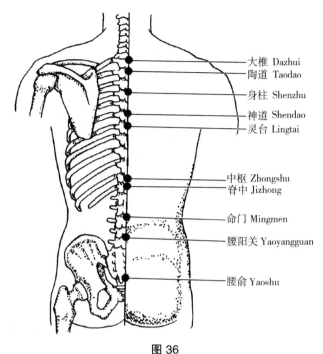

图 36
Figure 36

3. 命门（DU4）

定位：第 2 腰椎棘突下的凹陷中。

主治：虚损腰痛，阳痿，遗尿，遗精，月经不调，带下，尿频，泄泻，不育，不孕。

4. 脊中（DU6）

定位：第 11 胸椎棘突下的凹陷中。

主治：泄泻，黄疸，痔疾，癫痫，腰脊强痛。

5. 中枢（DU7）

定位：第 10 胸椎棘突下的凹陷中。

主治：腹胀满，胃痛，呕

3. Mingmen (DU4)

Location: The concavity in the infraspinous process of the L2.

Main indications: Consumptive disease, low back pain, impotence, enuresis, spermatorrhea, menoxenia, leukorrhea, micturition, diarrhea, infertility, and sterility.

4. Jizhong (DU6)

Location: The concavity in the infraspinous process of the T11.

Main indications: Diarrhea, jaundice, malaria, epilepsy, lumbar vertebra stiffness and pain.

5. Zhongshu (DU7)

Location: The concavity in the infraspinous process of the T10.

Main indications: Full sensation of the abdomen,

吐，黄疸，腰背痛。

6. 灵台（DU10）

定位：第 6 胸椎棘突下的凹陷中。

主治：背脊强痛，咳嗽，气喘，疔疮。

7. 神道（DU11）

定位：第 5 胸椎棘突下的凹陷中。

主治：心悸，心痛，癫痫，咳嗽，背脊强痛。

8. 身柱（DU12）

定位：第 3 胸椎棘突下的凹陷中。

主治：腰脊强痛，咳嗽，气喘，癫痫。

9. 陶道（DU13）

定位：第 1 胸椎棘突下的凹陷中。

主治：头痛项强，疟疾，发热，喘咳，腰脊强痛。

10. 大椎（DU14）

定位：第 7 颈椎棘突下的凹陷中。

主治：热病，感冒，疟疾，咳嗽，癫痫，风疹，项背强痛。

stomachache, vomiting, jaundice, and low back pain.

6. Lingtai (DU10)

Location: The concavity in the infraspinous process of the T6.

Main indications: Backbone stiffness and pain, cough, asthma, hard furuncle.

7. Shendao (DU11)

Location: The concavity in the infraspinous process of the T5.

Main indications: Palpitation, angina, epilepsy, cough, backbone stiffness and pain.

8. Shenzhu (DU12)

Location: The concavity in the infraspinous process of the T3.

Main indications: Lumbar vertebra stiffness and pain, cough, asthma, and epilepsy.

9. Taodao (DU13)

Location: The concavity in the infraspinous process of the T1.

Main indications: Headache, stiff neck, malaria, fever, short of breath, cough, lumbar vertebra stiffness and pain.

10. Dazhui (DU14)

Location: The concavity in the infraspinous process of the C7.

Main indications: Fever, cold, malaria, cough, epilepsy, rubella, neck and back stiffness and pain.

电热针的治疗原则

辨证论治

电热针治疗疾病,以中医基础理论为指导,运用中医诊断学、经络学、腧穴学以及刺法灸法学等知识和电热针的方法,根据患者具体病情进行辨证施治。中医临床常用的辨证方法有:八纲辨证、六经辨证、脏腑辨证、卫气营血辨证、三焦辨证、经络辨证六种。辨证论治,是中医治病的精华。电热针工作者,是在中医整体观念的指导下,在全面掌握和运用这些基本辨证方法中,将临床所见的不同证候,进行归纳、分析,进行辨证论治。在电热针临床实践中,将八纲、六经、脏腑、卫气营血、三焦和经络的辨证方法紧密结合起来,融会贯通。分析病性是属寒还是属热、属虚还是属实、属阴还是属阳,病位在表还是在里,在经还是在络,在脏还是在腑。然后确定

Therapeutic principles of the electrothermal acupuncture therapy

Treatment for syndrome differentiation

Electrothermal acupuncture therapy is based on the guidance of Traditional Chinese Medicine theory and the knowledge of Traditional Chinese Medicine diagnostics, meridian science, science of acupoint and acupuncture, moxibustion technique as well as electrothermal acupuncture therapy. The treatment is administered according to the actual illness condition of the patient. Common methods used in clinical Traditional Chinese Medicine practice for syndrome differentiation consist of 6 approaches including eight principles, six channels, Zang-Fu (visceral) theories, Wei/Qi/Ying/Blood stages, triple burner syndromes and meridian theories. Treatment based on syndrome differentiation is the essence of Traditional Chinese Medicine. Under the comprehensive guidance of Traditional Chinese Medicine and following the understanding/practicing basic syndrome differentiation approaches, the electrothermal acupuncture therapy practitioner is able to perform induction and analysis to differentiate syndromes and administer treatments based on different clinical manifestations. In the clinical practice of electrothermal acupuncture therapy, it is necessary to combine the syndrome differentiation approaches (i.e. eight principles, six channels, Zang-Fu theory, Wei/Qi/

治疗大法，按处方配穴，按方施术。采用补法或泻法，或补泻兼施，以通其经络，调其气血，使脏腑、气血、阴阳趋于调和，经络恢复平稳，达到"阴平阳秘，精神乃治"。

一、八纲辨证

八纲，即阴阳、表里、寒热、虚实，是辨证论治的总纲领，是以望、闻、问、切四诊所获得的资料为依据，对病变的病位、病性、正邪关系等情况进行综合分析，将其归纳为阴、阳、表、里、寒、热、虚、实八类证候而进行电热针治疗的一种方法。而这八类证候可以用阴阳两纲加以概括，即表证、热证、实证为阳证，里证、寒证、虚证为阴证。

二、脏腑辨证

脏腑辨证是以脏腑学说为基础，将四诊所获得的证候

Ying/Blood stages, three burner syndromes and meridian theory) to achieve mastery. Disease particular analysis includes cold-heat, deficiency-excess, Yin-Yang, mild-severe, meridian-collateral, Zang-Fu. The practitioner will decide the therapeutic regimen, locate proper acupoints, and apply prescriptions. The adoption of either tonifying or attenuating or both may soothe meridian, regulate Qi and blood, reconcile Zang-Fu and Qi-blood with Yin-Yang, and stabilize meridians to achieve "Yin-Yang equilibrium and good health and spirits".

I. Eight principles of syndrome differentiation

Eight principles (i.e. Yin-Yang, mild-severe, Cold-Heat, deficiency-excess) are the general principles of treatment for syndrome differentiation. Based on the information derived from the four traditional Chinese diagnostic methods (observation, listening, inquiry and palpation), the practitioner may conduct a comprehensive analysis on the location, feature and healthy/evil energy relationship of the illness, classify the disease as based on eight principles (i.e. Yin, Yang, mild, severe, Cold, Heat, deficiency and excess), and then perform electrothermal acupuncture therapy accordingly. These eight principles can be generally classified as two major sub-categories (Yin and Yang); that is, mild, heat and excess are Yang syndromes while severe, cold and deficiency are Yin syndromes.

II. Zang-Fu theories for syndrome differentiation

Zang-Fu theories for syndrome differentiation are based on Zang-Fu theory and make a comprehensive

和体征进行综合分析，从而对病变所在的脏腑部位、性质及正邪的盛衰做出诊断，进行治疗的一种辨证论治方法。脏腑与经络在生理上相互联系，在病理上密切相关。它包括肺病证、大肠病证、脾病证、胃病证、心（包）病证、小肠病证、肾病证、膀胱病证、三焦病证、肝胆病证。

三、气血辨证

气血辨证就是根据患者不同的证候分析气血一系列的变化，将其分析辨证为气病证、血病证和气血同病证。

气病证中又分为虚、实两大类。"虚"指气之不足，表现为功能低下或衰退，有气虚、气陷之分；"实"指气的有余，表现为功能亢进与太过，有气滞、气逆之别。

血病证归纳起来有血虚、血瘀和出血三个方面。出血可因气不摄血、血热妄行、阴虚火旺和瘀血内积导致。

气为阳，血为阴，气为

analysis on syndromes as well as signs derived from four diagnostic methods. This is an approach for syndrome differentiation to make diagnosis based on the location, nature and rise and fall of the healthy and evil of the lesion visceral organs, and subsequently prescribe treatment. Zang-Fu theory is closely related to the meridian theory in terms of physiology as well as pathology. Zang-Fu theories for syndrome differentiation depict syndromes concerning lungs, large intestine, spleen, stomach, heart (pericardium), small intestine, kidneys, bladder, three Jiaos, liver and gallbladder.

III. Qi-blood stages for syndrome differentiation

Qi-blood stages for syndrome differentiation is to differentiate a series of Qi-blood changes based on different syndromes of the patients, and divide those syndromes into diseases of Qi, blood and Qi-plus-blood.

Qi-related syndromes can be divided into deficiency and excess two major subtypes. "Deficiency" refers to insufficient Qi, hypofunction or impairment as representations, and can be divided into Qi deficiency and Qi collapsed caused by exhaustion; by contrast, "excess" refers to excessive Qi, uses hyperfunctional or irritation, and can be divided into Qi stasis and reversed flow of Qi.

Blood (Hematology) disease can be summarized in three aspects, including blood deficiency, blood stasis and bleeding. Bleeding may be caused by Qi failing to control blood, hemopyretic bleeding, hyperactivity of fire due to Yin deficiency and the accumulation of blood stasis.

Qi belongs to Yang and blood belongs to Yin; Qi as

血帅，血为气母，两者互相联系，相互依存。气能生血，能摄血，气行则血行，气滞则血凝。有形之血生于无形之气，无形之气必须依附于有形之血存在于体内。气与血生理上联系密切，也可导致病理上的气血同病，如气血两虚、气随血脱、气虚血瘀、血虚血瘀、气滞血瘀。

四、经络辨证

经络辨证，是以经络学说为指导，根据经络的循行部位和脏腑络属关系辨认经络病证的一种辨证方法。

经络以经脉为主体，因而在辨证时要以经脉的病证记载为主要依据。在电热针临床上，可根据病证所在的脏腑经络部位选穴配方。

（一）十二经脉病症

十二经脉，每一条经脉都有一定的循行路径和所属络的脏腑。如果发生病变，各有不同的病症。其病证表现可分属

commander of blood and blood as mother of Qi; Qi and blood are both connected, related and depend on each other. Qi can generate blood and accumulate blood, so smooth Qi improves blood circulation but Qi stasis causes blood coagulation. Visible blood is generated from invisible Qi; that is, invisible Qi must rely on the blood to accumulate in human bodies. Qi and blood are physiologically close related. In other words, Qi and blood may simultaneously cause pathological conditions, including Qi-blood deficiency, Qi desertion due to blood deficiency, blood stasis due to Qi deficiency, blood stasis due to blood deficiency and blood stasis due to Qi stagnation.

Ⅳ. Meridian theory

The use of syndrome differentiation is based on the guidance of meridian theories, which is one of the syndrome differentiation approaches on the basis of meridian circulatory pathways as well as the correlations with the visceral organs (Zang-Fu).

The meridian theory is primarily based on the meridian system, and therefore syndrome differentiation is based on meridian-related manifestations. In the clinical practice of electrothermal acupuncture therapy, the selection of acupoints on visceral organs or meridian channels should be in accordance with the prescriptions.

(Ⅰ) Syndromes related to 12 meridians

In the 12 meridians, each one consists of its unique circulation pathways and corresponding visceral organs. If there are any pathological changes, different syndromes may appear accordingly. The syndromes can be

2个方面：一为本经的脏或腑的生理功能失常，二为本经循行部位的病症。简述如下：

1. 手太阴肺经病症

咳嗽，气喘，咯血，咽喉肿痛，胸部胀满，缺盆部、肩背及手臂内侧前缘痛等。

2. 手阳明大肠经病症

鼻衄，鼻流清涕，齿痛，咽喉肿痛，颈肩前、上肢外侧前缘痛，肠鸣腹痛，泄泻，下赤白等。

3. 足阳明胃经病症

肠鸣，腹胀，水肿，胃脘痛，呕吐，善饥，鼻衄，口㖞，咽喉肿痛，胸腹及下肢外侧缘痛，发热，发狂等。

4. 足太阴脾经病症

嗳气，呕吐，胃脘痛，腹胀，便溏，黄疸，身重无力，舌根强痛，股膝内侧肿胀、厥等。

5. 手少阴心经病症

心痛，心悸，胁痛，失眠，盗汗，咽干口渴，上臂内侧痛，手心热等。

divided into two aspects: One is related to syndromes caused by Zang, Fu or physiological dysfunctions, another one is the syndromes related to the circulation channels. The syndromes are summarized as follows:

1. Syndromes relate to Tai-Yin Lung Meridian of Hand

Cough, asthma, hemoptysis, sore throat and swelling, breast engorge, Quepen acupoint, shoulder, back and anteromedial arm pain, etc.

2. Syndromes relate to Tai-Yang Large Intestine Meridian of Hand

Epistaxis, thin nasal discharge, toothache, sore throat and swelling, anterior neck and shoulder pain, anterolateral upper limb pain, borborygmus, abdominal pain, diarrhea, dysentery with red and white feces, etc.

3. Syndromes relate to Yang-Ming Stomach Meridian of Foot

Borborygmus, abdominal distention, edema, epigastric pain, vomiting, bulimia, epistaxis, mania, etc.

4. Syndromes relate to Tai-Yin Spleen Meridian of Foot

Belching, vomiting, epigastric pain, abdomen distention, loose stools, jaundice, heavy body weakness, stiff tongue and pain, medial groin and knee swelling, cold limbs, etc.

5. Syndromes relate to Shao-Yin Heart Meridian of Hand

Angina, palpitation, costalgia, insomnia, sweating, dry mouth and thirsty, inner upper arm pain, feverish palm, etc.

6. 手太阳小肠经病症

耳聋，目黄，咽喉痛，颊肿，少腹胀痛，肩臂外侧后缘痛。

7. 足太阳膀胱经病症

小便不利，遗尿，癫狂，疟疾，目痛，迎风流泪，鼻塞流涕，衄血，头痛，颈背腰臀部及下肢后面疼痛等。

8. 足少阴肾经病症

遗尿，尿频，遗精，阳痿，月经不调，气喘，咯血，舌干，咽喉肿痛，水肿，腰脊痛，股内侧后缘痛，下肢无力，足心热等。

9. 手厥阴心包经病症

心疼，心悸，心烦，胸闷，面赤，腋下疼，癫狂，上肢拘急，手心热等。

10. 手少阳三焦经病症

腹胀，水肿，小便不利，耳聋，耳鸣，目外眦、耳后痛，肩、臂、肘外侧痛等。

6. Syndromes relate to Tai-Yang Small Intestine Meridian of Hand

Deaf, jaundice eyes, sore throat, buccal swelling, low abdominal pain, posterolateral shoulder and arm pain.

7. Syndromes related to Tai-Yang Bladder Meridian of Foot

Dysuria, enuresis, manic-depressive psychosis, malaria, pain of eyes, epiphora with wind, nasal congestion and running nose, bleeding from five aperture or subcutaneous tissue, headache, neck, back and low back pain, posterior pain of lower extremities, etc.

8. Syndromes relate to Shao-Yin Kidney Meridian of Foot

Enuresis, frequent urination, nocturnal emission, asynodia, menoxenia, asthma, hemoptysis, dry tongue, sore throat and swelling, edema, low back pain, posteromedial groin pain, lower extremity asthenia, feverish soles, etc.

9. Syndromes relate to Jue-Yin Pericardium Meridian of Hand

Chest distress, palpitation, upset, chest pain, red face, subaxillary pain, manic-depressive psychosis, upper extremity spasm, feverish palms, etc.

10. Syndromes relate to Shao-Yang Three-Jiao Meridian of Hand

Abdomen distention, edema, dysuria, deaf, tinnitus, outer canthus, ear pain, lateral shoulder, arm, elbow pain, etc.

11. 足少阳胆经病症

头痛，目外眦痛，颔痛，目眩，口苦，缺盆部肿痛，腋下痛，胸胁、股及下肢外侧痛等。

12. 足厥阴肝经病症

腰痛，胸满，少腹痛，疝气，巅顶痛，咽干，呕逆，遗尿，小便不利，精神失常等。

（二）奇经八脉病症

奇经八脉具有加强经脉之间的联系，调节正经气血的作用，与肝、肾等脏及女子胞、脑髓等奇恒之腑的联系较为密切，失调则为病。根据其循行部位和生理特点，略述如下：

1. 任脉病症

带下，月经不调，不孕，疝气，遗精，遗尿，尿闭，胃脘及小腹痛，阴部痛等。

2. 督脉病症

脊柱强痛，角弓反张，癫痫。

3. 冲脉病症

腹内拘急而痛，月经不调，不孕，不育，气喘等。

11. Syndromes relate to Shao-Yang Gallbladder Meridian of Foot

Headache, outer canthus, jaw pain, dizziness, bitter taste, Quepen acupoint swelling and pain, axillary pain, chest pain and costalgia, lateral groin and lower extremity pain, etc.

12. Syndromes relate to Jue-Yin Liver Meridian of Foot

Waist pain, chest fullness, low abdomen pain, herniation, parietal headache, dry mouth, retching and hiccup, enuresis, dysuria, mental disorder, etc.

(Ⅱ) Syndromes related to 8 extraordinary vessels

Eight extraordinary vessels may strengthen the connections between the meridians, and regulate Qi and blood. Because their close connections with extraordinary Zang (e.g. liver, kidneys, etc.) and Fu (e.g. uterus, brain matter, etc.), dysregulation of Zang-Fu may cause disease. The circulation pathways and locations are briefly described as follows:

1. Syndromes related to Ren channel

Leukorrhea, menoxenia, sterility, herniation, nocturnal emission, enuresis, anuresis, epigastric and lower abdomen pain, genital pain, etc.

2. Syndromes related to Du channel

Spine stiffness and pain, opisthotonus, epilepsy.

3. Syndromes related to Chong channel

Intra-abdominal spasm and pain, menoxenia, sterility, infertility, asthma, etc.

4. 带脉病症

腹部胀满，腰部迟缓无力，带下，子宫下垂，下肢痿软等。

5. 阳跷脉病症

癫痫，不眠，目内眦赤痛，腰背痛，下肢痉挛，足外翻等。

6. 阴跷脉病症

癫痫，失眠，少腹痛，腰髋连阴中痛，下肢痉挛，足内翻等。

7. 阳维脉病症

恶寒发热等表证。

8. 阴维脉病症

胸痛，心痛，胃痛等里证。

（三）十五络脉病症

十五络脉主要分布于体表，以加强表里两经的联系，渗灌各部的气血。络脉的病证，可以补充经脉病症的不足。简述如下：

1. 手太阴络脉病症

手腕、手掌部发热，呼吸气短，遗尿，尿频。

2. 手少阴络脉病症

胸膈胀满，虚不能言。

4. Syndromes related to Belt channel

Abdomen distention, waist slow and weakness, leukorrhea, hysteroptosis, lower extremities atrophy and weakness, etc.

5. Syndromes relate to Yangqiao channels

Epilepsy, sleepless, inner canthus red and pain, low back and waist pain, lower extremities spasm, foot eversion, etc.

6. Syndromes relate to Yinqiao channels

Epilepsy, insomnia, low abdomen pain, waist, hip and pudendal pain, lower extremities spasm, foot inversion, etc.

7. Syndromes related to Yang-wei channels

Exterior syndromes such as aversion to cold with fever.

8. Syndromes related to Yin-wei channels

Interior syndromes such as chest pain, angina, stomachache, etc.

(3) Syndromes related to 15 collaterals

The 15 collaterals primarily distribute on the body surface to strengthen the connections between the two interior and exterior meridians in order to perfuse Qi and blood to different body parts. Syndromes relate to collaterals are the supplements to syndromes relate to meridians. The syndromes are briefly described as follows:

1. Syndromes related to Tai-Yin Collaterals of Hand

Feverish wrist and palm, short of breath, enuresis, frequent urination.

2. Syndromes related to Shao-Yin Collaterals of Hand

Chest and diaphragm distention, speechless.

3. 手厥阴络脉病症

心痛，心烦。

4. 手阳明络脉病症

齿痛，耳聋，牙齿酸冷，胸膈闷塞不畅。

5. 手太阳络脉病症

关节纵缓，肘部痿酸，皮肤生疣。

6. 手少阳络脉病症

肘关节拘挛，肘关节迟缓不收。

7. 足阳明络脉病症

癫狂，足胫部肌肉萎缩、松弛，咽部肿痛，突然喑哑。

8. 足太阳络脉病症

鼻塞，鼻流清涕，头痛，背痛，鼻出血。

9. 足少阳络脉病症

足部厥冷，下肢瘫痪，不能起立。

10. 足太阴络脉病症

腹内绞痛，霍乱吐泻。

11. 足少阴络脉病症

尿潴留，腰痛，心烦，胸闷。

3. Syndromes related to Jue-Yin Collaterals of Hand

Angina, upset.

4. Syndromes related to Yang-Ming Collaterals of Hand

Toothache, deaf, sore weak teeth, feeling chest stuffiness.

5. Syndromes related to Tai-Yang Collaterals of Hand

Joint impairment, elbow atrophy and soreness, skin wart.

6. Syndromes related to Shao-Yang Collaterals of Hand

Elbow joint constraint, muscle atrophy and motor impairment.

7. Syndromes related to Yang-Ming Collaterals of Foot

Manic-depressive psychosis, foot shin muscle atrophy and slacking, sore throat and swelling, sudden dumb.

8. Syndromes related to Zu Tai-Yang Collaterals

Nasal congestion, thin nasal discharge, headache, back pain, epistaxis.

9. Syndromes related to Shao-Yang Collaterals of Foot

Cold limbs, lower extremities paralysis, cannot stand up.

10. Syndromes related to Tai-Yin Collaterals of Foot

Abdominal cramp, cholera-induced vomiting and diarrhea.

11. Syndromes related to Shao-Yin Collaterals of Foot

Urine retention, low back pain, upset, chest tight-

12. 足厥阴络脉病症

阳强不倒，阴部瘙痒，睾丸肿胀，疝气。

13. 任脉络之病症

腹部皮肤胀痛、瘙痒。

14. 督脉络之病症

脊柱强直，头部沉痛，摇头。

15. 脾之大络病症

遍身疼痛，四肢关节松软无力。

12. Syndromes related to Jue-Yin Collaterals of Foot

Predominant Yang causing slacking, genital itching, testicle swelling, herniation.

13. Syndromes related to Ren channels

Abdomen skin stretching, pain and itching.

14. Syndromes related to Du channels

Spine stiffness, heavy head and headache, head shaking.

15. Syndromes related to Large Splenic Collateral

Systemic pain, four limbs joints loose and weakness.

下篇　临床论治　Part II: Clinical Treatment

内科疾病

Medical illness

慢性支气管炎

支气管受到细菌、病毒的感染或物理、化学因素的刺激，以及过敏、气候变化异常等因素引起的炎症称支气管炎，常以咳嗽、咯痰或喘促为主要症状。支气管炎是一种常见病、多发病，临床有急性和慢性之分。急性者可发于任何年龄，慢性者以成年人多见。慢性气管炎如果治疗不及时，可并发肺气肿、肺源性心脏病，严重影响工作与生活，甚至危及生命。

中医认为，本病属于"咳嗽""痰饮"等范畴。如因外邪从口鼻皮毛而入，肺气壅遏不宣，清肃失令，则起病较急，

Chronic Bronchitis

Bronchial infection-induced inflammation caused by bacteria, virus, physical/chemical stimulants, allergy or climate abnormalities is called bronchitis. The primary and common symptoms of bronchitis include cough, phlegm and shortness of breath. Bronchitis is a common and frequently-occurring disease, which can be classified as acute and chronic in clinical practice. Acute bronchitis may occur at any age, while chronic bronchitis often occurs in adults. If the treatment for chronic bronchitis is not in time, there is a possibility to develop emphysema and cor pulmonale, or even life-threatening and severely affecting work and daily living.

The Traditional Chinese Medicine practitioner believes that such disease is closely related to syndromes such as "cough" and "phlegm-fluid retention". If lung congestion without dispersion is caused by foreign

类似急性气管炎，有风寒、风热、燥热之分，多为实证。如因内脏失调，或脾虚失运，痰湿犯肺；或因肝火犯肺，灼津成痰；或肾阳不足，命门火衰，气失摄纳，肺失宣降，则发病缓慢，类似慢性气管炎，多为虚证或虚中夹实证，有脾虚、肝火、肾虚之分。

一、诊断及辨证要点

1. 湿痰犯肺，症见咳嗽痰多，痰白而黏，胸脘满闷，苔白腻，脉濡滑。

2. 肾气失纳者，症见咳嗽痰少，不易咳出，形瘦，气不得续，汗出，肢冷，舌淡，脉沉细数。

3. 有长期反复咳嗽病史，秋、冬天气寒冷时复发或加重，早晚咳嗽剧烈，痰多为白色清晰或黏液。

pathogens inspiration through mouth and nose, and thus impair depurative descending of lung Qi, the symptoms are usually acute like acute bronchitis. Such disease consists of subtypes including wind-cold, wind-heat and dryness-heat common cold, which is mostly excess disease. The disease may be caused by internal organs dysregulation; or phlegm dampness invading lungs may be caused by spleen deficiency or dysregulation; or liver fire invading lungs may be caused by fluid retention and thus formulates phlegm; or the disease may develop slowly like chronic bronchitis caused by kidney Yang insufficiency, declined of vital gate fire, lost Qi and food intake, disperse and lower the Qi in the lungs. All of these symptoms are most deficiency symptoms, or deficient plus excessive symptoms. Among these, spleen deficiency, liver fire or kidney deficiency may be included.

I. Key Points for Diagnosis and Syndrome Differentiation

1. For phlegm dampness invading lungs, the symptoms include coughing, productive, white and sticky phlegm, chest and epigastrium fullness and distress, whitish and glossy tongue fur, soft pulse.

2. For patients with kidney deficiency and lost, the symptoms are coughing, less phlegm but difficult to expel, thin body figure, insufficient Qi, sweating, cold limbs, pale tongue, pulse slow, thready and rapid.

3. For patients with long-term repetitive cough history, cold weather in fall and winter may induce disease relapse or aggravation easily, the symptoms are sever cough in the morning and evening, productive, white and

4. 两肺听诊呼吸音粗糙，或散在干、湿性啰音（以肺底部较多）；若为慢性喘息性支气管炎可听到哮鸣音。

5. 血液检查显示，白细胞总数及中性粒细胞百分率在急、慢性支气管炎继发细菌感染时可增高，病毒感染时可减少或不升高。

二、治疗方法

【痰湿犯肺证】

治法 健脾化湿，清痰利肺。

处方 肺俞（BL13）、太渊（LU9）、丰隆（ST40）、太白（SP3）、章门（LR13）。

方义 原穴为本脏真气所输注，故取肺经原穴太渊与脾经原穴太白，配合肺俞和脾经募穴章门，以运脾土而利肺气。因脾为生痰之源，肺为储痰之器，脾肺同取，乃标本合治之意。丰隆是足阳明胃经的络穴，以运中焦脾胃之气，使气引津布，痰湿得化。

sticky phlegm.

4. The auscultation on both lungs shows coarse breathing sound or diffusive dry or wet rales (mostly in the lower lobes), but for chronic asthmatic bronchitis, wheezing sound is observed.

5. The hematology test results show that the white blood cell count and the percentage of neutrophil cells may be increased during either acute or chronic bronchitis with subsequent bacterial infection, but those data may be decreased or unchanged while viral infection.

II. Therapeutic Methods

[Phlegm Dampness]

Therapeutic method: Invigorate spleen for eliminating dampness, and to remove phlegm to moisten lung.

Prescription: Feishu (BL13), Taiyuan (Lu9), Fenglong (ST40), Taibai (SP3), Zhangmen (LR13).

Mechanism of prescription: The Yuan acupoint is perfused by the original visceral and real Qi; hence the treatment for the Yuan acupoint from Lung Meridian Taiyuan and the Yuan acupoint from Spleen Meridian Taibai, along with Feishu and Mu acupoint from the Spleen Zhangmen may transport spleen circulation and thus facilitate the Qi in lungs. The spleen is the source of phlegm, and the lung is the reservoir. Therefore, treat the spleen and the lung at the same time is the approach to cure the symptoms and the disease. Fenglong is a collateral acupoint of the Yang-Ming Stomach Meridian of Foot, which can accumulate the Qi of the spleen and the stomach through regulating the acupoint Middle Jiao,

配穴 胸脘痞闷加内关、膻中；纳差加足三里、中脘。

方法 电热针治疗。

操作 选定穴位，常规皮肤消毒。以电热针斜刺肺俞 0.6～0.8 寸、直刺丰隆 0.7 寸、平刺章门 0.7 寸。然后接通电热针仪，电流量为 60mA，以患者有舒适温热或酸胀感为度。另配以毫针平刺太渊 0.5 寸、太白 0.5 寸，采用提插补法，均留针 40 分钟。

疗程 每日 1 次，30 次为 1 个疗程，疗程间可休息 3 天。

【肾虚失纳证】

治法 补肾纳气，定喘止咳。

处方 天突（RN22）、肾俞（BL23）、太溪（KI3）、气海（RN6）。

方义 天突为任脉之会穴，平喘止咳。肾俞为肾经背俞穴，能益肾补气。太溪是肾经原穴，乃本经之气所灌注，能补肾纳气。气海系元气之海，有补肾虚、益元气之功。

direct the Qi to Jinbu and thereby eliminate the phlegm dampness.

Matching points: For patients with chest and epigastric fullness and distress, add Neiguan and Danzhong; for patients with anorexia, add Zusanli and Zhongwan.

Method: Electrothermal acupuncture treatment.

Operations: Selecting the relevant acupoints, perform routine skin disinfection. Using electrothermal acupuncture needles, obliquely puncture into Feishu for 0.6~0.8", vertically into Fenglong for 0.7", and horizontally into Zhangmen for 0.7". Turn on the electrothermal acupuncture equipment, apply a current of 60mA to each acupoint, and the limit is that the patient feels comfortable, warm or soreness and swelling. In addition, using filiform needles, horizontally puncture into Taiyuan and Taibai for 0.5", and then leaving the needles in for 40 minutes.

Therapeutic course: Treat once a day, 30 times for a course, and a break of 3 days between courses.

[Kidney Deficiency and Lost]

Therapeutic method: Invigorate kidney, supply Qi, relieve short of breath and stop coughing.

Prescriptions: Acupoints of Tiantu (RN22), Shenshu (BL23), Taixi (KI3), Qihai (RN6).

Mechanism of prescription: Tiantu is a confluent acupoint of Ren channel, which can relieve short of breath and stop coughing. Shenshu is the Back-Shu acupoint of Kidney Meridian, which benefits kidney and nourishes Qi. Taixi is the Yuan acupoint of Kidney Meridian, where the location of Qi perfusion from the

诸穴共用，补肾纳气，定喘止咳。

配穴 食少乏力者加足三里、中脘；痰多者加丰隆；动则汗出者加阴郄。

方法 电热针治疗。

操作 选定穴位，常规皮肤消毒。以电热针斜刺肾俞0.8寸、直刺丰隆0.8寸、直刺足三里0.8寸。然后接通电热针仪，电流量60mA，以患者有舒适温热及胀感为度。另配以毫针靠胸骨柄内侧缓慢进针天突0.8寸，进针太溪0.6寸，直刺气海0.7寸，采用提插补法，均留针40分钟。

疗程 每日1次，10次为1个疗程。疗程间可以休息3天。

三、注意事项

1.气管炎尤其是老年患者，多同时伴有支气管扩张、肺气肿、哮喘等疾患，针灸治

original Meridian, and is able to invigorate kidney and supply Qi. The sea of Qi is the sea of vitality, which has the functions of kidney insufficiency invigoration and vitality energizing. Applying treatment on all acupoints may invigorate kidney, supply Qi, relieve short of breath and stop coughing.

Matching points: For patients eat less and weak, add Zusanli and Zhongwan. For patients with productive sputum, add Fenglong; for patients sweat easily when moving, add Yinxi.

Method: Electrothermal acupuncture treatment.

Operations: Selecting the relevant acupoints, perform routine skin disinfection. Using electrothermal acupuncture needles, obliquely puncture into Shenshu for 0.8", vertically into Fenglong and Zusanli for 0.8". Turn on the electrothermal acupuncture equipment, apply a current of 60mA to each acupoint, and the limit is that the patient feels comfortable, warm and swelling. In addition, using filiform needles, slowly puncture into Tiantu for 0.8" near medial side of the sternum, puncture into Taixi for 0.6", vertically into Qihai for 0.7" through lifting and thrusting tonifying, and then leaving the needles in for 40 minutes.

Therapeutic course: Treat once a day, 10 times for a course, and a break of 3 days during a course.

III. Precautions

1.Bronchitis is often accompanied by bronchiectasis, emphysema and asthma, particularly in senior patients. The application of acupuncture therapy should

疗的同时要配合药物治疗，以提高疗效。

2.避免受凉，预防感冒，戒烟。

四、典型病例

冯某，女，46岁，家庭妇女，北京人。

主诉：咳喘反复发作5年余，近1个月加重。病史：患者5年前因吃海鱼后发病，呼吸急促，喉间喘鸣，张口抬肩，不能平卧，呈强迫坐位，呼气性呼吸困难，经抢救治疗而缓解。之后四季均有发作，但秋、冬季节易发，咳喘多与接触过敏食物（鱼、虾、蟹），以及寒冷刺激关系密切。经过多种方法反复治疗至今未愈。

刻下症：1个月前因受风寒，诱发咳喘，自服治疗咳喘的药物（具体不详）后未见明显改善，咳嗽痰多，不易咳出，强迫坐位，呼吸困难，遂到我科就诊。纳可，眠差，二

be combined with medicinal therapy to enhance curative effects.

2. Avoid chillness, prevent from catching cold, quit smoking.

IV. Typical Case

Feng, female, 46 years old, housewife, residence: Beijing.

Self-reported symptoms: Cough and short of breath repeatedly for more than 5 years, and the symptoms are aggravated in the late one month. Medical history: The patient developed the symptom five years ago after she consumed marine fish. The symptoms included short of breath, stridor over pharynx, shoulder elevation with mouth open and failure of remain supine. The patient was forced to remain upright position and displayed short of breath. The above symptoms were relieved after receiving our treatment. Afterward, the disease episodes occurred in all four seasons, particularly frequent in fall and winter. The short of breath and asthma symptoms were closely related to the contact with anaphylactic food (e.g. fish, shrimp or crab) as well as the stimulation of cold weather. However, after receiving multiple approaches and repetitive treatments, the patient was not yet cured.

Current symptoms: The patient caught a cold one month ago and triggered short of breath and asthma. However, the symptoms were not significantly improved after the patient self-medicated with drugs for short of breath and asthma (the specificity unknown). Moreover, the phlegm became productive and sticky, difficult to ex-

便通畅，舌淡，脉沉细。

查体：双肺底闻及散在小水泡音。二尖瓣区及主动脉瓣第二听诊区闻及三级收缩期杂音。

辅助检查：胸片示"双肺纹理增粗"。白细胞计数：$11\times10^9/L$。

【诊断依据】

1. 中年女性，咳喘已5年之久。每遇寒冷季节及食用鱼、虾、蟹即可诱发。

2. 发作与进食海鱼、虾、蟹及寒冷刺激有关。

3. 查体：在二尖瓣区及主动脉瓣第二听诊区闻及三级收缩期杂音。

4. 辅助检查：胸片示"双肺纹理增粗"。白细胞计数为：$11\times10^9/L$。

5. 长期气短喘息，自汗心悸，神疲乏力，食少便溏，面色白。

【证治分析】

病因 饮食所伤。

病机 肺脾两虚。

pel, so the patient displayed difficult breathing and was forced to remain upright position. The patient therefore came to our clinic for medical assistance. Acceptable intake, poor sleep, smooth urination defecation, pale tongue, pulse slow, thready and rapid.

Physical examination: Small crackle sound dispersed over bilateral lung base. 3rd degree systolic murmur over mitral valve and aortic valve the 2nd auscultation area.

Auxiliary examination: Chest X-ray shows "bilateral lung marking thickening". White blood cells count: $11\times10^9/L$.

[Diagnostic Basis]

1. Middle-aged female, has had shortness of breath and cough for 5 years. The symptom is induced in cold weather or when the patient consumes fish, shrimp or crab.

2. The trigger of the syndrome is closely related to the consumption of fish, shrimp and crab, or the stimulation of cold weather.

3. Physical examination: 3rd degree systolic murmur over mitral valve and aortic valve the 2nd auscultation area.

4. Auxiliary examination: Chest X-ray shows "bilateral lung marking thickening". White blood cells count: $11\times10^9/L$.

5. Long-term short of breath, self sweating, palpitation, fatigue and weakness, eat less and loose stool, pale complexion.

[Syndrome-treatment Analysis]

Etiology: Caused by the food.

Pathogenesis: Lung and spleen deficiency.

证候分析 肺主气,肺虚则气失所主,故气短而喘、语声低微。肺气虚、卫外不固,则自汗、心悸,脾主肌肉四肢,脾虚则神疲乏力、食少便溏。气血不能上荣于面,则面色白。舌脉为气虚之象。

病位 肺、脾。

病性 虚性。

西医诊断 肺源性心脏病、慢性支气管炎。

中医诊断 喘证、咳嗽。

治法 补气健脾,益肺定喘。

方法 电热针治疗(温补法)。

处方 以手太阴肺经穴、背部腧穴为主。肺俞、脾俞、足三里、膏肓、定喘、太渊。

方义 脾俞、足三里可健脾益气;肺俞、膏肓、定喘三穴相伍,可平喘理肺;太渊是肺经的原穴,属土,有益肺平喘的作用,达到补土生金的目的。

配穴 心悸者加神门、内关;便溏者加关元、命门。

Syndrome analysis: Lung controls Qi, so deficiency of lung results in Qi lost, leading to short of breath and weak voice. Lung deficiency, leading to poor energy and thus fails to protect the body, self sweating, palpitation. The spleen controls muscles and four limbs, spleen deficiency leads to fatigue, weakness, poor appetite and loose stool. Qi and blood cannot support facial circulation, leading to pale complexion. Tongue shows Qi deficiency.

Lesion location: Lung, spleen.

Disease nature: Deficiency.

The diagnosis of Western Medicine: Cor pulmonale and chronic bronchitis.

The diagnosis of Traditional Chinese Medicine: Short of breath and cough.

Therapeutic method: Nourish Qi, tonify spleen, benefit lung and stop short of breath.

Method: Electrothermal acupuncture treatment (warm tonifying).

Prescription: Acupoints based on the Tai-Yin Lung Meridian of Hand and the back acupoints. Feishu, Pishu, Zusanli, Gaohuang, Dingchuan, Taiyuan.

Mechanism of prescription: Acupoints Pishu and Zusanli can invigorate spleen and benefit Qi; Feishu, Gaohuang and Dingchuan three acupoints can relieve short of breath and soothe lungs; Taiyuan is the Yuan acupoint of the Lung Meridian, with soil nature, can benefit lungs and stop short of breath, achieving the goals of supplying soil and generate gold.

Matching acupoint: For patients with palpitation, add Shenmen, Neiguan; for patients with loose stool, add

Guanyuan, Mingmen.

操作 选定穴位，皮肤常规消毒后，电热针直刺足三里 0.7 寸，直刺内关、太渊各 0.6 寸，直刺定喘 0.6 寸，斜刺（针尖向脊柱）肺俞、脾俞、膏肓各 0.8 寸。然后接通电热针仪，每穴分别给予 50mA 的电流量，太渊、内关给予 30mA 的电流量，以患者感到温热或胀感之舒适为度，留针 40 分钟。（注：每次选 3 组穴位给予电热针，余者用毫针，可轮流交替使用。）

Operations: Selecting the relevant acupoints, perform routine skin disinfection. Using electrothermal acupuncture needles, vertically puncture into Zusanli for 0.7", vertically into Neiguan, Taiyuan and Dingchuan for 0.6", obliquely into (with the needle tip towards spine) Feishu, Pishu and Gaohuang for 0.8". Turn on the electrothermal acupuncture equipment, apply a current of 50mA to each acupoint, for Taiyuan and Neiguan 30mA, and the limit is that the patient feels comfortable, warm and swelling, leaving the needle in for 40min. (Note: Select 3 pairs of acupoints for electrothermal acupuncture treatment each time, and treat the other acupoints with filiform needles. Both types of needles can be used in turn.)

疗程 每日 1 次，30 次为 1 个疗程，疗程间可休息 3～5 天，视病情再进入第 2 个疗程的治疗。一般 2～3 个疗程即可。

Therapeutic course: Treat once a day, 30 times for a course, and start the treatment for second series after a break of 3-5 days. Generally requires 2-3 treatment series.

【生活调摄】

1. 嘱患者在治疗期注意保暖，注意防寒，防止感冒。

2. 注意不接触可能诱发喘证的物质及食物，躲避可能诱发本病的环境。

3. 要适当配合体育锻炼，增强抵抗力。

4. 在施术过程中，必须注意电热针的针刺方向、深度，避免造成气胸。

[Lifestyle Change and Health Maintenance]

1. Ask the patient to keep warm, prevent from cold or catching cold during the treatment.

2. Pay attention not to eat or contact with materials or food that may induce short of breath, and avoid living in an environment full of triggering factors.

3. Have appropriate physical exercise to reinforce immune system.

4. Pay attention to the direction and depth of the electrothermal needles during application to avoid causing pneumothorax.

支气管哮喘

支气管哮喘是常见的呼吸道过敏性疾病，属于中医"哮""喘""痰饮"等范畴。其主要病因为"痰"，内因是伏痰在肺，外因为外感风寒、饮食、劳倦或情志而诱发，其中与气候变化最为密切。

发作时，痰随气升、痰气交阻、气道不利、肺失升降，而致呼吸困难，喉中有哮鸣声。若反复发作，久延不愈，寒痰伤阳，热痰伤阴，可导致肺、脾、肾三脏皆虚，而表现出本虚标实的证候。

一、诊断及辨证要点

1. 虚证喘而气微，动则喘甚，咳痰无力，气怯声低，舌苔白滑，脉细弱。

2. 寒证喘而气粗，痰白清稀，鼻流清涕，形寒肢冷，舌苔薄滑，脉沉弱。

Asthma

Asthma is a common respiratory hypersensitivity disease. Traditional Chinese Medicine believes that this disease belongs to the range of "croup", "wheezing", "phlegm-fluid retention". The primary etiology is "phlegm". The intrinsic causative factor is the insidious phlegm in the lung, while the extrinsic causative factors are the exotic cold, food, fatigue or sentiment. Of which, the weather is the most closely related factor.

At the onset, the sputum rises with the air and causes airway obstruction, which is disadvantageous to airway fluency and thus induces air ascending/descending abnormalities. It finally leads to dyspnea and wheezing in the throat. If the disease occurs repeatedly and persists for a long time without being cured, the cold phlegm may hurt Yang Qi. The heat phlegm may then hurt Yin Qi, leading to lung, spleen and kidney deficiency, and thus displaying symptoms of asthenia in origin and asthenia in superficiality.

I. Key Points for Diagnosis and Syndrome Differentiation

1. Deficiency syndrome: Dyspnea and Qi weak, severe short of breath when moving, unable to cough out sputum, Qi frightened and weak voice, tongue fur whitish and glossy, pulse thin and weak.

2. Cold syndrome: Dyspnea and Qi strong, phlegm whitish, clear and thin, thin nasal discharge, cold body and limbs, tongue fur thin and glossy, pulse deep and weak.

3. 既往有哮喘反复发作史或过敏史。

4. 发作大多在夜间，发作时突然胸闷，呼吸困难，喉间哮鸣，痰难咯出，不能平卧。发作将止时，咳吐白色泡沫痰液。

5. 发作时胸部听诊，两肺布满哮鸣音。

6. 血液检查显示，白细胞总数增加，嗜酸性粒细胞百分率升高。

7. 胸部放射线检查正常，久病年老者可有肺气肿改变。

8. 夜间突发气喘不能平卧时，应注意与心源性哮喘相鉴别。后者常伴有心悸、发绀、咳嗽、咯血性泡沫痰，查体可有心脏扩大、瓣膜区杂音、肺部湿啰音等阳性体征。

二、治疗方法

【虚证】

治法 补肾健脾，固肺止哮。

处方 太渊（LU9）、太溪（KI3）、肺俞（BL13）、膏肓（BL43）、足三里（ST36）、肾俞（BL23）。

方义 肺经原穴太渊、肾

3. Patients who have history of repeated asthma or allergy.

4. The onset is often during the night. The patient may feel sudden chest pain and short of breath, has croup sound in the throat, hard to cough out phlegm, and cannot remain supine. At the end of the onset, the patient may cough whitish bubbles and sputum.

5. Chest auscultation at the onset of the asthma may find croup and wheezing distributing all over both lungs.

6. The blood test results show increase of white blood cell counts and elevation of eosinophil percentages.

7. Normal chest X-ray result, but senior patients with long-term asthma may have emphysema lesions.

8. The patient may have sudden nocturnal asthma attack and thus cannot lie down. Should pay attention to differentiate from cor pulmonale. The latter often accompanies with palpitation, cyanosis, cough, hemoptysis with foam phlegm. Physical examination shows Yang syndromes such as cardiomegaly, heart murmur at valve zones and rales over the lungs.

II. Therapeutic Methods

[Deficiency Syndrome]

Therapeutic method: Tonify kidney, strengthen spleen, consolidate lung and stop asthma.

Prescription: Taiyuan (LU9), Taixi (KI3), Feishu (BL13), Gaohuang (BL43), Zusanli (ST36), Shenshu (BL23).

Mechanism of prescription: Apply acupuncture

经原穴太溪，针之以充肺肾之气。肺俞、膏肓调养肺气。取肾俞以纳肾气，取足三里调和胃气，胃气和则水谷精微上归于肺，肺气充沛则可固护皮毛，防御风寒。诸穴共用，可以充实肺、脾、肾之气，元气固密，哮喘自趋平安。

配穴 汗多者加阴郄、复溜；饮食欠佳者加中脘、脾俞。

方法 电热针治疗。

操作 选定穴位，常规皮肤消毒。以电热针直刺足三里0.8寸、直刺肾俞0.7寸、斜刺肺俞0.6寸。然后接通电热针仪，电流量60mA，以患者有舒适温热或酸胀感为度。另配以毫针平刺太渊0.5寸、直刺太溪0.5寸、斜刺膏肓0.6寸。采用提插补法，均留针40分钟。

疗程 每天1次，10次为1个疗程。疗程间可休息3天。

therapy on the Yuan acupoint Taiyuan of Lung Meridian and the Yuan acupoint Taixi of Kidney Meridian to supply the Qi of the lung and kidney. Use acupoints Feishu and Gaohuang to regulate the Qi of the lung. Apply to acupoint Shenshu to inspire kidney and to acupoint Zusanli to regulate stomach. Once the stomach is soothed, and the essential substance from foodstuff is absorbed and micro-return to the Lung Meridian, the lung Qi is enriched to consolidate skin and hair and protect from cold and wind. Applying treatment on all acupoints may invigorate the Qi of the lung, spleen and kidney, consolidate Qi, and therefore relieve asthma.

Matching points: For people with heavy sweat, add Yinxi and Fuliu; for people with poor appetite, add Zhongwan, Pishu.

Method: Electrothermal acupuncture treatment.

Operations: Select relevant acupoints, perform routine skin disinfection. Using electrotheraml acupuncture needles, vertically puncture into Zusanli for 0.8", vertically puncture into Shenshu for 0.7", and obliquely into Feishu for 0.6". Turn on the electrothermal acupuncture equipment, apply a current of 60mA to each acupoint. The limit is that the patient feels comfortable, warm or sore and swelling. Additionally, using filiform acupuncture needles, horizontally puncture into Taiyuan for 0.5", vertically puncture into Taixi for 0.5", and obliquely into Gaohuang for 0.6". Apply the method of lifting-thrusting tonifying needling. Leave the needles in for 40 minutes.

Therapeutic course: Once a day, 10 times for a series. Rest for 3 days between series.

【寒证】

治法 温阳散寒平喘。

处方 大椎（DU14）、风门（BL12）、身柱（DU12）、天突（RN22）。

方义 大椎、身柱为督脉穴，督脉总督一身阳气。大椎为手足三阳与督脉之会，故针刺大椎及身柱有振奋阳气的作用；风门又称热府，系足太阳膀胱经与督脉之会，因风邪多从此而入故名，善祛风散寒；天突为降气平喘之要穴。诸穴合用，可取温阳散寒平喘之功。

配穴 痰多者加丰隆；食少者加足三里。

方法 电热针治疗。

操作 选定穴位，常规皮肤消毒，以电热针直刺大椎 0.7 寸、直刺身柱 0.7 寸、斜刺风门 0.7 寸、直刺丰隆 0.8 寸。然后接通电热针仪，给予电流量 60mA。另配以毫针靠胸骨柄内侧刺入天突 0.7 寸（不留

[Cold Syndrome]

Therapeutic method: Warm Yang, disperse cold and relieve asthma.

Prescription: Dazhui (DU14), Fengmen (BL12), Shenzhu (DU12), Tiantu (RN22).

Mechanism of prescription: Dazhui and Shenzhu are acupoints of Du Collateral. The Du Collateral governs the systemic Yang Qi. Dazhui is the convergent acupoint of the Arm and Leg Triple Yang Meridian and the Du Collateral. Therefore, applying acupuncture therapy to Dazhui and Shenzhu may invigorate Yang Qi. Fengmen is also called Refu, which is the convergent acupoint of the Zu Tai Yang Bladder Meridian and the Du Collateral. The acupoint is named due to its accessibility of wind evil, and therefore the treatment for this acupoint may expel wind and remove cold. Tiantu is a key acupoint to depress Qi and relieve asthma; if applying treatment to all acupoints together, can achieve the effects of warm Yang, disperse cold and relieve asthma.

Matching points: For people with productive phlegm, add Fenglong; for people with poor appetite, add Zusanli.

Method: Electrothermal acupuncture treatment.

Operations: Selecting the relevant acupoints, perform routine skin disinfection. Using electrothermal acupuncture needles, vertically puncture into Dazhui, Shenzhu for 0.7", respectively; obliquely into Fengmen for 0.7", and vertically puncture into Fenglong for 0.8". Then turn on the electrothermal acupuncture equipment, apply a current of 60mA to each acupoint. Additionally,

针），其余穴位留针 40 分钟。

疗程 每天 1 次，10 天为 1 个疗程，疗程间可休息 3 天。

三、注意事项

1. 针刺背部腧穴，尤其是电热针较毫针粗，更要掌握好针刺方向，手法要轻、细，不宜直刺和提插、捻转，以免造成气胸。

2. 在哮喘发作期，应选择灸法，要求患者节制房事；缓解期用电热针治疗，严防感冒。

3. 应不吃或少吃容易发生过敏的食物，如虾、鱼、螃蟹、黄花菜等；禁烟、酒；还要少吃有刺激性的食物，如辣椒、八角、茴香、胡椒；咸味过重之食品，亦应少吃。

4. 哮喘发作严重者，应注意配合输氧及药物治疗，以提高疗效。对于针灸治疗效果较差的个别患者，要改用其他疗

using filiform acupuncture needles, near the medial side of the sternum, puncture into Tiantu for 0.7" (without leaving the needle in); but retain other needles in other acupoints for 40 minutes.

Therapeutic course: Once a day, 10 times for a course. Rest for 3 days between courses.

III. Precautions

1. When applying acupuncture therapy to the acupoints on the back, because of the electrothermal acupuncture needle is thicker than the filiform needle, please pay attention to ensure the direction of acupuncture therapy with light and smooth maneuver, and avoid direct puncture, lifting-and-thrusting or rotating to prevent from pneumothorax.

2. During the asthma attack, moxibustion is the first choice of treatment. The patient is also required to abstain from sexual activities. During the relief period, electrothermal acupuncture therapy will be applied. In the meantime, the patient is required to avoid catching cold.

3. Abstain from or eat less allergic food, including shrimps, fish, crab or daylily, etc. Do not smoke or drink, eat less stimulant spices such as chilly, star anise, fennel or pepper. Over salty food should also be avoided.

4. For people who have severe asthma attack, oxygenation accompanying with medicinal product therapy is required to enhance therapeutic efficacies. For individuals who response to acupuncture therapy poorly, other

法治之。

四、典型病例

王某，女，54岁，家庭妇女，北京人。

主诉：哮喘反复发作3年余，近1个月加重。病史：患者3年前因吃海鱼发病，之后每遇冷即会发作，尤其在冬季易发，哮喘发作多与寒冷及鱼虾食物有关，发作时喉中哮鸣有声，呼吸困难，甚至不能平卧。经治不愈，近期反复发作。

刻下症：因受风寒，平素自汗、怕风，经常感冒，每因天冷气候变化或寒冷刺激而诱发，发作前频繁喷嚏，鼻流清涕，继而咳喘发作。既往有海鱼、虾过敏史，进餐后就会发病。

查体：两肺呼吸音粗，有喘鸣音，双肺底可闻及散在性中、小水泡音。

辅助检查：胸片示"双肺纹理增粗"。白细胞计数：

therapeutic approaches should be considered.

IV. Typical Case

Wang, female, 54 years old, housewife, residence: Beijing.

Chief complaint: Repeated asthma attack for more than 3 years, and the syndrome aggravated in the past month. Medical history: The patient started to have the first asthma attack due to fish 3 years ago; since then, she suffered from asthma when cold weather or cold food. The attack is more frequent during winter, that is, the asthma is closely related to cold weather or food including fish or shrimp. During the attack, wheezing sound was found accompanying with short of breath. The patient couldn't even lie down. She received treatments for a while but the illness hasn't been cured. Moreover, she suffered from repeated occurrence frequently lately.

Current symptoms: The patient suffered from wind cold, so sweated a lot and was afraid of wind, and caught a cold frequently. Her asthma was induced almost every day due to cold weather or cold stimulants. She sneezed a lot with thin nasal mucus prior to asthma attack, and then started the attack. The patient had allergic history against sea fish and shrimps; that is, her asthma attack occurs if she consumed such food.

Physical examination: Coarse breathing sounds over bilateral lungs accompanying with wheezing. In addition, medium/insignificant disseminated crackles also heard at the bottom of bilateral lungs.

Auxiliary examination: The chest X-ray showed "bilateral lung texture thickening". White blood cell

$12×10^9$/L。

【诊断依据】

1. 中年女性，起病后慢性过程已3年之久，反复发作。

2. 咳喘与气候寒冷及食物（海鱼、虾）有密切关系。

3. 既往无特殊病史。

4. 体检可闻及哮鸣音，双肺底可闻及大、小水泡音。

5. 胸片示"双肺纹理增粗"。白细胞计数：$12×10^9$/L。

【证治分析】

病因 肺气虚亏。

病机 寒痰内伏，屡感风寒，失去表散，则寒邪入肺脏，使上焦津液不布，凝聚而感寒痰，内伏肺与膈上，因外感而触发。

证候分析 肺主气，外合皮毛，肺气虚弱，卫外不固，故汗出而恶风，且易感冒，故每遇气候变化而诱发。肺气虚弱不能化津，痰饮蕴肺，故气短声怯，咳痰清稀色白，鼻寒喷嚏乃风寒外束之象。舌脉为肺虚之象。

count: $12×10^9$/L.

[Diagnostic Basis]

1. A middle-aged female has chronic disease progression for 3 years since the first attack, and with repeated occurrence.

2. The cough and asthma is closely related to cold weather as well as cold food (e.g. sea fish and shrimps).

3. No previous special medical history documented.

4. Wheezing is found during physical examination, and significant/insignificant crackles are found at the bottom of bilateral lungs.

5. Chest X-ray showed "bilateral lung texture thickening". White blood cell count: $12×10^9$/L.

[Syndrome-treatment Analysis]

Etiology: Lung Qi deficiency.

Pathogenesis: Insidious cold phlegm, repeatedly feel wind cold, lose cold removing ability, so cold evils enters the lung, and Upper Jiao accumulation, causes cold phlegm inside the lung and on the diaphragm. The symptom can be triggered by external factors.

Syndrome analysis: Lung governs Qi, associating the skin and hair. If Lung Qi becomes deficient, the defense against foreign matter may be weaken, and thus result in sweating, generate evil wind, prone to cold, and the symptom is triggered easily when the weather is changed. Deficient lung Qi fails to transform into liquid, and results in phlegm accumulation in the lungs. The patient may display short of breath and weak voice, produce thin/clear/whitish phlegm, and sneeze when encountering cold. All of which are the signs of dyspnea due to wind-cold evil. The tongue showed signs of lung deficiency.

病位 肺。

Lesion location: Lung.

病性 虚性。

Disease nature: Deficiency.

西医诊断 支气管哮喘、慢性支气管炎。

The diagnosis of Western Medicine: Bronchial asthma and chronic bronchitis.

中医诊断 哮病、咳嗽。

The diagnosis of Traditional Chinese Medicine: Asthma and cough.

治法 温肺散寒，补益肺气，化痰止哮。

Therapeutic method: Warm lung, disperse cold, tonify lung Qi, dilute phlegm and stop asthma.

方法 电热针治疗、艾灸治疗。

Method: Electrothermal acupuncture treatment and moxibustion.

（1）电热针治疗

(1) Electrothermal acupuncture therapy

处方 定喘（EX-B1）、膏肓（BL43）、肺俞（BL13）、太渊（LU9）、风门（BL12）。

Prescription: Dingchuan (EX-B1), Gaohuang (BL43), Feishu (BL13), Taiyuan (LU9), Fengmen (BL12).

方义 定喘是止哮喘之经验穴；膏肓主治虚劳咳嗽哮喘，多用于慢性哮喘；太渊是手太阴经之土穴，配肺俞补土生金，以求治本；风门可疏风宣肺。

Mechanism of prescription: Dingchuan is the experience acupoint for asthma treatment; the major function of Gaohuang is to treat deficiency, fatigue, cough and asthma, which is mostly used for the treatment for chronic asthma. Taiyuan is the soil acupoint of the TaiYin Meridian of Hand, a matching point with Feishu, which supplement soil in order to generate gold for a permanent cure; Fengmen can be used to expel wind and open the inhibited lung energy.

配穴 食少乏力加足三里、中脘；痰多加丰隆；动则汗出加阴郄；咳嗽胁痛加支沟、中脘；胸脘痞满加膻中、天突。

Matching points: For people with poor appetite, add Zusanli and Zhongwan. For people with productive phlegm, add Fenglong. For people with easy sweating during the movement, add Yinxi, for people with cough accompanying flank pain, add Zhigou and Zhongwan. For people with chest fullness, add Danzhong and Tiantu.

操作 选定穴位，皮肤常

Operations: Selecting the relevant acupoints, per-

form routine skin disinfection. Using electrothermal acupuncture needles, vertically puncture into Dingchuan for 0.6", obliquely puncture (with the needle tip towards spine) into Feishu, Gaohuang and Fengmen for 0.6", respectively. Turn on the electrothermal acupuncture equipment, apply a current of 40mA to each acupoint. The limit is that the patient feels warm or swelling comfortable. Leave the needles in for 40 minutes. As for matching points, using electrothermal acupuncture needles, vertically puncture into Zusanli, Zhongwan, Zhigou, Fenglong and applying a current of 50mA to each acupoint; and horizontally puncture into Danzhong and Tiantu and applying a current of 40mA to each acupoint, the limit is that the patient feels warm or swelling comfortable. Leave the needles in for 40 minutes. (Note: select 3 pairs of acupoints each time, and use alternately.)

Therapeutic course: Once a day, 20 times for a course.

Therapeutic process: The patient was cured after a therapeutic course. The patient then received another therapeutic course to consolidate the efficacy. 1-year follow-up, no recurrence.

(2) Moxibustion

Prescription: Feishu (BL13), Pishu (BL20), Shenshu (BL23), Dazhui (DU14).

Matching points: For people with excessive asthma, add Shuifen and Fenglong; for people with deficient asthma, add Guanyuan; for people with Heat asthma, add Lieque and Fenglong; for people with cold asthma, add Zhongwan, Zusanli and Gaohuang.

操作 每日选2个穴，用艾条悬灸，每穴灸15分钟，以巩固疗效，预防再发。缓解期用此法可有预防作用。

疗程 每天1次，20次为1个疗程。

【生活调摄】

1. 治疗过程中，针刺背部腧穴时要掌握好进针的方向和深度，手法要轻，不宜进深，避免造成气胸。

2. 在缓解期，嘱患者注意预防感冒。

3. 避免吃容易发生过敏的食物，如油菜、黄花菜、鱼、虾、螃蟹等；烟、酒也应禁用；还应少吃刺激性食物，如辣椒、茴香、胡椒等。对甘肥滋腻之品、咸味过重之物应少吃或不吃为好。

4. 哮喘发作期，严重者应配合输氧及药物治疗。

支气管扩张症

支气管扩张症（简称支扩）是指支气管解剖结构上出现的不可复原性的扩张和变形，或有化脓性病变。常因急性感染病（流行性感冒）并发支气管肺炎处理不当，以及肺

Operations: Select 2 acupoints every day and use moxibustion over the skin, 15 minutes for each acupoint to consolidate therapeutic efficacies and prevent from recurrence. Use this approach during relieving period can prevent the disease from reoccurrence.

Therapeutic course: Once a day, 20 times for a course.

[Lifestyle Change and Health Maintenance]

1. When applying acupuncture therapy to the acupoints on the back, ensure the direction and depth of acupuncture therapy with light and smooth maneuver, and avoid too deep of a puncture to prevent pneumothorax.

2. During the relieving period, ask the patient to prevent from catching cold.

3. Abstain from allergic food, including rape, daylily, fish, shrimps, fish, crab, etc. Do not smoke or drink, eat less stimulant spices such as chilly, fennel or pepper. Eat less or abstain from sweet, greasy or over salty food.

4. During severe asthma attack, oxygenation accompanying with medicinal product therapy is required.

Bronchiectasis

Bronchiectasis refers to irreversible anatomical and structural dilation and deformity of bronchus or suppurative lesions. The common causes include acute infections (e.g. flu) combined with bronchitis but with poor management, tuberculosis, empyema, chronic bronchitis, bronchial asthma, etc. Such disease can be triggered at

结核脓肿、慢性支气管炎、支气管哮喘等引起。一年四季均可发病,以成年人为多见。

一、诊断及辨证要点

1. 邪热壅肺者,咳嗽或哮喘,痰黄黏稠或咳吐脓血,气味腥臭,或恶寒发热,舌质红,苔黄腻,脉滑数。

2. 肺寒不宣者,咳嗽或喘息胸闷,咳吐白痰,质稀或黏稠,形寒肢冷。咳嗽反复发作,经久不愈,尤其是晨起或体位改变时,咳出大量白色痰,舌苔白润,脉紧。

3. 发病特点是反复发作性咳嗽、咯痰、咯血、支气管壁组织破坏及管腔扩张。

4. 肺下叶听诊有湿啰音。

5. 胸片可见肺纹理粗糙,或有轨道状、卷发圈状阴影,支气管造影显示气管扩张病变。

four seasons, and mostly seen in adults.

I. Key Points for Diagnosis and Syndrome Differentiation

1. For people with syndrome of pathogenic heat congesting lung, they often cough or have asthma with yellowish sticky phlegm or hemoptysis with pus. The phlegm is smelly and with fish stench. For people with evil cold and thus have fever, their tongue appears to be reddish with yellowish and thick tongue fur as well as superficial and rapid pulse.

2. People with lung Qi dispersion failure may cough, short of breath and have chest pain, generate whitish, thin or sticky phlegm with cold body and limbs. Repeated cough not cured even being treated for a long time. Cough large amount whitish phlegm especially wake up in the morning or change body positions, tongue fur whitish and wet, and rapid pulse.

3. The feature is repeated cough, productive cough, hemoptysis, damaged bronchial walls and lumen dilatation.

4. Wet rales heard at the lower lobes of the lungs through auscultation.

5. Chest X-ray shows thick and rough lung texture, or with track-shape or hair-circle-shape shadow. The bronchography shows bronchial dilatation lesions.

II. Therapeutic Methods

[Syndrome of Pathogenic Heat Congesting Lung]

Therapeutic method: Clear heat and purge lung, lower adverse Qi and stop cough.

Prescription: Tiantu (RN22), Lieque (LU7), Feishu (BL13), Chize (LU5), Quchi (LI11).

Mechanism of prescription: Tiantu is the convergent acupoint of the Ren Collateral, which can benefit the throat and regulate lung Qi. Lieque is one of the convergent acupoints of the eight meridians, which has efficacies of clearing lung heat and dredging the throat and diaphragm. Feishu can regulate lung Qi. Chize is the He acupoint of the lung meridian, which can disperse the heat of lung gold. Quchi is the He acupoint of the Yang-Ming Large Intestine Meridian of Hand, which can cause diarrhea and achieve the goal of lung heat clearance. If applied all acupoints all together, the effects of clearing heat and purging lungs, depressing adverse Qi and stopping cough.

Matching point: For people with significant hemoptysis, add Yuji and Ganshu; for people with Yin deficiency such as heat flush and cold sweat, add Taixi and Sanyinjiao; for people with productive phlegm, add Zusanli and Fenglong.

Method: Electrothermal acupuncture treatment.

Operations: Selecting acupoints, perform routine skin disinfection. Using electrothermal acupuncture needles, obliquely puncture into Ganshu for 0.6", vertically puncture into Zusanli for 0.8", vertically into Fenglong

针仪,给予电流量60mA。另配以毫针刺入天突0.6寸(靠胸骨柄内侧),平刺列缺0.5寸,直刺曲池0.6寸,直刺尺泽0.7寸,均留针40分钟。

疗程 每天1次,20次为1个疗程。

【肺寒不宣证】

治法 温肺益气,化痰降浊。

处方 天突(RN22)、肺俞(BL13)、中脘(RN12)、膻中(RN17)、膏肓(BL43)。

方义 肺俞为肺气所输注的部位,能输泻肺气。天突顺气化痰、降逆平喘。膻中为气之会穴,中脘为胃之募穴,二穴相配能顺气和胃,化痰降浊。膏肓穴有温养肺气之功。五穴共奏温肺益气、化痰降浊之功。

配穴 纳少、乏力者加足三里;动则汗出、四肢欠温者加阴郄、后溪。

方法 电热针治疗。

for 0.7", and turn on the electrothermal acupuncture equipment, apply a current of 60mA. Additionally, using the filiform needles, puncture into Tiantu for 0.6" (close to the medial side of the sternum), horizontally into Lieque for 0.5", vertically into Quchi for 0.6", vertically into Chize for 0.7", leaving the needles in for 40 minutes.

Therapeutic course: Once a day, 10 times for a course.

[Syndrome of Non-dispersion Cold Lung Qi]

Therapeutic method: Warm lung and tonify Qi, dissolve phlegm and depress turbidity.

Prescription: Tiantu (RN22), Feishu (BL13), Zhongwan (RN12), Danzhong (RN17), Gaohuang (BL43).

Mechanism of prescription: Feishu is the entrance of lung Qi, which can release lung Qi. Tiantu can smooth the Qi, dissolve phlegm, depress adverse Qi and relieve dyspnea. Danzhong is the convergent acupoint of the Qi, Zhongwan is the Mu acupoint of the stomach, treatment for both of the acupoints can smooth the Qi, soothe stomach, dissolve phlegm and depress turbidity. Gaohuang has the effects of warming and nourishing the lung Qi. Treatment for all five acupoints can warm the lung, supply the Qi, dissolve the phlegm, and depress the turbidity.

Matching points: For people with poor intake or weak, add Zusanli; for people with excessive sweat during movement but cold in four limbs, add Yinxi and Houxi.

Method: Electrothermal acupuncture treatment.

Operations: Selecting acupoints, perform routine skin disinfection. Using electrothermal acupuncture needles, obliquely puncture into Feishu and Gaohuang for 0.7", vertically puncture into Zusanli for 0.8", and turn on the electrothermal acupuncture equipment, apply a current of 60mA. Additionally, using the filiform needles, vertically puncture into Zhongwan for 0.8", horizontally into Danzhong for 0.7", puncture into Tiantu for 0.7" (close to the medial side of the sternum), vertically into Houxi and Yinxi for 0.5", leaving the needles in for 40 minutes.

Therapeutic course: Once a day, 10 times for a course with a break of 3 days between courses.

III. Precautions

1. Bronchiectasis is often the results of repeated lung diseases, is a chronic condition hard to be cured. The Chinese herbal treatment in combination with Western medicinal product treatment is required if the patient displayed severe hemoptysis or infectious symptoms.

2. Avoid excessive eating or consume cold food or bitter and cold medicinal products, which may damage the lung Yang and result in lung cold and lung Qi dispersion failure.

3. Pay attention to eat less or avoid spicy, hot, greasy, sweet, alcohol or food with heavy taste in order to prevent from generating heat and product phlegm, and thus damage the lung collateral.

IV. Typical Case

Hu, female, 36 years old, employee, residence: Beijing.

Chief complaint: Cough and productive cough for a year with repeated occurrence, and the syndrome aggravated lately with hemoptysis. Medical history: After suffering from lobular pneumonia 1 year ago, the patient had sequelae of cough with whitish phlegm, sometimes even saw hemoptysis. After being examined by several medical institutes, the patient was diagnosed of "bronchiectasis". Symptomatic treatment was thereby recommended.

Current symptoms: Cough with large amount of whitish phlegm, sometimes hemoptysis or phlegm with fresh blood, accompanying with mild dyspnea, chest tightness, cold body and limbs, repeated cough, cough large amount of thin or sticky whitish phlegm especially when wake up in the morning or change body positions. The patient used to be physically healthy without any medical histories to be noted.

Physical examination: Coarse breathing sounds over bilateral lungs with wet rales over the right lower lob. 2nd degree systolic murmur over mitral valve and aortic valve the 2nd auscultation area.

Auxiliary examination: The chest X-ray showed "lung texture thickening and irregular with track-shape shadows". White blood cell count: $13\times10^9/L$.

[Diagnostic Basis]

1. A middle-aged woman with large amount whitish phlegm cough for 1 year, sometimes with hemoptysis.

2. Mostly caused by cold or consumption of cold food, aggravating by coughing, sometimes even cause

咳喘。

3. 既往有大叶性肺炎病史，从而遗留咳嗽。

4. 查体：两肺呼吸音粗，右肺下叶有湿性啰音。

5. 辅助检查：胸片示"肺纹理粗乱，有轨道状阴影"。白细胞计数：13×10⁹/L。

【证治分析】

病因　痰饮内伏。

病机　屡感风寒，先于表散，则寒邪入肺脏，长期饮食生冷，伤及肺气，使上焦津液不布，凝聚而成寒痰，内伏肺上，因外感而触发。

证候分析　肺主气，外合皮毛，肺气虚弱，卫外不固，故寒邪易入肺脏，长期食生饮冷，伤及脾胃，脾为生痰之源，肺为储痰之器，脾虚肺弱，故津液不布，而生成寒痰，呈大量白痰，舌脉为肺寒不宣之象。

病位　肺。

病性　寒性。

西医诊断　支气管扩张症、

cough-asthma.

3. Previous medical history of lobular pneumonia and thus leads to consequences of cough.

4. Physical examination: Coarse breathing sounds over bilateral lungs with wet rales over the right lower lob.

5. Auxiliary examination: The chest X-ray showed "lung texture thickening and irregular with track-shape shadows". White blood cell count: $13×10^9$/L.

[Syndrome-treatment Analysis]

Etiology: Insidious phlegm-fluid retention.

Pathogenesis: Suffering from wind cold repeatedly before the cold could be expelled to the body surface, so the evil cold enters into the lung. Long-term consuming raw or cold food will also damage the lung Qi, makes the Upper Jiao fluid accumulation and thus aggregate into cold phlegm, retain in the lung. Such evil cold can be triggered by foreign factors.

Syndrome analysis: The lung governs Qi, associating the skin and hair, so deficient and weak lung Qi may result in poor defense, and consequently allows cold evil entering the lung. In addition, consuming raw and cold food for a long time may damage the spleen and stomach. The spleen is the source of phlegm, and the lung is the reservoir, deficient spleen and weak lung leads to body fluid retention and therefore becoming cold phlegm. The patient may have large amount of whitish phlegm and the tongue shows lung deficiency with fluid accumulation.

Lesion location: Lung.

Disease nature: Cold.

The diagnosis of Western Medicine: Bronchiecta-

慢性支气管炎。

中医诊断 哮喘、咳嗽。

治法 温肺益气，化痰降浊。

方法 电热针治疗。

处方 天突（RN22）、肺俞（BL13）、中脘（RN12）、膻中（RN17）、膏肓（BL43）。

方义 肺俞是肺气所输注的部位，能输泻肺气；天突顺气化痰，降逆平喘；膻中是气之会穴，中脘是胃之募穴，二穴相配，顺气和胃，化痰降浊；膏肓穴有温养肺气之功效。诸穴共用，可奏温肺益气，化痰降浊之功。

配穴 纳少、乏力者加足三里；动则汗出、四肢欠温者加阴郄、后溪。

操作 选定穴位，皮肤常规消毒。电热针直刺中脘、足三里各0.7寸，平刺天突、膻中各0.7寸，斜刺（针尖向脊柱）肺俞、膏肓各0.8寸，直

sis or chronic bronchitis.

The diagnosis of Traditional Chinese Medicine: Asthma or cough.

Therapeutic method: Warm the lung, supply the Qi, dissolve the phlegm and depress the turbidity.

Method: Electrothermal acupuncture treatment.

Prescription: Tiantu (RN22), Feishu (BL13), Zhongwan (RN12), Danzhong (RRN17), Gaohuang (BL43).

Mechanism of prescription: Feishu is the entrance of lung Qi, so it is the location for lung Qi to enter and exit. Tiantu can smooth the Qi and dissolve the phlegm depress the adverse Qi and relieve the asthma. Danzhong is the convergent acupoint of the Qi, Zhongwan is the Mu acupoint of the stomach, treatment for both of the acupoints can smooth the Qi, soothe the stomach, dissolve the phlegm and depress the turbidity. Gaohuang has the effect of warming and nourishing the lung Qi. If the treatment applied to all acupoints all together may achieve the efficacies of warming the lung, invigorating the Qi, dissolving the phlegm and depressing the turbidity.

Matching points: For people with less intake and weak, add Zusanli; for people with excessive sweat during movement but four limbs cold, add Yinxi and Houxi.

Operations: Selecting the relevant acupoints, perform routine skin disinfection. Using electrothermal acupuncture needles, vertically puncture into Zhongwan and Zusanli for 0.7" respectively, horizontally puncture into Tiantu and Danzhong for 0.7", obliquely puncture (with

刺阴郄、后溪各 0.7 寸，接通电热针仪器，每个穴位分别给予 50mA 的电流量，以温热或胀之舒适为度，留针 40 分钟。（注：每日 1 次，每次选 3 组穴，分组交替应用。）

疗程 20 次为 1 个疗程，疗程期间可休息 5 天。

治疗过程 症状缓解较快，但因病程较久，还要多巩固治疗 1 个疗程，该患者共治疗 50 次后结束治疗。随访至今已 7 年未见复发。

原发性高血压

高血压是以体循环动脉血压升高为主要表现的临床综合征，是最常见的心血管疾病。成人正常血压为 ≥140/90mmHg，超过上述指数者则为高血压。本病与长期精神紧张、高盐饮食、大量吸烟有关，且有遗传倾向。

本病多归于中医"眩晕""头痛"等范畴。总因七情所伤，烦躁易怒，或饮食不节，过食辛辣厚味，导致肝阳上亢，痰湿内阻，日久阳盛于上，阴亏于下，以致阴阳失调而发。

the needle tip towards spine) into Feishu and Gaohuang for 0.8", vertically puncture into Yinxi and Houxi for 0.7". Turn on the electrothermal acupuncture equipment, apply a current of 50mA to each acupoint. The limit is that the patient feels warm or swell and comfortable. Leave the needles for 40 minutes. (Note: Select 3 pairs of acupoints each time, and use once a day alternately.)

Therapeutic course: 20 times for a course, a break of 5 days between courses.

Therapeutic process: The symptoms can be relieved quickly, but 1 additional consolidation therapy is required due to its long disease course. The patients received 50 times of acupuncture treatments in total during the course. 7-year follow-up to date, no recurrence.

High Blood Pressure

High blood pressure is a comprehensive clinical symptom caused primarily by the increase of aterial blood pressure of the systemic circulation, which is the most common cardiovascular disease. The normal blood pressure in adults is ≥140/90mmHg, anyone above such value is defined as hypertensive. This disease is closely related to long-term stress, high-salt diet and large amount of smoking, and it is also inheritive.

This disease is mostly categorized in the scope of "vertigo" or "headache" in Traditional Chinese Medicine. Caused by seven emotions, become agitated and irritative, or excessive eating, lots of spicy and heavy taste, leading to liver Yang hyperactivity, damp phlegm and interior obstruction. When it becomes chronic condition, the Yang Qi is excessive, and the Yin Qi is deficient, and

一、诊断及辨证要点

1. 肝阳上亢者，症见头目胀痛，心烦易怒，面红目赤，口苦胁痛，睡眠不宁，大便干结，舌红少苔或苔薄黄，脉弦。

2. 痰湿阻滞者，症见头重头痛，头晕发昏，心烦欲吐，少食多眠，腹泻痞满胖质淡，苔白腻或厚腻，脉弦滑。

3. 气血不足者，症见眩晕，动则加剧，劳累即发，面色白，唇甲不华，心悸少寐，神疲懒言，饮食减少，舌质淡，苔薄白，脉细弱。

4. 肝肾阴虚者，症见头晕眼花，目涩而干，耳鸣耳聋，腰酸腿软，足跟痛，夜尿频，舌红无苔，脉沉细尺弱。

5. 常见症状有头晕、头痛、头胀、眩晕、耳鸣、心悸、面红、烦躁、失眠等。

6. 血压在 140/90mmHg 以上者。

therefore results in Yin-Yang imbalance.

I. Key Points for Diagnosis and Syndrome Differentiation

1. For people with Liver Yang hyperactivity, their symptoms include headache, eye swelling and pain, agitated and upset, red face, red eyes, bitter taste, flank pain, sleepless, constipation, red tongue with less fur or thin yellowish fur, string pulse.

2. For people with wet phlegm obstruction, their common symptoms include heavy head, headache, dizziness, syncope, agitated and upset, poor appetite, sleepiness all the time, diarrhea and abdoman distention, fat tongue but light texture, whitish, thick and sticky tongue fur, slippery pulse.

3. For patients with Qi and blood deficiency, their common symptoms include vertigo, which is aggravated during movements, triggered by tiresome, pale complexion, lack of blood on the lips or nails, palpitation, sleepless, fatigue and talk less, decrease appetite, light tongue texture, whitish tongue fur and think and weak pulse.

4. For patients with liver and kidney Yin deficiency, their common symptoms include dizziness, dry eyes, tinnitus, deaf, low back pain and weak lower extremities, heel pain, nocturia, red tongue without fur, deep and slow and weak pulse.

5. Common symptoms include dizziness, headache, head swelling, vertigo, tinnitus, palpitation, red face, agitation and insomnia, etc.

6. Patients with blood pressure above 140/90mmHg.

二、治疗方法

【肝阳上亢证】

治法 平肝潜阳，滋阴降火。

处方 风池（GB20）、行间（LR2）、侠溪（GB43）。

方义 风池为足少阳胆经之穴，能疏浮阳而治眩晕；行间为足厥阴肝经之荥穴，与足少阴胆经之侠溪穴合用，为表里配穴法，有平肝潜阳、清降肝火之功。三穴共用，可收潜阴治阳、平降肝火之功效。

配穴 目赤者加关冲；面较灼热者加内庭；心悸者加内关、足三里；不寐者加神门。

方法 毫针治疗。

操作 选定穴位，常规皮肤消毒。针刺风池穴时，进针向后斜刺0.5寸，直刺行间0.6寸，直刺侠溪0.6寸并向后斜刺，直刺神门0.5寸，直刺内关0.5寸，直刺足三里0.8寸，留针30分钟。

疗程 20次为1个疗程，

II. Therapeutic Method

[Syndrome of Liver Yang Hyperactivity]

Therapeutic method: Calm the liver, suppress the Yang, nourish the Yin and suppress the fire.

Prescription: Fengchi (GB20), Xingjian (LR2), Xiaxi (GB43).

Mechanism of prescriptions: Fengchi is the acupoint of the Shao-Yang Gallbladder Meridian of Foot, which can dredge Yang hyperactivity and thus treat dizziness; Xingjian is the Xing point of the Jue-Yin Liver Meridian of Foot, if treated together with the Xiaxi acupoint, the acupoint of the Shao-Yin Gallbladder Meridian of Foot, is the superficies-interior points combination. The purpose is to calm the liver, suppress the Yang, and suppress the liver fire. If applied in all three acupoints, it can achieve the effeciency of suppressing Yin, treating Yang, and calming liver fire.

Matching points: For people with red eyes, add Guanchong. For people with hot face, add Neiting; for people with palpitations, add Neiguan and Zusanli. For people with sleeplessness, add Shenmen.

Method: Filiform therapy.

Operations: Selecting acupoints, perform routine skin disinfection. Using filiform needles, obliquely puncture downward into Fengchi for 0.5", Xingjian for 0.6", Xiaxi for 0.6", vertically puncture into Shenmen for 0.5", Neiguan for 0.5", zusanli for 0.8", leaving the needles in for 30 minutes.

Therapeutic course: 20 times for a course. A break

疗程期间可休息 5 天。

【痰湿阻滞证】

治法 健脾和胃，除湿化痰。

处方 中脘（RN12）、内关（PC6）、丰隆（ST40）、解溪（ST41）。

方义 本方以和中化浊为主，取中脘、丰隆以运中而化痰浊，中运健则湿浊消，湿除则痰自化。配内关清心火、和胃气，合解溪以益胃气。四穴合用，可调和脾胃，除湿化痰。

配穴 头重如裹者加头维。

方法 毫针治疗。

操作 选定穴位，常规皮肤消毒。提插泻法，直刺中脘0.5 寸，直刺内关 0.5 寸，直刺丰隆 0.8 寸，针尖向足跟部直刺解溪 0.5 寸，均留针 30 分钟。

疗程 每天 1 次，10 次为 1 个疗程，疗程间可以休息 3 天。

of 5 days between courses.

[Syndrome of Wet Phlegm Obstruction]

Therapeutic method: Invigorate spleen, soothe the stomach, remove dampness and dissolve phlegm.

Prescription: Zhongwan (RN12), Neiguan (PC6), Fenglong (ST40), Jiexi (ST41).

Mechanism of prescription: The method is based on neutralization and removing turbidity, so select Zhongwan and Fenglong to transport the central Qi and therefore dissolve phlegm and turbidity. Good central Qi circulation may eliminate dampness and turbidity, and thereby automatically dissolve the phlegm due to the removal of dampness. Matching with Neiguan to clear the heart fire, soothe stomach Qi; combining with Jiexi to invigorate stomach Qi. If applied in four acupoints together, can regulate and soothe spleen and stomach, remove dampness and dissolve phlegm.

Matching points: For people with heavy head like being wrapped, add Touwei.

Method: Filiform therapy.

Operations: Selecting the relevant acupoints, perform routine skin disinfection. Using lifting-thrusting and attenuating method, vertically puncture into Zhongwan, Neiguan for 0.5", vertically puncture into Fenglong for 0.8", and then the tip of the needle pointing toward the heel and vertically puncture into Jiexi for 0.5", leaving the needles in for 30 minutes.

Therapeutic course: 10 times for a course. A break of 3 days between courses.

[Syndrome of Qi and Blood Deficiency]

Therapeutic method: Invigorate the spleen and tonify the stomach, supply the Qi and improve blood circulation.

Prescription: Pishu (BL20), Shenshu (BL23), Guanyuan (RN4), Zusanli (ST36), Baihui (DU20).

Mechanism of prescription: Starting from supplementing the spleen and stomach, select Pishu and Shenshu to tonify yuan Qi, Zusanli to transport fluid, generate energy and transform into blood; Baihui and Guanyuan belong to Ren and Du Collaterals, which can invigorate Qi to improve blood circulation, supply Qi and blood, and recover the blood pressure.

Matching points: For people with palpitations, add Neiguang; for people with sleepless, add Shenmen; for people with tinnitus, add Tingguan.

Method: Electrothermal acupuncture treatment.

Operations: Selecting the relevant acupoints, perform routine skin disinfection. Using electrothermal acupuncture needles, obliquely puncture into Pishu for 0.7", vertically puncture into Shenshu for 0.6", vertically puncture into Zusanli for 0.8". Turn on the electrothermal acupuncture equipment, apply a current of 60mA. Additionally, using the filiform needles, horizontally puncture into Baihui for 0.5", vertically puncture into Guanyuan for 0.6", vertically puncture into Neiguan for 0.5", puncture (toward the ear lobe) into Tonggong for 0.5", vertically puncture into Shenmen for 0.5", leaving the needles in for 40 minutes.

Therapeutic course: 20 times for a course. A break

疗程期间可休息 5 天。

【肝肾阴虚证】

治法 补肝益肾，滋阴降火。

处方 肝俞（BL18）、肾俞（BL23）、三阴交（SP6）、太溪（KI3）、神门（HT7）。

方义 肝俞、肾俞滋补肝肾、调理冲任；三阴交是贯通肝、脾、肾三经的要穴，可以补益三阴虚损、清泻虚火；太溪滋肾阴；神门镇心安神。

配穴 头晕、头鸣者加百会；清热盗汗者加然谷。

方法 电热针治疗。

操作 选定穴位，常规皮肤消毒。电热针斜刺肝俞 0.6 寸，斜刺肾俞 0.6 寸，直刺三阴交 0.5 寸。然后接通电热针仪，电流量 65mA。另配以毫针直刺太溪 0.5 寸，直刺神门 0.3 寸，均留针 40 分钟。

疗程 20 次为 1 个疗程，疗程期间可休息 5 天。

三、注意事项

1. 注意饮食要规律，低

of 5 days between courses.

[Syndrome of Liver Kidney Yin Deficiency]

Therapeutic method: Tonifying liver, invigorating kidney, nourishing Yin and suppressing fire.

Prescription: Ganshu (BL18), Shenshu (BL23), Sanyinjiao (SP6), Taixi (KI3), Shenmen (HT7).

Mechanism of prescription: Ganshu and Shenshu nourish liver and kidney, regulate Chongren; Sanyinjiao is the key acupoint communicate the three meridians of liver, spleen and kidney, which can tonify the deficiency of three Yins, disperse deficiency fire. Taixi nourishes kidney Yin; Shenmen calms the mind.

Matching points: For people with dizziness or tinnitus, add Baihui; for people with heat and cold sweat, add Rangu.

Method: Electrothermal acupuncture treatment.

Operations: Selecting the relevant acupoints, perform routine skin disinfection. Using electrothermal acupuncture needles, obliquely puncture into Ganshu and Shenshu for 0.6", vertically puncture into Sanyinjiao for 0.5". Turn on the electrothermal acupuncture equipment, apply a current of 65mA. Additionally, using the filiform needles, vertically puncture into Taixi for 0.5", vertically puncture into Shenmen for 0.3", leaving the needles in for 40 minutes.

Therapeutic course: 20 times for a course. A break of 5 days between courses.

III. Precautions

1. Keep regular meals, low-salt and low-fat diet,

盐、低脂；少食刺激性食物，如辣椒、胡椒、烟酒等皆禁用。

2. 大便保持通畅，避免增加腹压。

3. 洗浴时不要用过高的水温泡澡，淋浴较适合。

4. 如发现头痛（突然剧烈头痛）、头晕、烦躁、血压急骤升高者，立即去医院治疗，避免高血压危象，预防脑血管意外发生。

5. 注意心态要平和，避免发怒及焦急，易引发脑血管意外。

四、典型病例

王某，女，62岁，退休人员，北京人。

主诉：眩晕，动则加剧，劳累即发，心悸少寐已4年之久，近日加重。病史：患者4年前因头晕、心悸到医院检查，发现血压高（170/100mmHg），从此开始服用降压药、降血脂药。近日症状加重，劳累即头晕加重，活动受限制。

刻下症：饮食减少，心悸不寐，神疲乏力，劳累即犯

eat less or avoid stimulants such as chilly, pepper, smoke and alcohol, etc.

2. Regulate defecation to avoid the increase of abdominal pressure.

3. Avoid bath with over-heated water, shower is more appropriate.

4. If suffered from headache (sudden or drastic headache), dizziness, agitation or sudden blood pressure rise, an emergent medical assistance in the hospital is required to avoid risks of high blood pressure and prevent from cerebrovascular accident.

5. Keep peaceful mind because agitation and anger may induce high blood pressure. Keep regular lifestyle and daily schedule.

IV. Typical Case

Wang, female, 62 years old, retiree, residence: Beijing.

Chief complaint: Dizziness aggravated with movements or fatigue, and with palpitation as well as insomnia for 4 years, the symptoms have aggravated lately. Medical history: The patient went to the hospital for examination 4 years ago for dizziness and palpitation, the results showed high blood pressure (170/100mmHg), she started to receive anti-hypertensive and anti-hyperlipidemia drug therapy ever since. The symptoms have been aggravated lately. Recently, as the patient felt fatigue, the symptom of headache has aggravated, limiting her activities.

Current symptoms: Poor appetite, palpitation, insomnia, tiresome and fatigue. If fatigue, the symptoms

病，时有头晕、耳鸣、口苦，尤其饭后就有睡意，稍有活动即心慌加重。

查体：血压 164/94mmHg（服降压药中）。二尖瓣区及主动脉瓣第二听诊区闻及二级收缩期杂音。

辅助检查：胸片示"左心室肥大"。心电图检查大致正常。血脂高。

【诊断依据】

1. 老年女性，眩晕 4 年之久。

2. 多在劳累之诱因下发病，眩晕耳鸣，心悸不寐。

3. 既往无特殊病史记载。

4. 查体：胸片示"左心室肥大"。心电图检查大致正常。血脂高。

5. 血压在 140/90mmHg 以上。

【证治分析】

病因　阴虚阳亢。

病机　风阳上扰，肝阴暗耗，肝阳升动，上扰清窍，发为眩晕。

证候分析　肝阳亢逆无制，上扰清窍，则眩晕耳鸣，头痛且胀；肝性失柔则易怒，肝火扰动心神可见失眠多梦；

occurred, accompanying with headache, tinnitus, bitter taste, sleepiness after meals, and significant palpitation with mild activities.

Physical examination: Blood pressure was 164/94mmHg (under the treatment of anti-hypertensive drugs). 2nd degree systolic murmur over mitral valve and aortic valve the 2nd auscultation area.

Auxiliary examination: The chest X-ray showed "left ventricle hypertrophy". The results of EKG exam showed generally normal. Hyperlipidemia.

[Diagnostic Basis]

1. Senior woman, suffered from vertigo for 4 years.

2. Mostly fatigue may trigger the incidence with symptoms including vertigo, tinnitus, palpitation and insomnia.

3. No specific medical histories.

4. Physical examination: Chest X-ray shows "left ventricle hypertrophy". The results of EKG exam showed generally normal. Hyperlipidemia.

5. Blood pressure above 140/90mmHg.

[Syndrome-treatment Analysis]

Etiology: Yin deficiency and Yang hyperactivity.

Pathogenesis: Hyperactivity of Fengyang, silent liver Yin consumption, liver Yang rises and is hyperactive, and consequently disturbs clear awakens called dizziness.

Syndrome analysis: Liver Yang hyperactivity, disturbs clear awaken, and thus causes dizziness and tinnitus, headache; patient's liver Yin nature may lose and become agitated, liver fire bothers mind and thus results in insomnia and dreamful. Liver Yang hyperactivity displays red face and red eyes, tongue fur yellowish, pulse shows strong liver fire.

Lesion location: Liver.

Disease nature: Excessive.

The diagnosis of Western Medicine: High blood pressure.

The diagnosis of Traditional Chinese Medicine: Upper hyperactivity vertigo.

Therapeutic method: Calm the liver, suppress Yang, and purge liver and gallbladder.

Method: Electrothermal acupuncture treatment.

Prescription: Primarily based on the Zu Jue Yin Liver Meridian and the Zu Shao Yang Gallbladder Meridian. Ganshu (BL18), Xingjian (LR2), Fengchi (GB20), Xiaxi (GB43).

Mechanism of prescription: Fengchi is the acupoint of the Zu Shao Yang Gallbladder Meridian, which can convey and disperse Yang deficiency and thus cure dizziness; Xingjian is the Xing point of Zu Jue Yin Liver Meridian, associates with the Xiaxi acupoint of the Zu Shao Yang Gallbladder Meridian, and forms superficies-interior points combination, which can calm the liver, suppress Yang, purge liver and gallbladder. If applied all acupoints all together can calm the liver, suppress Yang, and purge liver and gallbladder.

Matching points: For people with red eyes, add Guanchong for bloodletting; for people with insomnia and dreamful, add Shenmen and Sanyinjiao.

Operations: Selecting the relevant acupoints, perform routine skin disinfection. Using electrothermal acu-

下缘刺入 0.7 寸，直刺行间 0.6 寸，直刺侠溪 0.6 寸并向后斜刺，斜刺（针尖向脊柱）肝俞 0.7 寸，接通电热针仪，每个穴位分别给予 40mA 的电流量，以患者感到温胀为度，留针 40 分钟。另配以毫针放血关冲，直刺神门、三阴交各 0.6 寸，留针 40 分钟。

疗程 每日 1 次，留针 40 分钟，30 次为 1 个疗程。疗程间可休息 5 天，若无不适，亦可连续治疗，症状消退后还要巩固治疗 1 个疗程，可隔日治疗 1 次。

治疗过程 该患者治疗 1 个疗程后症状消失，治疗经过顺利，无反复。追踪观察 3 年，未见复发。

【生活调摄】

1. 饮食要有规律，低盐低脂，少食或不吃有刺激性的食物，如辣椒、胡椒、烟、酒等。

2. 嘱患者心志要平和，焦急、生气均会诱发高血压，生活要规律，按时作息。

3. 若遇有突发剧烈头痛、

puncture needles, vertically puncture into contralateral medial inferior rim of the orbit for 0.7", vertically puncture into Xingjian for 0.6", vertically and then obliquely posterior puncture into Xiaxi for 0.6", obliquely puncture (with the needle tip towards spine) into Ganshu for 0.7". Turn on the electrothermal acupuncture equipment, apply a current of 40mA to each acupoint. The limit is that the patient feels warm and swell. Leave the needles in for 40 minutes. Additionally, using the filiform needle for bloodletting at Guanchong, vertically puncture into Shenmen and Sanyinjiao for 0.6" respectively. Leave the needle in for 40 min.

Therapeutic course: Once a day. Leave the needle in for 40min, 30 times for a course. A break of 5 days between courses. If no discomfort, continuous treatment is allowed. An additional consolidation treatment course is needed after the symptoms are relieved, the treatment frequency may be once every other day.

Therapeutic process: After receiving a therapeutic course, the symptoms disappeared. The treatment process was smooth without recurrence. 3-year follow-up, no recurrence.

[Lifestyle Change and Health Maintenance]

1. Keep regular meals, low-salt and low-fat diet, eat less or avoid stimulants such as chilly, pepper, smoke and alcohol, etc.

2. Ask the patient to keep peaceful mind because agitation and anger may induce high blood pressure. Keep regular lifestyle and daily schedule.

3. If suffered from sudden or drastic signs of high

头晕、血压急骤升高等高血压危象之表现，应采取联合疗法，预防脑血管意外发生。

低血压

低血压又称体质性低血压，常见于体质较虚弱的人，女性多见，并有家族遗传倾向。多数原发性低血压无明显自觉症状，仅有血压低于90/50mmHg。部分人可因血压过低而引起头晕、头痛、心前区不适、疲劳、心悸、胸闷、气短等症，甚至昏厥，严重影响工作。

中医认为，本病多因先天禀赋不足、后天失养、思虑过度导致气血衰少，气虚阳弱，推动无力，气血不能通达四肢而引发，相当于中医"眩晕""怔忡"等范畴。

一、诊断及辨证要点

1. 气血不足者，症见怔忡，眩晕，面色萎黄，食欲不振，神疲乏力，爪甲不荣，肢体麻木，妇女月经量少、色

blood pressure such as headache, dizziness or sudden blood pressure rise, a combined therapy is recommended to prevent cerebrovascular accidents.

Low Blood Pressure

Low blood pressure is also called "constitutional low blood pressure", which is commonly seen in people with weaker constitutions, mostly in women, and has the tendency of family genetic predisposition. Lots of people with primary low blood pressure are asymptomatic in addition to blood pressure below 90/50mmHg. Part of the population may suffer from dizziness, headache, precordial discomfort, fatigue, chest tightness, short of breath, etc. or even syncope due to low blood pressure, and thus severely affecting work performance.

The Traditional Chinese Medicine believes that low blood pressure mostly is caused by Qi-blood deficiency and insufficiency, Qi deficiency and Yang weak resulted from insufficiency of natural endowment, poor-nourishment after birth plus excess worry, and thereby the heart is too weak to generate sufficient cardiac output, so the Qi and blood fails to circulate to four limbs. The symptoms are similar to the scope of "vertigo" or "palpitation" in Traditional Chinese Medicine.

I. Key Points for Diagnosis and Syndrome Differentiation

1. People with insufficient Qi and blood often display syndromes of palpitation, dizziness, sallow complexion, poor appetite, tiresome and fatigue, malnutrition of the nails, limbs numbness, scanty and light colored

淡，甚则闭经，舌淡苔白，脉细弱。

2. 肝肾阴虚者，症见头晕目眩，耳鸣健忘，失眠多梦，咽干口燥，腰膝酸软，胁痛，五心烦热，颧红盗汗，男子遗精，女子经少，舌红少苔，脉细数。

3. 血压低于90/50mmHg。

4. 各种理化检查均未发现异常体征者。

二、治疗方法

【气血不足证】

治法 补气养血，宁心安神。

处方 肾俞（BL23）、脾俞（BL20）、足三里（ST36）、三阴交（SP6）、内关（PC6）。

方义 脾为后天之本，取脾俞、足三里、三阴交健脾补胃以调生化之源；内关补气养血，宁心安神。肾为先天之本，取肾俞补肾气，肾气旺则精血自充。

配穴 多汗者加阴郄；

period, or even amenorrhea, light and whitish tongue fur, weak and slow pulse.

2. People with liver and kidney Yin deficiency often have symptoms of dizziness and vertigo, tinnitus, amnesia, insomnia, dreamful, dry throat and mouth, soreness and weakness over lower back and the knees, flank pain, burning sensations of five centers, red cheeks and cold sweating, nocturnal emission, scanty period, red tongue with less fur, weak and slow pulse.

3. Refer to patients with blood pressure lower than 90/50mmHg.

4. People with no abnormalities after all kinds of physical and chemical examinations.

II. Therapeutic Methods

[Qi and Blood Insufficiency]

Therapeutic method: Tonifying Qi and nourishing blood, relieve mental stress and keep calm.

Prescription: Shenshu (BL23), Pishu (BL20), Zusanli (ST36), Sanyinjiao (SP36), Neiguan (PC6).

Mechanism of prescription: The spleen is the root of required nature, so treatment on the Pishu, Zusanli and Sanyinjiao can invigorate spleen, tonify stomach and regulate the source of biochemistry. The treatment on Neiguan can supply Qi, nourish blood, relieve mental distress and keep calm. The kidney is the root of congenital natures, so treatment on the Shenshu to nourish kidney Qi, once the kidney Qi is energized, the vitality and blood is supplemented automatically.

Matching points: For people with excessive sweat,

心悸、神思不宁者加百会、神门。

方法 电热针治疗。

操作 选定穴位，常规皮肤消毒。用电热针直刺肾俞0.6寸、斜刺脾俞0.6寸、直刺足三里0.8寸、直刺三阴交0.6寸、直刺内关0.5寸。接通电热针仪，给予电流量60mA，以温热或酸胀的舒适感觉为度，留针40分钟。

疗程 20次为1个疗程，疗程间可休息5天。

【肝肾阴虚证】

治法 补肝肾，益气血。

处方 肝俞（BL18）、肾俞（BL23）、关元（RN4）、太溪（KI3）。

方义 肝俞、肾俞滋补肝肾，调理冲任；关元为足三阴与任脉之会，用以补摄下焦元气；太溪滋阴泻火。

配穴 心悸者加内关；耳鸣者加听宫；盗汗者加然谷。

方法 电热针治疗。

add Yinxi; for people with palpitation or agitated mind, add Baihui and Shenmen.

Method: Electrothermal acupuncture treatment.

Operations: Selecting acupoints, perform routine skin disinfection. Using electrothermal acupuncture needles, vertically puncture into Shenshu for 0.6", obliquely puncture into Pishu for 0.6", vertically puncture into Zusanli for 0.8", vertically puncture into Sanyinjiao for 0.6", and vertically puncture into Neiguan for 0.5". Turn on the electrothermal acupuncture equipment, apply a current of 60mA to each acupoint. The limit is that the patient feels warm or sore and swelling comfortable. Leave the needle in for 40 min.

Therapeutic course: Once a day, 20 times for a course. A break of 5 days between courses.

[Syndrome of Liver and Kidney Deficiency]

Therapeutic method: Tonifying liver and kidney and supplying Qi and blood.

Prescription: Ganshu (BL18), Shenshu (BL23), Guanyuan (RN4), Taixi (KI3).

Mechanism of prescription: Ganshu and Shenshu tonifies and nourishes liver and kidney, regulates Chongren. Guanyuan is the convergent acupoint of the Three Yin Meridians of Foot and the Ren Collateral, which is used to supply and consume Lower Jiao Yuan Qi. Taixi nourishes Yin and expels fire.

Matching points: For people with palpitation, add Neiguan; for people with tinnitus, add Tinggong; for people with cold sweating, add Rangu.

Method: Electrothermal acupuncture treatment.

操作 选定穴位，常规皮肤消毒。用电热针直刺肝俞0.6寸，直刺肾俞0.6寸，直刺关元0.6寸，直刺太溪0.5寸。然后接通电热针仪，每穴给予60mA的电流量，以温热或酸胀而舒适为度，留针40分钟。

疗程 每天1次，10次为1个疗程，疗程间可休息3天。

三、注意事项

1. 对于急性低血压，在针刺急救的过程中，必须配合药物，尽快找到血压下降的原因，针对病因进行治疗。

2. 对于厥证、脱证等都应在针治过程中采取综合治疗，同时要针对病因进行抢救。

冠状动脉粥样硬化性心脏病

冠状动脉粥样硬化性心脏病，简称冠心病，是指冠状动脉因粥样硬化后造成管腔狭窄或阻塞而影响冠状动脉血液循环，导致心肌缺血缺氧而引起的心脏病变。临床表现多为胸闷窒息或有心绞痛，常伴有心悸、气短，多在剧烈活动、情

Operations: Selecting acupoints, perform routine skin disinfection. Using electrothermal acupuncture needles, vertically puncture into Ganshu, Shenshu and Guanyuan for 0.6", and vertically puncture into Taixi for 0.5". Turn on the electrothermal acupuncture equipment, apply a current of 60mA to each acupoint. The limit is that the patient feels warm or sore and swelling comfortable. Leave the needle in for 40 min.

Therapeutic course: Once a day, 10 times for a course. A break of 3 days between courses.

III. Precautions

1. For acute low blood pressure, if used acupuncture therapy for emergency treatment, the application of medicinal products is required. It is critical to sort out the reasons causing blood pressure decrease in order to treat based on the etiology accordingly.

2. For syncope and collapse syndromes, a comprehensive therapy is required during the acupuncture therapy. A treatment focusing on the etiology is also required at the same time.

Coronary Atherosclerotic Heart Diseases

Coronary atherosclerotic heart diseases, coronary heart diseases for short, refer to heart diseases caused by that coronary artery atherosclerosis leads to stenosis or obstruction of vascular lumen which affects the blood circulation of coronary arteries, therefore causes myocardial ischemia and hypoxia. The clinical manifestations normally include chest distress and angina, generally accompanying palpitation, shortness of breath, most of

绪激动、寒冷刺激时突发，持续数分钟，经过休息或服用血管扩张药逐渐缓解。严重者可出现肢冷汗出，引发心源性休克或心衰。本病是中老年人最常见的心血管疾病之一。它的发生常与精神、神经、内分泌、血液、遗传等因素有关。

中医认为，本病属于"胸痹""厥心痛""真心痛"等范畴。主要因素是忧思恼怒，导致气机不畅，气滞则血瘀，阻于经脉或胸阳痹阻所致。

一、诊断及辨证要点

1. 气滞血瘀者，症见心前区或胸骨后阵发性刺痛，痛引肩背，胸闷、气短，甚则汗出肢冷，舌质紫黯。

2. 胸阳痹阻者，症见胸闷气短，嗜睡身倦，面色白，舌淡苔白，脉弦滑或弦细。

3. 心脾两虚者，症见心胸憋闷，神疲乏力，失眠健忘，纳呆便溏，舌淡苔白，脉濡弱

which attack upon intense activities, emotional excitement, stimulation of cold and last for several minutes, and can be relieved after rest or administration of vasodilators. In severe cases there may be cold limbs and sweating, inducing cardiogenic shock or heart failure. This is the most common cardiovascular disease among elder people. Its incidence normally is associated with mental, neural, endocrine, blood, genetic factors, etc.

Traditional Chinese Medicine believes that this disease belongs to the range of "thoracic obstruction", "precordial pain with cold limbs", "angina pectoris", etc. The main causes are sad thoughts and anger, unsmooth Qi Dynamic, Qi stagnation leads to blood stasis in the meridians and channels or obstruction of chest Yang.

I. Key Points for Diagnosis and Syndrome Differentiation

1. For patients with Qi stagnation and blood stasis, symptoms include paroxysmal pricking of the precordium or posterior sternum which radiates to the shoulder and back, chest distress and shortness of breath, or even sweating and cold limbs in severe cases, dark purple tongue.

2. For patients with Yang stagnation in chest, symptoms include chest distress and shortness of breath, drowsiness and body fatigue, pale complexion, light tongue with whitish fur, taut and slippery or taut and thin pulse.

3. For patients with deficiency of both heart and spleen, symptoms include chest distress, mental fatigue and asthenia, insomnia and amnesia, poor appetite and

或结代。

4. 心阳暴脱者，症见胸前区剧烈疼痛，反复发作或持续不休，引起心悸，呼吸急迫，口唇由紫转白，冷汗淋漓，四肢厥逆，神昏，脉微欲绝。

5. 有心电图改变。

二、治疗方法

【气滞血瘀证】

治法　理气活血，通络止痛。

处方　太冲（LR3）、期门（LR14）、心俞（BL15）、厥阴俞（BL14）、内关（PC6）、通里（HT5）。

方义　太冲为肝经之输穴、原穴；期门是肝之募穴，二穴相配可疏肝行气。心俞、厥阴俞分别为心经和心包经的背俞穴，有活血化瘀之功；内关、通里分别为心经与心包经的络穴，四穴相配可宁心安神、活血通络、化瘀止痛。诸穴合用，可收理气活血、通络止痛之功效。

sloppy stool, light tongue with whitish fur, soft and weak pulse or irregular and regular intermittent pulse.

4. For patients with heart Yang collapse, symptoms include intense pain of prethoracic area which attacks repeatedly or continues endlessly, leading to palpitation, tachypnea, change of lip color from purple into white, dripping cold sweat, extremely cold limbs, coma, weak pulse which is about to disappear.

5. Changes seen in the ECG.

II. Therapeutic Methods

[Syndrome of Qi Stagnation and Blood Stasis]

Therapeutic method: regulate Qi and activate blood circulation, soothe collaterals and alleviate pain.

Prescription: Taichong (LR3), Qimen (LR14), Xinshu (BL15), Jueyinshu (BL14), Neiguan (PC6), Tongli (HT5).

Mechanism of prescription: Taichong is a Shu acupoint and Yuan acupoint of Liver; Qimen is a Mu acupoint of Liver, the match of these two can soothe liver and activate Qi. Xinshu, Jueyinshu are Back-Shu acupoints of the Heart Meridian and Pericardium Meridian respectively, can activate blood circulation and remove stasis; Neiguan, Tongli are collateral acupoints of the Heart Meridian and Pericardium Meridian respectively, the match of these four can tranquilize mind, activate blood circulation, remove stasis and alleviate pains. The combined use of these acupoints can regulate Qi and activate blood circulation, soothe collaterals and alleviate pain.

方法 电热针治疗。

操作 选定穴位，常规皮肤消毒后，用电热针刺心俞、厥阴俞、期门，给予电流量60mA，以温热或酸胀而舒适感为度。另配以毫针刺入内关0.5寸、通里0.5寸，均留针40分钟。

疗程 每日1次，10次为1个疗程。

【胸阳痹阻证】

治法 温阳通络，豁痰止痛。

处方 足三里（ST36）、丰隆（ST40）、脾俞（BL20）、三阴交（SP6）、膻中（RN17）、关元（RN4）。

方义 足三里为足阳明经之合穴，用之和中；丰隆为足阳明经之络穴，用之化痰；脾俞是脾经之背俞穴，与足三阴经之交会穴三阴交合用，可健脾和血；膻中、关元可温心阳而益心肾。诸穴共用，温阳通络，豁痰止痛。

方法 电热针治疗。

操作 选定穴位，施以常

Method: Electrothermal acupuncture treatment.

Operations: Selecting acupoints, perform routine skin disinfection, then Using electrothermal acupuncture needles, puncture into Xinshu, Jueyinshu, Qimen, and give a current of 60mA, while the limit is that the patient feels partial warm or sore and swollen as well as comfortable. Additionally, using filiform needles, puncture into Neiguan for 0.5", Tongli for 0.5", leave the needles in for 40 minutes for both.

Therapeutic course: Once a day, 10 times for a course.

[Syndrome of Yang Stagnation in Chest]

Therapeutic method: Warm Yang and dredge collaterals, disperse phlegm and alleviate pains.

Prescription: Zusanli (ST36), Fenglong (ST40), Pishu (BL20), Sanyinjiao (SP6), Danzhong (RN17), Guanyuan (RN4).

Mechanism of prescription: Zusanli is the He acupoint from Yang-Ming Meridian of Foot, it can harmonize Middle Jiao; Fenglong is a collateral acupoint from Yang-Ming Meridian of Foot which can disperse phlegm; Pishu is a Back-Shu acupoint from Spleen Meridian, it can invigorate spleen and regulate blood when being matched with the confluent acupoint Sanyinjiao of the three-Yin Meridians of Foot; Danzhong, Guanyuan can warm heart Yang, tonify heart and kidney. The combined use of these acupoints can warm Yang and dredge collaterals, disperse phlegm and alleviate pains.

Method: Electrothermal acupuncture treatment.

Operations: Selecting acupoints, perform routine

规皮肤消毒。电热针直刺足三里 0.8 寸、直刺三阴交 0.6 寸、平刺膻中 0.7 寸、直刺关元 0.8 寸。然后接通电热针仪，给予电流量 60mA。以温热或酸胀舒适感觉为度。另配以毫针直刺丰隆 0.8 寸，均留针 40 分钟。

疗程 每天 1 次，10 次为 1 个疗程，疗程间可休息 3 天，再继续施术。

【心脾两虚证】

治法 补心健脾，养血安神。

处方 内关（PC6）、心俞（BL15）、足三里（ST36）、三阴交（SP6）。

方义 内关是心经之络穴，心俞为心经的背俞穴，足三里是足阳明胃经之合穴，三阴交是足三阴经之交会穴，四穴合用可补益心脾，益气养血安神。

方法 电热针治疗。

操作 选定穴位，施以常规皮肤消毒。电热针直刺足三里 0.8 寸、直刺三阴交 0.7 寸、直刺内关穴 0.6 寸。然后接通电热针仪，给予电流量 60mA，

skin disinfection. Using electrothermal acupuncture needles, vertically puncture into Zusanli for 0.8", Sanyinjiao for 0.6", horizontally puncture into Danzhong for 0.7", vertically puncture into Guanyuan for 0.8". Turn on the electrothermal acupuncture equipment, apply a current of 60mA. The limit is that the patient feels partial warm or sore and swollen as well as comfortable. Additionally, using filiform needles, vertically puncture into Fenglong for 0.8", leaving the needles in for 40 minutes.

Therapeutic course: Once a day, 10 times for a course. Rest for 3 days between courses and continue the treatment.

[Syndrome of Deficiency of the Heart and Spleen]

Therapeutic method: Replenish heart and invigorate spleen, nourish blood and tranquilize mind.

Prescription: Neiguan (PC6), Xinshu (BL15), Zusanli (ST36), Sanyinjiao (SP6).

Mechanism of prescription: Neiguan is a collateral acupoint of the Heart Meridian, Xinshu is the Back-Shu acupoint of the Heart Meridian, and Zusanli is a He acupoint from Yang-Ming Stomach Meridian of Foot, Sanyinjiao is the confluent acupoint of the three Yin Meridian of Foot, the match of these four can tonify heart and spleen, nourish Qi and blood as well as tranquilize mind.

Method: Electrothermal acupuncture treatment.

Operations: Selecting the relevant acupoints, perform routine skin disinfection. Using electrothermal acupuncture needles, vertically puncture into Zusanli for 0.8", Sanyinjiao for 0.7", puncture into Neiguan for 0.6". Turn on the electrothermal acupuncture equipment, apply

以温热或胀感而舒适为度。另配以毫针斜刺心俞0.7寸，均留针40分钟。

疗程 每天1次，10次为1个疗程，疗程间可休息3天。

三、注意事项

1. 针灸治疗过程中，要在严密的观察下进行治疗，如遇有病情较重者，应采取综合治疗。

2. 冠心病患者要避免摄入过多含大量胆固醇和脂肪酸类的肉食，必须合理安排饮食，注意适量。

3. 注意避免过度紧张、劳累，要适量活动，但要劳逸结合。

四、典型病例

韩某，男，67岁，退休工人，北京人。

主诉：心胸隐痛，久发不愈，心烦少寐，头晕、耳鸣已3年之久，近日加重。病史：患者近3年不断出现心前区隐隐作痛，反复发作，心烦不寐，服用药物后症状不减。

刻下症：头晕耳鸣，胸闷

a current of 60mA, and the limit is that the patient feels partial warm or swelling and comfortable. Additionally, using filiform needles, vertically puncture into Fenglong for 0.7", leaving the needles in for 40 minutes.

Therapeutic course: Once a day, 10 times for a course. Rest for 3 days between courses.

III. Precautions

1. During acupuncture treatment, the treatment should be done under strict observation, and for severe cases, a comprehensive therapy should be adopted.

2. Patients with coronary heart diseases should avoid intake too much food containing lots of cholesterol and fatty acids, and must reasonably arrange their diet, note that eat appropriate amount of food.

3. Note to avoid over-tension and overstrain, do appropriate amount of exercises, alternate work with rest.

IV. Typical Case

Han, male, 67 years old, retiree, residence: Beijing.

Self-reported symptoms: Dull of the heart pain and chest for a long time without cure, vexation and insufficient sleep, dizziness and tinnitus for 3 years, which aggravated recently. Medical history: The patient suffered from repeated onset of dull pain in the precordium, vexation and sleeplessness in the recent 3 years, and the symptoms were not relieved after medicine treatment.

Current symptoms: Dizziness and tinnitus, chest

气短，腰酸膝软，倦怠少力，时有心悸盗汗，舌红苔少，脉弦细。

查体：二尖瓣区及主动脉瓣第二听诊区闻及二级收缩期杂音。血压 164/100mmHg。

辅助检查：心电图示"T 波低平，S-T 段压低"。平板运动试验阳性。

【诊断依据】

1. 老年男性，发病 3 年，症见心前区隐隐作痛，头晕耳鸣，心悸盗汗，腰膝酸软，胸闷气短等，一直用药控制，症状时好时坏，反复发作。

2. 心电图示"T 波低平，S-T 段压低"。平板运动试验阳性。

3. 虽在服药，但血压仍在（140～160）/（100～90）mmHg 之间，始终未恢复正常。

【证治分析】

病因　年老体虚。

病机　年过半百，肾气渐衰，如肾阳虚衰，则不能温煦五脏之阳，可致心气不足，心胸失养而酿成本病。

distress and shortness of breath, aching lumbus and limp knees, fatigue and weakness, frequent palpitation and sweating at night, red tongue with less fur, string and thin pulse.

Physical examination: Grade 2 systolic noise at mitral valve area and second aortic valve area. Blood pressure 164/100 mmHg.

Auxiliary examination: ECG showed "low and flat T wave, depressed S-T segment". Positive in treadmill exercise test.

[Diagnostic Basis]

1. Old male, the disease had been lasted for 3 years, symptoms include dull pain in the precordium, dizziness and tinnitus, palpitation and sweating at night, aching lumbus and limp knees, chest distress and shortness of breath, etc. He accepted medication control, however the condition was not stable and the symptoms repeatedly onset.

2. ECG showed "low and flat T wave, depressed S-T segment". Positive in treadmill exercise test.

3. He was under medicine treatment but the blood pressure was still between (140-160)/(100-90) mmHg, which had not returned to normal.

[Syndrome-treatment Analysis]

Etiology: Old age and deficiency.

Pathogenesis: The patient's age was over 50 years old. His kidney Qi was becoming more and more deficient. For deficiency and depletion of kidney Yang, the Yang of five Zangs cannot be warmed, leading to ineffi-

证候分析 心气虚弱，鼓动无力，血滞心脉，故见胸闷隐痛，时作时好，心悸盗汗，倦怠懒言；心阴虚，故见心烦不寐；肾阴虚，故见头晕耳鸣，腰酸膝软；水不涵木，肝阳偏亢，故见头晕。舌脉均为阴血虚亏，心脉瘀阻之象。

病位 心、肾。

病性 阴虚。

西医诊断 冠状动脉粥样硬化性心脏病、高血压。

中医诊断 胸痹心痛、眩晕。

治法 滋阴益肾，养心止痛。

方法 电热针治疗。

处方 以手少阴心经、足少阴肾经穴为主。心俞（BL15）、肾俞（BL23）、神门（HT7）、太溪（KI3）、三阴交（SP6）、内关（PC6）。

方义 心俞、内关、肾俞、太溪补益心肾；神门补心除烦；三阴交养血滋阴。

ciency of the heart Qi, nourishment loss of the heart and chest and causing the disease.

Syndrome analysis: Deficient heart Qi, weak heartbeat, blood stagnation in the heart channels, therefore caused chest distension and dull pain that attack from time to time, palpitation and sweating at night, tiredness and laziness of speaking; heart Yin deficiency caused vexation and sleeplessness; kidney Yin deficiency caused dizziness and tinnitus, soreness and weakness of waist and knees; Water not nourishing Wood and hyperactivity of liver Yang caused dizziness. The pulse condition of tongue all indicated depletion and deficiency of Yin-blood, obstruction of the heart channels.

Lesion location: Heart, kidney.

Lesion nature: Yin deficiency.

The diagnosis of Western Medicine: Coronary atherosclerotic heart diseases, high blood pressure.

The diagnosis of Traditional Chinese Medicine: Chest obstruction and heart pain, vertigo.

Therapeutic method: Nourish Yin and tonify kidney, nourish heart and alleviate pains.

Method: Electrothermal acupuncture treatment.

Prescription: Mainly focus on acupoints of the Shao-Yin Heart Meridian of Hand and Shao-Yin Kidney Meridian of Foot. Xinshu (BL15), Shenshu (BL23), Shenmen (HT7), Taixi (KI3), Sanyinjiao (SP6), Neiguan (PC6).

Mechanism of prescription: Xinshu, Neiguan, Shenshu, Taixi can tonify heart and kidney; Shenmen can replenish heart and treat anxiety; Sanyinjiao can tonify blood and nourish Yin.

配穴 胸闷纳呆者加足三里、中脘；便秘者加天枢、照海。

操作 选定穴位，皮肤常规消毒。电热针斜刺（针尖向脊柱）心俞、肾俞各 0.7 寸，直刺三阴交、内关、足三里、中脘、天枢、照海、太溪、神门各 0.7 寸，接通电热针仪，每个穴位分别给予 40mA 的电流量，以患者感到温胀为度，留针 40 分钟。（注：每次选 3 组穴，轮流交替应用。）

疗程 每日 1 次，20 次为 1 个疗程。疗程间可休息 5～10 天，再进行第 2 个疗程的治疗。症状消退后，再巩固治疗 1 个疗程，可隔日治疗 1 次。

治疗过程 该患者疗效较好，治疗过程中未再发病。随访至今已 15 年之久，未见复发。

【生活调摄】

1. 饮食要有节制，不能过饱，要低盐低脂，避免摄入刺激性食物，如辛辣之品，多吃蔬菜水果。

2. 保持心志平和，避免过劳及焦急，注意生活起居规

Matching acupoints: For chest distress and anorexia, add Zusanli, Zhongwan. For constipation add Tianshu, Zhaohai.

Operations: Selecting the relevant acupoints, perform routine skin disinfection. Using electrothermal acupuncture needles, obliquely puncture (with the needle tip towards spine) into Xinshu, Shenshu for 0.7" respectively, vertically puncture into Sanyinjiao, Neiguan, Zusanli, Zhongwan, Tianshu, Zhaohai, Taixi, Shenmen for 0.7" respectively. Turn on the electrothermal acupuncture equipment, apply a current of 40mA to each acupoint, and the limit is that the patient feels warm and swollen, leaving the needles in for 40 minutes. (Note: select 3 pairs of acupoints each time, and use alternately.)

Therapeutic course: Once a day, 20 times for a course. Start the treatment for the second course after a break of 5-10 days. After the symptoms disappeared, perform another 1 course for consolidation which can perform once every two days.

Therapeutic process: The patient got relatively good efficacies, and no onset occurred during the treatment. There has been 15 years of follow-up to date, no recurrence seen.

[Lifestyle Change and Health Maintenance]

1. Have controlled diet, do not eat too much, have food with low salt and fat, avoid to intake stimulating food such as spicy food, eat more vegetables and fruits.

2. Keep peaceful mood and mind, avoid overstrain and anxiety, have regular lifestyle and enough sleep.

律，睡眠要充足。

3. 要适当锻炼，如散步、户外活动。

风湿性心脏病

风湿性心脏病（风心病）是指急性风湿性心脏病遗留下来的心脏瓣膜病变，故又称"风湿性心脏瓣膜病"。病变部位以二尖瓣和主动脉瓣最为多见，形成瓣口狭窄或关闭不全，或两者同时存在，导致血流动力学改变，出现心脏杂音，心功能代偿不全，心脏增大或充血性心力衰竭等症状。发病季节多在秋、冬二季，女性多于男性，发病年龄以 20～40 岁青壮年为多见。

中医认为，本病属于"心痹""惊悸""水肿""咳喘"等范畴。多因气血不足，心失所养；或情志刺激，心气郁结；或气滞血瘀，心脉痹阻，加之风寒湿热之邪乘虚而入，合而为病。发病部位在心，但与肺、脾、肾有关。

一、诊断及辨证要点

1. 气滞血瘀者，症见心悸

3. Do appropriate exercises, such as walking, outdoor activities.

Rheumatic Heart Diseases

Rheumatic heart diseases (RHD) refer to heart valvular diseases left by acute rheumatic heart diseases, so also called as "rheumatic valvular heart diseases". The most common lesion locations are mitral and aortic valve. The formation of valve orifice stenosis or incompetence or the presence of both two, cause changes in hemodynamics, the occurrence of symptoms such as cardiac murmur, cardiac incompensation, cardiac enlargement or congestive heart failure. The high-occurrence season of this disease are autumn and winter, and the number of female patients are more than that of males, the most common onset age is 20-40 years old.

Traditional Chinese Medicine believes that this disease belongs to the range of "heart obstruction", "palpitation", "edema", "cough and asthma", etc. Most are caused by insufficient Qi-blood, nourishment loss of the heart; or emotional stimulation, stagnation of the heart Qi; or Qi stagnation and blood stasis, obstruction of the heart channels, plus swooping in of Damp-Heat toxins, together lead to this disease. The lesion location is heart, but the disease is related to lung, spleen and kidney.

I. Key Points for Diagnosis and Syndrome Differentiation

1. For patients with Qi stagnation and blood stasis,

气促，头晕眼花，胸闷心痛，咳嗽咯血，唇紫甲灰，两颧紫红，全身浮肿，舌质青紫或有瘀斑，脉细数或结代。

2. 心血不足者，症见心悸，动则尤甚，气短自汗，头晕眼花，神疲乏力，面色苍白或萎黄，舌质淡胖有齿痕，脉细或濡弱。

3. 心肾阳虚者，症见心悸，浮肿，咳嗽喘急，动则加重，甚则不能平卧，手足不温，面色晦暗，舌质淡，苔白薄，脉沉细或结代。

4. 心电图异常。

二、治疗方法

【气滞血瘀证】

治法　疏肝理气，活血散结。

处方　内关（PC6）、间使（PC5）、通里（HT5）、神门（HT7）、心俞（BL15）、厥阴俞（BL14）、血海（SP10）、太冲（LR3）、期门（LR14）、章门（LR13）。

symptoms include palpitation and shortness of breath, dizziness, chest distress and heart pain, cough and hemoptysis, purple lips and gray fingernails, purplish red cheekbones, systemic edema, cyanoze tongue or ecchymosis on the tongue, thin and rapid pulse or irregular and regular intermittent pulse.

2. For patients with insufficiency of the heart's blood, symptoms include palpitation which aggravates with movement, shortness of breath and spontaneous sweating, dizziness, mental fatigue and asthenia, pale or sallow complexion, light and fat tongue with teeth prints, thin or soft and weak pulse.

3. For patients with Yang deficiency of the heart and kidney, symptoms include palpitation, edema, cough and excessive panting which aggravates with movement, or in severe cases unable to lie on the back, non-warm limbs, gloomy complexion, light tongue with whitish and thin fur, deep and thin or irregular and regular intermittent pulse.

4. Abnormal ECG.

II. Therapeutic Methods

[Syndrome of Qi Stagnation and Blood Stasis]

Therapeutic method: Soothe liver and regulate Qi, activate blood circulation and disperse stagnation.

Prescription: Neiguan (PC6), Jianshi (PC5), Tongli (HT5), Shenmen (HT7), Xinshu (BL15), Jueyinshu (BL14), Xuehai (SP10), Taichong (LR3), Qimen (LR14), Zhangmen (LR13).

方义 内关、间使分别为手厥阴心包经的原穴、经穴，通里、神门分别是手少阴心经的络穴、原穴，心俞为心之背俞穴，厥阴俞为心包之背俞穴，诸穴均可协调心经气机，起宁心安神、镇惊止悸的作用。血海是足太阴脾经穴，是治疗气滞血瘀的要穴。太冲、期门、章门分别是足厥阴肝经的原穴、募穴、会穴，可收疏肝理气、活血散结之功效。

配穴 心绞痛或胸痛彻背者加膻中、巨阙、郄门；晕厥者加人中、足三里、涌泉；咯血者加孔最、膈俞；风湿者加风池、大椎。

方法 毫针治疗（泻法）。

操作 选定穴位，常规皮肤消毒。直刺内关 0.5 寸，直刺间使 0.5 寸，直刺通里 0.4 寸，直刺神门 0.4 寸，向脊柱侧斜刺心俞 0.6 寸，向脊柱侧斜刺厥阴俞 0.6 寸，斜刺期门 0.5 寸，向前下方斜刺章门 0.6 寸。留针 30 分钟。

Mechanism of prescription: Neiguan and Jianshi are Yuan acupoint and meridian acupoint of Jue-Yin Pericardium Meridian of Hand respectively, Tongli and Shenmen are meridian acupoint and Yuan acupoint of Shao-Yin Heart Meridian of Hand respectively, Xinshu is the Back-Shu acupoint of the heart, Jueyinshu is the Back-Shu acupoint of Pericardium, these acupoints all can regulate Qi dynamic of the Heart Meridian, to tranquilize mind, relieve convulsion and stop palpitation. Xuehai is the meridian acupoint of Tai-Yang Spleen Meridian of Foot, is an important acupoint for treatment of Qi stagnation and blood stasis. Taichong, Qimen, Zhangmen are the Yuan acupoint, Mu acupoint and confluent acupoint from Jue-Yin Liver Meridian of Foot, they can soothe liver and regulate Qi, activate blood circulation and disperse stagnation.

Matching acupoints: For angina or chest pain radiating toward back add Danzhong, JuQue, Ximen. For coma add Renzhong, Zusanli, Yongquan. For hemoptysis add Kongzui, Geshu. For rheumatism add Fengchi, Dazhui.

Method: Filiform needle acupuncture treatment (attenuating).

Operations: Selecting the relevant acupoints, perform routine skin disinfection. Vertically puncture into Neiguan for 0.5", Jianshi for 0.5", Tongli and Shenmen for 0.4", obliquely puncture toward spine into Xinshu for 0.6", Jueyinyu for 0.6", Qimen for 0.5", obliquely puncture toward anterior and inferior direction into Zhangmen for 0.6". Leave the needles in for 30 minutes.

疗程 每天 1 次，10 次为 1 个疗程，疗程间可休息 3 天。

【心血不足证】

治法 补气养血，宁心安神。

处方 内关（PC6）、间使（PC5）、大陵（PC7）、通里（HT5）、神门（HT7）、心俞（BL15）、脾俞（BL20）、气海（RN6）、足三里（ST36）、三阴交（SP6）。

方义 内关、间使、大陵分别是手厥阴心包经的原穴、经穴、输穴，可镇惊止悸。通里、神门分别是手少阴心经的络穴、原穴，可宁心安神。心俞是心之背俞穴，脾俞是脾之背俞穴，能补益心脾，治疗气血不足。气海是任脉之穴，又名"丹田"，可调益周身之气。足三里是足阳明胃经的合穴，三阴交是足太阴脾经的交会穴，两穴皆可补养气血，收宁心安神之功。

配穴 气短者加定喘、膻中、肺俞；失眠者加郄门、太溪。

方法 电热针治疗（补法）。

Therapeutic course: Once a day, 10 times for a course. Rest for 3 days between courses.

[Syndrome of the Heart Blood Deficiency]

Therapeutic method: Replenish Qi and nourish blood, soothe one's mood and calm the mind.

Prescription: Neiguan (PC6), Jianshi (PC5), Daling (PC7), Tongli (HT5), Shenmen (HT7), Xinshu(BL15), Pishu(BL20), Qihai (RN6), Zusanli (ST36), Sanyinjiao (SP6).

Mechanism of prescription: Neiguan, Jianshi and Daling are the Yuan acupoint, meridian acupoint, Shu acupoint from Jue-Yin Pericardium Meridian of Hand respectively, they can relieve convulsion and stop palpitation. Tongli, Shenmen are the collateral acupoint and Yuan acupoint from Shao-Yin Heart Meridian of Hand respectively, they can soothe one's mood and calm the mind. Xinshu is the Back-Shu acupoint of the heart, Pishu is a Back-Shu acupoint of Spleen, they can tonify heart and spleen to treat Qi-blood deficiency. Qihai is an acupoint of Ren Channel, also called 'Dantian', can tonify Qi of the whole body. Zusanli is a He acupoint from Yang-Ming Stomach Meridian of Foot, Sanyinjiao is the confluent acupoint from Tai-Yin Spleen Meridian of Foot, the two both can replenish Qi and nourish blood to soothe one's mood and calm the mind.

Matching acupoints: For shortness of breath, add Dingchuan, Danzhong, Feishu. For insomnia add Ximen, Taixi.

Method: Electrothermal acupuncture treatment

下篇 临床论治 Part II: Clinical Treatment

操作 选定穴位，常规皮肤消毒。直刺内关0.6寸，直刺间使0.6寸，向脊柱侧斜刺心俞0.8寸，向脊柱侧斜刺脾俞0.8寸，直刺足三里0.8寸，直刺三阴交0.6寸。然后接通电热针仪，给每个穴位的电流量是60mA。另配以毫针直刺大陵0.4寸，直刺通里0.4寸，直刺神门0.5寸，直刺气海0.6寸，均留针40分钟。（注：每次电热针刺6穴，毫针刺2～3穴即可。）

疗程 每天1次，10次为1个疗程，疗程间休息3天。

【心肾阳虚证】

治法 振奋心阳，宁心安神。

处方 内关（PC6）、间使（PC5）、通里（HT5）、神门（HT7）、心俞（BL15）、厥阴俞（BL14）、肾俞（BL23）、命门（DU4）。

方义 内关、间使分别为手厥阴心包经的原穴、经穴，可有镇心安神之功。通里、神门分别为手少阴心经的络穴、原穴，能振奋心阳，宁心止惊。心俞是心之背俞穴，厥阴俞是心包之背俞穴，肾俞

(tonification).

Operations: Selecting relevant acupoints, perform routine skin disinfection. Vertically puncture into Neiguan for 0.6", Jianshi for 0.6", obliquely puncture toward spine into Xinshu for 0.8", Pishu for 0.8", vertically puncture into Zusanli for 0.8", Sanyinjiao for 0.6". Turn on the electrothermal acupuncture equipment, apply a current of 60mA to each acupoint. Additionally, using filiform needles, vertically puncture into Daling for 0.4", Tongli for 0.4", Shenmen for 0.5", Qihai for 0.6", leaving the needles in for 40 minutes. (Note: each time, puncture 6 acupoints with electrothermal needles and 2-3 acupoints with filiform needles.)

Therapeutic course: Once a day, 10 times for a course. Rest for 3 days between courses.

[Syndrome of Yang Deficiency of the Heart]

Therapeutic methods: Promote heart Yang, soothe one's mood and calm the mind.

Prescription: Neiguan (PC6), Jianshi (PC5), Tongli (HT5), Shenmen (HT7), Xinshu (BL15), Jueyinshu (BL14), Shenshu (BL23), Mingmen (DU4).

Mechanism of prescription: Neiguan, Jianshi are the Yuan acupoint and meridian acupoint from Jue-Yin Pericardium Meridian of Hand respectively, they can soothe one's mood and calm the mind. Tongli, Shenmen are the collateral acupoint and Yuan acupoint from Shao-Yin Heart Meridian of Hand respectively, they can promote heart Yang, pacify mood and stop convulsion. Xinshu

· 179 ·

是肾之背俞穴，皆可调补心肾之阳。命门是督脉之穴，可调理及补养周身之阳气。诸穴共用，可收振奋心阳、宁心安神之效。

配穴 水肿者加水分、曲泉、阴陵泉、中极；阳虚欲脱者加膻中、气海、足三里。

方法 电热针治疗（补法）。

操作 选定穴位，常规皮肤消毒。电热针向脊柱侧斜刺心俞 0.8 寸，向脊柱侧斜刺肾俞 0.8 寸，直刺足三里 0.7 寸。然后接通电热针仪，给每个穴位 60mA 的电流量，以温热舒适或酸胀感觉为度。另配以毫针直刺内关 0.5 寸、直刺间使 0.5 寸、直刺通里 0.5 寸、直刺神门 0.4 寸、向脊椎侧斜刺厥阴俞 0.6 寸、直刺阳陵泉 0.6 寸、直刺水分 0.5 寸、直刺曲泉 0.5 寸、直刺命门 0.6 寸，均留针 40 分钟。（注：每次电热针选 6 穴，毫针选 3～4 穴。）

疗程 每天 1 次，10 次为 1 个疗程，疗程间休息 3 天。

is the Back-Shu acupoint of the heart, Jueyinshu is the Back-Shu acupoint of Pericardium, Pishu is a Back-Shu acupoint of Spleen, these acupoints all can tonify Yang of the heart and kidney. Mingmen is an acupoint of Du Channel, it can tonify and nourish Yang Qi of the whole body. The combined use of these acupoints can promote heart Yang, soothe one's mood and calm the mind.

Matching acupoints: For edema add Shuifen, Ququan, Yinlingquan, Zhongji. For Yang deficiency up to collapse add Danzhong, Qihai, Zusanli.

Method: Electrothermal acupuncture treatment (tonification).

Operations: Selecting the relevant acupoints, perform routine skin disinfection. Using electrothermal acupuncture needles, obliquely puncture towards spine into Xinshu for 0.8", Shenshu for 0.8", vertically puncture into Zusanli for 0.7". Then turn on the electrothermal acupuncture equipment, apply a current of 60mA to each acupoint, and the limit is that the patient feels partial warm or sore and swollen as well as comfortable. Additionally, using filiform needles, vertically puncture into Neiguan for 0.5", Jianshi for 0.5", Tongli for 0.5", Shenmen for 0.4", obliquely puncture toward spine into Jueyinshu for 0.6", Yanglingquan for 0.6", Shuifen for 0.5", Ququan for 0.5", Mingmen for 0.6", leaving the needles in for 40 minutes. (Note: Each time, choose 6 acupoints for treatment with electrothermal needles and 3-4 acupoints for treatment with filiform needles.)

Therapeutic course: Once a day, 10 times for a course. Rest for 3 days between courses.

三、注意事项

1. 注意饮食宜清淡，选择富有营养又容易消化的食物，不要过咸。

2. 生活要规律，注意适当锻炼身体，坚持饭后散步，但不宜过量。

3. 预防外感，可在流感季节点按风池、足三里穴，或艾灸曲池和足三里穴，每穴10分钟，每日1次。

病毒性心肌炎

病毒性心肌炎是指外感病毒侵犯心脏后，引起心肌细胞变性坏死或心肌间质炎性改变的一种疾病。

中医认为，本病属于"心悸""怔忡""心痹"等范畴。

一、诊断及辨证要点

1. 发病多在春、秋季，男性多于女性，可见于各年龄层，成人发病年龄以20～30岁者居多。

2. 潜伏期为10天左右。临床表现不尽相同，轻者可无明显症状或有神疲乏力、气

III. Precautions

1. Have light diet, select food that abundant of nutrition and easy to digest, do not eat salty food.

2. Keep regular lifestyle, do appropriate exercises, adhere to walk after meals but do not take too much.

3. To prevent exogenous diseases, spot-press the acupoints Fengchi, Zusanli in the flu season, or apply moxibustion to Quchi and, Zusanli, or apply moxibustion to Quchi and Zusanli 10 minutes for each acupoint, once a day.

Viral Myocarditis

Viral myocarditis refers to the disease that the invasion of exogenous viruses into heart induces degeneration and necrosis of myocardial cells or inflammatory changes of myocardial matrix.

Traditional Chinese Medicine believes that this disease belongs to the range of "cardiopalmus", "palpitation", "heart obstruction".

I. Key Points for Diagnosis and Syndrome Differentiation

1. The high-occurrence season of this disease are spring and autumn, and the number of male patients are more than that of females, seen across all age ranges, the most common onset age of adults is 20-30 years old.

2. The latent period is around 10 days. The clinical manifestations vary; in slight cases there may be no obvious symptoms or manifestations like mental fatigue

短、胸闷等表现；重者可出现心悸、怔忡、头晕、四肢厥冷、面色苍白或发绀、唇指青紫、血压下降、脉结代无力或微弱等虚阳外脱等危重之象。

3. 不同程度的心功能不全，心电图异常（出现心动过速、心律不齐等临床体征）。

4. 多由素体虚弱，心阳不振或心血不足，又累积外感、外邪所致。临床上多为虚证或虚实夹杂证。

二、治疗方法

【心阳虚证】

治法　补益气血，振奋心阳。

处方　内关（PC6）、俞府（KI27）、膻中（RN17）、列缺（LU7）、厥阴俞（BL14）、心俞（BL15）、足三里（ST36）。

方义　内关是手厥阴心包经的原穴，俞府是足少阴肾经之穴，两穴可以交通心肾，宁心安神。膻中是任脉气会穴，心包之募穴，可补益气血，镇惊止悸。列缺是手太阴肺经之络穴，又通任脉，可以驱除外

and asthenia, shortness of breath, chest distress; in severe cases there may be critical symptoms like palpitation and cardiopalmus, dizziness, extremely cold limbs, pale complexion or cyanosis, cyanotic lips and fingers, decline of blood pressure, irregular and regular intermittent and weak pulse or weak and slight pulse, outward going of deficient Yang.

3. Various degrees of cardiac function insufficiency, abnormal ECG (clinical signs such as tachycardia and dysrhythmia can be seen).

4. Most are caused by body weakness, weakness of the heart Yang or insufficiency of the heart blood, plus the accumulation of exogenous infections and exogenous toxins. In clinics, most are deficiency syndromes or syndromes of intermingled deficiencies and excess.

II. Therapeutic Methods

[Syndrome of Yang Deficiency of the Heart]

Therapeutic method: Tonify Qi-blood, promote heart Yang.

Prescription: Neiguan (PC6), Shufu (KI27), Danzhong (RN17), Lieque (LU7), Jueyinshu (BL14), Xinshu (BL15), Zusanli (ST36).

Mechanism of prescription: Neiguan is a Yuan acupoint from Jue-Yin Pericardium Meridian of Hand, Shufu is an acupoint from Shao-Yin Kidney Meridian of Foot, these two can eliminate obstructions of transportation between heart and kidney, soothe one's mood and calm the mind. Danzhong is the confluent acupoint of Ren Channel and a Mu acupoint of Pericardium Merid-

邪，通调血脉。厥阴俞是心包之背俞穴，心俞是心之背俞穴，能取振奋心阳、疏通气机、宁心安神之功。足三里是足阳明胃经的合穴，可以补养气血，又能宁心。

配穴 心阳虚者加肾俞；气阴两虚者加神门、三阴交；心脉痹阻者加三阴交、膈俞。

方法 电热针治疗（温补法）。

操作 选定穴位，常规皮肤消毒。用电热针向椎体方向斜刺心俞0.8寸，向椎体方向斜刺厥阴俞0.8寸，直刺足三里0.8寸，向下斜刺大椎0.8寸，向椎体方向斜刺膈俞0.8寸。接通电热针仪，给予每个穴位60～70mA的电流量。另配以毫针直刺内关0.5寸，斜刺列缺0.5寸，斜刺俞府0.5寸，向下斜刺膻中0.5寸，均留针40分钟。

疗程 每天1次，10天为1个疗程，疗程间可以休息

ian, it can tonify Qi-blood, relieve convulsion and stop palpitation. Lieque is a collateral acupoint from Tai-Yin Lung Meridian of Hand and connected with Ren Channel, it can expel exogenous pathogenic factors, eliminate obstructions and regulate blood channels. Jueyinshu is a Back-Shu acupoint of Pericardium, Xinshu is a Back-Shu acupoint of the heart, they can promote heart Yang, soothe Qi dynamic, and calm the mind. Zusanli is a He acupoint from Yang-Ming Stomach Meridian of Foot, it can replenish Qi and nourish blood.

Matching acupoints: For deficiency of the heart Yang, add Shenshu. For deficiency of both Qi and Yang add Shenmen, Sanyinjiao. For obstruction of the heart vessel blockage stasis, add Sanyinjiao, Geshu.

Method: Electrothermal acupuncture treatment (warm tonifying).

Operations: Selecting the relevant acupoints, perform routine skin disinfection. Using electrothermal acupuncture needles, obliquely puncture toward vertebral bodies into Xinshu for 0.8", Jueyinshu for 0.8", vertically puncture into Zusanli 0.8", obliquely puncture downward into Dazhui for 0.8", obliquely puncture toward vertebral bodies into Geshu for 0.8". Turn on the electrothermal acupuncture equipment, apply a current of 60-70mA to each acupoint. Additionally, using filiform needles, vertically puncture into Neiguan for 0.5", obliquely puncture into Lieque for 0.5", Shufu for 0.5", obliquely puncture downward into Danzhong for 0.5", leaving the needles in for 40 minutes.

Therapeutic course: Once a day, 10 days as a course. Rest for 3 days between courses.

3天。

三、注意事项

1. 患者在急性期时，要注意休息；在恢复期和慢性期时，可适当进行身体锻炼，但必须注意不能过劳。

2. 在治疗期间，选择容易消化、富含维生素和蛋白质的食物。不能进餐过饱。要少食多餐。

3. 戒除烟酒嗜好。

心律失常

心律失常，又称心律不齐、心律紊乱，是指心脏冲动的起源和节律、传递顺序及冲动在心脏各部位的传导中任何一个环节发生异常者。

中医认为，本病属于"心悸""怔忡"等范畴。有的文献以迟脉、数脉、促脉、结脉、代脉等名之。综其病因为：情志失常、肝失疏泄、血行日趋障碍等，病发于心。

一、诊断及辨证要点

1. 心气虚者，症见心悸，

III. Precautions

1. Patients should pay attention to rest during the acute period. They can do appropriate exercises during the recovery period and the chronic period, but must not overstrain their bodies.

2. During treatment, choose food that is easy to digest, abundant of vitamins and proteins. Do not eat until too full. Have more meals a day but less food at each.

3. Quit smoking and drinking.

Arrhythmia

Arrhythmia, also called dysrhythmia or cardiac arrhythmia, refers to abnormalities of cardiac impulse origin and rhythm, transfer order and impulse that occur at any link during conduction between various cardiac parts.

Traditional Chinese Medicine believes that this disease belongs to the range of "cardiopalmus", "palpitation". In some literatures it is named as delay pulse, rapid pulse, abrupt pulse, irregularly intermittent pulse, and regularly intermittent pulse. Etiology: Emotional disorders, loss of liver soothing and dredging, increasing disorders of blood circulation, and leading to diseases originated from the heart.

I. Key Points for Diagnosis and Syndrome Differentiation

1. For patients with deficiency of the heart Qi,

气短乏力，活动后尤甚，胸闷气短，疲倦自汗，面色白，舌苔薄白，脉细弱。

2. 心阴虚者，症见心悸怔忡，失眠健忘，五心烦热，咽干舌燥，时有汗出，舌红少津，脉细数。

3. 心阳虚者，症见心悸，心中常惕惕而动，心胸发闷，形寒肢冷，自汗，乏力，舌苔薄白或舌体胖嫩，脉细数或结代。

4. 心脉瘀阻者，症见心悸气短，心前区疼痛或不适，或痛及肩背，或痛引上臂内侧，口唇、面色、指甲青紫，舌质黯红，舌边有瘀斑，脉涩或沉弦而缓或结代。

二、治疗方法

【气滞血瘀】

治法 调整气机，活血止痛。

处方 心俞（BL15）、内关（PC6）、神门（HT7）。

方义 心俞是心经之气输

symptoms include palpitation, shortness of breath and asthenia which aggravates after exercises, chest distress and shortness of breath, fatigue and spontaneous sweating, pale complexion, thin and whitish tongue fur, thin and weak pulse.

2. For patients with deficiency of the heart Yin, symptoms include palpitation and cardiopalmus, insomnia and amnesia, dysphoria in chest with palms-soles, dry throat and tongue, sweating from time to time, red tongue and less fluid, thin and rapid pulse.

3. For patients with deficiency of the heart Yang, symptoms include palpitation, perturbing, distress of chest, cold body and limbs, spontaneous sweating, asthenia, thin and whitish tongue fur or fat and tender tongue, thin and rapid or irregular and regular intermittent pulse.

4. For patients with obstruction of the heart channels, symptoms include palpitation and shortness of breath, pain or discomfort of precordium, or pain radiated to the shoulder and back, or pain radiated to the interior upper arms, purple lips, complexion and fingernails, dark red tongue with ecchymosis on the edge, uneven pulse or deep, taut and slow pulse, or irregular and regular intermittent pulse.

II. Therapeutic Methods

[Qi Stagnation and Blood Stasis]

Therapeutic method: Regulate Qi Dynamic, activate blood and alleviate pain.

Prescription: Xinshu (BL15), Neiguan (PC6), Shenmen (HT7).

Mechanism of prescription: Xinshu is the acu-

注于背部的腧穴，是治疗心脏病的主要穴位。内关是八脉交会穴之一，属心包经，有调整气机、活血止痛的作用，被称为"心宝""冠心病救星"。神门是心经的原穴，有宁心神的作用。针刺温补上述三穴，可以调气活血，抚心宽胸，使心悸、脉结代能得到缓解。

配穴 心气虚者加膻中、列缺；心阴虚者加三阴交、太冲；心阳虚者加素髎、大椎、关元；心血瘀阻者加膈俞、膻中；期前收缩（早搏）者加三阴交；心动过速者加足三里；心动过缓者加素髎、通里；房颤者加膻中、曲池；高血压者加曲池、风池；心绞痛者加神堂、膻中。

方法 电热针治疗（温补法）。

操作 选择穴位，常规皮肤消毒。用电热针向椎体方向斜刺心俞、膈俞各0.8寸，直刺足三里、三阴交各0.7寸，直刺关元0.7寸，直刺曲池0.8寸。接通电热针仪，分别给予

point located on the back, into where the Qi of the Heart Meridian infuses, it is the main acupoint for treatment of the heart diseases. Neiguan is one of the confluent acupoints of eight Channels and belongs to Pericardium Meridian, it can regulate Qi Dynamic, activate blood and alleviate pain, therefore this acupoint is called as "treasure for heart", "savior for coronary heart diseases". Shenmen is a Yuan acupoint of the Heart Meridian, it can tranquillize heart and mind. Needle acupuncture with the method of warm tonification on the three acupoints above can regulate Qi and activate blood, pacify mood and relieve chest stuffiness, so as to relieve palpitation, irregular and regular intermittent pulse.

Matching acupoints: For deficiency of the heart Qi add Danzhong, Lieque; For deficiency of the heart Yin add Sanyinjiao, Taichong. For deficiency of the heart Yang add Suliao, Dazhui, Guanyuan. For heart blood obstruction add Geshu, Danzhong. For ventricular premature contraction (premature beat) add Sanyinjiao. For tachycardia add Zusanli. For bradycardia add Suliao, Tongli. For atrial fibrillation add Danzhong, Quchi; For high blood pressure, add Quchi, Fengchi. For angina add Shentang, Danzhong.

Method: Electrothermal acupuncture treatment (warm tonifying).

Operations: Selecting the relevant acupoints, perform routine skin disinfection. Using electrothermal acupuncture needles, obliquely puncture toward vertebral bodies into Xinshu and Geshu for 0.8" respectively, vertically puncture into Zusanli, Sanyinjiao for 0.7", Guanyuan for 0.7", Quchi for 0.8". Turn on the electro-

每个穴位 60～65mA 的电流量。另配以毫针直刺内关 0.5 寸，直刺神门 0.4 寸，斜刺膻中、列缺各 0.5 寸，直刺通里 0.4 寸，斜刺神堂 0.5 寸，斜刺素髎 0.3 寸，均留针 40 分钟。

疗程 每天 1 次，10 次为 1 个疗程，疗程间可休息 3 天。

三、注意事项

1. 稳定情绪，坚定治疗信心，这是取得治疗效果的关键。

2. 严重心律失常者，要配合药物综合治疗，亦求以根治为要。

3. 要求患者配合治疗，生活要有规律，心态平衡，注意劳逸结合，必须休息治疗。

4. 饮食宜清淡，合理饮食，进餐不宜过饱，要少食多餐。

5. 忌烟酒嗜好。

心脏神经官能症

心脏神经官能症，又称心血管神经官能症，是心血管系统功能失调的一种病症。临床

---

thermal acupuncture equipment, apply a current of 60-65mA to each acupoint. Additionally, using filiform needles, vertically puncture into Neiguan for 0.5", Shenmen for 0.4", obliquely puncture into Danzhong and Lieque for 0.5" respectively, vertically puncture into Tongli for 0.4", obliquely puncture into Shentang for 0.5", obliquely puncture into Suliao for 0.3", leaving the needles in for 40 minutes.

Therapeutic course: Once a day, 10 times for a course. Rest for 3 days between courses.

III. Precautions

1. Stabilize mood and firm confidence in treatment, which is the key to achieve good efficacies.

2. For patients with severe arrhythmia, it is required to apply medication as well, and the key point is radical cure.

3. Ask patients to cooperate with the treatment, keep regular lifestyle and mental balance, pay attention to alternate work with rest, and must have rest to receive treatment.

4. Have light and reasonable diet, do not eat too much, have more meals a day but less food at each.

5. Quit smoking and drinking.

Cardiac Neurosis

Cardiac neurosis, also called cardiovascular neurosis, is a kind of cardiovascular system dysfunctions. Main clinical manifestations include dyspnea (sighing

表现以呼吸困难（呈叹息样呼吸）、心悸、疲倦、心前区隐痛、眩晕等为主症。多因劳累和精神紧张等因素而加重，同时并发其他系统的神经官能症。

中医认为，本病与"心悸""怔忡"等相似。特点是时作时止，时轻时重。思虑过度、经常生气的人易发此病。病位在心，但与肝气不舒、脾气不充有关。

一、诊断及辨证要点

1. 虚者，症见心悸怔忡，气短胸闷，自汗，疲乏无力，舌质淡嫩，苔薄白，脉细沉。

2. 心血不足者，兼见头晕、目眩、健忘、失眠。

3. 阴火虚旺者，兼见面色苍白、畏寒肢冷。

4. 实者，症见心悸怔忡，受惊易发作，心烦易怒，口干口苦，便秘，尿赤，舌苔黄腻，脉滑弦或滑数。

respiration), palpitation, fatigue, dyspnea in the precordium, vertigo. Most will aggravate due to factors like fatigue and psychentonia, while simultaneously occur neurosis of other systems.

Traditional Chinese Medicine believes that this disease is similar to "cardiopalmus", "palpitation". The feature is intermittent attack, and varying severities. Patients who worry beyond measure and often get angry are vulnerable to this disease. The lesion location is heart, but the disease is associated with obstruction of liver Qi and insufficiency of the spleen Qi.

I. Key Points for Diagnosis and Syndrome Differentiation

1. For patients with deficiency, symptoms include palpitation and cardiopalmus, shortness of breath and chest distress, spontaneous sweating, fatigue and asthenia, light and tender tongue with thin and whitish fur, thin, and deep pulse.

2. For patients with heart blood insufficiency, there also are symptoms like dizziness, vertigo, amnesia, and insomnia.

3. For patients with deficient exuberance of Yin Fire, there are also symptoms like pale complexion, intolerance of cold and extreme chilliness.

4. For patients with excess syndrome, symptoms include palpitation and cardiopalmus which are easy to attack after being frightened, vexation and irritability, dry and bitter mouth, constipation, yellow and greasy tongue

fur, slippery and taut or slippery and rapid pulse.

二、治疗方法

【虚证】

治法 养血益气，定悸安神。

处方 心俞（BL15）、内关（PC6）、间使（PC5）、神门（HT7）。

方义 心悸多为虚证，病位在心，故取心经背部之腧穴，取心俞以宁心安神；内关是心包经之络穴，可防治心血管系统的疾病；间使是心包经之经穴，是主治心悸、心痛的常用穴；神门是心经之原穴，是防治心脏病的保健穴之一。四穴配伍，有调整心脏阴阳，使其趋于平衡并增强心气的作用。

配穴 气血不足者加膈俞、脾俞、足三里、三阴交；阴虚火旺者加太溪、复溜、肾俞、太冲；心阳虚弱者加关元、气海。

方法 电热针治疗（温补法）。

操作 选定穴位，常规皮肤消毒。用电热针向椎体方向

II. Therapeutic Methods

[Deficiency syndromes]

Therapeutic method: Nourish blood and tonify Qi, calm down palpitation, and pacify mind.

Prescription: Xinshu(BL15), Neiguan(PC6), Jianshi(PC5), Shenmen (HT7).

Mechanism of prescription: Most of palpitation cases are deficiency syndromes, the lesion location is in the heart, so use the acupoint Xinshu on the back, which from Heart Meridian, to soothe one's mood and calm the mind; Neiguan is a collateral acupoint from Pericardium Meridian, can prevent and treat disease of cardiovascular system; Jianshi is a meridian acupoint from Pericardium Meridian, is a commonly used acupoint for treatment of palpitation and heart pains; Shenmen is a Yuan acupoint from Heart Meridian, it is one of the care acupoints for prophylaxis and treatment of cardiac diseases. The match of these four acupoint can regulate Yin-Yang balance of the heart and strengthen heart Qi.

Matching acupoint: For Qi-blood insufficiency add Geshu, Pishu, Zusanli, Sanyinjiao. For Yin deficiency and Fire exuberance, add Taixi, Fuliu, Shenshu, Taichong. For deficiency and weakness of the heart Yang add Guanyuan, Qihai.

Method: Electrothermal acupuncture treatment (warm tonifying).

Operations: Selecting the relevant acupoints, perform routine skin disinfection. Using electrothermal acu-

斜刺心俞、膈俞、脾俞、肾俞各 0.8 寸，直刺足三里 0.8 寸，直刺三阴交 0.7 寸，直刺复溜 0.7 寸，直刺关元、气海各 0.8 寸，直刺间使 0.7 寸。接通电热针仪，给予每个穴位 60～80mA 的电流量。另配以毫针直刺内关 0.6 寸，直刺太冲、太溪各 0.5 寸，直刺神门 0.4 寸，均留针 40 分钟。

疗程 每日 1 次，10 次为 1 个疗程。疗程间可休息 3 天，再进行第 2 个疗程的治疗。

【实证】

治法 宽胸理气，化痰安神。

处方 心俞（BL15）、丰隆（ST40）、神道（DU11）、郄门（PC4）。

方义 取心俞以安神；丰隆是足阳明胃经的络穴，有化痰祛湿之效；神道是络穴，有治疗心悸、心痛之长；郄门是心包经的郄穴，有防治心脏病之功能。诸穴共用，可奏化痰安神之功效。

配穴 口苦者加尺泽、胆俞；便秘者加足三里、天枢；心烦易怒者加肝俞、太溪、百会。

puncture needles, obliquely puncture toward vertebral bodies into Xinshu, Geshu, Pishu, Shenshu for 0.8" respectively, vertically puncture into Zusanli for 0.8", Sanyinjiao and Fuliu for 0.7", vertically puncture into Guanyuan, Qihai for 0.8" respectively, Jianshi for 0.7". Turn on the electrothermal acupuncture equipment, apply a current of 60-80mA to each acupoint. Additionally, using filiform needles, vertically puncture into Neiguan for 0.6", vertically puncture into Taichong and Taixi for 0.5" respectively, Shenmen for 0.4", leaving the needles in for 40 minutes.

Therapeutic course: Once a day, 10 times for a course. Start the treatment for the second course after a break of 3 days.

[Excess Syndrome]

Therapeutic method: Relieve chest distress and regulate Qi, disperse phlegm and tranquillize mind.

Prescription: Xinshu (BL15), Fenglong (ST40), Shendao (DU11), Ximen (PC4).

Mechanism of prescription: Use Xinshu to tranquillize mind; Fenglong is a collateral acupoint from Yang-Ming Stomach Meridian of Foot, it can disperse phlegm and remove Damp; Shendao is a collateral acupoint, it can treat palpitation and heart pains; Ximen is a Xi acupoint from Pericardium Meridian, it is effective in prophylaxis and treatment of cardiac diseases. The combined use of these acupoints can disperse phlegm and tranquillize mind.

Matching acupoints: For bitter mouth add Chize, Danshu. For constipation add Zusanli, Tianshu. For vexation and irritability add Ganshu, Taixi, Baihui.

方法 毫针治疗（泻法）。

操作 选定穴位，常规皮肤消毒。用毫针向椎体方向斜刺心俞、神道、胆俞、肝俞，每个穴位分别刺入 0.8 寸，直刺丰隆、足三里、三阴交各 0.7 寸，直刺天枢 0.8 寸，直刺郄门 0.8 寸，平刺百会 0.5 寸，直刺太溪 0.4 寸，均留针 30 分钟。

疗程 每日 1 次，10 次为 1 个疗程。

三、注意事项

对器质性心脏病引起的心律不齐，若针治效果欠佳时，一定要配合中、西药物治疗。

四、典型病例

李某，女，51 岁，技术员，北京人。

主诉：胸闷、气短、心悸不安、失眠健忘已有 3 年之久，近日加重。病史：患者退休后，因思虑过度，继而出现心悸不安，失眠健忘，时有纳少胸闷，头晕乏力，气短多汗，经多家医院诊治始终不愈。

Method: Filiform needle acupuncture treatment (attenuating).

Operations: Selecting the relevant acupoints, perform routine skin disinfection. Using filiform needles, obliquely puncture toward vertebral bodies into Xinshu, Shendao, Danshu, Ganshu for 0.8" respectively, vertically puncture into Fenglong, Zusanli, Sanyinjiao for 0.7" respectively, vertically puncture into Tianshu for 0.8", Ximen for 0.8", horizontally puncture into Baihui for 0.5", vertically puncture into Taixi for 0.4", leaving the needles in for 30 minutes.

Therapeutic course: Once a day, 10 times for a course.

III. Precautions

For dysrhythmia caused by organic heart diseases, if the efficacies of acupuncture treatment are poor, then the treatment must be done in combination with Chinese Herb Medicine and Western Medicine treatments.

IV. Typical Case

Li, female, 51 years old, technician, residence: Beijing.

Self-reported symptoms: Chest distress and shortness of breath, palpitation and disturbance, insomnia and amnesia for 3 years, which aggravated recently. Medical history: After retirement, due to worry beyond measure, the patient suffered from palpitation and disturbance, insomnia and amnesia, poor appetite and chest distress from time to time, dizziness and asthenia, shortness of breath and hydrosis, and she was not cured after diagno-

刻下症：心慌失眠，胸闷气短，面色白，头晕乏力，纳少，二便通畅，舌质淡，苔白，脉细涩。

查体：二尖瓣区及主动脉瓣第二听诊区闻及二级收缩期杂音。

辅助检查：未见异常。

【诊断依据】

1. 中年女性，处于阴阳失调之际。

2. 退休在家，突然脱离群体，感到孤独、失落，思虑过度，情绪低落。

3. 既往无特殊病史记载。

【证治分析】

病因　心脾两虚。

病机　因思虑过度，劳伤心脾，使气血生化不足，心血耗伤，渐至心失所养，发为心悸。

证候分析　脾失运化之权，气血化源不足，故纳少胸闷，头晕乏力，气短易汗。心血不足，则心悸。神明失养，神不守舍，则失眠健忘。心其华在面，气血虚，故面色白，舌淡红，脉细弱。

sis and treatment by several hospitals.

Current symptoms: Palpitation and insomnia, chest distress and shortness of breath, pale complexion, dizziness and asthenia, less food intake, smooth urination and defecation, light tongue with white fur, thin and uneven pulse.

Physical examination: Grade 2 systolic noise at mitral valve area and second aortic valve area.

Auxiliary examination: No abnormalities.

[Diagnostic Basis]

1. Middle-aged female, in the period that Yin and Yang disharmony.

2. Retied at home, suddenly left group, felt lonely, lost, worried too much beyond measure, down in spirits.

3. No previous recorded special medical history.

[Syndrome-treatment Analysis]

Etiology: Deficiency of the heart and spleen.

Pathogenesis: Deeply worried, impairment of the heart and spleen, led to insufficiency of Qi-blood generation and transformation, consumption and impairment of the heart blood, gradually led to nourishment loss of the heart and presented as palpation.

Syndrome analysis: Spleen lost the governance on transportation and transformation, the transportation source of Qi-blood was insufficient, therefore caused less food intake and chest distress from time to time, dizziness and asthenia, shortness of breath and hydrosis. heart blood deficiency causes palpitation. Nourishment loss of mind and consciousness, mind loosing, caused insomnia and amnesia. The prosperity of the heart is presented at the face, therefore deficiency of Qi-blood caused pale complexion, light and red tongue as well as thin and weak pulse.

病位 心、脾。

病性 气血虚。

西医诊断 心脏神经官能症。

中医诊断 心脾两虚型心悸。

治法 养血益气,定悸安神。

方法 电热针治疗。

处方 以足阳明胃经穴、背俞穴为主。心俞（BL15）、膈俞（BL17）、脾俞（BL20）、巨阙（RN14）、足三里（ST36）。

方义 心俞、巨阙为俞募配穴,功在调补心气,定悸安神;血之会膈俞可补血养心;气血之生成,赖水谷精微所化,故取脾俞、足三里健中焦以助气血化生。

配穴 腹胀、便溏者加上巨虚、天枢；心气虚者加膻中、列缺。

操作 选定穴位,皮肤常规消毒。电热针斜刺（针尖向脊柱）心俞、膈俞、脾俞各

Lesion location: Heart, spleen.

Disease nature: Deficiency of Qi-blood.

The diagnosis of Western Medicine: Cardiac neurosis.

The diagnosis of Traditional Chinese Medicine: Palpitation with deficiency of the heart and spleen.

Therapeutic method: Nourish blood and tonify Qi, calm down palpitation and pacify mind.

Method: Electrothermal acupuncture treatment.

The prescription focused on meridian acupoints and Back-Shu acupoints from Yang-Ming Stomach Meridian of Foot. Xinshu(BL15), Geshu (BL17), Pishu (BL20), Juque (RN14), Zusanli (ST36).

Mechanism of prescription: Xinshu and Juque are use for the method of Shu-Mu acupoints combination, their effects are to tonify heart Qi, calm down palpitation and pacify mind; the confluent acupoint of blood, Geshu, can replenish blood and nourish heart, the generation of Qi-blood is the transformation of food essence, so use Pishu, Zusanli to reinforce Middle Jiao, so as to promote transformation and generation of Qi-blood.

Matching acupoints: For abdominal distension and sloppy stool add Juxu, Tianshu. For deficiency of the heart Qi, add Danzhong, Lieque.

Operations: Selecting the relevant acupoints, perform routine skin disinfection. Using electrothermal acupuncture needles, obliquely puncture (with the needle

0.8寸，直刺足三里、上巨虚、天枢各0.7寸，平刺膻中、列缺各0.7寸，接通电热针仪，每个穴位分别给予50mA的电流量，留针40分钟。（注：每次选3组穴轮流交替应用。）

疗程 每日1次，20次为1个疗程，疗程间如无不适，可连续治疗2个疗程，或者休息7天再进行治疗。

治疗过程 该患者治疗过程中，疗效较好，针治20次后症状基本消失，又巩固治疗1个疗程。

【生活调摄】

1. 稳定患者情绪，回避忧思，注意调和情志。

2. 本病针灸疗效好，不但能减轻和控制症状，而且完全可以治愈。

慢性胃炎

慢性胃炎是以胃黏膜的特异性慢性炎症为主要病理变化的常见病。其发病原因与免疫因素或幽门括约肌舒缩功能紊乱及胆汁返流有关。急性胃炎反复发作，可以引发慢性胃炎。本病可分为浅表性胃炎、

tip towards spine) into Xinshu, Geshu, Pishu for 0.8" respectively, vertically puncture into Zusanli, Shangjuxu, Dianshu for 0.7" respectively, horizontally puncture into Danzhong, Lieque for 0.7" respectively. Turn on the electrothermal acupuncture equipment, apply a current of 50mA to each acupoint, leaving the needles in for 40 minutes. (Note: select 3 pairs of acupoints each time, and use alternately.)

Therapeutic course: Treat once a day, 20 times for a course, and if no discomfort, perform 2 continuous courses, or continue the treatment after 7-day rest.

Therapeutic course: The patient got relatively good efficacies during treatment, and the symptoms basically disappeared after 20 times of treatment, and the patient received another 1 treatment course to consolidate the efficiency.

[Lifestyle Change and Health Maintenance]

1. Stabilize patient emotion, avoid worries and sorrow, pay attention to regulate mood.

2. The acupuncture treatment has good efficacies for this disease. It can not only relieve and control the symptoms, but also completely cure the disease.

Chronic Gastritis

Chronic gastritis is a common disease that its main pathogenic change is specific chronic inflammation of gastric mucosa. Its causes are associated with immune factors or contraction and relaxation dysfunction of pyloric sphincter and bile reflex. The repeated onset of acute gastritis can induce chronic gastritis. This disease can be divided into 4 types: superficial gastritis, atrophic

萎缩性胃炎、糜烂性胃炎及肥厚性胃炎4种（型）。临床以浅表性胃炎为多见，浅表性胃炎可以转变成萎缩性胃炎，或与萎缩性胃炎并存。

本病发病率随年龄的增长而增高，根据统计，青年人发病率占20%，而60岁以上的老人则为57%～80%。其萎缩性改变、肠上皮化和非典型性增生等病理改变可以恶变，又称为癌前病变，因而引起人们的广泛重视。

慢性胃炎患者，临床有消化不良、上腹部灼痛、胀痛或隐痛、食欲不振、恶心嗳气等症状，可间歇出现或长期存在。胃出血者可有吐血或柏油便（柏油样黑便）。

中医认为，本病属于"胃脘痛""胃痞"等范畴。多因饮食不节，情志失调，劳倦过度，久病体弱所致。其发病与脾、胃、肝等脏腑功能失调有关。由于本病病程较长，易于反复，故表现出虚实相兼、寒热夹杂等复杂证候。临床可分为肝胃不和、脾胃虚寒、胃阴不足3种证型。

gastritis, erosive gastritis and hypertrophic gastritis. Superficial gastritis is more common clinically, and superficial gastritis can change into atrophic gastritis or coexist with atrophic gastritis.

The incidence rate of this disease increases with age. According to the statistics, the incidence of young people accounts for 20%, while that of the elderly over 60 years old is 57% to 80%. The pathogenic changes of this disease, like atrophic changes, intestinal metaplasia and atypical hyperplasia, can undergo malignant transformation, which also called precancerous lesions, therefore it should attract wide attention.

For patients with chronic gastritis, clinical symptoms include dyspepsia, burning-like pain, swelling pain or dull pain of the upper abdomen, poor appetite, nausea and blenching, which can occur intermittently or exist persistently. For patients with gastrorrhagia there may be hematemesis or tarry stool (asphalt-like black stool).

Traditional Chinese Medicine believes that this disease belongs to the range of "epigastric pain", "stomach fullness". Most likely it is caused by intemperate diet, emotional disorders, overfatigue, weak body due to long-term disease. Its incidence is associated with dysfunctions of organs like spleen, stomach, liver. Since this disease has a relatively long course and is easy to reoccur, therefore it presents complex syndromes like intermingled deficiency and excess, intermingled Cold and Heat. It can be divided into 3 syndrome types clinically: disharmony between spleen and stomach, deficiency-Cold of the spleen and stomach, stomach Yin insufficiency.

一、诊断及辨证要点

1. 肝胃不和者,症见胃脘胀痛,痛连两胁,纳差嗳气,呃逆酸苦,大便不畅,每因情绪不畅而痛作,苔多薄白,脉弦。

2. 脾胃虚寒者,症见胃脘部隐隐作痛,神疲乏力,四肢欠温,纳食减少,大便溏薄,舌质淡,苔白腻,脉虚弱。

3. 胃阴不足者,症见胃脘灼痛,口燥咽干,纳差嘈杂,手足烦热,大便干结,舌红少津,脉细数。

4. 胃镜检查可明确诊断。

(1) 浅表性胃炎。根据胃镜所见,可以分为单纯、糜烂和出血3型,主要表现为:①黏膜水肿,斑点状充血和细微的红白相间;②黏膜皱裂,顶端浅样充血;③条片状灰白色稠液黏附于黏膜表面,不易脱落;④黏膜斑点状充血或糜烂。以③④两项对诊断较为可靠。病变多以弥漫性分布,多

I. Key Points for Diagnosis and Syndrome Differentiation

1. For patients with disharmony between spleen and stomach, symptoms include epigastric swelling pain which radiates to the two side of ribs, poor appetite and blenching, sour and bitter hiccoughing, unsmooth defecation, the pain often onset due to bad mood, excessive and thin and white tongue fur, taut pulse.

2. For patients with deficiency-Cold of the spleen and stomach, symptoms include epigastric dull pain, mental fatigue and asthenia, cold limbs, reduced food intake, sloppy and thin stool, light tongue with white and greasy fur, weak pulse.

3. For patients with stomach Yin insufficiency, symptoms include epigastric burning-like pain, dry mouth and throat, poor appetite and noise, restless heat of hands and feet, dry and hard stool, red tongue with less fluid, thin and rapid pulse.

4. The disease can be definitely diagnosed by gastroscopy examination

(1) Superficial gastritis: according to what is seen in the gastroscopy exam, it can be divided into 3 types, simple, erosive and hemorrhagic ones, the main manifestations include: ① edema, mottled congestion and slight checked pattern with red and white of the mucosa; ② mucosa fissure, shallow congestion on the top; ③ strip-like gray thick liquid attaches to the mucosal surface, which is hard to peel off; ④ spotted congestion or erosion of the mucosa. ③ and ④ are relatively reliable in the diagnosis. Most lesions show diffuse distributions,

发于胃窦部。组织活检发现病变浅表，淋巴细胞和炎细胞的浸润大多限于胃小凹水平以上的浅层固有膜，有时也可以遍及黏膜全层；上皮有变性、再生、增生等变化，肠上皮化生不多见，腺体一般正常，黏膜厚度正常。

（2）慢性萎缩性胃炎和胃萎缩。在镜下可见的主要表现：①失去正常黏膜的橘红色，代以苍灰色，且色调不均匀；②黏膜呈现明显的红白相间，有较大片的苍白区；③黏膜皱襞细小，甚至平坦，反光度增强，黏膜下血管显露；④有时可见散在不规则的颗粒或结节，为增生性改变；⑤杂以浅表糜烂或出血。以上表现常呈局限（灶）性分布，其周围黏膜常有浅表性胃炎的改变。根据萎缩与浅表性改变程度不同又有浅表萎缩性胃炎与萎缩浅表性胃炎之别。或组织检查发现黏膜层有炎性及纤维化，腺体广泛破坏，腺体损失半数以上，出现肠上皮化生或假幽门腺化生。黏膜层变薄，黏膜肌层增厚。有时可合并腺窦增生而使黏膜层变厚，称为"过

and most are originated from the gastric antrum. Tissue biopsy showed superficial lesions, and lymphocyte and inflammatory cell infiltration is limited to the superficial inherent membrane above the level of gastric pit, sometimes the infiltration may distribute across the whole mucosal layer. There are changes of degeneration, regeneration, hyperplasia in the epithelium, and intestinal metaplasia is not common, while glands generally are normal, the thickness of the mucosa is normal.

(2) Chronic atrophic gastritis and lipogastry: main manifestations can be seen under the gastroscopy: ① the orange color of normal mucosa is replaced by the color of gray, and the tone is not even; ② the mucosa shows obvious pattern of red alternating with white, with large area of pale region; ③ the duplicature becomes thinner or even flat, the reflectance increases, the submucosal blood vessels expose; ④ sometimes scattered irregular particles or nodules can be seen, which are proliferative changes; ⑤ mixing with superficial erosion or bleeding. The above symptoms normally distribute locally, and there often are changes of superficial gastritis in the surrounding mucosa. According to the different degrees of atrophic and superficial changes, it is again divided into superficial gastritis and atrophic superficial gastritis. Or in the tissue biopsy it is found that there are inflammation and fibrillation in the mucosal layer, extensive damage of glands, and more than a half of the glands are lost, there is intestinal metaplasia or pseudopyloric metaplasia. The mucosal layer becomes thinner and the muscular layer of mucosa becomes thicker. Sometimes there also occurs sinus-gland proliferation which makes the mucosa thicker,

形成"，萎缩性胃炎进一步发展成为胃黏膜萎缩时，黏膜内炎症浸润几乎消失，胃固有腺体明显萎缩，甚至消失，并且被修复后的纤维组织和残存的其他间质成分所代替。

（3）慢性糜烂性胃炎（黏膜糜烂）：在胃镜下可分为2型。①持续型：呈乳头状隆起，为慢性增殖性病变，可3～5年不消退，或发展成为有蒂息肉，又称疣状胃炎；②消失型：为炎性渗出性病变，一般数月内消退。主要表现为胃炎黏膜区出现多个疣状、膨大皱襞状或丘疹样隆起，直径5～10mm，顶端可见黏膜缺损或脐样凹陷，中心部有糜烂；隆起周围多无红晕，但常伴有大小相仿的红斑。以上病变多分布于胃窦部。持续型胃炎黏膜隆起较多，中央凹陷小；消失型则隆起不明显，中央凹陷小而面积较大。形态上应与息肉和Ⅱa+c型早期胃癌鉴别。

（4）肥厚性胃炎（胃黏膜皱裂肥厚）："肥厚性胃炎"是胃镜下的诊断，在组织病理学上并无黏膜及上皮细胞的肥大性改变。胃镜下的表现有：①皱襞隆起处柔软、圆钝、光

called "peramorphosis". When the atrophic gastritis develops further into atrophy of gastric mucosa, the inflammatory infiltration within the mucosa almost disappears, the inherent glands in the stomach atrophy obviously or even disappear, and are replaced by repaired fibrous tissues or remaining other stromal components.

(3) Chronic erosive gastritis (mucosal erosion): under the gastroscopy it can be divided into two types. ① persistent type: it is a chronic proliferative lesion which shows papillary uplift, and it may not subside for 3-5 years or develops into the polyp with stem, also called verrucous gastritis; ② disappearing type: it is a kind of inflammatory exudative lesions, which may subside within several months. The main manifestations include: several verrucous, swollen folds or papuloid uplifts with a diameter of 5-10mm, and mucosa defects or notch-like pit on the top as well as erosion in the center can be seen; normally there is no flush but erythema with similar size around the uplift. Most of the above lesions are located in the gastric antrum. Persistent uplifts are more common, the center pit is small. The uplift in the cases of disappearing type is not obvious, while the center pit is small but the area is big. It should be identified from polypus and Ⅱa+c early gastric cancer.

(4) Hypertrophic gastritis (hypertrophy of gastric mucosal folds): "hypertrophic gastritis" is the diagnosis made under the gastroscopy, and there are no hypertrophic changes of mucosa and epithelial cells in the respect of histopathology. The manifestations seen under the gastroscopy include: ① the uplifted part of folds are

滑，呈铺路形状，脑回状或海绵结节状，正常充气下并不消失；②皱襞顶部可有充血、糜烂和出血；③皱襞之间的间隙狭小，呈龟裂状；④间隙凹陷处可有较多清淡黏膜附着。

胃镜下见到的皱襞粗大有以下几种情况：①十二指肠球部溃疡活动期：高胃酸分泌和胃壁肌层紧张度增加，以致皱襞粗大，多于溃疡活动期后消失；②胃泌素病：胃黏膜增粗及皱襞粗大的发生与大量胃泌素的积放和高胃酸分泌状态有关；③胃巨皱襞症（Menetrier病）：此为一种原因不明的常见病，其黏膜皱襞肥大只限于黏膜，且以胃体部大弯较为显著。

二、治疗方法

【脾胃不和证】

治法　疏肝和胃，降逆止呕。

处方　中脘（RN12）、足三里（ST36）、期门（LR14）、内关（PC6）、阳陵泉（GB34）。

方义　取胃之募穴中脘，胃之合穴足三里，以疏通胃气

soft, rounded, smooth, and are like pavements, gyrus or sponge nodules, and do not disappear with normal inflation; ② there may be congestion, erosion and bleeding at the top of folds; ③ the gaps between folds are narrow and ramous; ④ there may be more clear and light mucosa attached at the recess of the gaps.

The hypertrophy of gastric folds under the gastroscopy are as followed: ① the active period of the ulcers at the duodenal bulb: the high gastric acid secretion and the increased tension of the gastric muscular layers cause the hypertrophy of folds, most of which disappear after the active period of the ulcers; ② gastrin diseases: the incidence of hypertrophy of gastric mucosa and folds is associated with the accumulation and release of large amount of gastrin and high gastric acid secretion status; ③ giant gastric folds disease (Menetrier's disease): this is a common disease with causes unknown, and its hypertrophic mucosal folds are only limited within the mucosa, and is most obvious at the greater curvature of stomach.

II. Therapeutic Methods

[Syndrome of Disharmony Between Spleen and Stomach]

Therapeutic method: Soothe the liver and harmonize the stomach, reduce negative energy and stop vomiting.

Prescription: Zhongwan (RN12), Zusanli (ST36), Qimen (LR14), Neiguan (PC6), Yanglingquan (GB34).

Mechanism of prescription: Use the Mu acupoint Zhongwan from Stomach Meridian, the He acupoint

而升清降浊；取心包之络穴内关，以开胸脘之郁结，配肝之募穴期门，胆之合穴阳陵泉，以平肝胆之逆气。诸穴合用，肝得条达，胃得和降，诸症自除。

配穴 脘痞胀满加脾俞、公孙；嗳气吞酸加肝俞、胆俞、丘墟。

方法 毫针治疗（泻法）。

操作 选定穴位，皮肤常规消毒。直刺中脘 0.8 寸，直刺足三里 0.8 寸，直刺内关 0.5 寸，斜刺期门 0.5 寸，直刺阳陵泉 0.5 寸，提插泻法。

疗程 每天 1 次，留针 30 分钟，10 天后为 1 个疗程，连续治疗 5～6 个疗程。

【脾胃虚寒证】

治法 温中散寒，健脾和胃。

处方 脾俞（BL20）、胃俞（BL21）、中脘（RN12）、

Zusanli from Stomach Meridian, to soothe stomach Qi, ascend lucidity and descend turbidity. Use the collateral acupoint Neiguan from Pericardium Meridian to disperse stagnation in the chest and abdomen, and match it with the Mu acupoint Qimen from Liver Meridian, the He acupoint Yanglingquan from Gallbladder Meridian, to calm down the reversed Qi of liver and gallbladder. The combined use of these acupoints can achieve organized access of liver, harmonization and descending of stomach, then various symptoms can be resolved naturally.

Matching acupoints: For epigastric fullness and distention add Pishu, Gongsun. For belching and acid swallowing add Ganshu, Danshu, Qiuxu.

Method: Filiform needle acupuncture treatment (attenuating).

Operations: Selecting the relevant acupoints, perform routine skin disinfection. Vertically puncture into Zhongwan for 0.8", Zusanli for 0.8", Neiguan for 0.5", obliquely puncture into Qimen for 0.5", vertically puncture into Yanglingquan for 0.5", use the method of lifting-thrusting and attenuating.

Therapeutic course: Once a day, leave the needles in for 30 minutes, 10 times for a course. Treat continuously for 5-6 courses.

[Syndrome of Deficiency-Cold of Spleen and Stomach]

Therapeutic method: Warm Middle Jiao and disperse Cold, invigorate spleen and regulate stomach.

Prescription: Pishu (BL20), Weishu (BL21), Zhongwan (RN12), Zhangmen (LR13), Zusanli (ST36),

章门（LR13）、足三里（ST36）、内关（PC6）。

方义 取脾之募穴章门配脾俞，胃之募穴中脘配胃俞，以温中散寒，健脾和胃；取心包之络穴内关，胃之合穴足三里，以理气宽中，和胃止痛。诸穴合用，共奏健脾益气，温中散寒之功。

配穴 脾虚食积者加璇玑、公孙；脾虚泄泻者加天枢、大肠俞。

方法 电热针治疗（补法）。

操作 选定穴位，皮肤常规消毒。向脊柱侧斜刺脾俞0.8寸，向脊柱侧斜刺胃俞0.8寸，直刺中脘0.6寸，向前方斜刺章门0.8寸，直刺足三里0.8寸，直刺内关0.6寸，然后接通电热针仪，每个穴位给予电流量60～80mA，以温热或胀感舒适为度，留针40分钟。

疗程 每天1次，10次为1个疗程，连续治疗90天。

Neiguan (PC6).

Mechanism of prescription: Use the Mu acupoint Zhangmen of spleen to match with Pishu, use the Mu acupoint Zhongwan of the stomach to match with Weishu, so as to warm spleen and stomach for dispelling cold, invigorate spleen and harmonize stomach. Use the collateral acupoint Neiguan from Pericardium Meridian and the He acupoint Zusanli of the stomach to loosen Middle Jiao and regulate Qi, harmonize stomach and alleviate pains. The use of the combination of these acupoints can invigorate spleen and tonify Qi, warm spleen and stomach for dispelling cold.

Matching acupoints: For spleen deficiency and food accumulation add Xuanji, Gongsun. For spleen deficiency and diarrhea, add Tianshu, Dachangshu.

Method: Electrothermal acupuncture treatment (tonifying).

Operations: Selecting the relevant acupoints, perform routine skin disinfection. Obliquely puncture toward spine into Pishu for 0.8", obliquely puncture toward spine into Weishu for 0.8", vertically puncture into Zhongwan for 0.6", obliquely puncture forward into Zhangmen for 0.8", vertically puncture into Zusanli for 0.8", vertically puncture into Neiguan for 0.6". Then turn on the electrothermal acupuncture equipment, apply a current of 60-80mA to each acupoint, and the limit is that the patient feels warm or swelling and comfortable, leaving the needles in for 40 minutes.

Therapeutic course: Once a day, 10 times for a course, continuously treat for 90 days.

【胃阴不足证】

治法 养阴和胃，健脾益气。

处方 中脘（RN12）、胃俞（BL21）、幽门（KI21）、三阴交（SP6）、章门（LR13）、足三里（ST36）、太溪（KI3）。

方义 取胃之募穴中脘配胃俞，胃之合穴足三里，足三阴之交会穴三阴交，肾之募穴幽门，以健脾和胃，使脾为胃行其津液；配肝之募穴章门，以疏肝理气，和胃降逆，配胃之原穴太溪，以滋阴降火益胃。诸穴合用，共奏健胃益气，养阴和胃之功。

配穴 胃脘灼痛者加悬钟、厉兑；便血者加血海。

方法 电热针治疗（补法）。

操作 选定穴位，常规皮肤消毒。直刺中脘0.6～0.8寸，向脊柱侧斜刺胃俞0.8寸，直刺幽门0.6寸（不得深刺），直刺三阴交0.8寸，向前下方斜刺章门0.6寸；直刺足三里0.8

[Syndrome of the Stomach Yin Insufficiency]

Therapeutic method: Nourish Yin and harmonize the stomach, invigorate spleen and tonify Qi.

Prescription: Zhongwan (RN12), Weishu (BL21), Youmen (KI21), Sanyinjiao (SP6), Zhangmen (LR13), Zusanli (ST36), Taixi (KI3).

Mechanism of prescription: Use the Mu acupoint Zhongwan to match with Weishu, the He acupoint Zusanli of Stomach, the confluent acupoint Sanyinjiao of the three Yin meridians of Foot, the Mu acupoint Youmen of Stomach to invigorate spleen and harmonize the stomach, to facilitate spleen to transport fluid for stomach. Match with the Mu acupoint Zhangmen of Liver to soothe liver and regulate Qi, harmonize the stomach to reduce negative energy; match with the Yuan acupoint Taixi of the Stomach to nourish Yin, reduce Fire and tonify stomach. The use of the combination of these acupoints can invigorate stomach and tonify Qi, nourish Yin and harmonize the stomach.

Matching acupoints: For burning-like epigastric pain, add Xuanzhong, Lidui. For bloody stool add Xuehai.

Method: Electrothermal acupuncture treatment (tonifying).

Operations: Selecting the relevant acupoints, perform routine skin disinfection. Vertically puncture into Zhongwan for 0.6-0.8", obliquely puncture toward spine into Weishu for 0.8", vertically puncture into Youmen (deep puncture is forbidden) for 0.6", vertically puncture into Sanyinjiao for 0.8", obliquely puncture toward ante-

寸，然后接通电热针仪，每个穴位给予电流量 60mA，以温热或酸胀而舒服为度。另配以毫针直刺太溪 0.5 寸，留针 40 分钟。

疗程 每天 1 次，10 次为 1 个小疗程，连续治疗 90 天为 1 个大疗程，即可结束治疗。

三、注意事项

1. 慢性胃炎之胃脘部疼痛，针灸治疗一般多能立即止痛。疼痛缓解或症状消失后亦还要坚持治疗，方可收到较好的远期疗效。

2. 凡虚证、寒证或秋冬季节寒带地区患者多选用电热针治疗效果较好；实证、热证可选用毫针治疗；过饥、过饱、嗜酒者不宜选用针灸治疗。

3. 治疗期间调理饮食，食物以清淡容易消化为宜，忌辛辣、油腻、生冷、粗糙之品。

四、典型病例

马某，女，52 岁，技术员，

rior inferior direction into Zhangmen for 0.6"; vertically puncture into Zusanli for 0.8". Then turn on the electrothermal acupuncture equipment, apply a current of 60mA to each acupoint, and the limit is that the patient feels warm or sore and swollen and comfortable. Additionally, using filiform needles, vertically puncture into Taixi for 0.5", leaving the needles in for 40 minutes.

Therapeutic course: Once a day, 10 times for a course, continuous treatment for 90 days as a major course, then end the treatment.

III. Precautions

1. For epigastric pain of the chronic gastritis, pain can normally be alleviated immediately by the acupoint treatment. It is necessary to adhere to the treatment after pain relief or disappearance of symptoms, so as to get better long-term efficacies.

2. For patients with deficiency syndromes, Cold syndromes, patients that had the disease onset in the autumn and winter, or patients who are located in frigid areas, choose electrothermal acupuncture treatment to achieve better efficacies. For excess syndrome and Heat syndrome choose filiform needling treatment. For patients with over-hunger, over-satiety and drunkards, acupuncture treatment is not appropriate.

3. During treatment, regulate diet, better to have light diet and have food that easy to digest, do not eat spicy, greasy, raw, cold and rough food.

IV. Typical Case

Ma, female, 52 years old, technician, residence:

北京人。

主诉：胃脘冷痛，吐清水6个多月。病史：患者6个月前因吃冷食过量，从而胃脘冷痛，时有呕吐清水，怕冷喜暖，不渴，经过治疗亦时好时坏，不能吃冷食。

刻下症：胃脘冷痛，吃冷食后加重，得温后缓解，时有腹痛，舌淡苔白，脉细。

查体：未见异常。

辅助检查：胃镜示"慢性胃炎"。

【诊断依据】

1. 中老年女性，胃脘冷痛半年之久，不能吃冷食，经治不愈，时轻时重。

2. 胃镜证实为慢性胃炎。

3. 素体脾胃虚弱，又饮食不节，多饮寒食冷，致胃脘痛反复发作。

【证治分析】

病因 脾胃虚寒。

病机 素体脾胃虚弱，饮食不节，导致脾阳不足，中焦虚寒，胃脘失于温养。

Beijing.

Self-reported symptoms: Epigastric cold pain, vomiting clear water for more than 6 months. Medical history: 6 months ago, the patient eat too much cold food therefore suffered from epigastric cold pain and vomited clear water from time to time, was afraid of cold and preferred to warm, didn't feel thirty, and the symptoms still recurred from time to time after treatments, she couldn't eat cold food.

Current symptoms: Epigastric cold pain that was aggravated after intake of cold food while got relieved after being warmed, frequent abdominal pain, light tongue with white fur, thin pulse.

Physical examination: No abnormalities.

Auxiliary examination: Gastroscopy indicated "superficial gastritis".

[Diagnostic Basis]

1. Aged female, epigastric cold pain for a half year, unable to eat cold food, unhealed by treatment, the severity varied from time to time.

2. The chronic gastritis was confirmed by the gastroscope exam.

3. Spleen and stomach weakness plus intemperate diet and excessive intake of cold food and drinks, caused the repeated onset of the epigastric pain.

[Syndrome-treatment Analysis]

Etiology: Deficiency-Cold of the spleen and stomach.

Pathogenesis: Spleen and stomach weakness plus intemperate diet caused spleen Yang insufficiency, deficiency-Cold of Middle Jiao, loss of nourishment of the

epigastric pain part.

证候分析 脾胃虚寒，病属正虚，故胃痛绵绵，以空腹为甚，进食则缓，寒得温而散，气得按而行，故喜热喜按，脾虚中寒，水不运化而上逆，故泛吐清水，中阳不振，故神疲乏力，手足不温，舌淡，脉沉细，皆为脾胃虚弱，中阳不足之象。

Syndrome analysis: Deficiency in the Cold of the spleen and stomach, the disease belongs to the range of weakened body resistance, and therefore causes endless stomachaches. This is aggravated by an empty stomach and gets relieved after food intake. Cold will disperse with warm, Qi will moves after pressing, therefore the patient prefers to warm and pressing; deficiency-Cold of the spleen and stomach, Water cannot be transported and transformed and goes up reversely, therefore vomit clear water; weakness of Middle Yang causes mental fatigue and asthenia, cold limbs, light tongue, deep and thin pulse; all the above are symptoms of the spleen and stomach weakness, insufficiency of Middle Yang.

病位 脾、胃。

Lesion location: Spleen, stomach.

病性 虚寒。

Disease nature: Deficiency and cold.

西医诊断 慢性胃炎。

The diagnosis of Western Medicine: Chronic gastritis.

中医诊断 胃脘痛。

The diagnosis of Traditional Chinese Medicine: Epigastric pain.

治法 温中散寒，健脾和胃。

Therapeutic method: Warm Middle Jiao and disperse Cold, invigorate spleen and regulate stomach.

方法 电热针治疗。

Method: Electrothermal acupuncture treatment.

处方 脾俞（BL20）、胃俞（BL21）、中脘（RN12）、足三里（ST36）、内关（PC6）、章门（LR13）。

Prescription: Pishu (BL20), Weishu (BL21), Zhongwan (RN12), Zusanli (ST36), Neiguan (PC6), Zhangmen (LR13).

方义 取脾之募穴章门配脾俞，胃之募穴中脘配胃俞，以温中散寒，健脾和胃；取心包经之络穴内关，胃之合

Mechanism of prescription: Use the Mu acupoint Zhangmen of Spleen to match with Pishu, use the Mu acupoint Zhongwan of the Stomach to match with Weishu, so as to warm spleen and stomach for dispelling

穴足三里，以宽中理气，和胃止痛，诸穴共用，取其健脾益气，温中散寒之功能。

配穴 脾虚食积加璇玑、公孙；脾虚泄泻加天枢、大肠俞、三阴交。

操作 选定穴位，皮肤常规消毒。电热针直刺足三里、三阴交、中脘、内关各 0.7 寸，斜刺脾俞、胃俞、大肠俞、章门各 0.7 寸，然后接通电热针仪，每个穴位分别给予 50mA 的电流量，以患者感温热、胀而舒适为度，留针 40 分钟。（注：每次选取 3 组穴给予电热针治疗，交替轮流使用。其余穴位毫针治疗，每次 40 分钟。）

疗程 每日 1 次，30 次为 1 个疗程。

治疗过程 该患者在治疗过程中，效果明显，8 次后症状基本消失。因患者病程较长，故需治疗 2 个月，以达根治。经过 2 个月的治疗，胃镜复查示"浅表性胃炎"，自觉症

cold, invigorate spleen and harmonize stomach. Use the collateral acupoint Neiguan from Pericardium Meridian and the He acupoint Zusanli of the Stomach to loosen Middle Jiao and regulate Qi, harmonize stomach and alleviate pains. The combined use of these acupoints can invigorate spleen and tonify Qi, warm spleen and stomach for dispelling cold.

Matching acupoints: For spleen deficiency and food accumulation add Xuanji, Gongsun. For spleen deficiency and diarrhea add Tianshu, Dachangshu, Sanyinjiao.

Operations: Selecting the relevant acupoints, perform routine skin disinfection. Using electrothermal acupuncture needles, vertically puncture into Zusanli, Sanyinjiao, Zhongwan, Neiguan for 0.7" respectively, obliquely puncture into Pishu, Weishu, Dachangshu, Zhangmen for 0.7" respectively. Then turn on the electrothermal acupuncture equipment, apply a current of 50mA to each acupoint, and the limit is that the patient feels warm or swell and comfortable, leaving the needles in for 40 minutes. (Note: select 3 pairs of acupoints for electrothermal acupuncture treatment each time, use alternately. Treat others with filiform needles 40 minutes each time.)

Therapeutic course: Once a day, 30 times for a course.

Therapeutic process: The patient acquired obvious efficacies during the treatment, and her symptoms basically disappeared after 8 times of treatment. Since the disease course of this patient was long, so treat 2 months to affect a radical cure. After 2 months of treatment, the re-examination of gastroscopy indicated "superficial gas-

状全部消失，临床治愈出院。随访2年未见复发。

【生活调摄】

1. 注意饮食规律，节制饮食，忌食生冷、辛辣食品，注意饮食卫生。

2. 胃脘部注意保温。

3. 治疗期间，令患者保持心情舒畅并积极配合治疗，方能根治。

4. 饭后坚持散步，以助消化，锻炼身体，增强体质。

胃下垂

胃下垂是指胃的位置低于正常，甚者垂入盆腔的一种消化道疾病。胃下垂发生的原因有先天性与后天性之分。先天性胃下垂多见于先天性无力型体质，多和其他脏器如肾等同时下垂。后天性胃下垂多由于某种原因导致腹壁张力弛缓，腹压下降，胃体失去支撑而致。如妇人新产后，或大量放腹水之后，或腹腔巨大肿瘤摘除后等；也有胸廓变形或长期上肢负重而引起胃体下垂者。

中医认为，本病属于"胃

tritis", and subjective symptoms all disappeared. The patient was clinically cured and discharged from the hospital. Following the next two year, no recurrence occurred.

[Lifestyle Change and Health Maintenance]

1. Keep regular diet and control diet, do not eat raw and cold, spicy food, pay attention to diet hygiene.

2. Keep warm for stomach and abdomen area.

3. During treatment, make patients keep good mood and cooperate with treatments actively, so as to affect a radical cure.

4. Having a walk after meals to promote digestion and keep physical exercising to strengthen physique.

Gastroptosis

Gastroptosis refers to a digestive tract disease that the location of the stomach is lower than normal, or even the stomach droops into the pelvic cavity. The causes of gastroptosis are divided into congenital ones and acquired ones. Congenital gastroptosis is mostly seen in patients with congenital weakness, and normally the stomach droops down together with other organs like kidneys. For acquired gastroptosis, in most cases it's caused by that abdominal wall tension relaxation and decline of abdominal pressure due to some reasons lead to loss of support of the stomach. For example, after new delivery of women, after discharge of large amount of ascites, or after excision of large tumors in the abdominal cavity. In some cases, the gastroptosis is caused by thoracic deformity or long-term load-bearing of the upper limbs.

Traditional Chinese Medicine believes that this dis-

下""胃缓"的范畴。多见于先天禀赋薄弱，身体瘦削之人。其病因与长期饮食不节或劳役过度等有关。

一、诊断及辨证要点

1. 临床可见腹胀，上腹疼痛，食欲不振，时有呕吐，便秘等消化道症状。

2. 多见于 20～40 岁的青壮年，女性多于男性，并属先天性无力体质者。

3. 经 X 线检查证实胃下垂。

4. 脾虚气陷证，症见脘腹痞满，嗳气不舒，倦怠少力，形体消瘦，胃纳减少，胃脘疼痛，食后腹胀下坠，或呕吐，平卧时症状减轻，大便秘结，舌淡苔薄白，脉虚弱少力。

5. 气机阻滞证，症见脘痞腹胀，餐后坠胀更甚，水饮内停，呕吐清水痰涎，胃内有振水声，舌淡苔薄白，脉沉细无力。

ease belongs to the ranges of "ventroptosis" "down-bearing stomachache". Most are seen in patients with inadequate inherent endowment and thin body. The causes of this disease may be associated with long-term intemperate diet or overstrain.

I. Key Points for Diagnosis and Syndrome Differentiation

1. Digestive tract symptoms include abdominal distension, pain of the upper abdomen, poor appetite, frequent vomiting, constipation can be seen clinically.

2. Most are seen in young adults of 20-40 years old who have congenital weak constitution, more female patients than male ones.

3. Gastroptosis is confirmed by the X-ray examination.

4. Syndrome of the spleen deficiency and Qi collapse, symptoms include abdominal fullness and distention, uneasy blenching, fatigue and weakness, thin body, reduced food intake, epigastric pain, distension and falling down of the abdomen or vomiting after meals, which can be relieved when lying on the back, constipation, light tongue with thin and whitish fur, weak pulse.

5. Syndrome of Qi Dynamic obstruction, symptoms include abdominal fullness and distention, aggravated bearing-down and distention, internal water retention, vomit with clear water and phlegm and saliva, succession sound within the stomach, light tongue with thin and whitish fur, deep and thin and weak pulse.

二、治疗方法

【脾虚气陷证】

治法 健脾益胃，补气升提。

方法 电热针治疗、艾灸治疗。

（1）电热针治疗

处方 足三里（ST36）、中脘（RN12）、梁门（ST21）、气海（RN6）、关元（RN4）、胃上穴、脾俞（BL20）、胃俞（BL21）、百会（DU20）。

方义 足三里是胃之合穴，是治疗胃病的重要腧穴，可以调理脾胃，补益胃气；中脘为胃经募穴，是胃气汇聚之处，又为腑之会穴；梁门属胃经要穴，邻近胃腑，有健脾胃、助运化的作用，二穴合用以补益脾胃之气，而滋生化之源；气海是生成元气之海，关元能培元固本，二穴合用以补益元气，元气旺盛则胃自可升提；胃上穴位于下脘旁开4寸处，是治疗胃下垂的要穴，有升举下陷、益气提胃的作用。脾俞、胃俞属背俞穴，是脾胃脏腑之气所输注之地，可健脾强胃，补中益气；百会是督脉与三阳经气之交会穴，有升阳

II. Therapeutic Methods

[Syndrome of Spleen Deficiency and Qi Collapse]

Therapeutic method: Invigorate spleen and tonify stomach, invigorate and ascend Qi.

Method: Electrothermal acupuncture treatment, moxa-moxibustion treatment.

(1) Electrothermal acupuncture treatment.

Prescription: Zusanli (ST36), Zhongwan (RN12), Liangmen (ST21), Qihai (RN6), Guanyuan(RN4), Weishang Acupoint, Pishu (BL20), Weishu (BL21), Baihui (DU20).

Mechanism of prescription: Zusanli is a He acupoint of the Stomach, an important acupoint for treatment of stomach diseases, it can regulate spleen and stomach, tonify stomach Qi; Zhongwan is a Mu acupoint of the Stomach Meridian, the convergence place of stomach Qi as well as a confluent acupoint of Fu which locates near the stomach Fu, it can invigorate spleen and stomach, promote transportation and transformation. The match of these two can replenish Qi of the spleen and stomach so as to nourish the source of generation and transformation. Qihai is the sea for generation of vital Qi, Guanyuan can reinforce vital essence and foundation, the match of these two can replenish vital Qi, and the thriving of vital Qi can ascend the stomach naturally. The Weishang Acupoint locates at 4" from the acupoint Xiawan, is an important acupoint for treatment of gastroptosis, it can ascend up collapse, tonify Qi and ascend stomach. Pishu, Weishu are Back-Shu acupoints, are the infusion places

补气之功，阳气旺盛则升举有力。诸穴共用，可奏健脾益胃、补气升提之效。

配穴 呕吐者加内关；便秘者加大肠俞；气滞脘痞、满腹坠胀者，加公孙、天枢；停饮者加天枢、阴陵泉；气血两亏者加三阴交、内关。

操作 选定穴位，皮肤常规消毒。电热针直刺胃上穴 0.8 寸，直刺足三里、中脘、梁门、气海、关元各 0.7 寸，平刺百会 0.7 寸，然后接通电热针仪，每个穴位分别给予 50mA 的电流量，以患者感到温胀舒适为度，留针 40 分钟。（注：每次选 3 组穴，与胃上穴交替轮流使用；配穴要根据需要进行选择，主要依症状来选择穴位。）

疗程 每日 1 次，留针 40 分针，60 次为 1 个疗程，一般 2～3 个疗程即可。

of Zang Qi and Fu Qi of the spleen and stomach and spleen, can invigorate spleen and strengthen stomach, replenish Middle Jiao and tonify Qi. Baihui is the confluent acupoint of Du Channel and Qi of three Yang meridians, it can ascend Yang and replenish Qi, and exuberant Yang Qi can promote powerful ascending and lifting. The combined use of these acupoints can invigorate spleen and tonify stomach, invigorate and ascend Qi.

Matching acupoints: For vomiting add Neiguan. For constipation add Dachangshu. For Qi stagnation and epigastric fullness, bearing-down distension and fullness of abdomen, add Gongsun, Tianshu. For fluid retention add Tianshu, Yinlingquan. For depletion of Qi and blood add Sanyinjiao, Neiguan.

Operations: Selecting the relevant acupoints, perform routine skin disinfection. Using electrothermal acupuncture needles, vertically puncture into Weishang Acupoint for 0.8", vertically puncture into Zusanli, Zhongwan, Liangmen, Qihai, Guanyuan for 0.7" respectively, horizontally puncture into Baihui for 0.7". Turn on the electrothermal acupuncture equipment, apply a current of 50mA to each acupoint, and the limit is that the patient feels warm and swollen as well as locally comfortable, leaving the needles in for 40 minutes. (Note: Choose 3 pairs of acupoint each time, use alternatively with Weishang Acupoint; choose matching acupoints based on needs, and choose acupoints mainly depending on symptoms.)

Therapeutic course: Once a day, leave the needles in for 40 minutes, 60 times for a course. Generally treat for 2-3 courses.

（2）艾灸疗法

处方 百会（DU20）、足三里（ST36）、中脘（RN12）、脾俞（BL20）、气海（RN6）。

配穴 重度下垂入盆腔者，加灸关元；久病体弱、眩晕、失眠、心悸者，加灸三阴交。

操作 百会、脾俞选用艾条灸，每次 10～15 分钟。足三里、中脘、气海选用艾炷灸，每穴 5～7 壮，隔日 1 次。

疗程 每日或隔日 1 次，20 次为 1 个疗程。本法可单独应用，也可与体针配合，先针后灸或先灸后针均可。

三、注意事项

1. 治疗过程中，应少食多餐，宜食易消化的食物，避免暴饮暴食，勿过食肥甘油腻的食品，餐后宜平卧 30 分钟。

2. 令患者多锻炼身体，引导患者多做腹肌运动，以提高和巩固疗效。

3. 针灸治疗后应平卧休息 30 分钟。

(2) Moxa-moxibustion therapy.

Prescription: Baihui (DU20), Zusanli (ST36), Zhongwan (RN12), Pishu(BL2O), Qihai (RN6).

Matching acupoints: For severe gastroptosis with the stomach drooping into the pelvic cavity, add Guanyuan. For weak body due to long-term disease, vertigo, insomnia, palpitation, add Sanyinjiao.

Operations: Use moxa-stick moxibustion for Baihui and Pishu, 10-15 minutes each time. Use moxa-cone moxibustion for Zusanli, Zhongwan, Qihai, 5-7 times per day, once every other day.

Therapeutic course: Once a day or every two days, 20 times for a course. This method can be used alone or together with body acupuncture, moxibustion after acupuncture or acupuncture after moxibustion are both allowable.

III. Precautions

1. During treatment, have more meals a day but less food each time, better to eat food that easy to be digested, avoid to eat and drink too much, do not eat fat, sweet and greasy food, it is better to lie on the back for 30 minutes after meals.

2. Instruct patients to do more exercises, guide them to do more abdominal muscle movements so as to improve and consolidate efficacies.

3. Patients should lie on the back for 30 minutes to rest after acupuncture treatment.

幽门梗阻

幽门梗阻是指由于幽门部痉挛、水肿、狭窄而引起胃神经功能障碍的一种消化道病症。

中医认为，本病属于"胃反""反胃"等范畴。多因酒食不节，情绪失调，劳倦伤中等因素，损伤脾胃，健运失调所致。

一、诊断及辨证要点

1. 脾胃虚寒者，症见脘腹痞胀，宿食不化，朝食暮吐，神疲乏力，食少便溏，苔白质淡，脉沉细。

2. 中焦积热者，症见脘腹胀满，宿食不化，朝食暮吐，暮食朝吐，吐出物混浊酸臭，口渴便秘，舌红，苔黄腻，脉滑数。

3. 痰浊内阻者，症见脘腹胀满，朝食暮吐，暮食朝吐，吐出物有大量痰涎水液，或头

Pylorochesis

Pylorochesis refers to a disease of digestive tract which caused by neurological dysfunction of stomach due to spasm, edema and stenosis of pylorus area.

Traditional Chinese Medicine believes that this disease belongs to the category of "regurgitation", "gastric disorder causing nausea". Most are caused by spleen and stomach impairment, dysfunction of the spleen in transportation, which due to intemperate diet and drinking, mood disorders, fatigue impairing vitality essence.

I. Key Points for Diagnosis and Syndrome Differentiation

1. For patients with deficiency-Cold of the spleen and stomach, symptoms include abdominal fullness and distension, indigestion, eating in the morning but vomiting in the evening, mental fatigue and asthenia, less food intake and sloppy stool, white fur and light tongue, deep and thin pulse.

2. For patients with Heat accumulation in Middle Jiao, symptoms include abdominal fullness and distension, indigestion, eating in the morning but vomiting in the evening, eating in the evening but vomiting in the next morning, turbid and acidic odor vomit, thirsty and constipation, red tongue with yellow and greasy fur, slippery and rapid pulse.

3. For patients with internal phlegm turbid retention, symptoms include abdominal fullness and distension, eating in the morning but vomiting in the evening, eating

晕，或上腹有痞块，心下悸动，舌苔白滑，脉弦滑。

4. 瘀血停滞者，症见脘腹胀满刺痛，上腹积块坚硬，推之不移，宿食不化，朝食暮吐，暮食朝吐，或吐黄沫，或吐褐色浊液，舌质黯红，或有瘀点，脉弦滑。

二、治疗方法

【脾胃虚寒证】

治法 温中散寒，健脾和胃。

处方 足三里（ST36）、中脘（RN12）、天枢（ST25）、梁门（ST21）、脾俞（BL20）、胃俞（BL21）、膈俞（BL17）。

方义 足三里是胃之合穴，中脘是胃的募穴，两穴合用，远近相配，能健脾益胃，通降胃气，有温中止呕之效。脾俞、膈俞、胃俞均属于背俞穴，能调补脾胃之气，与中脘合用，俞募相配，可使脾胃强健，水谷腐熟而运化。天枢、梁门亦是胃经腧穴，能健脾益

in the evening but vomiting in the next morning, a lot of phlegm and saliva fluid within the vomit, or dizziness, or lump within the upper abdomen, heart throbbing, white and slippery tongue fur, taut and slippery pulse.

4. For patients with static blood stagnation, symptoms include abdominal fullness and distension and prickling, hard lump within the upper abdomen which does not move by pushing, indigestion, eating in the morning but vomiting in the evening, eating in the evening but vomiting in the next morning, or vomiting yellow foam, or vomiting brown turbid fluid, dark red tongue, or with petechia, taut and slippery pulse.

II. Therapeutic Methods

[Syndrome of Deficiency-Cold of Spleen and Stomach]

Therapeutic method: Warm Middle Jiao and disperse Cold, invigorate spleen and regulate stomach.

Prescription: Zusanli (ST36), Zhongwan (RN12), Tianshu (ST25), Liangmen (ST21), Pishu (BL20), Weishu (BL21), Geshu (BL17).

Mechanism of prescription: Zusanli is a He acupoint of the Stomach, Zhongwan is a Mu acupoint of the Stomach, the match of these two is a match of distal and proximal acupoints, can invigorate spleen and tonify stomach, soothe and descend stomach Qi, so as to warm Middle Jiao and stop vomiting. Pishu, Geshu, Weishu are all Back-Shu acupoints, can tonify spleen and stomach Qi. If it is used with Zhongwan, the match of Shu acupoint and Mu acupoint can strengthen spleen and stom-

气，和胃降逆，循经取之，可补益脾胃，通降气机。诸穴共用，有健脾益胃，温中降逆之功。

配穴 谷食不化者加下脘；大便溏泻者加三阴交；呕吐者加内关；腹中冷痛者加关元。

方法 电热针治疗（温补法）。

操作 选定穴位，常规皮肤消毒。电热针直刺足三里0.8寸，直刺中脘0.7寸，向脊椎方向斜刺脾俞、胃俞、膈俞各0.8寸，直刺天枢0.8寸，斜刺梁门0.7寸，直刺三阴交0.7寸，直刺关元0.8寸，直刺下脘0.7寸，直刺内关0.6寸。然后接通电热针仪，每个穴位分别给予电流量60～70mA，留针40分钟。

疗程 每天1次，或早、晚各1次，10次为1个疗程，休息3天后再进行第2个疗程的治疗。

ach, digest grains and transport as well transform them. Tianshu and Liangmen are also acupoints of the Stomach Meridian, they can invigorate spleen and tonify Qi, regulate stomach and reduce negative energy. If select these acupoint according to the meridians, can nourish spleen and stomach as well as soothe and descend Qi Dynamic. The combined use of these acupoints can invigorate spleen and tonify stomach, warm Middle Jiao and reduce negative energy.

Matching acupoints: For indigestion of grains add Xiawan. For sloppy stool add Sanyinjiao. For vomiting add Neiguan. For cold and pain within the abdomen add Guanyuan.

Method: Electrothermal acupuncture treatment (warm tonifying).

Operations: Selecting the relevant acupoints, perform routine skin disinfection. Using electrothermal acupuncture needles, vertically puncture into Zusanli for 0.8", Zhongwan for 0.7", obliquely puncture toward spine into Pishu, Weishu, Geshu for 0.8" respectively, vertically puncture into Tianshu for 0.8", Liangmen for 0.7", Sanyinjiao for 0.7", Guanyuan for 0.8", Xiawan for 0.7", Neiguan for 0.6". Then turn on the electrothermal acupuncture equipment, apply a current of 60-70mA to each acupoint, leaving the needles in for 40 minutes.

Therapeutic course: Treat once a day or once in the morning and in the afternoon respectively, 10 times for a course, and start the treatment for the second course after a break of 3 days.

【中焦积热证】

治法 清胃泻热，降逆止呕。

处方 中脘（RN12）、内庭（ST44）、上巨虚（ST37）、外陵（ST26）、商阳（LI1）。

方义 胃募穴中脘泻之以清热和胃，降逆止呕；内庭是胃经荥穴，可清胃泻热；上巨虚属下合穴，能清热和胃；商阳属大肠经井穴，能清泻阳明，其泻热之力宏大，三穴共用，可清泻胃中积热。外陵属胃经腧穴，有和胃消胀、理气降逆之功。诸穴共用，共奏清胃泻热，降逆止呕之功。

配穴 胃热内盛口渴者加解溪；热盛口中酸臭者加合谷；腹痛胀甚者加梁丘；大便秘结者加大巨。

方法 毫针治疗（泻法）。

操作 选定穴位，常规皮肤消毒。毫针直刺中脘 0.8 寸，

[Syndrome of Heat Accumulation in Middle Jiao]

Therapeutic method: Clear stomach and disperse Heat, reduce negative energy and stop vomiting.

Prescription: Zhongwan (RN12), Neiting (ST44), Shangjuxu (ST37), Wailing (ST26), Shangyang (LI1).

Mechanism of prescription: Use the acupoint of the Stomach Meridian, Zhongwan, to clear Heat and harmonize the stomach, reduce negative energy and stop vomiting; Neiting, a Xing acupoint of the Stomach Meridian, can clear stomach and disperse Heat; Shangjuxu, a Lower He acupoint, can clear Heat and harmonize the stomach; Shangyang, a Jing acupoint of Large Intestine Meridian, can clear and disperse Yang-Ming, and its effect of Heat dispersing is very great. The match of these three can clear and disperse the accumulated Heat within the stomach. Wailing, an acupoint of the Stomach Meridian, can tonify stomach and disperse distention, regulate Qi and reduce negative energy. The combined use of these acupoints can clear stomach and disperse Heat, reduce negative energy and stop vomiting.

Matching acupoints: For thirstiness due to internal exuberance of stomach Heat, add Jiexi. For Heat exuberance leading to acidic odor in the mouth, add Hegu. For severe abdominal distension and pains add Liangqiu. For constipation add Daju.

Method: Filiform needle acupuncture treatment (attenuating).

Operations: Selecting the relevant acupoints, perform routine skin disinfection. Using filiform needles,

斜刺内庭 0.5 寸，直刺上巨虚 0.8 寸，直刺商阳 0.3 寸（毫针速刺不留针），直刺外陵 0.8 寸，直刺解溪 0.4 寸，直刺梁丘 0.7 寸，直刺大巨 0.8 寸。提插泻法，留针 30 分钟。

疗程　每天 1 次或 2 次（早、晚各 1 次），10 次为 1 个疗程，休息 3 天后再进行第 2 个疗程的治疗。

【痰浊内阻证】

治法　健脾胃化痰饮，和胃气降呕逆。

处方　中脘（RN12）、丰隆（ST40）、章门（LR13）、公孙（SP4）。

方义　中脘调补脾胃之气，化湿消食；丰隆祛痰降逆，胃募中脘配丰隆以和胃化痰。章门健脾益胃而化痰饮；公孙健脾益肾。脾募章门，配公孙以健脾蠲饮。诸穴合用，可奏健脾胃化痰饮，和胃气降呕逆之功效。

vertically puncture into Zhongwan for 0.8", obliquely puncture into Neiting for 0.5", vertically puncture into Shangjuxu for 0.8", Shangyang for 0.3" (rapid puncture with filiform needle, do not leave the needle in), vertically puncture into Wailing for 0.8", Jiexi for 0.4", Liangqiu for 0.7", Daju for 0.8". Method of lifting-thrusting and attenuating, leaving the needles in for 30 minutes.

Therapeutic course: Treat once or twice (one in the morning, and one in the afternoon) a day, 10 times for a course, and start the treatment for the second course after a break of 3 days.

[Syndrome of Internal Phlegm Turbid Retention]

Therapeutic method: Invigorate spleen and stomach, disperse phlegm and retained fluid, harmonize the stomach Qi and descend counterflow.

Prescription: Zhongwan (RN12), Fenglong (ST40), Zhangmen (LR13), Gongsun (SP4).

Mechanism of prescription: Zhongwan can tonify Qi of the spleen and stomach, disperse Damp and remove food accumulation; Fenglong can disperse phlegm and descend adverse energy. The match of Zhongwan and Fenglong from Stomach Meridian can harmonize the stomach and disperse phlegm. Zhangmen can invigorate spleen and tonify stomach so as to disperse phlegm and retained fluid; Gongsun can invigorate spleen and tonify kidney. Match the acupoint Zhangmen of Spleen Meridian with Gongsun to invigorate spleen and remove retained fluid. The combined use of these acupoints can invigorate spleen and stomach, disperse phlegm and retained fluid, harmonize the stomach Qi and descend

配穴 恶心呕吐多发者加内关；上腹痞块者加梁门；心下悸动者加上脘；眩晕者加解溪。

方法 电热针温补法加毫针泻法。

操作 选定穴位，常规消毒。电热针直刺中脘 0.8 寸，直刺公孙 0.7 寸，斜刺梁门 0.7 寸，然后接通电热针仪，每个穴位分别给予电流量 50～60mA。另配以毫针直刺丰隆 0.6 寸，斜刺章门 0.8 寸，直刺内关 0.6 寸，均施提插泻法，留针 40 分钟。

疗程 每天 1 次，10 次为 1 个疗程，疗程间休息 3 天后再进行第 2 个疗程的治疗。

【瘀血停滞证】

治法 健脾益气，活血化瘀，和胃降逆。

处方 膈俞（BL17）、中脘（RN12）、章门（LR13）、脾俞（BL20）。

方义 血之会膈俞是祛瘀要穴，有开胃利膈、活血化

counterflow.

Matching acupoints: For frequent onset of nausea and vomiting add Neiguan. For lumps in the upper abdomen add Liangmen. For heart throbbing add Shangwan. For vertigo add Jiexi.

Method: Electrothermal acupuncture treatment (warm tonifying) plus filiform needle treatment (attenuating).

Operations: Selecting the relevant acupoints, perform routine disinfection. Using electrothermal acupuncture needles, vertically puncture into Zhongwan for 0.8", Gongsun for 0.7", obliquely puncture into Liangmen for 0.7". Turn on the electrothermal acupuncture equipment, apply a current of 50-60mA to each acupoint. Additionally, using filiform needles, vertically puncture into Fenglong for 0.6", obliquely puncture into Zhangmen for 0.8", vertically puncture into Neiguan for 0.6", using the method of lifting-thrusting and attenuating for all. Leave the needles in for 40 minutes.

Therapeutic course: Treat once a day, 10 times for a course, and start the treatment for the second course after a break of 3 days.

[Syndrome of Static Blood Stagnation]

Therapeutic method: Invigorate spleen and tonify Qi, activate blood circulation and remove stasis, regulate stomach and reduce negative energy.

Prescription: Geshu (BL17), Zhongwan (RN12), Zhangmen (LR13), Pishu (BL20).

Mechanism of prescription: The confluent acupoint of blood, Geshu, is an important acupoint for

瘀之功；胃之募穴中脘是治胃病之要穴，能补脾和胃；章门是脾之募，又是脏之合穴，脾胃之气通于此，有疏导脾胃之气，活血化瘀消积的作用；脾俞是背俞穴，能健脾益气，培中和胃，俞募穴相配，健脾益胃，化瘀消积，和胃降逆。

配穴 脘腹胀满者加梁门；胃中灼热者加太溪；吐血便血者加血海；身体虚弱者加肾俞、关元。

方法 毫针治疗（泻法）。

操作 选定穴位，常规消毒。毫针直刺中脘 0.7 寸，向脊柱方向斜刺膈俞、脾俞、肾俞各 0.7 寸，斜刺章门 0.6 寸，直刺内关 0.6 寸，直刺梁门 0.6 寸，直刺血海 0.6 寸，直刺太溪 0.5 寸，留针 30 分钟。

疗程 每天 1 次，每次选 4～5 组穴，10 次为 1 个疗程，

removing stasis, it can open stomach and benefit diaphragm, activate blood circulation and remove stasis. The Mu acupoint Zhongwan of the Stomach is an important acupoint for treatment of stomach diseases, it can replenish spleen and harmonize the stomach; Zhangmen is a Mu acupoint of the Spleen as well as the He acupoint of Zang, through where the Qi of stomach and spleen passes, it can soothe Qi of stomach and spleen, activate blood circulation and remove stasis as well as disperse accumulated food; Pishu is a Back-Shu acupoint, it can invigorate spleen and tonify Qi, reinforce Middle Jiao and harmonize the stomach, the match of Shu acupoint and Mu acupoint can invigorate spleen and tonify stomach, remove stasis and disperse accumulations, harmonize the stomach and reduce negative energy.

Matching acupoints: For abdominal distension add Liangmen. For burning-like feeling within the stomach add Taixi. For hematemesis and bloody stool add Xuehai. For weak body add Shenshu, Guanyuan.

Method: Filiform needle acupuncture treatment (attenuating).

Operations: Selecting the relevant acupoints, perform routine disinfection. Using filiform needles, vertically puncture into Zhongwan for 0.7", obliquely puncture toward spine into Geshu, Pishu, Shenshu for 0.7" respectively, obliquely puncture into Zhangmen for 0.6", vertically puncture into Neiguan for 0.6", Liangmen for 0.6", Xuehai for 0.6", Taixi for 0.5", leaving the needles in for 30 minutes.

Therapeutic course: Treat once a day, choose 4-5 pairs of acupoints each time, 10 times for a course, and

如无不适，可进行第2个疗程的治疗。

三、注意事项

1. 积极治疗导致幽门梗阻的原发病变，如胃及十二指肠溃疡、慢性胃炎等。同时，尽快做胃部检查，排除胃部肿瘤，以免延误手术治疗。

2. 注意对此患者，针灸治疗只起配合治疗作用，必须尽快查找病因，给予相应的根除治疗方法。

3. 治疗中注意观察病情的变化，切勿延误治疗。

胆道疾病及结石症

胆道疾病常见的有急性胆囊炎、胆道蛔虫症、胆结石等。多见于青壮年，女性多于男性。胆道疾病多由于胆道梗阻、胆汁滞留、肠道细菌感染所致。胆结石则由胆红素或胆固醇的代谢障碍，或胆道中的异物等所引起。而胆系感染与胆结石又常同时存在，相互为因果。

中医认为，本病属于"胁痛""腹痛""黄疸""结胸发黄""胆火"等范畴。多因情志抑郁、肝胆郁结、疏泄失常；

start the treatment for the second course if no discomfort.

III. Precautions

1. Actively treat the primary lesion which causes the pylorochesis, like stomach and duodenal ulcers, chronic gastritis, etc. While do stomach check to exclude stomach tumors, so as to avoid delay of surgery treatments.

2. Note that for such patients, acupuncture treatment is an adjuvant therapy only, must find the cause and perform corresponding cure method.

3. During treatment, note that observe changes of conditions, do not delay the treatment.

Biliary Tract Diseases and Lithiasis

Common biliary tract diseases include acute cholecystitis, ascariasis of biliary tract, cholelithiasis, etc. More common in young adults, more women than men. Biliary tract diseases mostly are caused by biliary tract obstruction, cholestasis, intestinal bacterial infections. While cholelithiasis is caused by metabolic disorders of bilirubin or cholesterol, or foreign bodies in the biliary tract. And biliary infections and cholelithiasis are often coexisting, interacting as both cause and effect.

Traditional Chinese Medicine believes that this disease belongs to the category of "hypochondriac pain", "abdominal pain", "icteric", "knotted chest with jaundice", "gallbladder fire", etc. Most are caused by

或过食肥腻、内蕴湿热、阻于肝胆、胆汁排泄不畅；或因蛔虫上扰，致胆气不通，胆汁外溢肌肤等而引发。若胆汁久蕴，则凝结而成砂石。

emotional depression, stagnation of liver and gallbladder, disorders of soothing and dredging; or intake of too much fatty food, internal accumulation of Damp-Heat, obstruction of liver and gallbladder, unsmooth excretion of bile; or ascariasis; lead to obstruction of gallbladder Qi, overflooding of bile over skin. After long-term accumulation, the bile will coagulate into gall stone.

一、诊断及辨证要点

1. 胆道系急性感染者，临床表现是寒战高热，右上腹痛，呈持续性或阵发性加剧，黄疸，胆囊区触痛，或伴反跳痛，墨菲征阳性，或伴消化不良症状。

2. 以血象中性粒细胞增多与核左移为特征。慢性者右上腹常隐痛或钝痛，脂餐后加重。

3. 胆结石临床可无症状，但若嵌顿于胆道则可见胆绞痛，阻塞性黄疸，或胆道感染症状。痛剧时常伴有恶心、呕吐，缺少食欲。

4. 可借助 X 线、胆 B 超检查，能明确诊断。

5. 气郁者，症见右上腹隐痛，闷胀，时有窜痛，伴口苦咽干，食少腹胀，舌苔微腻或

I. Key Points for Diagnosis and Syndrome Differentiation

1. For patients of acute infections, clinical manifestations include shiver and high fever, pain of right upper abdomen, which aggravate persistently or paroxysmally, icteric, haphalgesia, or accompanying rebound tenderness, positive Murphy's sign, or accompanying dyspepsia.

2. Its characteristics are neutrophilic leukocytosis and neutrophil shift to left in the hemogram. Patients of chronic infections suffer from frequent dull pain which will be aggravated after intaking fatty food.

3. For cholelithiasis, there may be no symptoms clinically, however if the gall stone is incarcerated in the biliary tract then there can be symptoms of cholecystalgia, obstructive jaundice, or biliary tract infections. In cases of intensive pains, there are often accompanied nausea, vomiting and lack of appetite.

4. The disease can be definitely diagnosed by X-ray examination and biliary B ultrasound examination.

5. For patients with Qi stasis, symptoms include dull pain and distension of the right upper abdomen with frequent scurrying pain, accompanying bitter mouth and

薄白。

6.湿热者，症见胁脘绞痛，阵发性加剧，拒按，伴口苦纳呆，寒战交热，恶心呕吐，便秘尿黄，甚者神昏谵语，舌红绛，苔黄糙，脉弦数或细数。

二、治疗方法

【肝胆湿热证】

治法 疏肝利胆，清热利湿。

方法 电热针、艾灸治疗。

（1）电热针治疗

处方 胆俞（BL19）、肝俞（BL18）、日月（GB24）、期门（LR14）、阳陵泉（GB34）、胆囊（EX-LE6）、太冲（LR3）。

方义 本证为肝胆失于疏泄所致。以通降下行为顺，根据"六腑以通为用""不通则痛"的原理，取肝、胆背俞穴，疏泄肝胆热邪；阳陵泉是胆经合穴，太冲为肝经原穴，二者合用，可疏利肝胆，理气解郁；期门为肝之募穴，日月为胆之募穴，二穴可疏局部经气；胆囊穴是治疗肝胆疾病之经验穴。诸穴共用，能收疏肝

dry mouth, less food intake and abdominal distension, slightly greasy or thin and white tongue fur.

6. For patients with Damp-Heat, symptoms include hypochondriac and epigastric angina with paroxysmal aggravation, refusal to pressing, chills alternating hot, nausea and vomiting, constipation and yellow urine, or in severe cases, coma and delirium, dark red tongue with yellow and rough fur, taut and rapid or thin and rapid pulse.

II. Therapeutic Methods

[Syndrome of Damp-Heat of Liver and Gallbladder]

Therapeutic method: Soothe liver and reinforce gallbladder, clear Heat and remove Damp.

Method: Electrothermal acupuncture treatment, moxa-moxibustion treatment.

(1) Electrothermal acupuncture treatment

Prescription: Danshu (BL19), Ganshu (BL18), Riyue (GB24), Qimen (LR14), Yanglingquan (GB34), Dannang (EX-LE6), Taichong (LR3).

Mechanism of prescription: The syndrome is caused by the loss of soothing and dredging of liver and gallbladder. The smooth circulation refers to descending and downward flowing, according to the principle "smooth six Fu can function normally" and "stagnation leading to pain", use Back-Shu acupoints of Liver and Gallbladder Meridians to disperse Heat toxins of liver a gallbladder; Yanglingquan is a He acupoint of Gallbladder Meridian, Taichong is a Yuan acupoint of Liver Meridian, the match of these two can soothe liver and gallbladder, regulate Qi and remove stasis; Qimen is a

利胆、清热利湿、理气止痛、排石之功效。

配穴 气郁者，加行间；湿热者，加足三里、阴陵泉、三阴交；脓毒者，加大椎、内关、足临泣、关冲、委中、十宣，点刺放血；绞痛者，加合谷、郄门；呕吐者加内关；发热者加曲池、大椎。

操作 选定穴位，皮肤常规消毒。电热针斜刺（针尖向脊柱）胆俞、肝俞各0.7寸，直刺阳陵泉、足三里、阴陵泉、三阴交、曲池各0.8寸，直刺大椎、内关、足临泣各0.7寸，接通电热针仪，每个穴位分别给予40mA的电流量，留针40分钟，关冲、委中、十宣点刺放血。

疗程 每日1次，10次为1个疗程。

（2）艾灸疗法

处方 阳陵泉（GB34）、期门（LR14）、日月（GB24）、肝俞（BL18）、胆俞（BL19）、太冲（LR3）、支沟（SJ6）。

Mu acupoint of Gallbladder meridian, Riyue is a Mu acupoint of Liver, these two can soothe local meridian Qi. The acupoint Dannang is an experienced acupoint for treatment of liver and gallbladder diseases. The combined use of these acupoints can soothe liver and reinforce gallbladder, clear Heat and remove Damp, regulate Qi and alleviate pains, remove calculus.

Matching acupoints: For Qi stasis, add Xingjian; For Damp-Heat, add Zusanli, Yinlingquan, Sanyinjiao. For sepsis add Dazhui, Neiguan, Zulinqi, Guanchong, Weizhong, Shixuan, use pricking blood therapy. For angina add Hegu, Ximen. For vomiting add Neiguan. For pyrexia add Quchi, Dazhui.

Operations: Selecting the relevant acupoints, perform routine skin disinfection. Using electrothermal acupuncture needles, obliquely puncture (with the needle tip towards spine) into Danshu, Ganshu for 0.7" respectively, vertically puncture into Yanglingquan, Zusanli, Yinlingquan, Sanyinjiao, Quchi for 0.8" respectively, vertically puncture into Dazhui, Neiguan, Zulinqi for 0.7" respectively. Turn on the electrothermal acupuncture equipment, apply a current of 40mA to each acupoint, and use pricking blood therapy for Guanchong, Weizhong and Shixuan, leave the needle in for 40 minutes.

Therapeutic course: Once a day, 10 times for a course.

(2) Moxa-moxibustion therapy

Prescription: Yanglingquan (GB34), Qimen (LR14), Riyue (GB24), Ganshu (BL18), Danshu(BL19), Taichong (LR3), Zhigou (SJ6).

配穴 发热者加大椎、曲池、合谷；绞痛者加丘墟、足三里；胸腹胀满者加膈俞、内关、丰隆。

操作 每次选3～4个穴，每穴用艾条悬灸15～20分钟，每日1次。或每穴用艾炷灸3～5壮，每日灸2次。

疗程 每日1次，10次为1个疗程。

三、注意事项

1. 忌食辛辣、油腻之品，保持大便通畅，饮食有节，心态平和。

2. 治疗胆结石时，配合中药治疗会有较好的疗效。

3. 遇胆道感染患者，除针灸治疗之外，还要配合中、西药物共同治疗，减少患者的痛苦，缩短疗程。

腹痛

腹痛是临床常见的一种症状，主要由于腹内脏器病变而引起，也可由胸部疾患（如肺炎、胸膜炎、心绞痛）放射而来。因此，腹痛涉及的疾病范围很广，必须认真鉴别，明确

Matching acupoints: For pyrexia, add Dazhui, Quchi, Hegu. For angina add Qiuxu, Zusanli. For distension of chest and abdomen, add Geshu, Neiguan, Fenglong.

Operations: Choose 3-4 acupoints each time, perform moxa-stick suspension-moxibustion on each acupoint for 15-20 minutes, once a day. Or use 3-5 cones of moxa-cone moxibustion for each acupoint, twice a day.

Therapeutic course: Once a day, 10 times for a course.

III. Precautions

1. Do not eat spicy and greasy food, keep smooth defecation, regular diet and peaceful mind.

2. For treatment of cholelithiasis, it will be better efficacious if performed in combination with Chinese Herb Medicine treatment.

3. For patients with biliary tract infection, there should be a combination of Chinese Herb Medicine treatment and Western Medicine treatment in addition to acupuncture treatment, so as to reduce patients' pain and shorten treatment course.

Abdominal Pain

Abdominal pain is a clinically common symptom, which is mainly caused by intra-abdominal organ diseases, or caused by radiation of chest diseases (such as pneumonia, pleuritis, angina).Therefore, abdominal pain involves a wide range of diseases and must be carefully identified as well as clearly diagnosed for correct treat-

诊断，才能正确治疗。

中医认为，腹痛的发生与受寒、饮食不节、情志刺激及素体脏腑阳虚等有关。其病机有虚实，但以实为主。实证，因湿热、食积、气滞血瘀、寒积等导致腑气通降失常，气血运行受阻。虚证，因脏气虚寒、气血不能温养所致。

一、诊断及辨证要点

1. 详细询问病史，注意腹痛部位、性质、时间与饮食的关系，以及其他并发症状，结合体检和必要的实验室检查，作出鉴别诊断。

2. 凡有恶寒、发热等全身症状，或恶心、呕吐、腹泻等消化道症状，先于腹痛或与腹痛同时出现的，多属内科疾患。结合下列不同的部位可分别考虑不同的疾病。

3. 上腹部疼痛伴恶心呕吐的，多属胃部疾病；右上腹部疼痛伴发热、恶寒、恶心、呕吐或腹泻，或黄疸，多属肝胆

ments.

Traditional Chinese Medicine believes that occurrence of abdominal pains is associated with catching a cold, intemperate diet, emotional stimulations and Yang deficiency of the body, etc. Its pathogenesis is divided into two types, deficiency and excess ones, among which the excess domain. Excess syndrome: Circulation and flowing down failure of Fu Qi, obstruction of Qi-blood circulation caused by Damp-Heat, retention of food, Qi stagnation and blood stasis, accumulation of Cold, etc. Deficiency syndrome: Caused by Zang Qi deficiency and cold, failure of Qi-blood nourishment.

I. Key Points for Diagnosis and Syndrome Differentiation

1. Get a detailed medical history, note the relation between site of abdominal pain, time and diet, as well as other concurrent symptoms, combine them with results of physical examination as well as other necessary lab examinations to make a differential diagnosis.

2. In cases there are systemic symptoms such as aversion to cold, pyrexia, or digestive tract symptoms such as nausea, vomiting, diarrhea, which occur before or simultaneously with abdominal pains, normally these cases belong to the range of medical diseases. Different diseases can be considered in combination with the following different parts.

3. For upper abdominal pain accompanying nausea and vomiting, most belong to stomach diseases. For right upper abdominal pain, accompanying pyrexia, aversion to cold, nausea, vomiting or diarrhea, or icteric, most

系统疾病；脐周围或左下腹部疼痛，伴恶寒、发热、恶心、呕吐、腹泻而局部有压痛症状者，属胃肠道炎症；脐周围阵发性疼痛而无明显压痛者，多属肠寄生虫疾病；右下腹痛，如有反复发作，除外阑尾炎，应考虑肠结核。

4. 以腹痛为主症，且病情严重，腹部切诊有明显压痛部位，伴有腹肌紧张或反跳痛，或触及包块者，应考虑急腹症。

5. 一般而言，持续性腹痛，多见于炎症及内出血；阵发性腹痛，多见于梗阻；持续性、伴阵发性加剧的疼痛，多见于炎症并有梗阻；钝痛和胀痛多见于炎症；绞痛多见于梗阻。

6. 除腹部外还应检查胸部，询问有无咳嗽、胸痛等其他症状，从而鉴别由于胸部疾病引起的放射性痛。

7. 凡妇女患者应询问月经史，鉴别痛经、输卵管炎、盆腔炎、宫外孕等妇科疾病。

8. 寒凝腹痛者，症见遇温痛减，遇寒则甚，口不渴，四肢不温，大便溏薄或泄泻，腹

belong to liver and gallbladder diseases. For peri-umbilicus pain or left lower abdominal pain, accompanying aversion to cold, pyrexia, nausea, vomiting, diarrhea as well as local tenderness, belong to gastrointestinal inflammation. For peri-umbilicus paroxysmal pain without obvious tenderness, most belong to intestinal parasitic diseases. For right lower abdominal pain with recurrent attacks, exclude appendicitis and consider enterophthisis.

4. For abdominal pain as the main symptom and the conditions are severe, obvious tenderness can be found in the abdominal palpation, accompanying with tension of abdominal muscle or rebound tenderness, or palpated mass, acute abdominal diseases should be considered.

5. Generally, persistent abdominal pains are mostly seen in inflammation and internal hemorrhage. Paroxysmal abdominal pains are mostly seen in obstructions; persistent abdominal pains accompanying paroxysmal intensified pains are mostly seen in inflammation with obstruction. Dull pains and swelling pains are mostly seen in inflammation; angina is mostly seen in obstruction.

6. In addition to the abdomen, the chest should also be checked. Ask if any other symptom like cough, chest pain, so as to identify radiative pains caused by chest diseases.

7. For female patients, it is necessary to ask about their menstrual history, so as to identify gynecological diseases like dysmenorrhea, salpingitis, pelvic inflammation, and ectopic pregnancy.

8. For patients with abdominal pain due to cold stagnation, symptoms include pain relieving in warm environments and pain intensifying in cold environments,

中肠鸣，小便清利，苔白腻，脉沉紧。若兼表寒，则有恶寒发热。

9. 食滞腹痛者，症见脘腹胀痛，痛处拒按，痛则欲泻，大便臭秽，泻后痛减，厌食，恶心欲吐，嗳腐吞酸，舌苔腻，脉滑。

10. 阳虚腹痛者，症见腹痛绵绵，时作时休，喜热恶寒，痛时喜按，饥饿、劳累后加重，大便溏薄，兼见神疲、气短、怯寒、舌淡苔白、脉沉细。

11. 肝郁腹痛者，症见脘腹胀痛，痛处攻窜不定，或连及少腹及两胁，嗳气频作，常因情志所伤而发或加重，多躁善怒，苔薄白，脉沉弦。

二、治疗方法

【寒凝腹痛】

治法　温中散寒，理气止痛。

cold extremities, sloppy stool or diarrhea, intra-abdominal borborygmus, clear and disinhibited urine, whitish and greasy tongue fur, deep and tense pulse. If accompanied with exterior cold, then aversion to cold and pyrexia exist.

9. For patients with abdominal pain due to retention of food, symptoms include abdominal distention and pains, pressure-refused, desire of diarrhea when pain occurs, stool with foul smell, pain relief after diarrhea, anorexia, nausea and vomiting, putrid belching and acid swallowing, greasy tongue fur, slippery pulse.

10. For patients with abdominal pain due to Yang deficiency, symptoms include long-term abdominal pain which attacks intermittently, preference for warm and aversion to cold, preference for pressing when pain occurs, pain intensifying with hunger or tire, sloppy and thin stool, accompanying mental fatigue, shortness of breath, fear of cold, light tongue with white fur, deep and thin pulse.

11. For patients with abdominal pain due to liver stasis, symptoms include abdominal distention and pains, affected area changing uncertainly, sometimes involving lateral lower abdomen and both sides of the ribs, frequent belching, often occurs or is aggravated due to emotional causes, rattiness and irritability, thin and whitish tongue fur, deep and taut pulse.

II. Therapeutic Methods

[Abdominal Pain Due to Cold Stagnation]

Therapeutic method: Warm Middle Jiao and disperse Cold, regulate Qi and alleviate pains.

处方 中脘（RN12）、梁门（ST21）、大横（SP15）、足三里（ST36）、三阴交（SP6）、公孙（SP4）、合谷（LI4）。

方义 中脘、梁门、足三里、三阴交能温中和胃散寒，大横、公孙可健脾理气，佐以手阳明经之原穴合谷，既能散寒邪，又能调畅大肠气机。诸穴共用，可奏温中散寒、理气止痛之功效。

配穴 脐下痛者，加关元、中极；脐周痛者，加天枢、气海；侧腹痛者，加带脉、归来、太冲、阳陵泉。

方法 电热针治疗。

操作 选定穴位，皮肤常规消毒。电热针直刺中脘、梁门、大横、合谷各0.6寸，直刺足三里、三阴交各0.7寸，接通电热针仪，每个穴位分别给予30～40mA的电流量，以患者感到温热及舒适为度，留针40分钟。

疗程 每天1次，5天为1个疗程，留针40分钟。疗程间休息2～3天，根据病情再决定是否进行第2个疗程的

Prescription: Zhongwan (RN12), Liangmen (ST21), Daheng (SP15), Zusanli (ST36), Sanyinjiao (SP6), Gongsun (SP4), Hegu (LI4).

Mechanism of prescription: Zhongwan, Liangmen, Zusanli, Sanyinjiao can warm Middle Jiao, tonify stomach and disperse Cold, Daheng, Gongsun can invigorate spleen and regulate Qi, and they can disperse Cold toxins as well as regulate Qi Dynamic of the large intestine when being matched with the Yuan acupoint Hegu from Yang-Ming Meridian of Hand. The use of combination of these acupoints can warm Middle Jiao and disperse Cold, regulate Qi and alleviate pains.

Matching acupoints: For subumbilical pains add Guanyuan, Zhongji. For periumbilical pains add Tianshu, Qihai. For lateral abdominal pains add Daimai, Guilai, Taichong, Yanglingquan.

Method: Electrothermal acupuncture treatment.

Operations: Selecting the relevant acupoints, perform routine skin disinfection. Using electrothermal acupuncture needles, vertically puncture into Zhongwan, Liangmen, Daheng, Hegu for 0.6" respectively, vertically puncture into Zusanli, Sanyinjiao for 0.7" respectively. Turn on the electrothermal acupuncture equipment, apply a current of 30-40mA to each acupoint, and the limit is that the patient feels warm and locally comfortable, leaving the needles in for 40 minutes.

Therapeutic course: Treat once a day, 5 times for a course, leaves the needles in for 40 minutes. Rest for 2-3 days between courses, decide if perform the second course depending on the disease conditions. Generally

治疗。一般治疗1～2个疗程即可。

【食滞腹痛】

治法 化食导滞，调理胃肠。

处方 中脘（RN12）、天枢（ST25）、气海（RN6）、足三里（ST36）、三阴交（SP6）、内庭（ST44）。

方义 中脘通理脾胃、消食导滞，气海行气止痛，二穴相伍，善治脘腹胀痛；天枢、足三里、三阴交可通腑理气、健脾和胃化食；内庭为治疗伤食之经验效穴。诸穴共用，可奏化食导滞、调理胃肠之功。

方法 电热针治疗。

操作 选定穴位，皮肤常规消毒。电热针直刺中脘、气海、天枢、足三里、三阴交各0.7寸，斜刺内庭0.6寸，接通电热针仪，每个穴位分别给予30mA的电流量，以达舒适为度，留针40分钟。

疗程 每天1次，5天为

cured after 1-2 courses.

[Abdominal Pain due to Retention of Food]

Therapeutic method: Promote digestion and disperse stagnation, tonify stomach and intestine.

Prescription: Zhongwan (RN12), Tianshu (ST25), Qihai (RN6), Zusanli (ST36), Sanyinjiao (SP6), Neiting (ST44).

Mechanism of prescription: Zhongwan soothes and tonifies spleen and stomach as well as promotes digestion and disperses stagnation, while Qihai activates Qi and alleviates pains, the match of these two can treat abdominal distention and pains; Tianshu, Zusanli and Sanyinjiao can soothe Fu organs and regulate Qi, invigorate spleen, tonify stomach and promote digestion; Neiting is a well-known effective acupoint for treatment of impairment by overeating. The use of combination of these acupoints can promote digestion and disperse stagnation, tonify stomach and intestine.

Method: Electrothermal acupuncture treatment.

Operations: Selecting the relevant acupoints, perform routine skin disinfection. Using electrothermal acupuncture needles, vertically puncture into Zhongwan, Qihai, Tianshu, Zusanli, Sanyinjiao for 0.7" respectively, obliquely puncture into Neiting for 0.6". Turn on the electrothermal acupuncture equipment, apply a current of 30mA to each acupoint, and the limit is that the patient feels locally comfortable, leaving the needles in for 40 minutes.

Therapeutic course: Treat once a day, 5 times for

1个疗程，留针40分钟。疗程间休息2～3天，根据病情再决定是否进行第2个疗程的治疗。一般治疗1～2个疗程即可。

【阳虚腹痛】

治法 温补肾阳，健脾理气。

处方 脾俞（BL20）、肾俞（BL23）、胃俞（BL21）、中脘（RN12）、气海（RN6）、章门（LR13）、足三里（ST36）、三阴交（SP6）。

方义 取脾胃之俞募穴以健脾和中、益气养血；肾俞、关元、气海均为补肾要穴，三穴合用，可温补元阳；足三里、三阴交二穴合用，可调和中气，健脾扶正。诸穴共用，可取温补肾阳、健脾理气之效。

方法 电热针治疗。

操作 选定穴位，皮肤常规消毒。电热针斜刺（针尖向脊柱）脾俞、胃俞、肾俞各0.7寸，直刺中脘、气海、足三里、三阴交各0.7寸，平刺章门0.7寸，接通电热针仪，每个穴位分别给予40mA的电流

a course, leaves the needles in for 40 minutes. Rest for 2-3 days between courses, decide if perform the second course depending on the disease conditions. Generally cured after 1-2 courses.

[Abdominal Pain Due to Yang Deficiency]

Therapeutic method: Warm and tonify kidney Yang, invigorate spleen and regulate Qi.

Prescription: Pishu(BL20), Shenshu(BL23), Weishu(BL21), Zhongwan (RN12), Qihai (RN6), Zhangmen (LR13), Zusanli (ST36), Sanyinjiao (SP6).

Mechanism of prescription: Selecting the relevant acupoint Shu and mu acupoints of Spleen and Stomach Meridians to invigorate spleen and regulate Middle Jiao, tonify Qi and nourish blood; Shenshu, Guanyuan, Qihai are all important acupoints for kidney replenishment, the combination of these three acupoints can warm and nourish Yuan Yang; the combination of Zusanli and Sanyinjiao can regulate Middle-Jiao Qi, tonify Qi and strengthen vital Qi. The use of combination of these acupoints can warm and tonify kidney Yang, invigorate spleen and regulate Qi.

Method: Electrothermal acupuncture treatment.

Operations: Selecting the relevant acupoints, perform routine skin disinfection. Using electrothermal acupuncture needles, obliquely puncture (with the needle tip towards spine) into Pishu, Weishu, Shenshu for 0.7" respectively, vertically puncture into Zhongwan, Qihai, Zusanli, Sanyinjiao for 0.7" respectively, horizontally puncture into Zhangmen for 0.7". Turn on the electro-

量，以达穴下有胀或温热感觉且舒适为度，留针 40 分钟。

疗程 每天 1 次，5 天为 1 个疗程，留针 40 分钟。疗程间休息 2～3 天，根据病情再决定是否进行第 2 个疗程的治疗。一般治疗 1～2 个疗程即可。

【肝郁腹痛】

治法 疏肝解郁，行气止痛。

处方 膻中（RN17）、太冲（LR3）、气海（RN6）、内关（PC6）、阳陵泉（GB34）、足三里（ST36）。

方义 膻中为气之会穴，功于理气；气海是肓之源，为三焦通行之道，功于通气止痛；足三里配阳陵泉，效在疏肝利胆、调和中气；内关与太冲同属厥阴经，二穴相伍，可疏肝解郁、调畅情志。诸穴共用，可奏疏肝解郁、行气止痛之功效。

方法 电热针治疗。

操作 选定穴位，皮肤常规消毒。电热针直刺气海、阳

thermal acupuncture equipment, apply a current of 40mA to each acupoint, and the limit is that the patient feels swelling or warm and comfortable under acupoints, leaving the needles in for 40 minutes.

Therapeutic course: Treat once a day, 5 times for a course, leaves the needles in for 40 minutes. Rest for 2-3 days between courses, decide if perform the second course depending on the disease conditions. Generally cured after 1-2 courses.

[Abdominal Pain Due to Liver Stasis]

Therapeutic method: Soothe liver Qi stagnation, activate Qi and alleviate pains.

Prescription: Danzhong (RN17), Taichong (LR3), Qihai (RN6), Neiguan (PC6), Yanglingquan (GB34), Zusanli (ST36).

Mechanism of prescription: Danzhong is a confluent acupoint of Qi, it can regulate Qi; Qihai is the origin of the region between the heart and the diaphragm as well as the passway of three Jiaos, it can soothe Qi and alleviate pains; the match of Zusanli and Yanglingquan can soothe liver and reinforce gallbladder, regulate Middle-Jiao Qi; Neiguan and Taichong are both belong to Jue-Yin Meridian, the match of these two can soothe liver Qi stagnation, regulate emotions. The use of combination of these acupoints can soothe liver Qi stagnation, activate Qi and alleviate pains.

Method: Electrothermal acupuncture treatment.

Operations: Selecting the relevant acupoints, perform routine skin disinfection. Using electrothermal

陵泉、足三里各 0.8 寸，直刺内关 0.6 寸，平刺膻中 0.7 寸，斜刺太冲 0.7 寸。然后接通电热针仪，每个穴位分别给予 40mA 的电流量，以患者感到胀而舒适为度，留针 40 分钟。

疗程 每天 1 次，5 天为 1 个疗程，留针 40 分钟。疗程间休息 2～3 天，根据病情再决定是否进行第 2 个疗程的治疗。一般治疗 1～2 个疗程即可。

三、注意事项

1. 针治腹痛时，选腹部穴位要注意针刺的深度及角度，避免伤及内脏。

2. 治疗过程中，令患者注意调理饮食，避免烟酒刺激，忌食肥甘、辛辣之品，勿过饥过饱。严重者应禁食或给予半流食。

3. 对急腹症患者，要在严密的观察下配合中、西药物综合治疗。必要时采取紧急措施，绝不能延误病情，注意患者的安全。

acupuncture needles, vertically puncture into Qihai, Yanglingquan, Zusanli for 0.8" respectively, vertically puncture into Neiguan for 0.6", horizontally puncture into Danzhong for 0.7", obliquely puncture into Taichong for 0.7". Then turn on the electrothermal acupuncture equipment, apply a current of 40mA to each acupoint, and the limit is that the patient feels swell and comfortable, leaving the needles in for 40 minutes.

Therapeutic course: Treat once a day, 5 times for a course, leaves the needles in for 40 minutes. Rest for 2-3 days between courses, decide if perform the second course depending on the disease conditions. Generally cured after 1-2 courses.

III. Precautions

1. For acupuncture treatment of abdominal pains, attentions should be paid to depth and angles of needle puncture when selecting acupoints, so as to avoid organ damages.

2. During treatment, ask patients pay attention to diet regulation, avoid stimulations from tobacco and alcohol, do not eat fat and sweet, spicy food, do not be too hungry or eat too much. In severe cases, patients should be on fasting or be fed with semiliquid diets.

3. For patients with acute abdominal diseases, in combination of Chinese Herb Medicine and Western Medicine treatments under close observation are required. Take emergency measures if necessary, must not delay the illness, and pay attention to patient safety.

肠麻痹

肠麻痹是由于腹壁受某种刺激或电解质紊乱，使肠壁肌肉活动受到抑制或肠管处于麻痹状态，肠蠕动减弱或消失的一种病症。

中医认为，本病属于"腹胀""臌胀"的范畴。多由气滞、津枯、气虚等原因而致大肠传导失司，腑气不通，气聚作胀，或术后脏腑功能尚未恢复，气机逆乱而成。针治的目的重在行气导滞、调和胃肠、补中气。

一、诊断及辨证要点

1. 临床表现为高度腹胀、无矢气、肠鸣音减弱或消失，伴纳呆、神疲、焦虑、便秘。

2. 多发生于弥漫性腹膜炎，或手术后腹膜出血或感染等。

3. X线检查可见大量积气，无液平面或梗阻现象。

4. 实验室检查，血象正常

Enteroparalysis

Enteroparalysis is a disease caused by inhibited intestine wall muscle activities or numbness status of intestinal canal, weakening or disappearance of bowel movements due to certain irritation of abdominal wall or electrolyte disturbance.

Traditional Chinese Medicine believes that this disease belongs to the range of "abdominal distension", "meteorism". Most are caused by disorders of large intestine transmission, obstruction of Fu Qi, Qi gathering causing distension due to Qi stagnation, depletion of fluid, Qi deficiency, or organs functions have not yet recovered postoperatively, causing disorders of Qi Dynamic. The purpose of acupuncture treatment is to activate Qi and remove stagnation, tonify intestines and stomach, replenish Middle-Jiao Qi.

I. Key Points for Diagnosis and Syndrome Differentiation

1. The clinical manifestations include high-level abdominal distension, no flatus, reduction or disappearance of bowel sound, accompanying anorexia, mental fatigue, anxiety, constipation.

2. Most are seen in diffuse peritonitis, or postoperative retroperitoneal hemorrhage or infections, etc.

3. Large amount of accumulated gas can be seen in the X-ray examination, and no signs of fluid levels or obstruction.

4. Lab examination: Normal hemogram or leukocy-

或白细胞增多。

二、治疗方法

【脾虚气滞证】

治法 理气导滞。

处方 大肠俞（BL25）、天枢（ST25）、中脘（RN12）、足三里（ST36）、上巨虚（ST37）。

方义 本病是因大肠传导失司、腑气不通所致。取大肠经之背俞穴大肠俞与大肠经之募穴天枢相配，行气导滞，调理肠胃，恢复大肠传导功能；选腑之会穴中脘、大肠经下合穴上巨虚，取其运中通腑，以复中焦升降之职；加足三里、内庭以和胃降逆、通导腑气。诸穴共用，共收理气导滞之功。

配穴 脐下痛者，加关元、中极；脐周痛者，加气海；侧腹痛者，加带脉、归来、太冲、阳陵泉。

方法 电热针治疗。

操作 选定穴位，皮肤常规消毒。电热针斜刺（向脊柱方向）大肠俞 0.7 寸，直刺天枢

tosis.

II. Therapeutic Methods

[Syndrome of Spleen Deficiency and Qi Stagnation]

Therapeutic method: Regulate Qi and remove stagnation.

Prescription: Dachangshu(BL25), Tianshu (ST25), Zhongwan (RN12), Zusanli (ST36), Shangjuxu (ST37).

Mechanism of prescription: This disease is caused by disorders of large intestine transmission, obstruction of Fu Qi. Use the Back-Shu acupoint Dachangshu of Large Intestine to match the Mu acupoint Tianshu of Large Intestine, so as to activate Qi and remove stagnation, tonify intestines and stomach, recover the transmission function of large intestine; choose the confluent acupoint of Fu, Zhongwan, and the He acupoint Shangjuxu from Large Intestine Meridian to transport Middle-Jiao Qi and soothe Fu, so as to recover the function of Middle-Jiao ascending and descending; add Zusanli, Neiting to regulate stomach and descend adverse energy, soothe Fu Qi. The use of combination of these acupoints can regulate Qi and remove stagnation.

Matching acupoints: For subumbilical pains add Guanyuan, Zhongji. For periumbilical pains add Qihai. For lateral abdominal pains add Daimai, Guilai, Taichong, Yanglingquan.

Method: Electrothermal acupuncture treatment.

Operations: Selecting the relevant acupoints, perform routine skin disinfection. Using electrothermal acupuncture needles, obliquely puncture (toward spine)

0.8寸、中脘0.7寸，直刺上巨虚、足三里各0.8寸，向上斜刺内庭0.7寸。然后接通电热针仪，给予大肠俞20mA的电流量，分别给予天枢、中脘、上巨虚、足三里40mA的电流量，给予内庭30mA的电流量，以患者感到舒适为度，留针40分钟。

疗程 每日1次，一般3～5次即可恢复常态。

三、注意事项

1. 针灸治疗本病，以单纯动力性肠麻痹效果较好。

2. 对合并腹腔炎症或感染者，要配合药物共同治疗。

3. 治疗过程中，要注意适当禁食或进流质饮食，视病情而定。

4. 必须慎重诊断，除外梗阻性肠麻痹，以免误诊。

慢性腹泻（肠炎）

慢性腹泻又称"久泻"，大多由于消化不良、慢性肠炎、肠功能紊乱、结肠过敏、溃疡性结肠炎以及肠结核等引起。

into Dachangshu for 0.7", vertically puncture into Tianshu for 0.8", Zhongwan for 0.7", vertically puncture into Shangjuxu, Zusanli for 0.8' respectively, obliquely puncture upward into Neiting for 0.7". Then turn on the electrothermal acupuncture equipment, apply a current of 20mA to Dachangshu, a current of 40mA to Tianshu, Zhongwan, Shangjuxu, Zusanli respectively, a current of 30mA to Neiting, and the limit is that the patient feels comfortable, leaving the needles in for 40 minutes.

Therapeutic course: Once a day, generally return to normal conditions after 3-5 treatments.

III. Precautions

1. For acupuncture treatment of this disease, better efficacy can be seen in simple dynamic enteroparalysis.

2. For patients with concurrent abdominal inflammation or infection, treatment in combination with medicines is required.

3. During treatment, pay attention to appropriate fasting or liquid diet, depending on patient condition.

4. The diagnosis must be done with cautions to exclude obstructive enteroparalysis, so as to avoid misdiagnosis.

Chronic Diarrhea (Enteritis)

Chronic diarrhea is also called "long-term diarrhea", most of which are caused by dyspepsia, chronic colitis, bowel dysfunction, adaptive colitis, ulcerative colitis and enterophthisis, etc.

中医认为，脾肾阳虚、外感时邪、饮食不节或肝气郁结等，都可导致腹泻反复发作，久则脾虚胃弱，运化功能失调，脾病及肾，脾肾两虚，病情更为迁延。

Traditional Chinese Medicine believes that Yang deficiency of spleen and kidney, affecting of seasonal pathogenic factors, intemperate diet or liver Qi stagnation, etc., all may cause repeated onset of diarrhea, long time of which can cause spleen deficiency and stomach weakness, disorder of transportation and transformation functions, expanding of spleen disease to kidney, spleen and kidney deficiency, and further delay of conditions.

一、诊断及辨证要点

I. Key Points for Diagnosis and Syndrome Differentiation

1. 本病主证为大便次数增多，粪质稀薄，反复发作，病程较长。

1. The main symptoms of this disease are increased defecation frequency, thin stool, repeated onset and relatively long disease course.

2. 询问有无痢疾既往史，注意大便性质，要与慢性痢疾相鉴别。

2. Ask if there is any previous history of dysentery, pay attention to stool properties to identify this disease from chronic dysentery.

3. 如便秘与腹泻交替发生，或伴有腹痛和不规则低热，询问有无结核病史，右下腹部有无压痛与包块，结合红细胞沉降率、胃肠钡餐透视、X线、大便检查以及辅助检查，诊断有无肠结核。

3. If constipation and diarrhea occurs alternatively, or accompanying abdominal pain or irregular lower fever, ask if any medical history of enterophthisis, if any tenderness and mass of right lower abdomen, and make diagnosis on the presence of enterophthisis in combination with erythrocyte sedimentation rate, gastrointestinal barium meal fluoroscopy, X-ray examination, stool examination and auxiliary examinations.

4. 中年以上患者，全身健康状况较差，大便带血者应考虑除外肠癌。

4. For middle-aged or older patients with poor general health status and bloody stool, exclusion of intestinal cancer should be considered.

5. 发作与精神情绪有关，并伴有失眠、头晕等症。各项检查均无特殊发现，多属肠功

5. The onset of this disease is associated with mental and emotional conditions, and is accompanied with insomnia, dizziness, etc. No special findings in all exam-

能紊乱或结肠过敏。

6. 脾胃虚弱者，症见大便溏薄，或时泻时溏，内夹消化不良的食物，面色萎黄，食欲不振，疲劳倦怠，舌淡苔白，脉缓或弱。

7. 肝郁乘脾者，每遇精神刺激、情绪紧张时，即腹痛腹泻，泻后痛缓，矢气频作，伴胸胁胀闷，嗳气食少，舌淡红，苔薄白，脉弦。

8. 肾阳虚衰者，每于黎明泄泻，腹部隐痛，肠鸣而泻，形寒肢冷，舌淡苔白，脉沉细。

二、治疗方法

【脾胃虚弱证】

治法 健脾益气。

方法 电热针治疗、艾灸治疗。

（1）电热针治疗

处方 天枢（ST25）、中脘（RN12）、足三里（ST36）、大肠俞（BL25）、脾俞（BL20）、章门（LR13）。

方义 天枢是大肠募穴，中脘是胃募穴，二者可调整肠

inations, most are belong to the range of bowel dysfunction or adaptive colitis.

6. For patients with spleen and stomach weakness, symptoms include sloppy and thin stool, or diarrhea and sloppy stool occurs alternatively, within which there is poor digested food; sallow complexion, poor appetite, fatigue and tiredness, light tongue with whitish fur, slow or weak pulse.

7. For patients with liver stasis restricting spleen, upon each mental stimulation and emotional tension, abdominal pain and diarrhea will occur, pain relieving after defection, frequent onset of flatus, accompanying distress of chest and ribs, belching and less food intake, light and red tongue with thin and whitish fur, taut pulse.

8. For patients with deficiency and depletion of kidney Yang, diarrhea occurs at every dawn, with dull pain of abdomen, defection after bowel sound, cold body and limbs, light tongue with whitish fur, deep and thin pulse.

II. Therapeutic Methods

[Syndrome of Spleen and Stomach Weakness]

Therapeutic method: Invigorate spleen and tonify Qi.

Method: Electrothermal acupuncture treatment, moxa-moxibustion treatment.

(1) Electrothermal acupuncture treatment

Prescription: Tianshu (ST25), Zhongwan (RN12), Zusanli (ST36), Dachangshu (BL25), Pishu (BL20), Zhangmen (LR13).

Mechanism of prescription: Tianshu is a Mu acupoint of Large Intestine, Zhongwan is a Mu acupoint of

胃运化和传导功能,止泻消胀;脾俞与章门分别是脾经的俞募穴,俞属阳,募属阴,俞募相配,阴阳相合,可以加强健脾益气的作用。再加胃经合穴足三里、大肠之背俞穴大肠俞,以鼓舞中气,调和腑之气机。诸穴共用,可使脾阳得伸,运化有数。

配穴 脾胃虚弱者,加胃俞、气海;肝郁乘脾者,加肝俞、行间;肾阳虚衰者,加肾俞、命门、关元、三阴交。

操作 选定穴位,皮肤常规消毒。电热针直刺天枢、中脘、足三里各 0.8 寸,斜刺章门 0.7 寸,向脊椎方向斜刺脾俞、大肠俞各 0.8 寸,直刺肾俞、命门、关元各 0.7 寸。然后接通电热针仪,每个穴位分别给予 50～60mA 的电流量,以患者感到温热舒适为度,留针 40 分钟。(注:每次选 3 组穴,每日 1 次,穴位轮流交替选用;肝俞、太冲用毫针施以

Stomach, and the two acupoints can be used to regulate transportation and transformation as well as transmission functions of intestines and stomach, eliminate diarrhea and disperse swelling. Pishu and Zhangmen are Shu acupoint and Mu acupoint of the Spleen respectively, Shu belongs to Yang, Mu belongs to Yin, and the match of Shu and Mu as well as Yin and Yang can enhance the efficacies of invigorating spleen and tonifying Qi. And add the He acupoint of Stomach Meridian, Zusanli and the Back-Shu acupoint Dachangshu of Large Intestine, to promote Middle-Jiao Qi, regulate Qi Dynamic of Fu. The use of combination of these acupoints can promote extension of spleen Yang as well as regular transportation and transformation.

Matching acupoints: For spleen and stomach weakness, add Weishu, Qihai. For liver stasis restricting spleen, add Ganshu, Xingjian. For deficiency and depletion of kidney Yang, add Shenshu, Mingmen, Guanyuan, Sanyinjiao.

Operations: Selecting the relevant acupoints, perform routine skin disinfection. Using electrothermal acupuncture needles, vertically puncture into Tianshu, Zhongwan, Zusanli for 0.8" respectively, obliquely puncture into Zhangmen for 0.7", obliquely puncture toward spine into Pishu, Dachangshu for 0.8" respectively, vertically puncture into Shenshu, Mingmen, Guanyuan for 0.7" respectively. Then turn on the electrothermal acupuncture equipment, apply a current of 50-60mA to each acupoint, and the limit is that the patient feels warm and comfortable, leaving the needles in for 40 minutes. (Notes: choose 3 pairs of acupoints each time, once a day, use acupoints alternately. Use filiform needles with attenuating method for Ganshu and Taichong, strong stimulation with no needles left.)

Therapeutic course: Treat once a day, leave the needles in for 40 minutes, 60 times for a course, and start the treatment for the second course after a break of 7-10 days. Generally cured after 1-2 courses.

(2) Moxa-moxibustion treatment

Prescription: Tianshu (ST25), Zhongwan (RN12), Zusanli (ST36), Weishu (BL21), Dachangshu (BL25).

Matching acupoints: For spleen and stomach weakness, add Pishu, Qihai. For deficiency and depletion of kidney Yang, add Mingmen, Shenshu. For liver stasis restricting spleen, add Pishu, Qimen, Taichong, Yanglingquan.

Operations: After selecting 3 pairs of acupoints, treat once a day, perform moxibustion for 10-15min each time. (Notes: If moxa-cone moxibustion is used, moxibustion of 3-5 cones are needed for each acupoint. For patients with deficiency of kidney Yang, ginger-separated moxibustion or aconite moxibustion can be selected.)

Therapeutic course: Treat once a day, leave the needles in for 40 minutes, 60 times for a course, and start the treatment for the second course after a break of 7-10 days. Generally cured after 1-2 courses.

III. Precautions

1. During treatment, patients are required to pay

意饮食卫生，勿进食生冷、油腻及刺激性食物。

2. 必须注意保温，切勿受湿受凉，尤其注意腹部保温。

3. 对于泄泻日久者，要注意是否有脱水现象，脱水者要适当给予补液。

慢性结肠炎

慢性结肠炎多指慢性非特异性溃疡性结肠炎，是直肠、结肠黏膜的表浅性、非特异性炎症性病变。

中医认为，本病属于"泄泻"的范畴。多因久病体虚或饮食不节、情志郁怒，导致脏腑功能失调而成。其病变脏腑主要在脾胃，但与肝肾关系密切，病机关键主要责之于脾虚湿盛。由于病程长，故形成久病多虚或虚中夹实的病机变化。临床多为脾胃虚弱证、脾肾阳虚证。

一、诊断及辨证要点

1. 临床以腹泻、腹痛、便血、里急后重、低热、贫血、消瘦等为主要症状。

attention to dietetic hygiene, do not eat raw and cold, greasy and stimulating food.

2. Attentions must be paid to keep warm, do not be affected by damp and cold, especially on the abdomen.

3. For patients with long-term diarrhea, note if there are any dehydration symptoms. If yes, a fluid infusion should be given to affected patients.

Chronic Colitis

Chronic colitis mostly refers to chronic non-specific ulcerative colonitis, is a superficial, non-specific, inflammatory pathological change of rectum and colon mucous membrane.

Traditional Chinese Medicine believes that this disease belongs to the range of "diarrhea". Most are caused by body weakness due to long-term disease or intemperate diet, depress or anger, leading to organ dysfunction. The main affected organs are spleen and stomach, but the disease is closely related to liver and kidney, and the main point of pathogenesis is spleen deficiency with overabundance of Damp. Due to long disease course, the pathogenesis changes of deficiency due to long-term disease or intermingled deficiency and excess syndromes. Spleen and stomach weakness, Yang deficiency of spleen and kidney are two syndromes mostly seen clinically.

I. Key Points for Diagnosis and Syndrome Differentiation

1. Main clinical symptoms include diarrhea, abdominal pain, bloody stool, tenesmus, lower fever, anemia, emaciation, etc.

2. The incidence of this disease is associated with immune abnormalities, psychiatric factors, inheritance and nonspecific infections, etc.

3. Main lesion sites include rectum, sigmoid colon, in severe cases the whole colon can be affected.

4. The age of onset is mainly on the 20-40 age bracket, the onset can be acute or chronic, symptoms can be slight or severe, mostly are chronic, repeated onset, with large harm to human health.

5. For syndrome of spleen and stomach weakness, symptoms include sometime sloppy stool with undigested whole grains, abdominal distention, reduced diet intake, increased defecation frequency with intake of few greasy food, sallow complexion, fatigue and weakness, light tongue with whitish fur, thin and weak pulse.

6. For syndrome of Yang deficiency of spleen and kidney, symptoms include diarrhea at dawn, defection after bowel sound, pain relief after diarrhea, accompanying cold body and limbs, soreness and weakness of waist and knees, abdominal distension, poor appetite, light tongue with whitish fur, deep and thin pulse.

7. If possible, enteroscopy can also be done to confirm the positions of the lesions.

II. Therapeutic Methods

[Syndrome of Spleen and Stomach Weakness]

Therapeutic method: Invigorate spleen and tonify Qi, remove Damp and stop diarrhea.

Prescription: Zhongwan (RN12), Tianshu (ST25), Zusanli (ST36), Shangjuxu (ST37), Yinlingquan (SP9),

上巨虚（ST37）、阴陵泉（SP9）、三阴交（SP6）。

方义 募穴是人体脏腑之气汇聚之处，故取胃募中脘、大肠募天枢，可以健脾益气，调整胃肠之气机，使运化传导功能得以恢复；上巨虚是胃经穴，乃足阳明之脉气所发之处，有固肠止泻之功能；脾与胃相表里，取三阴交、阴陵泉以疏调足太阴脾经之经气，使脾气得运，水精四布，小便通利，则湿从小便去而泄泻自然而愈。诸穴合用，共奏健脾益气、祛湿止泻之功效。

配穴 脾虚甚者，加脾俞、关元俞；脘腹胀满者，加公孙；肝郁气滞者，加肝俞、行间；湿蕴化热者，加内庭、曲池。

方法 电热针治疗。

操作 选定穴位，皮肤常规消毒。电热针直刺中脘、天枢各 0.7 寸，直刺足三里、上巨虚各 0.8 寸，直刺阴陵泉、三阴交各 0.7 寸，接通电热针仪，

Sanyinjiao (SP6).

Mechanism of prescription: Mu acupoints are the convergence place of human body Qi, so use Mu acupoints Zhongwan from Stomach, Tianshu from Large Intestine to invigorate spleen and tonify Qi, regulate the Qi Dynamic of stomach and intestines, so as to recover the transportation and transformation functions as well as transmission function; Shangjuxu is a meridian acupoint of Stomach, as well as the place from where channel Qi of Foot Yang-Ming originates, it can nourish intestines and stop diarrhea; spleen and stomach are exterior and interior organs corresponding to each other, so use Sanyinjiao, Yinlingquan to soothe and regulate meridian Qi of Tai-Yin Spleen Meridian of Foot, to promote transportation of spleen Qi, distribute of Water essence, soothe urination, then the Damp is removed through urine, then the disease can be cured naturally. The use of combination of these acupoints can invigorate spleen and tonify Qi, remove Damp and stop diarrhea.

Matching acupoints: For severe spleen deficiency, add Pishu, Guanyuanshu. For abdominal distention add Gongsun. For liver stasis and Qi stagnation add Ganshu, Xingjian. For Damp accumulation transforming into Heat, add Neiting, Quchi.

Method: Electrothermal acupuncture treatment.

Operations: Selecting the relevant acupoints, perform routine skin disinfection. Using electrothermal acupuncture needles, vertically puncture into Zhongwan, Tianshu for 0.7" respectively, Zusanli, Shangjuxu for 0.8" respectively, Yinlingquan, Sanyinjiao for 0.7" respec-

每个穴位分别给予 50～60mA 的电流量,以患者感到温热或胀而舒适为度,留针 40 分钟。(注:每次选 3～4 个穴位,交替应用。)

疗程 每日 1 次,留针 40 分钟,60 次为 1 个疗程,疗程间可休息 7～10 天,再继续第 2 个疗程的治疗。一般治疗 1～2 个疗程即可。

【脾肾阳虚证】

治法 温补脾肾,祛湿止泻。

方法 电热针治疗、艾灸治疗。

(1)电热针治疗

处方 中脘(RN12)、脾俞(BL20)、章门(LR13)、天枢(ST25)、肾俞(BL23)、足三里(ST36)。

方义 脾俞与章门分别为脾之俞募穴,俞募相配,有健脾益气之功;配大肠募穴天枢、胃之募穴中脘、胃经之合穴足三里,可振脾阳,使之运化有数;取肾俞以益命火、壮肾阳,助脾腐熟水谷。诸穴共用,可收温补脾肾、祛湿止泻之功效。

tively. Turn on the electrothermal acupuncture equipment, apply a current of 50-60mA to each acupoint, and the limit is that the patient feels warm or swelling and comfortable, leaving the needles in for 40 minutes. (Note: select 3-4 acupoints each time, and use alternately.)

Therapeutic course: Treat once a day, leave the needles in for 40 minutes, 60 times for a course, and start the treatment for the second course after a break of 7-10 days. Generally cured after 1-2 courses.

[Syndrome of Yang Deficiency of Spleen and Kidney]

Therapeutic method: Warmly tonify spleen and kidney, remove Damp and stop diarrhea.

Method: Electrothermal acupuncture treatment, moxa-moxibustion treatment.

(1) Electrothermal acupuncture treatment

Prescription: Zhongwan (RN12), Pishu (BL20), Zhangmen (LR13), Tianshu (ST25), Shenshu (BL23), Zusanli (ST36).

Mechanism of prescription: Pishu and Zhangmen are Shu acupoint and Mu acupoint of Spleen respectively, the match of Shu and Mu can invigorate spleen and tonify Qi; match them with Mu acupoints Tianshu from Large Intestine, Zhongwan from Stomach, and the He acupoint Zusanli from Stomach Meridian, to promote spleen Yang, regular transportation and transformation. Use Shenshu to nourish Life Fire, reinforce kidney Yang, help spleen to digest food. The use of combination of these acupoints can warmly tonify spleen and kidney, remove Damp and stop diarrhea.

Matching acupoints: For deficiency and depletion of kidney Yang, and soreness and weakness of waist and knees, add Mingmen, Guanyuan. For abdominal pain and borborygmus add Dachangshu. For patients who suffer from fullness of abdomen and refuse to eat, add Weishu, Sanyinjiao. For cold body and limbs add Qihai.

Operations: Selecting the relevant acupoints, perform routine skin disinfection. Using electrothermal acupuncture needles, vertically puncture into Zhongwan, Tianshu, Zusanli for 0.8" respectively, obliquely puncture toward anterior inferior direction into Zhangmen for 0.8", obliquely puncture (with the needle tip towards spine) into Pishu for 0.7", vertically puncture into Shenshu for 0.7", vertically puncture into Guanyuan, Qihai, Sanyinjiao for 0.7" respectively, obliquely puncture (with the needle tip towards spine) into Weishu, Dachangshu for 0.8" respectively, vertically puncture into Mingmen for 0.7". Then turn on the electrothermal acupuncture equipment, apply a current of 50-60mA to each acupoint, and the limit is that the patient feels warm or swelling and comfortable, leaving the needles in for 4 minutes. (Note: select 3-4 acupoints each time, and use alternately.)

Therapeutic course: Treat once a day, leave the needles in for 40 minutes, 60 times for a course, and start the treatment for the second course after a break of 7-10 days. Generally cured after 1-2 courses.

(2) Moxa-moxibustion treatment

Prescription: Tianshu (ST25), Zhongwan (RN12), Zusanli (ST36), Pishu (BL20).

脾俞（BL20）。

配穴 气短懒言，加气海；腹中冷痛、肠鸣即泻，加神阙、水分、合谷。

操作 选定穴位，用生姜切成半分厚薄片，中间扎些小孔，放置穴位上用艾炷灸之，使局部皮肤红晕即可。每日1次，每次灸20分钟。或用艾条灸之，每次选2个穴，每日1次，各穴灸15～20分钟。

疗程 每日1次，留针40分钟，60次为1个疗程，疗程间可休息7～10天，再继续第2个疗程的治疗。一般治疗1～2个疗程即可。

三、注意事项

1. 针灸治疗效果较好，若遇效果不明显者，需配合中药治疗。

2. 施灸时，必须注意观察，绝对不能发生烧烫伤。

3. 令患者注意腹部保暖，忌食生冷、油腻、刺激性食物。

四、典型病例

刘某，男，44岁，职员，

Matching acupoints: For short of breath and laziness of speak, add Qihai; For cold and pain within abdomen, diarrhea immediately after borborygmus, add Shenque, Shuifen, Hegu.

Operations: Selecting the relevant acupoints, cut gingers into thin slices with a thickness of half a centimeter, and puncture some small holes on ginger slices, put these slices on the acupoints and cauterize them with moxa cones till local skin flush occurs. Once a day, 20 minutes for each time. Or perform moxibustion with moxa sticks, select 2 acupoints each time, once a day, 15-20 minutes for each acupoint.

Therapeutic course: Treat once a day, leave the needles in for 40 minutes, 60 times for a course, and start the treatment for the second course after a break of 7-10 days. Generally cured after 1-2 courses.

III. Precautions

1. The efficacy of acupuncture treatment is better, and in cases that the effects are not obvious, then Chinese Herb Medicine treatment should be used as well.

2. During moxibustion, careful observation is required so as to strictly forbid burns and scald.

3. Ask patients pay attention to warm keeping of abdomen, do not eat raw and cold, greasy and stimulating food.

IV. Typical Case

Liu, male, 44 years old, employee, residence: Bei-

北京人。

主诉：慢性泄泻2年多，加重1个月。病史：患者近两年因工作需要应酬多，经常饮酒，逐渐出现间歇性腹泻，上腹部作胀，多为溏泻便（呈糊状），有时为稀水便，未引起重视，近1个月来上述症状加重，大便每日2次。

刻下症：大便呈糊状，水谷不化，稍进油腻之物则大便次数增多，饮食减少，脘腹胀满不适，面色萎黄，肢倦乏力，舌淡苔白，脉细弱。未见发热、恶心、呕吐，无尿频、尿急、尿痛、便秘，无呕血、便血及脓血便。平素体健，无其他病史记载。

查体：二尖瓣区及主动脉瓣第二听诊区闻及二级收缩期杂音。肠鸣音稍活跃，无气过水声。

辅助检查：未见异常。

【诊断依据】

1. 中年男性，慢性起病，慢性腹泻有2年之久。

2. 无明显诱因间歇性出现腹泻，上腹部作胀，大便多为糊状便，有时为稀水便，已有两年之久，症状与频繁饮酒

jing.

Self-reported symptoms: Chronic diarrhea for more than 2 years, which became aggravated for one month. Medical history: The patient often drank alcohol due at social engagements required by his job, so gradually developed intermittent diarrhea, upper abdominal distension, most sloppy stool (paste-like), sometimes thin water-like stool, which didn't attracted enough attention of the patient. The above symptoms became aggravated the past month, when the patient defecated twice a day.

Current symptoms: Paste-like stool, indigestion of water and grains, increased defecation frequency with intake of few greasy food, reduced diet intake, abdominal distention, sallow complexion, fatigue and weakness, light tongue with whitish fur, thin and weak pulse. No pyrexia, nausea, vomiting were seen, no frequent micturition, urgent micturition, painful micturition, constipation, no hematemesis, bloody stool and bloody purulent stool. Usually healthy, no other recorded medical history.

Physical examination: Grade 2 systolic noise in the mitral valve area and second aortic valve area. Slightly active bowel sound, no sound of gas going through water.

Auxiliary examination: No abnormalities.

[Diagnostic Basis]

1. Middle-aged male, slow onset, chronic diarrhea for 2 years.

2. Intermittent diarrhea occurred without obvious induced causes, upper abdominal distension, most paste-like stool, sometimes thin water-like stool, for two years. The symptoms were related to frequent drinking.

有关。

3. 既往无特殊病史记载。

4. 查体除肠鸣音稍活跃外，无明显阳性体征。

5. 血、尿、便常规正常。

【证治分析】

病因 饮食所伤。

病机 饮食过量，宿食内停，阻滞肠胃，传化失常，故腹部疼痛肠鸣，脘腹痞满。

证候分析 宿食不化，则浊气上逆，故嗳腐酸臭。宿食下注，则泻下臭如败卵。泻后腐浊外泄，故腹痛减轻。舌苔厚腻，脉滑，为宿食内停之象。

病位 脾、胃、大肠。

病性 虚性。

转归 泄泻有暴泻、久泻之别，其中暴泻的转归有三：一是治愈；二是反复发作而致脾虚；三是久泻脾虚而致脾肾俱虚。

西医诊断 慢性肠炎。

中医诊断 脾胃虚弱型泄泻。

3. No previous recorded special medical history.

4. Physical examination: No obvious positive signs except slightly active bowel sound.

5. Normal in blood, urine, stool routine tests.

[Syndrome-treatment Analysis]

Etiology: Caused by diet.

Pathogenesis: Excessive food intake, internal accumulation of food, causing intestines and stomach obstruction, disorders of transportation and transformation, therefore causing abdominal pain and borborygmus, abdominal distention.

Syndrome analysis: Indigestion of accumulated food leading to abnormal rising of turbid Qi, subsequently causing belching with fetid and acidic odor. The down-flow of accumulated food causes stool with the smell of rotten eggs. Rotten and turbid Qi is excreted with defection, therefore the abdominal pain is relieved. Thick and greasy tongue furs, slippery pulse, are symptoms of internal accumulation of food.

Lesion location: Spleen, stomach, large intestine.

Disease nature: Deficiency.

Prognosis of diarrhea is divided into fulminant diarrhea and chronic diarrhea, and the outcomes of fulminant diarrhea are three: One is cure, the second is repeated onset leading to spleen deficiency. The third one is long-term diarrhea leading to spleen deficiency, subsequently causing deficiency of spleen as well as kidney.

The diagnosis of Western Medicine: Chronic colitis.

The diagnosis of Traditional Chinese Medicine: Diarrhea of spleen and stomach weakness type.

治法 健脾益胃。

方法 电热针治疗、艾灸治疗。

（1）电热针治疗

处方 以脾胃经的经穴为主。天枢（ST25）、足三里（ST36）、上巨虚（ST37）。

方义 足三里和上巨虚分别是胃及大肠之下合穴，"合治内腑"，两穴均是治疗胃肠病之要穴，临床证明有显著效果。天枢是大肠募穴，关元是小肠募穴，属肠道疾病的就近取穴。其中，关元还对里急后重有效。阴陵泉、三阴交是脾经穴，可以清利胃肠湿热。合谷是大肠经原穴，对控制腹痛有良好的作用。恶心呕吐者加内关，有降逆止呕的作用；发热者加曲池，以清除邪热。

配穴 腹痛甚者加合谷、三阴交；恶心呕吐者加内关；发热者加曲池、大椎；里急后重者加关元。

操作 选穴定位，皮肤常规消毒。电热针直刺足三里、

Therapeutic method: Invigorate spleen and tonify stomach.

Method: Electrothermal acupuncture treatment, moxa-moxibustion treatment.

(1) Electrothermal acupuncture treatment

Prescription: Mainly use meridian acupoints from Spleen Meridian and Stomach Meridian. Tianshu (ST25), Zusanli (ST36), Shangjuxu (ST37).

Mechanism of prescription: Zusanli and Shangjuxu are lower He acupoints of Stomach and Large Intestine respectively, "He acupoints treat viscera diseases", the two acupoints are both important acupoints for treatment of gastrointestinal diseases, and their obvious efficacies have been proven clinically. Tianshu is a Mu acupoint of Large Intestine, Guanyuan is a Mu acupoint of Small Intestine, the use of these two belongs to the range of nearest acupoint selection for intestinal diseases. And Guanyuan also has effects on tenesmus. Yinlingquan, Sanyinjiao are meridian acupoints of Spleen Meridian, they can remove and disperse Damp-Heat of stomach and intestines. Hegu is a Yuan acupoint of Large Intestine Meridian, it has good effects on control of abdominal pains. Add Neiguan for patients with nausea and vomiting, to descend adverse energy and stop vomiting. For patients with pyrexia add Quchi to remove Heat toxins.

Matching acupoints: For severe abdominal pains add Hegu, Sanyinjiao. For nausea and vomiting add Neiguan. For pyrexia add Quchi, Dazhui. For tenesmus add Guanyuan.

Operations: Selecting the relevant acupoints, perform routine skin disinfection. Using electrothermal

天枢、上巨虚各 0.8 寸，接通电热针仪，每个穴位分别给予 50mA 的电流量，以温热或胀感舒适为度，留针 40 分钟。配合毫针治疗，留针 40 分钟。

疗程 每天 1 次，留针 40 分钟，10 次为 1 个疗程。疗程间可休息 3～5 天，再进行第 2 个疗程的治疗。一般需要治疗 2～3 个疗程。

治疗过程 患者至今病情稳定。

（2）艾灸治疗

处方 足三里（ST36）、天枢（ST25）、上巨虚（ST37）。

配穴 同电热针治疗。

操作 采用艾条灸，每次选用 2 个穴，每个穴艾条悬灸 15～20 分钟。

疗程 同电热针治疗。

【生活调摄】

1. 禁食生冷、油腻食物，注意饮食卫生。

2. 切勿受潮及受凉，注意腹部保暖。

3. 在治疗过程中，注意饮食要有节制，保持饮食规律

acupuncture needles, vertically puncture into Zusanli, Tianshu, Shangjuxu for 0.8" respectively. Turn on the electrothermal acupuncture equipment, apply a current of 50mA to each acupoint, and the limit is that the patient feels warm or swelling and comfortable, leaving the needles in for 40 minutes. Combine with filiform needles, leaving the needles in for 40 minutes.

Therapeutic course: Once a day, leave the needles in for 40 minutes, 10 times for a course. Start the treatment for the second course after a break of 3-5 days. Generally treat for 2-3 courses.

Therapeutic process: The patient's condition is stable so far.

(2) Moxa-moxibustion treatment

Prescription: Zusanli (ST36), Tianshu (ST25), Shangjuxu (ST37).

Matching acupoints: Same as the electrothermal acupuncture treatment.

Operations: Use moxa-stick moxibustion, select 2 acupoints each time, perform moxa-stick suspension-moxibustion on each acupoint for 15-20 minutes.

Therapeutic course: The same to electrothermal acupuncture treatment.

[Lifestyle Change and Health Maintenance]

1. Do not eat raw and cold, greasy food, pay attention to dietetic hygiene.

2. Do not be affected by Damp and Cold, pay attention to warm keeping of abdomen.

3. During treatment, note that diet should be controlled, keep regular diet and good mood.

营养障碍性水肿

营养障碍性水肿，是指体内营养物质长期摄入不足，恶病质的过度消耗，或因其他疾病引起的消化不良而导致的一种不同程度水肿的低蛋白血症。由于低蛋白血症使血浆胶体渗透压降低，皮下脂肪少，脂肪松弛，过多的水分从毛细血管渗出而存积于细胞间隙，故形成水肿。若合并维生素等缺乏，则水肿更为严重。临床多表现为精神萎靡，面白无华，饮食缺少，全身乏力，浮肿按之不起，初期常是轻度浮肿，仅局限于踝部、下肢、面部等，严重者则全身浮肿兼有腹水、胸腔积液，劳累和多食盐分者浮肿常加重。

中医认为，本病属于"阴水"的范畴。多因饮食习惯不良，偏食厌食，摄食过少，致脾气亏损；或病后及劳倦伤脾，脏腑功能失调，以致脾虚不能运化水湿，肾虚开合不利，水湿泛滥于肌肤引起。临床多为虚证。

Trophopathic Edema

Trophopathic edema refers to a hypoproteinemia with edema of varying degrees, which is caused by long-term insufficiency of nutrition intake and excessive consumption by cachexia, or dyspepsia due to other diseases. Since hypoproteinemia reduces the plasma colloid osmotic pressure, subcutaneous fat, causes looseness of fat, let excessive water exudes from capillaries and therefore form edema. The condition of edema will be more severe if concurrent vitamin deficiency and other deficiencies are exit. Normally the clinical manifestations include spiritlessness, pale and gloomy complexion, lack of food intake, systemic asthenia, swelling which do not rebound after being pressed, generally slight swelling at first which only limited to ankle, lower limbs, face and other parts, in severe cases there occurs asthenia accompanying ascites and hydrothorax, and in cases of tiredness and excessive intake of salt, the swelling generally aggravates.

Traditional Chinese Medicine believes that this disease belongs to the range of "Yin edema". Most are caused by bad dietary habits, dietary bias and anorexia, or too little food intake, leading to depletion and deficiency of spleen Qi; or spleen damage after diseases or fatigue, dysfunction of internal organs, causing spleen deficiency therefore unable to transportation and transformation Water-Damp as well as kidney deficiency therefore unsmooth opening and closing, over-flooding of Water-Damp upon the skin. Deficiency syndromes are

一、诊断及辨证要点

1. 脾胃气虚者，头面或四肢水肿，时肿时消，食欲缺少，倦怠少力，少气懒言，大便溏泻，舌淡苔白，脉弱缓。

2. 脾肾阳虚者，眼睑及全身水肿，腰以下肿甚，按之凹陷不起；腰腹胀满，腰酸腿软，食少便溏，小便短小，面色苍白，神疲肢冷，舌淡苔白滑，脉沉迟。

二、治疗方法

【脾肾阳虚证】

治法　健脾利湿，化气利水。

处方　脾俞（BL20）、胃俞（BL21）、三焦俞（BL22）、气海（RN6）、足三里（ST36）、三阴交（SP6）、水分（RN9）。

方义　取脾俞、胃俞培补中焦，以助健运；三焦俞以通调水道，气海以调畅气机，气机和畅，则水道通利；水分

mostly seen clinically.

I. Key Points for Diagnosis and Syndrome Differentiation

1. For patients with Qi deficiency of spleen and stomach, symptoms include edema of face or limbs, which onset time to time, lack of appetite, fatigue and weakness, short of breath and laziness of speak, sloppy stool, light tongue with whitish fur, weak and slow pulse.

2. For patients with Yang deficiency of spleen and kidney, symptoms include edema of eyelids and anasarca, which especially severe at parts under the waist, not rebounding after being pressed; waist and abdominal distention. Aching lumbus and limp legs, less food intake and sloppy stool, short and less amount of urination, pale complexion, mental fatigue and cold limbs, light tongue with white and smooth fur, deep and slow pulse.

II. Therapeutic Methods

[Syndrome of Yang Deficiency of Spleen and Kidney]

Therapeutic method: Invigorate spleen and remove Damp, transform Qi and soothe Water.

Prescription: Pishu (BL20), Weishu (BL23), Sanjiaoshu (BL22), Qihai (RN6), Zusanli (ST36), Shuifen (RN9).

Mechanism of prescription: Use Pishu, Weishu to replenish Middle Jiao to promote normal transportation. Use Sanjiaoshu to dredge and regulate Water channels. Use Qihai to regulate and soothe Qi Dynamic, and regu-

合利水邪，三穴合用可行气利水。足三里健脾化湿，助气血生化之源，促进脏腑功能恢复；三阴交导湿下行。诸穴共用可收健脾利湿，化气利水之效。

配穴 肾脾阳虚者加肾俞、太溪；脘腹胀满者加中脘；便溏泻者加天枢。

方法 电热针治疗（温补法）。

操作 选定穴位，常规皮肤消毒。电热针向脊柱方向斜刺脾俞、肾俞、胃俞、三焦俞各0.8寸，直刺气海0.8寸，直刺水分0.8寸，直刺足三里0.8寸，直刺三阴交0.7寸。接通电热针仪，每个穴位分别给予电流量60mA。另配以毫针刺太溪0.5寸，留针40分钟。（注：上述穴位分为两组，轮流交替使用。）

疗程 每天1次，10次为1个疗程，两个疗程间休息3天。

lated Qi Dynamic can promote unobstructed Water channels. Shuifen can remove Water toxins, the combination of these three acupoints can transform Qi and smooth Water. Zusanli can invigorate spleen and remove Damp, facilitate the source of generation and transformation of Qi-blood, promote the recovery of internal organ functions; Sanyinjiao can induce the down-flow of Damp. The use of combination of these acupoints can invigorate spleen and remove Damp, transform Qi and soothe Water.

Matching acupoints: For Yang deficiency of kidney and spleen add Shenshu, Taixi. For abdominal distention add Zhongwan. For sloppy stool add Tianshu.

Method: electrothermal acupuncture treatment (warm tonifying).

Operations: Prepare selected acupoints, perform routine skin disinfection. Using electrothermal acupuncture needles, obliquely puncture toward spine into Pishu, Shenshu, Weishu, Sanjiaoshu for 0.8" respectively, vertically puncture into Qihai and Shuifen for 0.8", Zusanli for 0.8", Sanyinjiao for 0.7". Turn on the electrothermal acupuncture equipment, apply a current of 60mA to each acupoint. Additionally, using filiform needles, vertically puncture into Taixi for 0.5", leaving the needles in for 40 minutes. (Note: Divide above acupoints into two groups for alternate use.)

Therapeutic course: Once a day, 10 times for a course. Rest for 3 days between two courses.

III. Precautions

1. Note that instruct patients to supplement protein, improve intake of nutritious food, remember that salt intake should be appropriate, do not develop dietary bias.

2. Avoid overstrain, pay attention to appropriate rest, alternate work with rest, keep regular lifestyle.

IV. Typical Case

Su, female, 32 years old, employee, residence: Beijing.

Self-reported symptoms: Puffy face and swollen limbs for 3 months, which became aggravated in the last 2 weeks. Medical history: The patient had healthy body before, then due to gradual weight increase, she started to control diet and take weight-reducing drugs in order to lose weight, then gradually developed ankle edema, which was slight at start and then diffused to face and lower limbs recently. In hospital examinations, no positive signs were found except low protein level, but symptoms like spiritlessness, abdominal distention and less food intake, mental fatigue and asthenia, short and less amount of urination, sloppy stool were occurred, and the edema aggravated with tiredness, and the treatment efficacy was poor.

Current symptoms: Pale complexion, swollen limbs, mental fatigue and asthenia, aggravated time to time, poor appetite and sleep, good urination and defection. Light tongue with white and smooth fur. Deep and thin pulse.

Physical examination: Grade 2 systolic noise at mitral valve area and second aortic valve area. Lower limbs and ankle swelling with pitting edema.

Auxiliary examination: Blood biochemical tests indicated "low protein".

[Diagnostic Basis]

1. Patients control diet by themselves, take antiobesity drugs.

2. Biochemical tests indicated "low protein".

3. Diagnose based on clinical symptoms and signs.

4. Dysfunctions of liver, spleen and kidney.

[Syndrome-treatment Analysis]

Etiology: Caused by diet, spleen deficiency and Damp obstruction.

Pathogenesis: Spleen deficiency and Damp retention due to diet control, overstrain, deficiency and depletion of spleen Qi, weakness of Middle Yang, incapability of Qi transformation and Water transportation, Water-Damp over-flooding upon skin leading to formation of edema.

Syndrome analysis: Spleen deficiency can lead to weakness of Middle Yang, disorder of normal transportation, Qi not transformed into Water, therefore cause over-flooding of Water toxins, face and lower limbs swelling can be seen, and Damp is Yin toxin with viscosity property, which can be more possible to impair spleen with tiredness, the swelling occurs and disappears repeatedly. Therefore the swelling aggravates with tiredness or in the afternoon; spleen deficiency can lead to

化，水湿不行而小便短少，舌淡苔白滑，脉沉细，为脾虚湿邪内蕴之象。

病位 肺、脾、肾。
病性 虚性。
西医诊断 营养障碍性水肿。

中医诊断 阴水。

治法 温运脾阳，气化利水。
方法 电热针治疗。
处方 脾俞（BL20）、足三里（ST36）、三阴交（SP6）、三焦俞（BL22）、胃俞（BL21）、气海（RN6）、水分（RN9）。

方义 取脾俞、胃俞培补中焦，以助运化；三焦俞以通调水道；气海以调畅气机，气机和畅，则水道通行；水分可分利水邪，三穴合用可行气利水；足三里健脾化湿，助气血生化之源，促进脏腑功能恢复；三阴交导湿下行，诸穴共用，可收湿运脾阳，气化利水

weak transportation and transformation, therefore causes abdominal distention and less food intake, sloppy stool. Spleen deficiencies can lead to non-warm-reinforcing of Yang, therefore causes pale complexion, mental fatigue and asthenia, non-transformation of Yang-Water, non-transportation of Water-Damp leading to short and less amount of urination, light tongue with white and smooth fur, deep and thin pulse. All the above are signs of internal retention of Damp toxin due to spleen deficiency.

Lesion location: Lung, spleen, kidney.
Disease nature: Deficiency.
The diagnosis of Western Medicine: Trophopathic edema.
The diagnosis of Traditional Chinese Medicine: Yin edema.
Therapeutic method: Warm and activate spleen Yang, transform Qi and soothe Water.
Method: Electrothermal acupuncture treatment.
Prescription: Pishu (BL20), Zusanli (ST36), Sanyinjiao (SP6), Sanjiaoshu (BL22), Weishu (BL21), Qihai (RN6), Shuifen (RN9).

Mechanism of prescription: Use Pishu, Weishu to replenish Middle Jiao to promote transportation and transformation. Use Sanjiaoshu to dredge and regulate Water channels. Use Qihai to regulate and soothe Qi Dynamic, and regulated Qi Dynamic can promote unobstructed Water channels; Shuifen can remove Water toxins, the combination of these three acupoints can transform Qi and smooth Water. Use Zusanli to invigorate spleen and disperse Damp, facilitate the source

之功效。

配穴 脘闷少食加中脘，和胃消胀；脾肾阳虚加肾俞、太溪，补肾温阳，以利开阖；便溏加天枢，调理肠腑。

操作 选定穴位，皮肤常规消毒。电热针直刺足三里、三阴交、水分、气海各0.7寸，斜刺（针尖向脊柱）脾俞、胃俞、三焦俞各0.8寸，接通电热针仪，每个穴位分别给予50mA的电流量，以患者感到温热或胀感为度，留针40分钟。（注：每次选3组穴给予电热针治疗，余者用毫针治疗。）

疗程 每日1次，10次为1个疗程，连续治疗3个疗程，疗程间可休息3天。

治疗过程 每日1次，连续治疗12次，患者症状缓解，浮肿消退，精神好转，饮食增加，二便正常，为继续巩固疗效，共治疗30次，随访1年未

of generation and transformation of Qi-blood, promote the recovery of internal organ functions; Sanyinjiao can induce the downward flow of Damp, the use of combination of these acupoints can warm and activate spleen Yang, transform the Qi and soothe the Water.

Matching acupoints: For chest distress add Zhongwan to regulate stomach and eliminate distension. For Yang deficiency of spleen and kidney add Shenshu, Taixi to replenish kidney and warm Yang so as to promote opening and closure. For sloppy stool add Tianshu, to tonify intestines.

Operations: Select the relevant acupoints, perform routine skin disinfection. Using electrothermal acupuncture needles, vertically puncture into Zusanli, Sanyinjiao, Shuifen, Qihai for 0.7" respectively, obliquely puncture (with the needle tip towards spine) into Pishu, Weishu, Sanjiaoshu for 0.8" respectively. Turn on the electrothermal acupuncture equipment, apply a current of 50mA to each acupoint, and the limit is that the patient feels warm or swell and comfortable, leaving the needles in for 40 minutes. (Note：Select 3 pairs of acupoints for electrothermal acupuncture treatment each time, and treat the other acupoints with filiform needles.)

Therapeutic course: Once a day, 10 times for a course. Continuously treat for 3 courses. Rest for 3 days between courses.

Therapeutic process: Once a day, continuously treat 12 times, the patient's symptoms were relieved, the swelling dispersed, mental status improved, food intake increased, with normal urination and defection, and the patient was received total 30 treatments in order to con-

见复发。

【生活调摄】

1. 饮食必须合理满足生理需要，多了解营养学方面的知识。

2. 减肥要选择对健康无害而有益于健康的方法；多增加体育锻炼，增强体质，提高自身免疫功能；合理安排生活。

3. 多食用蔬菜、水果，忌食膏粱厚味之品，饮食要清淡。

慢性肾小球肾炎

慢性肾小球肾炎，简称慢性肾炎，是一种常见的肾脏疾病。

中医认为，本病属于"水肿""腰痛""虚劳"等范畴。多因食饱劳倦等因素伤及脾胃，致使体内水精散布及气化功能发生障碍而发病。

一、诊断及辨证要点

1. 病程长，有蛋白尿、镜下血尿、水肿等临床症状，常伴有不同程度的肾功能损伤。

2. 多因患者自身免疫功能缺失所致。

solidate the efficacies, and there were no recurrence seen in a year of follow-up.

[Lifestyle Change and Health Maintenance]

1. The diet must be reasonable to meet physiological needs, learn more knowledge about nutriology.

2. Methods of losing weight which have no harm but benefits to health should be chosen; increase sports exercises to strengthen physical body, improve autoimmune functions; reasonably arrange life.

3. Eat more vegetables and fruits, do not eat greasy and surfeit flavor, fat rich food, have light diet.

Chronic Glomerulonephritis

Chronic glomerulonephritis, chronic nephritis for short, is a common kidney disease.

Traditional Chinese Medicine believes that this disease belongs to the category of "edema", "lumbago", "consumptive disease", etc. Most are caused by factors such as excessive food intake and fatigue impairing spleen and kidney, leading to Water essence diffusing within the body and disorder of Qi transformation.

I. Key Points for Diagnosis and Syndrome Differentiation

1. Long disease course, clinical symptoms include proteinuria, microscopic hematuria, edema; often accompanied with kidney dysfunctions of different degrees.

2. Most are caused by absence of autoimmune functions of the patient.

3. 部分患者是由急性肾炎演变而来，有肾炎病史。

4. 初病多足跗微肿，逐渐周身浮肿。腰以下肿甚，按之凹陷不易恢复，小便清利或短涩，常伴有腹胀、便溏、腰痛、腿酸软、畏寒肢冷等症状。

二、治疗方法

【脾肾阳虚证】

治法 健脾温肾，助阳利水。

处方 肾俞（BL23）、脾俞（BL20）、足三里（ST36）、三阴交（SP6）、气海（RN6）、水分（RN9）、太溪（KI3）。

方义 肾俞可温补肾阳，配足少阴肾经原穴太溪，以温肾固本，助阳利水。脾俞可温运脾阳，足三里可健脾培土振中阳，三阴交长于疏通脾经，为输布运化精液，三穴相配能健脾胃，促运化，祛水湿。温补气海以助阳化气，取水分以分利水邪。诸穴共用，能壮肾阳，健脾运，可收温阳化气利水之功效。

3. For some patients, the disease is developed from acute nephritis, with a history of nephritis.

4. At first it normally is slight swelling at the back of foot, then gradually develops into systemic swelling. Especially severe swelling at parts under the waist, not easy to rebound after being pressed, clear and disinhibited or short and pain urination, often accompanying symptoms such as abdominal distension, sloppy stool, waist pain, aching and limp legs, intolerance of cold and extreme chilliness.

II. Therapeutic Methods

[Syndrome of Yang Deficiency of Spleen and Kidney]

Therapeutic method: Invigorate spleen and warm kidney, promote Yang and soothe Water.

Prescription: Shenshu (BL23), Pishu (BL20), Zusanli (ST36), Sanyinjiao (SP6), Qihai (RN6), Shuifen (RN9), Taixi (KI3).

Mechanism of prescription: Shenshu can warm and tonify kidney Yang, and can warm kidney and strengthen foundation as well as promote Yang and soothe Water when being matched with the Yuan acupoint Taixi from Shao-Yin Kidney Meridian of Foot. Pishu can warm and activate spleen Yang, Zusanli can invigorate spleen, replenish Earth and prosper Middle-Jiao Yang, Sanyinjiao is good at soothe Spleen Meridian, distribute as well as transport and transform essence fluid, the match of these three can invigorate spleen and stomach, promote transportation and transformation, remove

Water-Damp. Use warm tonifying method for the acupoint Qihai to promote Yang and transform Qi, use Shuifen to remove Water toxins. The use of combination of these acupoints can strengthen kidney Yang, invigorate spleen and transportation, so as to warm Yang, transform Qi and disperse Water.

Matching acupoints: For abdominal distension add Zhongwan. For sloppy and thin stool add Tianshu, Yinlingquan.

Method: Electrothermal acupuncture treatment (warm tonifying).

Operations: Selecting the relevant acupoints, perform routine skin disinfection. Using electrothermal acupuncture needles, obliquely puncture toward spine into Pishu, Shenshu for 0.8" respectively, vertically puncture into Zusanli for 0.8", Sanyinjiao for 0.7", Zhongwan for 0.7", Tianshu for 0.7", Yinlingquan for 0.7". Turn on the electrothermal acupuncture equipment, apply a current of 60-80mA to each acupoint. Additionally, using filiform needles, vertically puncture into Taixi for 0.4", leaving the needles in for 40 minutes.

Therapeutic course: Once a day, 10 times for a course. Rest for 3 days between courses.

III. Precautions

1. The acupuncture therapy has good efficacies in treatments of hematuria, proteinuria, edema and other symptoms, however for patients with severe impairment of kidney, combination of Chinese Herb Medicine and Western Medicine treatments is required.

2. Patients with severe edema should rest in bed,

息，待病转好再离床活动，避免过劳。

3. 避免感冒、受寒、受潮湿，注意防止上呼吸道及泌尿系感染，注意盐摄入要适量及少饮水，还要注意少吃醋、虾、蟹及生冷食物。

四、典型病例

冯某，男，43岁，职员，北京人。

主诉：腰痛1年，全身浮肿3个月。病史：患者于1年前的秋季，夜临湿冷之地，自觉着凉，第2天发烧，腰痛，周身无力，腰酸腿软，经医院诊为"急性肾炎"，经治不适症状减轻，但未根治，始终腰痛，晨起上眼睑浮肿，近3个月全身水肿，尿少，怕冷，食欲不振，肢体无力，经中、西医诊治效果不明显。

刻下症：晨起眼睑浮肿，全身浮肿，腰部疼痛，活动后加重，纳差，时有恶心呕吐，眠差，二便通畅。舌质淡，苔白，脉沉细。

and get out of bed for activities after condition improvement, avoid overstrain.

3. Avoid catching a cold, being affected by Cold and Damp, note that avoid upper respiratory tract and urinary system infections. Note that salt intake should be appropriate and drink less water. Also, it should be noted that intake less vinegar, shrimps, crabs and other raw and cold food.

IV. Typical Case

Feng, male, 43 years old, employee, residence: Beijing.

Self-reported symptoms: Waist pain for 1 year, systemic dropsy for 3 months. Medical history: In the last autumn, the patient arrived at a damp and cold place at night, and felt that he caught a cold. The patient developed fever in the next day, accompanying waist pain, systemic weakness, aching lumbus and limp legs, and was diagnosed as "acute nephritis" by a hospital and his symptoms were relieved after treatment, but no radical cure achieved. He still had waist pain with upper eyelid swelling upon wake-up time at each morning. In the recent 3 months, he developed anasarca with symptoms like less urine, intolerance to cold, poor appetite, weakness of body and limbs, and little efficacies obtained after treatment of both Traditional Chinese Medicine and Western Medicine.

Current symptoms: Upper eyelid swelling in the morning, systemic swelling, waist pain, aggravated after activities, poor appetite, nausea and vomiting which occurring time to time, poor sleep, smooth urination and defection. Light tongue with white fur, deep and thin pulse.

查体：二尖瓣区及主动脉瓣第二听诊区闻及二级收缩期杂音。

辅助检查：血常规检查示红细胞计数 $2.94\times10^{12}/L$、白细胞计数 $5.2\times10^9/L$、血红蛋白 82g/L。尿常规检查示蛋白（++）、红细胞计数 2～3 个、白细胞计数 5～6 个。肾功能正常。

【诊断依据】

1. 中年男性，全身水肿 3 个月。

2. 血常规提示贫血。

3. 尿常规提示有蛋白、红细胞、白细胞、管型。

4. 1 年前有急性肾炎病史。

5. 腰酸腿软，周身无力，长期腰痛，有水肿病史。

【证治分析】

病因 阳虚水泛。

病机 肾阳亏虚，膀胱气化不利，开阖不利，水液内停，形成水肿。

证候分析 脾虚水肿，久延不愈，伤及肾阳，肾阳亏虚，水液不能排泄，其肿日趋加重。症见全身水肿，腹大胸满，水气上凌心肺，故卧喘促；肾阳不足，膀胱气化失

Physical examination: Grade 2 systolic noise at mitral valve area and second aortic valve area.

Auxiliary examination: Blood routine examination indicated erythrocyte $2.94\times10^{12}/L$, leukocyte $5.2\times10^9/L$, hemoglobin 82g/L. Urine routine examination indicated protein (++), erythrocyte 2-3, leukocyte 5-6. Normal kidney functions.

[Diagnostic Basis]

1. Middle-aged man, anasarca for 3 months.

2. Blood routine examination indicated anemia.

3. Urine routine examination indicated presence of proteins, erythrocytes, leukocytes, and casts.

4. History of acute nephritis one year ago.

5. Aching lumbus and limp legs, body weakness, long-term waist pain, history of edema.

[Syndrome-treatment Analysis]

Etiology: Yang deficiency and over-flooding of Water.

Pathogenesis: Depletion and deficiency of kidney Yang, bad Qi transformation of bladder, unsmooth opening and closing, internal retention of Water fluid, causing edema.

Syndrome analysis: Spleen deficiency and edema, which last for a long time, impaired kidney Yang and caused depletion and deficiency of kidney Yang, Water fluid couldn't be discharged out, therefore the edema became more and more severe. Symptoms included anasarca, big abdomen and chest distention, Water-Qi as-

常，则尿短少；肾阳虚衰，不能温煦，则畏寒肢冷，面色萎黄；舌淡胖，边有齿痕，苔白，脉沉细为阳气虚衰，水湿内盛之象。

病位 脾、肾。

病性 脾肾阳虚。

西医诊断 慢性肾炎。

中医诊断 水肿。

治法 温肾健脾，化气行水。

方法 电热针治疗。

处方 肾俞（BL23）、关元（RN4）、三焦俞（BL22）、脾俞（BL20）、足三里（ST36）、太溪（KI3）、三阴交（SP6）。

方义 肾俞温补肾阳，关元助阳气化，三焦俞调三焦气化功能，分利水肿；脾俞、足三里健脾以运水，扶正培元，健脾益气；太溪为肾之原穴，取之以滋补肾阴；三阴交为足三阴经交会穴，取之滋养肝、

cending to heart and lungs therefore caused shortness of breath when lying; deficiency of kidney Yang, Qi transformation disorder of bladder, causing shortness and less amount of urination; depletion and deficiency of kidney Yang couldn't warm the body, therefore cause intolerance of cold and extreme chilliness, sallow complexion; light and fat tongue with teeth prints at edge, whitish tongue fur, deep and thin pulse, these are symptoms of depletion and deficiency of Yang Qi, internal over-abundance of Water-Damp.

Lesion location: Spleen, kidney.

Disease nature: Yang deficiency of spleen and kidney.

The diagnosis of Western Medicine: Chronic nephritis.

The diagnosis of Traditional Chinese Medicine: Edema.

Therapeutic method: Warm kidney and invigorate spleen, transform Qi and transport Water.

Method: Electrothermal acupuncture treatment.

Prescription: Shenshu (BL23), Guanyuan (RN4), Sanjiaoshu (BL22), Pishu (BL20), Zusanli (ST36), Taixi (KI3), Sanyinjiao (SP6).

Mechanism of prescription: Shenshu can warm and tonify kidney Yang, Guanyuan can promote transformation of Yang Qi, Sanjiaoshu can regulate Qi transformation function of three Jiaos, remove edema; Pishu, Zusanli can invigorate spleen to transport Water, strengthen healthy Qi and reinforce vital essence, invigorate spleen and tonify Qi; Taixi is a Yuan acupoint of Kidney, it can

脾、肾。诸穴合用，可收滋阴清热利尿之功效。

配穴 血尿者加血海；心悸、失眠者加神门；小便不利者加水道；小腹胀满者加曲骨。

操作 选定穴位，皮肤常规消毒。电热针直刺关元、水分、足三里、三阴交各0.7寸，斜刺（针尖向脊柱）肾俞、脾俞、三焦俞各0.8寸，接通电热针仪，每个穴位分别给予电流量50mA，以患者感到温热或胀感而舒适为度，留针40分钟。（注：每次选3组穴轮流交替应用电热针，余穴给予毫针治疗，留针40分钟。）

疗程 每日1次，10次为1个疗程，中间休息3天，连续治疗3个疗程。

治疗过程 该患者治疗经过顺利，经过20次治疗后，症状基本消失，精神好转，体力增加。2个月后，全身浮肿消退，腰痛消失，血、尿常规复诊正常。2个月之前，每日治疗1次，2个月后基本痊愈，

nourish kidney Yin; Sanyinjiao is the confluent acupoint of three Yin meridians of Foot, it can nourish liver, spleen, kidney. The combination of these acupoints can be used to nourish Yin, clear Heat and promote urination.

Matching acupoints: For hematuria add Xuehai. For palpitation and insomnia add Shenmen. For unsmooth urination add Shuidao. For distension of lower abdomen add Qugu.

Operations: Selecting the relevant acupoints, perform routine skin disinfection. Using electrothermal acupuncture needles, vertically puncture into Guanyuan, Shuifen, Zusanli, Sanyinjiao for 0.7'' respectively, obliquely puncture (with the needle tip towards spine) into Shenshu, Pishu, Sanjiaoshu for 0.8'' respectively. Turn on the electrothermal acupuncture equipment, apply a current of 50mA to each acupoint, and the limit is that the patient feels warm or swelling and comfortable, leaving the needles in for 40 minutes. (Note: Select 3 pairs of acupoints to apply electrothermal acupuncture treatment each time, and treat the other acupoints with filiform needle, leaving the needles in for 40 minutes.)

Therapeutic course: Once a day, 10 times for a course. Rest for 3 days between courses. Continuously treat for 3 courses.

Therapeutic process: The treatment for this patient was successful, and his symptoms basically disappeared after 20 treatments, the mental status improved and the physical strength increased. After 2 months, his systemic swelling dispersed, the waist pain disappeared and the results from blood and urine routine retests were normal. Two months before, treated once a day, and the patient was basically cured after 2 months. The patient then received treatment once every two days to consolidate the efficacies. After 15 treatments, he was discharged from the hospital. 2-year follow-up, the patient could work and have daily life normally, with not any discomfort.

[Lifestyle Change and Health Maintenance]

1. During treatment, medicine treatment is not necessary for patients with obvious efficacies.

2. During treatment, keep light diet, pay attention to warm keeping and rest, avoid fatigue.

3. In severe cases, it is required to choose a comprehensive therapy with combination of acupuncture and medicine therapies for treatment.

Pyelonephritis

Pyelonephritis refers to local inflammation of kidney. Most are caused by ascending bacterial infections, among which the most common is E. Coli.

Traditional Chinese Medicine believes that this disease belongs to the range of "stranguria". Most are caused by unclear external genital organs, invasion of filthiness and turbidness toxins into bladder, or excessive intake of fat and sweet food leading to internal generation of Damp-Heat which downward flowing into bladder and causes Damp-Heat of bladder as well as irregular Qi transformation.

I. Key Points for Diagnosis and Syndrome Differentiation

1. For patients with Damp-Heat of bladder, symp-

赤热，尿时灼痛，急迫不爽，起痛较急，可伴发热，舌苔黄腻，脉滑数。

2. 阴虚邪恋者，症见小便黄赤，尿时灼热和疼痛，口渴欲饮，手足心热，腰酸明显，舌红少苔，脉细数。

3. 脾肾两虚者，病久不疗，常因劳倦或房事而诱发。症见小便余沥不尽，周身乏力，腰骶部重坠，腰痛绵绵，或伴有夜尿多，舌质偏淡，苔薄白，脉沉细。

4. 女性发病率偏高。主要临床表现为：腰痛、腰酸、尿频、尿急，有急性与慢性之分。急性肾盂肾炎起病急，可伴有发热、寒战、恶心、食欲不振等症状，体检时有上输尿管点或肋腰点压痛和肾区叩痛。慢性肾盂肾炎从急性者演变而来，常伴有乏力、低热、夜尿等症状。

toms include dark and hot urine, burning-like pain when urinating, urgent and unsmooth urination, acute onset of pain, may accompany pyrexia, yellow and greasy tongue fur, slippery and rapid pulse.

2. For patients with Yin deficiency and toxin accumulation, symptoms include yellow and dark urine, hot and burning-like pain when urinating, thirsty and desire of drinking, hot palms and sole centers, obvious waist soreness, red tongue with less fur, thin and rapid pulse.

3. For patients with spleen and kidney deficiency, the disease lasts for a long time and is hard to cure, which is normally induced by fatigue or excessive sexual intercourses. Symptoms include endless and dripping urine, systemic asthenia, bearing-down feeling at the lumbosacral portion, long-term waist pain, or accompanying excessive urine at night, light tongue with thin and whitish fur, deep and thin pulse.

4. The incidence rate is higher among females than that of males. Main clinical manifestations include: Lower back pain, lower back soreness, frequent micturition, urgent micturition, and are divided into acute ones and chronic ones. The onset of acute pyelonephritis is urgent, and it may be accompanied with symptoms like pyrexia, chills, nausea, poor appetite, and there will be tenderness at the point of upper urethra or the costolumbar point and percussion pain at the kidney area. Chronic pyelonephritis is developed from acute ones, normally is accompanied with symptoms like asthenia, lower fever and urination at night.

二、治疗方法

【膀胱湿热证】

治法 清热利尿通淋。

处方 膀胱俞（BL28）、中极（RN3）、阴陵泉（SP9）、委阳（BL39）。

方义 膀胱俞属膀胱经，为膀胱之气输注之处，中极为膀胱之募，两穴配合为俞募配穴法，可调整膀胱之气，疏利气机，利尿通淋；阴陵泉是脾经原穴，可健脾胃，助气化，以利小便；委阳是膀胱经穴，又是三焦之下合穴，能通三焦，利水道，清下焦湿热。诸穴共用，可收清热膀胱，利尿通淋之效。

配穴 小腹胀满者加曲骨；高烧者加合谷、曲池；两肋胀满、口苦者加行间；小便难解者加次髎、中极。

方法 毫针治疗（泻法）。

操作 选定穴位，常规皮肤消毒。用毫针向脊柱方向斜刺膀胱俞 0.6 寸，直刺阴陵泉

II. Therapeutic Methods

[Syndrome of Bladder Damp-Heat]

Therapeutic method: Clear heat and soothe urination, treat stranguria.

Prescription: Pangguangshu(BL28), Zhongji(RN3), Yinlingquan (SP9), Weiyang (BL39).

Mechanism of prescription: Pangguangshu belongs to Bladder Meridian, is the infusion place of bladder Qi, Zhongji is a Mu acupoint from Bladder Meridian, the match of these two acupoint is the method of Shu-Mu acupoints combination, which can regulate bladder Qi, soothe Qi Dynamic, soothe urination and treat stranguria; Yinlingquan is a Yuan acupoint of Spleen Meridian, it can invigorate spleen and stomach, promote Qi transformation, so as to soothe urination; Weiyang is a meridian acupoint of Bladder Meridian, as well as a He acupoint under the three Jiaos, it can dredge three Jiaos, soothe Water channels, clear Damp-Heat of Lower Jiao. The use of combination of these acupoints can clear Heat of bladder, soothe urination and treat stranguria.

Matching acupoints: For distension of lower abdomen add Qugu. For high fever add Hegu, Quchi. For distension of both sides of the chest, bitter taste, add Xingjian. For difficult urination add Ciliao, Zhongji.

Method: Filiform needle acupuncture treatment (attenuating).

Operations: Selecting the relevant acupoints, perform routine skin disinfection. Using filiform needles, obliquely puncture toward spine into Pangguangshu for

0.6 寸，直刺委阳 0.5 寸，直刺曲骨 0.5 寸，直刺合谷 0.5 寸，直刺曲池 0.6 寸，留针 30 分钟。

疗程 每天 1 次，10 天为 1 个疗程。若无不适，可进行第 2 个疗程的治疗；若有不适，可休息 3 天。

【阴虚邪恋证】

治法 通利水道，培元固本。

处方 肾俞（BL23）、膀胱俞（BL28）、中极（RN3）、三阴交（SP6）、太溪（KI3）、照海（KI6）。

方义 肾俞具有滋肾阴、益肾气、泻肾火、利水湿之功能；膀胱俞是膀胱之气转输之处，具有通利水道、培元固本之功，配膀胱之募中极，以疏利膀胱气机；太溪是肾经原穴，取之以滋补肾阴；三阴交是足三阴经交会穴，取之滋养肝、脾、肾；照海是八脉交会穴，是阴跷脉新生之处，有滋阴清热利尿的作用。诸穴配用，共收滋阴清热利尿之功效。

0.6", vertically puncture into Yinlingquan for 0.6", vertically puncture into Weiyang for 0.5", vertically puncture into Qugu for 0.5", Hegu for 0.5", Quchi for 0.6", leaving the needles in for 30 minutes.

Therapeutic course: Once a day, 10 days for a course. Start the treatment for the second course if there is no discomfort. If there is any discomfort, take a break for 3 days.

[Syndrome of Yin Deficiency and Toxin Accumulation]

Therapeutic method: Dredge water channels, reinforce vital essence and foundation.

Prescription: Shenshu (BL23), Pangguangshu (BL28), Zhongji (RN3), Sanyinjiao (SP6), Taixi (KI3), Zhaohai (KI6).

Mechanism of prescription: Shenshu can nourish kidney Yin, tonify kidney Qi, disperse kidney Fire, soothe Water-Damp; Pangguangshu is the transfer station for bladder Qi, which can dredge water channels, reinforce vital essence and foundation, and it can soothe and regulate the Qi Dynamic of bladder when being matched with the Mu acupoint Zhongji from Bladder Meridian; Taixi is a Yuan acupoint from Kidney Meridian, it can nourish kidney Yin; Sanyinjiao is the confluent acupoint of three Yin Meridians of Foot, it can nourish liver, spleen, kidney; Zhaohai is a confluent acupoint of eight channels, as well as the generation place of Yin-Qiao Channel, it can nourish Yin, clear Heat and promote urination. The combination of these acupoints can be used to nourish Yin, clear Heat and promote urination.

配穴 血尿者加血海；心悸者加神门。

方法 电热针治疗（温补法）。

操作 选定穴位，常规皮肤消毒。电热针向脊柱方向斜刺肾俞、膀胱俞各0.8寸，直刺中极0.7寸，直刺三阴交0.7寸。接通电热针仪，每个穴位分别给予电流量60～80mA。另配以毫针直刺太溪、照海各0.4寸，留针40分钟。

疗程 每天1次，10次为1个疗程。疗程间休息3天，再进行第2个疗程的治疗。

【脾肾两虚证】

治法 扶正培元，健脾益气。

处方 肾俞（BL23）、脾俞（BL20）、中极（RN3）、足三里（ST36）、气海（RN6）。

方义 肾俞补肾气，益元阳，气海是先天元气汇聚之处，主治脏气虚惫，真气不足，两穴合用，以补益脾肾，培补下焦；中极是膀胱之募，可调整膀胱经气，助阳利水；脾俞是脾气输注之处，配足三里，以扶正培元，健脾益气。诸穴合

Matching acupoints: For hematuria add Xuehai. For palpitation and insomnia add Shenmen.

Method: Electrothermal acupuncture treatment (warm tonifying).

Operations: Selecting the relevant acupoints, perform routine skin disinfection. Using electrothermal acupuncture needles, obliquely puncture toward spine into Shenshu, Pangguangshu for 0.8" respectively, vertically puncture into Zhongji for 0.7", Sanyinjiao for 0.7". Turn on the electrothermal acupuncture equipment, apply a current of 60-80mA to each acupoint. Additionally, using filiform needles, vertically puncture into Taixi, Zhaohai for 0.4" respectively, leaving the needles in for 40 minutes.

Therapeutic course: Once a day, 10 times for a course. Start the treatment for the second course after a break of 3 days.

[Syndrome of Spleen and Kidney Deficiency]

Therapeutic method: Strengthen healthy Qi and reinforce vital essence, invigorate spleen and tonify Qi.

Prescription: Shenshu (BL23), Pishu (BL2O), Zhongji (RN3), Zusanli (ST36), Qihai (RN6).

Mechanism of prescription: Shenshu can replenish kidney Qi and tonify Yuan Yang, Qihai is the convergence place of congenital Yuan Qi, which can mainly treat deficiency and weakness of visceral Qi, deficiency of genuine Qi, the match of these two acupoints can tonify spleen and kidney, nourish Lower Jiao; Zhongji is a Mu acupoint of Bladder Meridian, which can regulate meridian Qi of Bladder meridian, promote Yang

用，以达调补脾肾，培元固本之功效。

配穴 夜尿多者加关元；腰酸痛者加命门、气海；小便不利者加水道。

方法 电热针治疗（温补法）。

操作 选定穴位，常规皮肤消毒。电热针直刺肾俞 0.8 寸，向脊柱方向斜刺脾俞 0.8 寸，直刺中极、气海各 0.7 寸，直刺命门 0.8 寸，直刺水道 0.8 寸。接通电热针仪，每个穴位分别给予电流量 60～70mA，留针 40 分钟。

疗程 每天 1 次，10 天为 1 个疗程。若无不适，可进行第 2 个疗程的治疗。

三、注意事项

1. 针灸治疗血尿、蛋白尿、水肿等症状效果较好，但如肾功能损伤较重者，要配合中、西药物综合治疗。

2. 水肿严重者应卧床休

and soothe Water; Pishu is the infusion point of spleen Qi, which can strengthen healthy Qi and reinforce vital essence, invigorate spleen and tonify Qi when being matched with Zusanli. The use of combination of these acupoints can tonify spleen and kidney, reinforce vital essence and foundation.

Matching acupoints: For urorrhagia at night add Guanyuan. For pain and soreness of waist add Mingmen, Qihai. For unsmooth urination add Shuidao.

Method: Electrothermal acupuncture treatment (warm tonifying).

Operations: Selecting the relevant acupoints, perform routine skin disinfection. Using electrothermal acupuncture needles, vertically puncture into Shenshu for 0.8", obliquely puncture towards spine into Pishu for 0.8", vertically puncture into Zhongji, Qihai for 0.7" respectively, Mingmen for 0.8", Shuidao for 0.8". Turn on the electrothermal acupuncture equipment, apply a current of 60-70mA to each acupoint, leaving the needles in for 40 minutes.

Therapeutic course: Once a day, 10 days for a course. Start the treatment for the second course if there is no discomfort occurred.

III. Precautions

1. The acupuncture therapy has good efficacies in treatments of hematuria, proteinuria, edema and other symptoms, however for patients with severe impairment of kidney, combination of Chinese Herb Medicine and Western Medicine treatments is required.

2. Patients with severe edema should rest in bed,

息，待病转好再离床活动，避免过劳。

3. 避免感冒、受寒、受潮湿，注意防止上呼吸道及泌尿系感染，注意盐摄入要适量及少饮水，还要注意少吃醋、虾、蟹及生冷食物。

尿失禁

尿失禁是指尿液不能自主的排出，或不能控制而致的尿液淋漓不尽。

中医认为，本病属于"遗尿"的范畴。多因脾、肾、膀胱虚弱，固摄失常或脏腑功能失调，膀胱气化失司所致。

一、诊断及辨证要点

1. 真性尿失禁，是因为尿道括约肌因损伤或神经功能失调，丧失控制排尿的能力。临床常与肢体麻木、疼痛、感觉障碍、运动失常、神经反射异常等病症并存。

2. 假性尿失禁，是因为尿道阻塞（前列腺肥大、尿道狭窄）或膀胱收缩无力（脊髓损伤）等排尿障碍造成尿潴留、尿液外溢。临床可见尿急，排

and get out of bed for activities after condition improvement, avoid overstrain.

3. Avoid colds, to be affected by Cold and Damp, note that avoid upper respiratory tract and urinary system infections. Note that salt intake should be appropriate and drink less water. Also, it should be noted that intake less vinegar, shrimps, crabs and other raw and cold food.

Urinary Incontinence

Urinary incontinence refers to that urine cannot be discharged spontaneously, or endless urine due to failure of control.

Traditional Chinese Medicine believes that this disease belongs to the range of "enuresis". Most are caused by weakness of spleen, kidney and bladder, disorder of astringency securing or dysfunction of organs, irregular Qi transformation of bladder.

I. Key Points for Diagnosis and Syndrome Differentiation

1. Genuine urinary incontinence refers to that the urinary sphincter loses function of urination control due to injuries or dysfunction of nerves. It often clinically coexists with diseases like limb numbness and pain, disturbance of sensation, motor disorder, abnormal nerve reflex.

2. False urinary incontinence, caused by that urination disorders due to urinary tract obstruction (prostatic hyperplasia, urethrostenosis) or weak contractility of bladder (spinal cord injuries) lead to uroschesis and urine leakage. Clinical symptoms include urgent urination,

尿困难，小腹胀痛，膀胱区膨隆等症。

3. 压力性尿失禁，是因尿道括约肌松弛，当咳嗽、喷嚏、哭、笑等动作所致腹内压骤然增加时造成尿液外溢。多见于老年人、肥胖者、经产妇女等。

4. 针灸治疗尿失禁，必须明确诊断，治疗前找到致病原因，可取得较好的治疗效果。

二、治疗方法

【肾虚不固证】

治法　益肾助阳，摄约膀胱。

处方　肾俞（BL23）、膀胱俞（BL28）、三阴交（SP6）、关元（RN4）、中极（RN3）。

方义　肾俞、膀胱俞是足太阳膀胱经穴，又分别为肾与膀胱之背俞穴；中极、关元是任脉经穴，又分别是膀胱与小肠经之募穴。四穴合用，可共补下元，益肾助阳，摄约膀胱。三阴交是足太阴脾经穴，又是足太阳、足少阴、足厥阴交会穴，有健脾、调肝、益肾之功效，与上穴合用，相得益彰。

dysuresia, distension and pain of lower abdomen, bulge of bladder area, etc.

3. Stress urinary incontinence, refers to urine leakage caused by sudden increase of intra-abdominal pressure when coughing, sneezing, crying or laughing due to loosen urinary sphincter. Normally seen among elders, obese people and parous women.

4. Before acupuncture treatment for urinary incontinence, clear diagnoses are required to find the causes. The acupuncture therapy has relatively good efficacies for urinary incontinence.

II. Therapeutic Methods

[Syndrome of Kidney Deficiency and Insecurity]

Therapeutic method: Nourish kidney and promote Yang, regulate bladder.

Prescription: Shenshu (BL23), Pangguangshu (BL28), Sanyinjiao (SP6), Guanyuan (RN4), Zhongji (RN3).

Mechanism of prescription: Shenshu and Pangguangshu are meridian acupoints of Tai-Yang Bladder Meridian of Foot, and also are Back-Shu acupoints of Kidney and Bladder respectively; Zhongji and Guanyuan are meridian acupoints of Ren Channel as well as the Mu acupoint of Bladder and Small Intestine Meridians respectively, The use of the combination of these four acupoints can tonify lower origin, nourish kidney and promote Yang, regulate bladder. Sanyinjiao is a meridian acupoint from Tai-Yin Spleen Meridian of Foot, as well as the confluent acupoint of Tai-Yang Meridian of

Foot, Shao-Yin Meridian of Foot and Jue-Yin Meridian of Foot, it can invigorate spleen, regulate liver, tonify kidney. When it used with the above acupoints, they can complement each other.

配穴 肾虚者加气海、横骨、太溪；肝、脾、肾失调者加阴陵泉、足三里、中封、商丘。

Matching acupoints: For kidney deficiency add Qihai, Henggu, Taixi. For disorders of liver, spleen and kidney add Yinlingquan, Zusanli, Zhongfeng, Shangqiu.

方法 电热针治疗（温补法）。

Method: Electrothermal acupuncture treatment (warm tonifying).

操作 选定穴位，常规皮肤消毒。电热针向脊柱方向斜刺肾俞、膀胱俞各0.8寸，直刺中极、关元各0.8寸，直刺三阴交0.7寸，直刺横骨0.6寸，直刺足三里0.8寸。然后接通电热针仪，每个穴位分别给予60～80mA的电流量。另配以毫针直刺太溪、中封、商丘各0.4寸，留针40分钟。

Operations: Selecting the relevant acupoints, perform routine skin disinfection. Using electrothermal acupuncture needles, obliquely puncture toward spine into Shenshu, Pangguangshu for 0.8" respectively, vertically puncture into Zhongji, Guanyuan for 0.8" respectively, Sanyinjiao for 0.7", Henggu for 0.6", Zusanli for 0.8". Turn on the electrothermal acupuncture equipment, apply a current of 60-80mA to each acupoint. Additionally, using filiform needles, vertically puncture into Taixi, Zhongfeng, Shangqiu for 0.4" respectively, leaving the needles in for 40 minutes.

疗程 每天1次，10次为1个疗程。疗程间可休息3天，再进行第2个疗程的治疗。

Therapeutic course: Once a day, 10 times for a course. Start the treatment for the second course after a break of 3 days.

三、注意事项

III. Precautions

1. 造成尿失禁的原因不同，治疗效果也不同。若尿道括约肌损伤、脊髓神经损伤造成的尿失禁，效果欠佳；对功能性尿失禁疗效较好。

1. The treatment efficacy on urinary incontinence varies depending on different causes of the disease. For urinary incontinence caused by sphincter injuries of urinary tract and spinal nerve injuries, the efficacy is poor, while for functional urinary incontinence the efficacy is

2. For treatment of urinary incontinence, the acupuncture can also be done in combination with medicine treatment so as to improve efficacies.

Urethritis

Urethritis refers to inflammatory lesions of urinary tract caused by bacteria (Escherichia coli, streptococcus, staphylococcus) infections.

Traditional Chinese Medicine believes that this disease belongs to the category of "stranguria". Most are caused by downward flow of Damp-Heat or invasion of filthiness and turbidness. At the early phase, normally belong to excess syndrome, and develop into deficiency syndrome or syndrome of intermingled deficiency and excess after long-term delay without cure.

I. Key Points for Diagnosis and Syndrome Differentiation

1. For patients with excess syndrome, symptoms include damp and turbid urine like rice water, or with mucus, silk-like materials, severe itching or burning-like pain when urinating, distension of lower abdomen, yellow or yellow and greasy tongue fur, taut and rapid or deep and taut pulse.

2. For patients with deficiency syndrome, symptoms include unsmooth and endless urine, intermittent attack of frequent micturition, onset with fatigue, or even dropping of urine when urinating, light tongue with thin fur, deep and thin or thin and rapid pulse.

二、治疗方法

【实证】

治法 清热利湿。

处方 膀胱俞（BL28）、阴陵泉（SP9）、中极（RN3）、三阴交（SP6）。

方义 本病主因湿热下注所致，故取膀胱俞与中极以清热利湿，疏理膀胱气机。取脾经之合穴阴陵泉和脾经之经穴三阴交以健脾渗湿，兼调肝肾。四穴合用，共收清湿热、调三阴之功效。

配穴 湿热重者加足三里、归来。

方法 毫针治疗（泻法）。

操作 选定穴位，常规皮肤消毒。用毫针向脊柱方向斜刺膀胱俞 0.8 寸，直刺阴陵泉 0.5 寸，向下斜刺中极 3 寸，使针感到尿道处，直刺三阴交 0.7 寸，直刺足三里 0.6 寸，直刺归来 0.7 寸，留针 30 分钟。

疗程 每日 1 次，10 次为 1 个疗程。疗程间可不休息，

II. Therapeutic Methods

[Excess Syndrome]

Therapeutic method: Clear Heat and remove Damp.

Prescription: Pangguangshu (BL28), Yinlingquan (SP9), Zhongji (RN3), Sanyinjiao (SP6).

Mechanism of prescription: This disease is mainly caused by downward flow of Damp-Heat, therefore use Pangguangshu and Zhongji to clear Heat and remove Damp, soothe and regulate the Qi Dynamic of bladder. Use the He acupoint Yinlingquan of Spleen and the meridian acupoint Sanyinjiao of Spleen to invigorate spleen and excrete Damp as well as regulate liver and kidney. The use of the combination of these four acupoints can clear Heat and remove Damp, regulate the three Yins.

Matching acupoints: For severe Damp-Heat add Zusanli, Guilai.

Method: Filiform needle acupuncture treatment (attenuating).

Operations: Selecting the relevant acupoints, perform routine skin disinfection. Using filiform needles, obliquely puncture toward the spine into Pangguangshu for 0.8", vertically puncture into Yinlingquan for 0.5", obliquely puncture downward into Zhongji for 3", make the feeling of needle puncturing spread to the urinary tract, vertically puncture into Sanyinjiao for 0.7", Zusanli for 0.6", Guilai for 0.7", leaving the needles in for 30 minutes.

Therapeutic course: Once a day, 10 times for a course. Directly start the treatment for the second course

直接进行第 2 个疗程的治疗。

【虚证】

治法 益肾健脾，化湿利尿。

处方 关元（RN4）、三阴交（SP6）、肾俞（BL23）、脾俞（BL20）、足三里（ST36）、中极（RN3）、阴陵泉（SP9）。

方义 本病多由湿热滞留，耗伤气阴而致。故取任脉的关元、中极以益肾通淋；取膀胱经穴脾俞、肾俞以益肾健脾，化湿利尿；取脾经穴三阴交、阴陵泉以健脾渗湿；取胃经合穴足三里以健脾和胃，升降气机。诸穴共用，可奏健脾益肾，利湿通淋，调理气机之功效。

方法 电热针治疗（温补法）。

操作 选定穴位，常规皮肤消毒。电热针向脊柱方向斜刺肾俞、脾俞各 0.8 寸，直刺关元、中极各 0.7 寸，直刺足三里 0.8 寸，直刺三阴交 0.7 寸，直刺阴陵泉 0.7 寸。接通电热针仪，每个穴位分别给予

without break.

[Deficiency Syndrome]

Therapeutic method: Tonify kidney and invigorate spleen, remove Damp and facilitate urination.

Prescription: Guanyuan(RN4), Sanyinjiao (SP6),Shenshu (BL23), Pishu(BL20), Zusanli (ST36), Zhongji (RN3), Yinlingquan (SP9).

Mechanism of prescription: This disease is mostly caused by retention of Damp and Heat, consumption of Qi and Yin. Therefore use Guanyuan and Zhongji from Ren Channel to tonify kidney and treat stranguria. Use the meridian acupoints Pishu and Shenshu from Bladder Meridian to tonify kidney and invigorate spleen, remove Damp and facilitate urination. Use the meridian acupoints Sanyinjiao and Yinlingquan from Spleen Meridian to invigorate spleen and excrete Damp. Use the He acupoint Zusanli from Stomach Meridian to invigorate spleen and tonify stomach, ascend and descend Qi Dynamic. The use of combination of these acupoints can invigorate spleen, and tonify kidney, remove Damp and treat stranguria, regulate Qi Dynamic.

Method: Electrothermal acupuncture treatment (warm tonifying).

Operations: Selecting the relevant acupoints, perform routine skin disinfection. Using electrothermal acupuncture needles, obliquely puncture toward spine into Shenshu, Pishu for 0.8" respectively, vertically puncture into Guanyuan, Zhongji for 0.7" respectively, Zusanli for 0.8", Sanyinjiao for 0.7", Yinlingquan for 0.7". Turn on the electrothermal acupuncture equipment, apply a cur-

电流量 60～70mA，留针 40 分钟。

疗程 每日 1 次，10 天为 1 个疗程。疗程间可休息 3 天，再进行第 2 个疗程的治疗。

三、注意事项

1. 注意个人卫生。

2. 由淋双球菌引起的特异性尿道失禁，属于本病的范畴，应到性病科进行诊治。

3. 饮食上应注意禁忌或少食辛辣刺激性食品。

膀胱炎

膀胱炎是因细菌经尿道上行感染，或由肾炎下行感染，或因物理、化学因素刺激引起的膀胱黏膜红肿、浸润、甚或出血、溃疡以及坏死的一种病症。

中医认为，本病属于"淋证"的范畴。多由湿热蕴而下注，或秽浊之邪侵袭，膀胱气化失常而致。发病初期多是实证、热证，迁延日久则多演变成虚证或虚实夹杂证。

rent of 60-70 mA to each acupoint, leaving the needles in for 40 minutes.

Therapeutic course: Once a day, 10 days for a course. Start the treatment for the second course after a break of 3 days.

III. Precautions

1. Pay attention to personal hygiene.

2. The specific urethral incontinence caused by diplococcus reniformis belongs to the category of this disease, and the patients with this condition should visit STD department for diagnosis and treatment.

3. In the respect of diet, note that do not eat or eat less spicy and stimulating food.

Urocystitis

Urocystitis is a disease caused by ascending infections from bacteria through the urinary tract, or descending infections of nephritis, or swelling, infiltration or even bleeding, ulceration and necrosis of bladder mucous membrane due to physical or chemical irritations.

Traditional Chinese Medicine believes that this disease belongs to the range of "stranguria". Most are caused by accumulation and downward flow of Damp-Heat, or invasion of filthiness and turbidness toxins leading to Qi transformation disorders of bladder. At the early phase, normally belong to excess syndrome, heat syndrome, and develop into deficiency syndrome or syndrome of intermingled deficiency and excess after long-term delay.

一、诊断及辨证要点

1. 发病女性多于男性。

2. 实证者,小便热涩,尿意急迫,尿频,尿后带血,或尿时混浊、疼痛,少腹胀,发热恶寒,舌质红,苔黄,脉数。

3. 虚证者,尿痛、尿急、尿频反复发作或尿有余沥,神疲乏力,舌质淡,苔薄黄或少苔,脉沉细或细数。

二、治疗方法

【实证】

治法 清热,利湿,化浊。

处方 膀胱俞(BL28)、次髎(BL32)、小肠俞(BL27)、三焦俞(BL22)、阴陵泉(SP9)、中封(LR4)、然谷(KI2)。

方义 本病是膀胱病变,多由湿热、秽浊侵袭所致,故取膀胱经穴膀胱俞、次髎、小肠俞、三焦俞以清热利湿,利尿通淋,调理气机。脾经合穴阴陵泉能健脾渗湿,胃经穴然谷可益肾导赤,肝之经穴中封,能疏肝健脾,理气止痛。

I. Key Points for Diagnosis and Syndrome Differentiation

1. More common among females than among males.

2. For patients with excess syndrome, symptoms include hot urine and stranguria, urgent micturition, frequent micturition, bloody urine, or turbid urine with pain, distension of lateral lower abdomen, pyrexia and aversion to cold, red tongue with yellow fur, rapid pulse.

3. For patients with deficiency syndrome, symptoms include repeated attacks of painful micturition, urgent micturition, frequent micturition or endless urine, mental fatigue and asthenia, light tongue with thin and yellow or less fur, deep and thin or thin and rapid pulse.

II. Therapeutic Methods

[Excess Syndrome]

Therapeutic method: Clear Heat and remove Damp, relieve turbidity.

Prescription: Pangguangshu(BL28), Ciliao(BL32), Xiaochangshu(BL27), Sanjiaoshu(BL22), Yinlingquan(SP9), Zhongfeng (LR4), Rangu (KI2).

Mechanism of prescription: This disease is a kind of bladder pathological changes, which is mostly caused by invasion of Damp-Heat as well as filthiness and turbidness, so use the meridian acupoints Pangguangshu, Ciliao, Xiaochangshu and Sanjiaoshu from Bladder Meridian to clear heat and soothe urination, treat stranguria, and regulate Qi Dynamic. The He acupoint, Yinlingquan from Spleen Meridian can invigorate spleen and excrete

诸穴合用，可收清热利湿，通利膀胱，理气止痛之效。湿热清、小便利，则淋证自疗。

配穴 发热者加曲池；小腹胀痛者加曲泉、行间；恶心纳差者加足三里；尿中带血者加三阴交。

方法 毫针治疗（泻法）。

操作 选定穴位，常规皮肤消毒。用毫针向椎体方向斜刺膀胱俞、小肠俞、次髎、三焦俞各0.7寸，直刺阴陵泉0.6寸，直刺中封、然谷各0.4寸。提插泻法，留针30分钟。

疗程 每日1次，10天为1个疗程。疗程间可休息3天，再进行第2个疗程的治疗。

【虚证】

治法 补肾健脾，利尿通淋。

处方 中极（RN3）、关元（RN4）、肾俞（BL23）、水道（ST28）、曲泉（LR8）、三阴交（SP6）。

Damp, the meridian acupoint Rangu from Stomach Meridian can tonify kidney and dredge Red, the meridian acupoint Zhongfeng from Liver Meridian can soothe liver and invigorate spleen, regulate Qi and alleviate pains. The use of combination of these acupoints can clear Heat and remove Damp, soothe bladder, regulate Qi and alleviate pains. The stranguria can be cured naturally given that Damp-Heat is cleared and urination is smooth.

Matching acupoints: For pyrexia add Quchi. For distending pain of abdomen, add Ququan, Xingjian. For nausea and poor appetite add Zusanli. For bloody urine add Sanyinjiao.

Method: Filiform needle acupuncture treatment (attenuating).

Operations: Selecting the relevant acupoints, perform routine skin disinfection. Using filiform needles, obliquely puncture toward vertebral bodies into Pangguangshu, Xiaochangshu, Ciliao, Sanjiaoshu for 0.7" respectively, vertically puncture into Yinlingquan for 0.6", Zhongfeng, Rangu for 0.4". Method of lifting-thrusting and attenuating, leaving the needles in for 30 minutes.

Therapeutic course: Once a day, 10 days for a course. Start the treatment for the second course after a break of 3 days.

[Deficiency Syndrome]

Therapeutic method: Reinforce kidney and invigorate spleen, soothe urination, treat stranguria.

Prescription: Zhongji (RN3), Guanyuan (RN4), Shenshu (BL23), Shuidao (ST28), Ququan (LR8), Sanyinjiao (SP6).

方义 本证多为湿热滞留，耗伤阴液，阻滞气机而致。故取任脉中极、关元以益肾通淋，膀胱经穴肾俞可益肾利水。水道是足阳明胃经穴，能通调水道，三阴交是足太阴脾经穴，可健脾渗湿。联合曲泉能疏肝解郁，通调前阴。诸穴合用，共奏补肾健脾，利尿通淋之效。

配穴 湿热未清者加膀胱俞；尿中带血者加血海；遇劳即发者加气海、气海俞。

方法 电热针治疗（补法）。

操作 选定穴位，常规皮肤消毒。电热针直刺中极、关元各0.8寸，直刺曲泉0.8寸，直刺三阴交0.8寸，直刺水道0.7寸，直刺气海0.7寸，向椎体方向斜刺肾俞、气海俞、膀胱俞各0.8寸，直刺血海0.7寸。接通电热针仪，每个穴位分别给予电流量40mA，每次选3～4个穴施术，留针40分钟。

Mechanism of prescription: Most are caused by retention of Damp and Heat, consumption of Yin fluid, obstruction of Qi Dynamic. So use Zhongji and Guanyuan from Ren Channel to tonify kidney and treat stranguria, and the meridian acupoint Shenshu from Bladder Meridian can tonify kidney and soothe Water. Shuidao is a meridian acupoint from Yang-Ming Stomach Meridian of Foot, it can regulate Water channels; Sanyinjiao is a meridian acupoint from Tai-Yin Spleen Meridian of Foot, it can invigorate spleen and excrete Damp. They can soothe liver Qi stagnation, dredge and regulate external genitalia when being matched with Ququan. The use of combination of these acupoints can reinforce kidney and invigorate spleen, soothe urination, treat stranguria.

Matching acupoints: For patients with uncleared Damp-Heat add Pangguangshu. For bloody urine add Xuehai. For immediate attacks following fatigue add Qihai, Qihaishu.

Method: Electrothermal acupuncture treatment (tonifying).

Operations: Selecting the relevant acupoints, perform routine skin disinfection. Using electrothermal acupuncture needles, vertically puncture into Zhongji, Guanyuan for 0.8" respectively, Ququan for 0.8", Sanyinjiao for 0.8", Shuidao for 0.7", Qihai for 0.7", obliquely puncture toward vertebral bodies into Shenshu, Qihaishu, Pangguangshu for 0.8" respectively, vertically puncture into Xuehai for 0.7". Turn on the electrothermal acupuncture equipment, apply a current of 40mA to each acupoint, select 3-4 acupoints for treatment each time, leaving the needles in for 40 minutes.

疗程 每天1次,7次为1个疗程。疗程间休息3天,再进行第2个疗程的治疗。

三、注意事项

1. 注意个人卫生。

2. 饮食上应注意禁忌或少食辛辣刺激性食品。

老年痴呆症

老年痴呆是指老年期发生的原发性退行性脑病,并有脑组织特征性病理改变的一种精神病。一般认为大脑组织变性及一些外界因素,如感染、中毒、精神因素等可能是发病的有关因素。本病的病理变化是脑组织弥漫性萎缩和退化性改变,以缓慢进行性记忆力丧失和智能减退为主要临床特征。最先表现为性格改变,变得自私、主观、固执、注意力不集中,以后逐渐出现记忆力障碍和判断错误,由于猜疑和幻觉而导致冲动及破坏性行为,后期患者终日卧床,大小便不能自理。

中医认为,本病属于"痴呆""健忘""郁证""癫证""狂证"等范畴。人的生、长、壮、老与肾气的盛衰密切相

Therapeutic course: Once a day, 7 times for a course. Start the treatment for the second course after a break of 3 days.

III. Precautions

1. Pay attention to personal hygiene.

2. In the respect of diet, note that do not eat or eat less spicy and stimulating food.

Alzheimer's Disease

Alzheimer's disease is a kind of psychosis, it refers to the primary degenerative encephalopathy with characteristic pathological changes of brain tissues, which occurs in the gerontic period. It is generally believed that cerebral tissue degeneration and some external factors such as infections, intoxication, mental factors may be related factors for disease attacks. The pathological changes of this disease are diffuse atrophy and degenerative changes of cerebral tissues, the main clinical characteristics of which are slow progressive memory loss and hypophrenia. The earliest signs are personality changes, become selfish, subjective, stubborn, absent-minded, then the patient develops gradually impaired memory and misjudgment, as well as destructive behaviors like beating person, cursing due to suspension and illusion. In the later phase the patient becomes bedridden and develops urinary and fecal incontinence.

Traditional Chinese Medicine believes that this disease belongs to the range of "dementia", "amnesia", "depression syndrome", "quiet insanity", "manic psychosis", etc. The growth, development, strengthening and aging

关。肾主骨生髓，脑为髓之海，肾之精不足，髓不得上冲于脑，脑海不足则喜忘前言，智力和技巧显著减退。

of human are closely related to the prosperity and deficiency of kidney Qi. The kidney governs marrow generation of bones. The brain is the sea of marrow, deficiency of kidney essence causes the marrow to be unable to rise up to the brain, while the deficiency of brain sea causes amnesia, obvious degeneration of intelligence and skills.

一、诊断及辨证要点

1. 心脾两虚者，症见心悸梦扰，头晕纳差，神疲乏力，诸事善忘或神思错乱，善悲欲哭，舌质淡，苔少，脉细弱。

2. 肝肾亏虚者，症见头晕目眩，反应迟钝，健忘神疲，耳鸣耳聋，腰酸腿软，失眠口干，舌体干瘪，舌质暗淡，舌体震颤或痿软，脉沉细或弱。

3. 阴虚火旺者，症见兴奋多动，急躁易怒，面红目赤，多言善惊，毁物打人，不避亲疏，形瘦，舌红苔干，脉细数。

I. Key Points for Diagnosis and Syndrome Differentiation

1. For patients with deficiency of both heart and spleen, symptoms include palpitation and disturbed dreams, dizziness and poor appetite, mental fatigue and asthenia, amnesia and insanity, susceptible to sorrow and easy to cry, light tongue with less fur, thin and weak pulse.

2. For patients with depletion and deficiency of liver and kidney, symptoms include dizziness, slow response, amnesia and mental fatigue, tinnitus and deafness, aching lumbus and limp legs, insomnia and dry mouth, wizened tongue, dim tongue color, tremulous or flaccid tongue body, deep and thin or weak pulse.

3. For patients with hyperactivity of fire and Yin deficiency, symptoms include excitability and hyperactivity, irascibility, flushed face and congested eyes, garrulity, susceptible to fright, beating person and destroying things, acting with no difference upon close and distant relationships, skinny body, red tongue with dry fur, thin and rapid pulse.

二、治疗方法

【肾虚精亏，髓海不充】

治法　补肾气，益阴精。

处方　百会（DU20）、大椎（DU14）、风池（GB20）、肾俞（BL23）、命门（DU4）、神门（HT7）、哑门（DU15）。

方义　百会为督脉之穴，位于巅顶，有降清阳、醒脑开窍之功。哑门是督脉之穴，位于项中，取之以醒脑安神。临床证明，风池有活血化瘀之功效。大椎为诸阳之会，与百会、哑门穴相配，可有振奋阳气、醒脑开窍之功。"肾主骨生髓""脑为髓之海"，故取肾俞补肾滋阴，健脑益智。命门有益命火、补肾阴的作用。神门是心经之原穴，能降心火，安心神。诸穴共用，补肾气、益阴精，以充脑之物质基础，促进脑的功能。

配穴　心脾两虚配心俞、厥阴俞、脾俞、足三里；肝肾

II. Therapeutic Methods

[Kidney Deficiency and Essence Depletion, Insufficiency of Marrow Sea]

Therapeutic method: Replenish kidney Qi and strengthen Yin essence.

Prescription: Baihui (DU20), Dazhui (DU14), Fengchi (GB20), Shenshu (BL23), Mingmen (DU4), Shenmen (HT7), Yamen (DU15).

Mechanism of prescription: Baihui is an acupoint of Du Channel which locates on the top, it can ascend Qing-Yang, restore consciousness and induce resuscitation. Yamen is an acupoint of Du Channel which locates at the middle of neck, it can restore consciousness and calm mind. It has been proven clinically that Fengchi can activate blood circulation and remove stasis. Dazhui is the confluent acupoint of all Yangs, it can promote Yang Qi, restore consciousness and induce resuscitation when being matched with Baihui and Yamen. "The kidney governs marrow generation of bones", "the brain is the sea of marrow", therefore use Shenshu to replenish kidney and nourish Yin, invigorate brain and promote intelligence. Mingmen can nourish Life Fire, reinforce kidney Yin. Shenmen is a Yuan acupoint of Heart Meridian, it can calm down heart Fire, tranquillize mind. The use of combination of these acupoints can replenish kidney Qi, tonify Yin essence, so as to supplement cerebral material basis and promote cerebral functions.

Matching acupoints: For deficiency of both heart and spleen add Xinshu, Jueyinshu, Pishu, Zusanli. For

亏虚配脾俞、志室、太溪；有痰者，配丰隆、合谷、三阴交；阴虚火旺配人中、后溪、大钟。

方法 电热针治疗。

操作 选定穴位，皮肤常规消毒。电热针向上斜刺大椎0.6～0.7寸，直刺肾俞0.7～0.8寸，直刺命门0.7寸，直刺足三里0.6～0.8寸。接通电热针仪，每个穴位分别给予电流量50～60mA，留针40分钟。另配以毫针补法，留针40分钟。

疗程 每日1次，30次为1个疗程，疗程间休息7～10天。

三、注意事项

1. 注意本病应与老年期发生的中毒性或症状性精神病、动脉硬化性精神病、额叶肿瘤引起的痴呆等症鉴别。

2. 对患者要注意生活上的照顾，防止因大小便不利或失禁及长期卧床引起的褥疮感染等并发症。

3. 本病的治疗要采取综合疗法，如中药、针灸、按摩、功能训练，必要的西药配合，发挥中、西医药的长处。这样

depletion and deficiency of liver and kidney add Pishu, Zhishi, Taixi. For phlegm add Fenglong, Hegu, Sanyinjiao. For hyperactivity of Fire and Yin deficiency add Renzhong, Houxi, Dazhong.

Method: Electrothermal acupuncture treatment.

Operations: Selecting the relevant acupoints, perform routine skin disinfection. Using the electrothermal acupuncture needles, obliquely puncture upward into Dazhui for 0.6-0.7", vertically puncture into Shenshu for 0.7-0.8", Mingmen for 0.7", Zusanli for 0.6-0.8". Turn on the electrothermal acupuncture equipment, apply a current of 50-60mA to each acupoint, leaving the needles in for 40 minutes. Additionally, use filiform needles with tonifying method, leave the needles in for 40 minutes.

Therapeutic course: Once a day, 30 times for a course. Rest for 7-10 days between courses.

III. Precautions

1. This disease should be differentiating from toxic or symptomatic psychosis, arteriosclerotic psychosis, dementia caused by frontal lobe tumors which may occur during gerontic period.

2. Pay attention to care of patients' daily life, avoid complications like bedsore infections which are caused by inconvenience of urination and defection or incontinence and bed-ridden.

3. For the treatment of this disease, a comprehensive therapy which combines Chinese Herb Medicine treatment, acupuncture treatment, massage, functional exercises together, as well as necessary Western Medi-

有利于患者减少痛苦，促进康复，提高疗效。

四、典型病例

韩某，男，69岁，职员，北京人。

主诉：健忘，善愁欲哭，神疲乏力5年，近日加重。病史：患者5年前发现糖尿病，逐渐体力差，性格改变，自私、固执，注意力不集中，经检查诊断为"痴呆症"。近两年发展较快，出现记忆力障碍和判断错误，多有猜疑和幻觉而导致破坏性行为，如骂人、打人，经治不见好转。

刻下症：遇事易忘，性格变化，固执，注意力难集中，行为乖戾，打人毁物，眠差，昼夜颠倒，纳食尚可，舌质红，苔黄厚腻，脉滑数。

查体：两肺呼吸音粗。二尖瓣区及主动脉瓣第二听诊区可闻及二级收缩期杂音。

辅助检查：头部核磁共振示"脑白质病变、脑萎缩、多发性脑梗死"。空腹血糖8.6mmol/L。尿糖（+++）。

cine treatment should be used to utilize the advantages of Traditional Chinese Medicine and Western Medicine. This approach can reduce patients' pain, promote recovery and improve efficacies.

IV. Typical Case

Han, male, 69 years old, employee, residence: Beijing.

Self-reported symptoms: Amnesia, susceptible to sorrow and easy to cry, mental fatigue and asthenia for 5 years, which became aggravated recently. Medical history: The patient was diagnosed as diabetes 5 years ago, since then the physical strength weakened gradually, the personality changed, became selfish, stubborn, absent-minded, and was diagnosed as "dementia" after examinations. The disease progressed relatively rapidly in recent two years, the patient developed impaired memory and misjudgment, and had destructive behaviors like beating person, cursing due to suspension and illusion.

Current symptoms: Amnesia, personality changes, stubborn, absent-minded, perverse behaviors, beating person and destroying things, poor sleep, day and night reversion, fair appetite, red tongue with yellow and thick and greasy fur, slippery and rapid pulse.

Physical examination: Coarse breath sounds in both lungs. Grade 2 systolic noise at mitral valve area and second aortic valve area.

Auxiliary examination: Head MRI indicated 'leukodystrophy, encephalanalosis, multiple cerebral infarction'. FBG 8.6 mmol/L. GLU (+++).

【诊断依据】

1. 老年男性，体弱多病，神志恍惚，言语错乱，善悲欲哭。

2. 头部核磁共振提示"脑白质病变、脑萎缩、多发性脑梗死"。

3. 消渴病史 5 年，空腹血糖 8.6mmol/L，尿糖（+++），服用降糖药治疗中。

4. 性格改变，自私、固执，喜怒无常，多因猜疑和幻觉而致，出现打人、骂人行为。

【证治分析】

病因 情志内伤，脏腑功能失调。

病机 情志内伤，导致脏腑功能紊乱，致痰气郁结，蒙蔽心窍，出现精神抑郁，表情淡漠，沉默痴呆。

证候分析 痴呆日久，心脾两虚，气血化源不足，心神失养，故可见神志恍惚、言语错乱等神志失常之症及心悸易惊，夜寐不安。脾气不足，故食少倦怠，舌淡，苔白，脉细。均为心脾两虚，气血不足之象。

病位 心、脾。

病性 虚性。

[Diagnostic Basis]

1. Old male, valetudinarianism, wandering in the mind, paraphasia, susceptible to sorrow and easy to cry.

2. Head MRI indicated "leukodystrophy, encephalanalosis, multiple cerebral infarction".

3. A 5-year history of symptom-complex of excessive eating, FBG 8.6mmol/L, GLU (+++), in treatment with antidiabetics.

4. Personality changes, selfish, stubborn, moodiness, most are caused by suspicion and illusion, with behaviors like beating person, cursing.

[Syndrome-treatment Analysis]

Etiology: Internal injuries caused by seven emotions, dysfunction of internal organs.

Pathogenesis: Internal injuries caused by seven emotions leading to dysfunction of internal organs, stasis of phlegm Qi, obstruction of sense organs, subsequently cause deprementia, apathia, silence and dementia.

Syndrome analysis: Long-term dementia causing deficiency of heart and spleen, insufficient transportation source of Qi-blood, nourishment loss of mind, therefore symptoms of delirium such as wandering in the mind and paraphasia can be seen, as well as palpitation and easy to be scared, disturbed sleep at night. Deficiency of spleen Qi causes less food intake and fatigue, light tongue with whitish fur, thin pulse. These are all symptoms of deficiency of heart and spleen, insufficiency of Qi-blood.

Lesion location: Heart, spleen.

Disease nature: Deficiency.

西医诊断 老年痴呆症、脑白质病变、多发性腔隙性脑梗死、脑萎缩、糖尿病。

中医诊断 痴呆、消渴。

治法 健脾养心，补气益血。

方法 电热针治疗。

处方 百会（DU20）、大椎（DU14）、风池（GB20）、肾俞（BL23）、命门（DU4）、神门（HT7）、心俞（BL15）、厥阴俞（BL14）、脾俞（BL20）、足三里（ST36）、三阴交（SP6）、哑门（DU15）。

方义 百会是督脉之穴，位于巅顶，有升清阳、醒脑开窍之功效；哑门为督脉之穴，位于项中，取之以醒脑安神；取风池有活血化瘀之功；大椎为诸阳之会，与百会、哑门相伍，可收振奋阳气、醒脑开窍之功效；"肾主骨生髓""脑为髓之海"，故取肾俞补肾滋阴，健脑益智；命门有益命火、补肾阳的作用；神门为心经之原穴，能降心火，安心神；脾俞、三阴交、足三里能健脾益气；心俞、厥阴俞能养心安神。

The diagnosis of Western Medicine: Alzheimer's disease, leukodystrophy, multiple lacunar cerebral infarction, encephalanalosis, diabetes.

The diagnosis of Traditional Chinese Medicine: Dementia, symptom-complex of excessive eating.

Therapeutic method: Invigorate spleen and nourish heart, replenish Qi and tonify blood.

Method: Electrothermal acupuncture treatment.

Prescription: Baihui (DU20), Dazhui (DU14), Fengchi (GB20), Shenshu (BL23), Mingmen (DU4), Shenmen (HT7), Xinshu (BL15), Jueyinshu (BL14), Pishu (BL20), Zusanli (ST36), Sanyinjiao (SP6), Yamen (DU15).

Mechanism of prescription: Baihui is an acupoint of Du Channel which locates on the top, it can ascend Qing-Yang, restore consciousness and induce resuscitation. Yamen is an acupoint of Du Channel which locates at the middle of neck, it can restore consciousness and calm mind; Fengchi can activate blood circulation and remove stasis. Dazhui is the confluent acupoint of all Yangs, it can promote Yang Qi, restore consciousness and induce resuscitation when being matched with Baihui and Yamen. "The kidney governs marrow generation of bones", "the brain is the sea of marrow", therefore use Shenshu to replenish kidney and nourish Yin, invigorate brain and promote intelligence. Mingmen can nourish Life Fire, reinforce kidney Yang. Shenmen is a Yuan acupoint of Heart Meridian, it can calm down heart Fire, tranquillize mind. Pishu, Sanyinjiao, Zusanli can invigo-

配穴 自汗气短加大椎、内关；肝肾亏虚加肝俞、志室、太溪；有痰者加丰隆、合谷、三阴交。

操作 选定穴位，皮肤常规消毒。电热针平刺百会0.7寸，斜刺风池、肾俞、心俞、厥阴俞、脾俞各0.7寸，直刺大椎、命门、足三里、三阴交、合谷、太溪、丰隆、内关各0.6寸。接通电热针仪，每个穴位分别给予电流量40mA，以患者感胀而舒适为度，留针40分钟。（注：每次选取3组穴给予电热针治疗，其余穴位用毫针治疗，留针40分钟。）

疗程 每日1次，30次为1个疗程，疗程间休息7～10天。

治疗过程 该患者在治疗过程中，配合服用中西药物、功能训练等综合治疗，针后3个月精神较好，情绪稳定，能与人交流，睡眠、饮食都较正常，不再哭闹、打人、骂人。改为隔日治疗1次，连续治疗半年之久，除记忆力差之外，

rate spleen and tonify Qi. Xinshu, Jueyinshu can nourish heart and tranquillize mind.

Matching acupoints: For spontaneous sweating and shortness of breath add Dazhui, Neiguan. For depletion and deficiency of liver and kidney, add Ganshu, Zhishi, Taixi. For phlegm add Fenglong, Hegu, Sanyinjiao.

Operations: Selecting the relevant acupoints, perform routine skin disinfection. Using electrothermal acupuncture needles, horizontally puncture into Baihui for 0.7", obliquely puncture into Fengchi, Shenshu, Xinshu, Jueyinshu, Pishu for 0.7" respectively, vertically puncture into Dazhui, Mingmen, Zusanli, Sanyinjiao, Hegu, Taixi, Fenglong, Neiguan for 0.6" respectively. Turn on the electrothermal acupuncture equipment, apply a current of 40mA to each acupoint, and the limit is that the patient feels swell and comfortable, leaving the needles in for 40 minutes. (Note：Select 3 pairs of acupoints for electrothermal acupuncture treatment each time, and treat the other acupoints with filiform needles, leaving the needles in for 40 minutes.)

Therapeutic course: Once a day, 30 times for a course. Rest for 7-10 days between courses.

Therapeutic process: During treatment, the patient was treated in combination with Chinese Herb Medicine and Western Medicine treatments as well as functional exercises. Three months after acupuncture, the patient got better vitality and stable mood, could communicate with others, sleep and diet became better, no more crying, beating and cursing. The therapy changed to treat once every two days for half a year continuously, the pa-

基本具备正常老年人的生活能力。8个多月后结束治疗，随访至今健在。

【生活调摄】

1. 要耐心说服，让患者能配合治疗是关键。

2. 要选取综合治疗法，将针灸、中药、西药、功能训练相结合，还要有对症治疗的方法。

3. 饮食调配合理，一定要满足患者病体之需要，忌辛辣油腻之类食物，定时定量。

4. 功能训练时，言语、听力、肢体等均按需要制订项目，有计划地进行，尽力求实效。

5. 切忌精神打击及刺激，减少精神负担。

脑卒中

脑卒中是脑部及颈部或支配脑的颈部动脉病变，引起脑局灶性血液循环障碍，导致急性或亚急性脑损伤的神经系统病变。本病多发生于中老年人，病前多有高血压、糖尿病、动脉硬化的病史。以偏瘫、失语、昏迷等为常见症状。治疗不及时常遗留较严重

tient basically restored normal elder life except for poor memory. The treatment ended 8 months later, follow-up till now, and the patient is still alive.

[Lifestyle Change and Health Maintenance]

1. The key point is patient persuasion to let patients cooperate with treatments.

2. Use comprehensive therapies, combine acupuncture, Chinese Herb Medicine, Western Medicine, and functional exercises together, and there also should be methods for symptomatic treatment.

3. Reasonable diet regulation, and the diet must meet the physiological needs of the body, do not eat spicy and greasy food, have diet at fixed time and with fixed amount.

4. In the respect of functional exercises, programs should be developed depending on needs for speaking, listening and limb movement exercises, and perform them as per a schedule so as to obtain real effects.

5. Mental attacks and stimulations are strictly forbidden, reduce mental stress.

Cerebrovascular Diseases

Cerebrovascular diseases are pathological changes of brain and neck or cervical arteries governing the brain, causing local blood circulation disorders of brain, nervous system disease inducing acute or subacute cerebral injuries. This disease is mostly seen in the middle and old aged, generally with medical histories of high blood pressure, diabetes, arteriosclerosis before the development of this disease. Common symptoms include semiplegia, aphasia, coma, etc. Normally severe sequelae will

的后遗症。脑血管病包括出血性及缺血性2大类，出血性脑血管病包括脑出血、蜘蛛网膜下腔出血；缺血性脑血管病包括脑血栓形成及脑栓塞。

中医认为，本病属于"中风""卒中"的范畴。多因忧思恼怒，饮食不节，恣酒纵欲等，以致阴阳失调，脏腑气偏，气血错落，肌肤筋脉失于濡养，阴亏于下，肝阳暴张，肝风内动，夹痰夹火，横窜经隧，蒙蔽清窍所致。其病多与心、肝、肾三脏阴阳失调密切相关，临床上常将中风分为中经络与中脏腑两大类。中经络者病位较浅，病情较轻，一般无神志改变；中脏腑者病位较深，病情较重，有神志不清的临床表现。

一、诊断及辨证要点

【中经络证】

1. 半身不遂，一侧肢体偏

be caused without timely treatment. Cerebrovascular diseases include two types, hemorrhagic ones and ischemic ones, while the hemorrhagic ones are further divided into cerebral hemorrhage and subarachnoid hemorrhage; the ischemic ones are divided into cerebral thrombosis and cerebral embolism.

Traditional Chinese Medicine believes that this disease belongs to the categories of "stroke" and "apoplexy". Most are caused by sad thoughts and anger, intemperate diet, excessive drinking and indulging in carnal pleasure without restraint, leading to imbalance between Yin and Yang as well as between Zang Qi and Fu Qi, disorders of Qi-blood, nourishment loss of tendons and channels, Yin deficiency of lower body, over-expending of liver Yang, internal movement of liver Wind with phlegm and Fire, blood over-flooding within meridian passways, obstruct sense organs. Most are related with imbalance of Yin and Yang in the heart, liver and kidney. Normally apoplexy is clinically divided into two types: apoplexy involving meridians and collaterals, apoplexy involving Zang and Fu. For patients with apoplexy involving meridians and collaterals, the condition is normally mild with no mind changes. For apoplexy involving Zang and Fu, the lesion is normally deep, and the condition is severe, with clinical presence of obnubilation.

I. Key Points for Diagnosis and Syndrome Differentiation

[Syndrome of Apoplexy Involving Meridians and Collaterals]

1. Hemiplegia, hemiplegia without use of one side

枯不用，或痿软无力，或麻木不仁，常有感觉异常，舌紫或有瘀斑，苔白，脉细或弦。

2. 口眼㖞斜，口角流涎，或伴有口眼瞤动，言语不利，舌淡苔白，脉弦细或弦缓。

【中脏腑证】

1. 闭证者，突然昏倒，不省人事，口噤不开，肢体强直，两手握固，大小便闭，舌红，苔黄腻，脉弦滑。

2. 脱证者，突然昏倒，不省人事，目合口开，鼻鼾息微，手撒肢冷，汗多不止，二便自遗，肢体瘫软，舌痿，脉细微欲绝。

二、治疗方法

【中经络证】

（1）半身不遂

治法 舒筋活络，调和气血。

处方 肩髃（LI15）、曲池（LI11）、外关（SJ5）、环跳（GB30）、足三里（ST36）、阳陵泉（GB34）、太冲（LR3）、太溪（KI3）。

of the body, or paralysis and weakness, or numbness, normally accompanying paresthesia, purple tongue or with ecchymosis, whitish tongue fur, thin or taut pulse.

2. Wry eyes and mouth, distortion of mouth corners, drooling from mouth corner, or accompanying movement of mouth and eyes, influent speaking, light tongue with whitish fur, taut and thin or taut and slow pulse.

[Syndrome of Apoplexy Involving Zang and Fu]

1. For patients with blockage syndrome, symptoms include sudden faint, being unconscious, trismus, stiff limbs and body, clenching of hands, no urination and defecation, red tongue with yellow and greasy fur, taut and slippery pulse.

2. For patients with collapse syndrome, symptoms include sudden faint, being unconscious, closed eyes and opened mouth, snoring and weak breathing, loosen hands and cold limbs, excessive and endless sweating, gatism, weak and limp body and limbs, flaccid tongue, string pulse which is about to disappear.

II. Therapeutic Methods

[Syndrome of Apoplexy Involving Meridians and Collaterals]

(1) Hemiplegia

Therapeutic method: Relax tendons and activate collaterals, regulate Qi-blood.

Prescription: Jianyu (LI15), Quchi (LI11), Waiguan (SJ5), Huantiao (GB30), Zusanli (ST36), Yanglingquan (GB34), Taichong (LR3), Taixi (KI3).

方义 肩髃是手阳明与阳跷脉之交会穴,曲池为手阳明之合穴,合谷是手阳明之原穴,足三里是足阳明之合穴。阳明乃多气多血之经,本方重取上下肢阳明经之要穴,目的在于通畅其气血,气行血畅,筋脉得养,肢体运动功能得以恢复。手少阳络穴外关,主治肘臂屈伸不利;足少阳交会穴环跳、筋会穴阳陵泉,可治疗下肢痿痹和足痉挛。诸穴共用,可收舒筋活络,调和气血之功。

配穴 肘部拘挛,加曲池;腕部拘挛,加大陵;膝部拘挛,加曲泉;踝部拘挛,加太溪;手指拘挛,加八邪;足趾拘挛,加八风。

方法 电热针治疗。

操作 选定穴位,皮肤常规消毒。电热针直刺肩髃 0.6~0.7 寸,直刺曲池 0.7~0.8 寸,直刺足三里 0.7~0.8 寸,接通电热针仪,每个穴位分别给予电流量 50~60mA,以患者舒适为度,留针 40 分钟。

Mechanism of prescription: Jianyu is the confluent acupoint of Yang-Ming Meridian and Yang-Qiao Channel of Hand, Quchi is a He acupoint from Yang-Ming Meridian of Hand, Hegu is a Yuan acupoint from Yang-Ming Meridian of Hand, Zusanli is a He acupoint from Yang-Ming Meridian of Hand. Yang-Ming Meridian is a meridian full of Qi and blood. This prescription uses important acupoints for Yang-Ming meridians of upper and lower limbs, aimed to soothe Qi-blood and movement functions of limbs can be recovered if the circulation of Qi and blood is smooth and unobstructed. Waiguan is a collateral acupoint of Shao-Yang Meridian of Hand, it mainly treats inconvenient flexing and stretching of elbow. The confluent acupoint Huantiao of Shao-Yang Meridian of Foot and the confluent acupoint Yanglingquan of tendons can treat lower limb paralysis and foot spasm. The use of combination of these acupoints can relax tendons and activate collaterals, regulate Qi-blood.

Matching acupoints: For elbow contracture add Quchi. For wrist contracture add Daling. For knee contracture add Ququan. For ankle contracture add Taixi. For finger contracture add Baxie. For toe contracture add Bafeng.

Method: Electrothermal acupuncture treatment.

Operations: Selecting the relevant acupoints, perform routine skin disinfection. Using electrothermal acupuncture needles, vertically puncture into Jianyu for 0.6-0.7", Quchi for 0.7-0.8", Zusanli for 0.7-0.8". Turn on the electrothermal acupuncture equipment, apply a current of 50-60mA to each acupoint, and the limit is that the patient feels comfortable, leaving the needles in for

下篇 临床论治 Part II: Clinical Treatment

40 minutes.

疗程 每日 1 次，30 次为 1 个疗程。疗程间可休息 7 天，然后进行第 2 个疗程的治疗。

Therapeutic course: Treat once a day, 30 times for a course. Start the treatment for the second course after a break of 7 days.

（2）口眼㖞斜

(2) Wry Eyes and Mouth

治法 舒筋通络。

Therapeutic method: Relax tendons and activate collaterals.

处方 地仓（ST4）、颊车（ST6）、承泣（ST1）、阳白（GB14）、攒竹（BL2）、合谷（LI4）、外关（SJ5）、风池（GB20）。

Prescription: Dicang (ST4), Jiache (ST6), Chengqi (ST1), Yangbai (GB14), Cuanzhu (BL2), Hegu (LI4), Waiguan (SJ5), Fengchi (GB20).

方义 口眼部是手足阳明经脉循行所过之处，取地仓、颊车、攒竹、承泣、阳白为局部取穴，直达病所，可通络活血以濡养面部肌肤；合谷为四总穴之一，主治面口疾病；内庭是足阳明荥穴，可疏导本经之经气；风池乃治风之要穴，针之可通络息风。本方旨在近调病变处之气血，远可疏导本经之经气，气血调畅病可自愈。

Mechanism of prescription: Mouth and eyes are exterior of where the Yang-Ming meridians and channels of hands as well as feet pass through, use the method of local acupoint selecting for Dicang, Jiache, Cuanzhu, Chengqi, Yangbai to make the effects of acupuncture reach lesions, they can dredge collaterals and activate blood so as to nourish facial muscles and skins; Hegu is one of the four command points, it is mainly used to treat face and mouth diseases; Neiting is a Xing acupoint of Yang-Ming Meridian of Foot, it can soothe the meridian Qi of this meridian; Fengchi is an important acupoint for treatment of Wind, it can dredge collaterals and claim wind. The purpose of this prescription is to regulate Qi-blood around lesions, soothe the meridian Qi of the interested meridian, and the disease will be cured naturally if Qi-blood circulation is unobstructed.

配穴 流涎加承浆；易怒加太冲；语言謇涩加廉泉、通里。

Matching acupoints: For hydrostomia add Chengjiang. For irritability add Taichong. For dysphasia add Lianquan, Tongli.

· 291 ·

方法　电热针治疗。

操作　选定穴位，皮肤常规消毒。电热针平刺地仓 0.6～0.7 寸，斜刺颊车 0.6～0.7 寸，直刺合谷 0.5 寸，直刺承泣 0.3 寸，斜刺阳白 0.3 寸，接通电热针仪，每个穴位分别给予电流量 50～60mA，以患者舒适为度，留针 40 分钟。

疗程　每日 1 次，30 次为 1 个疗程。疗程间可休息 7 天，然后进行第 2 个疗程的治疗。

【中脏腑证】

（1）闭证

治法　镇肝降逆，清心安神。

处方　人中（DU26）、十宣（EX-UE11）、太冲（LR3）、丰隆（ST40）、百会（DU20）。

方义　闭证乃中风急症，故急取十二井穴点刺放血，以决壅开闭，促其神志清醒。督脉连贯脑髓；百会位于巅顶，是督脉与三阳经的交会处，配人中以泻肝经之火，降上逆之血。泻肝经原穴太冲、心包经荥穴劳宫，可镇肝降逆，清心安神。方中取足阳明络穴丰隆，旨在振奋脾胃气机，蠲浊化痰。决壅开闭，镇肝潜阳，

Method: Electrothermal acupuncture treatment.

Operations: Selecting the relevant acupoints, perform routine skin disinfection. Using electrothermal acupuncture needles, horizontally puncture into Dicang for 0.6-0.7", obliquely puncture into Jiache for 0.6-0.7", vertically puncture into Hegu for 0.5", Chengqi for 0.3", obliquely puncture into Yangbai for 0.3". Turn on the electrothermal acupuncture equipment, apply a current of 50-60mA to each acupoint, and the limit is that the patient feels comfortable, leaving the needles in for 40 minutes.

Therapeutic course: Treat once a day, 30 times for a course. Start the treatment for the second course after a break of 7 days.

[Syndrome of Apoplexy Involving Zang and Fu]

(1) Blockage Syndrome

Therapeutic method: Calm liver and descend adverse energy, clear heart and tranquilize mind.

Prescription: Renzhong (DU26), Shixuan (EX-UE11), Taichong (LR3), Fenglong (ST40), Baihui (DU20).

Mechanism of prescription: Blockage syndrome is a kind of acute stroke, so quickly puncture into the Shierjing for pricking blood therapy, so as to remove obstruction and facilitate opening as well as closing, to promote sanity. Du Channel links up the brain marrow; Baihui locates on the top, is the confluent acupoint of Du Channel and three Yang meridians. When being matched with Renzhong, it can dredge the Fire of Liver Meridian, descend upward reverse blood. Perform attenuating puncture on the Yuan acupoint Taichong from Liver Meridian and the Xing acupoint Laogong from Pericardium Me-

清心醒神，涤浊化痰是本方的主要功能。

配穴 牙关紧闭者加地仓、颊车；失语者加通里、哑门；吞咽困难者加照海、天突。

方法 毫针治疗。

操作 选定穴位，皮肤常规消毒。十二井穴点刺放血，向上斜刺人中0.3寸，平刺百会0.5寸，直刺太冲0.5寸，直刺劳宫0.3寸，直刺丰隆0.8寸。

疗程 根据患者的病情变化，可每日治疗1次或间隔治疗2小时1次。

（2）脱证

治法 救阴回阳，固脱醒神。

处方 人中（DU26）、涌泉（KI1）、承浆（RN24）、关元（RN4）、神阙（RN8）、气海（RN6）。

方义 脱证是中风危候，方取人中，旨在开窍醒神，针

ridian can calm liver and descend adverse energy, clear heart and tranquilize mind. In the prescription, use the collateral acupoint Fenglong from Yang-Ming Meridian of Foot can prosper Qi Dynamic of spleen and stomach, eliminate turbidity and phlegm. The main effects of this prescription include remove obstruction and facilitate opening as well as closing, calm liver and suppress Yang, clear heart and induce resuscitation, eliminate turbidity and phlegm.

Matching acupoints: For trismus, add Dicang, Jiache. For aphasia add Tongli, Yamen. For dysphonia add Zhaohai, Tiantu.

Method: Filiform needle acupuncture treatment.

Operations: Selecting the relevant acupoints, perform routine skin disinfection. Using pricking blood therapy at the acupoint Shierjing, obliquely puncture upward into Renzhong for 0.3", horizontally puncture into Baihui for 0.5", vertically puncture into Taichong for 0.5", Laogong for 0.3", Fenglong for 0.8".

Therapeutic course: Treat once a day or once every 2 hours, depending on the patient condition.

(2) Collapse Syndrome

Therapeutic method: Rescue Yin and recover Yang, treat collapse and induce resuscitation.

Prescription: Renzhong (DU26), Yongquan (KI1), Chengjiang (RN24), Guanyuan (RN4), Shenque (RN8), Qihai (RN6).

Mechanism of prescription: Collapse syndrome is a critical syndrome in apoplexy, so use Renzhong to

补足少阴井穴涌泉、任脉交会穴承浆，以救欲竭之真阴。任脉交会穴关元，针之可补元阴元阳。命门为生命之根，温针可壮阳益肾。元神寄于神阙，温针可安神固脱。诸穴共用，可达救阴回阳、固脱醒神之目的。

配穴 虚汗不止者加阴郄；酣睡不醒者加申脉；小便不禁者加水道、三阴交、足三里。

方法 电热针治疗。

操作 选定穴位，皮肤常规消毒。电热针直刺关元、气海各0.7寸，直刺足三里0.8寸，直刺三阴交0.7寸，直刺涌泉0.6寸，接通电热针仪，每个穴位分别给予50~60mA的电流量，以胀感舒适为度，留针40分钟。另配以毫针斜刺人中0.3寸，向舌根方向斜刺承浆0.5寸，均用补法轻浅刺激，不留针。神阙隔盐灸10分钟。

induce resuscitation, and perform tonifying acupuncture on the Jing acupoint Yongquan of Shao-Yin Meridian of Foot as well as the confluent acupoint Chengjiang of Ren Channel so as to rescue the nearly depleted genuine Yin. Acupuncture of the confluent acupoint Guanyuan of Ren Channel can replenish Yuan Yin and Yuan Yang. Mingmen is the Root of Life, acupuncture with warm needling of this acupoint can strengthen Yang and tonify kidney. Primordial spirit is stored in the Shenque, acupuncture with warm needling of this acupoint can tranquilize mind and treat collapse. The use of combination of these acupoints can rescue Yin and recover Yang, treat collapse and induce resuscitation.

Matching acupoints: For persistent abnormal sweating due to general debility, add Yinxi. For drowsiness add Shenmai. For incontinence of urine add Shuidao, Sanyinjiao, Zusanli.

Method: Electrothermal acupuncture treatment.

Operations: Selecting the relevant acupoints, perform routine skin disinfection. Using electrothermal acupuncture needles, vertically puncture into Guanyuan and Qihai for 0.7" respectively, vertically puncture into Zusanli for 0.8", Sanyinjiao for 0.7", Yongquan for 0.6". Turn on the electrothermal acupuncture equipment, apply a current of 50-60mA to each acupoint, and the limit is that the patient feels comfortable, leaving the needles in for 40 minutes. Additionally, using filiform needles, vertically puncture into Renzhong for 0.3", obliquely puncture toward root of tongue into Chengjiang for 0.5", both using tonifying method with slight stimulation, do not leave the needle in. Perform salt suspension-moxibustion on Shenque for 10 minutes.

Therapeutic course: Once a day, leave the needles in for 40 minutes, 10 times for a course. Start the treatment for the second course after a break of 3-5 days.

III. Precautions

1. For patients with apoplexy involving viscera and organs in critical conditions, combination of Traditional Chinese Medicine and Western Medicine should be taken for timely rescue so as to rescue the patient out of danger as soon as possible.

2. For patients with apoplexy involving meridians and collaterals, it is necessary to perform acupuncture therapy as soon as possible, while instruct patients to do limb functional exercises, so as to facilitate function recovery of affected limbs and avoid sequelae.

3. When puncturing acupoints at chest and back area, it is necessary to control puncturing directions and use mild manipulation, and needles shouldn't be inserted too deep so as to avoid pneumothorax.

4. For patients with spontaneous bleeding tendency or poor blood coagulation function, tongue acupuncture therapy is not appropriate.

5. Pricking blood therapy on the acupoint Shierjing, stop the bloodletting as soon as the condition improved. The method is improper to be used for long time to avoid impairment of Qi-blood.

四、典型病例

案一 脑血栓

李某,男,74岁,技术员,北京人。

主诉:左半身不遂伴语言欠流利15天。病史:患者于15天前的夜晚受风寒,翌日晨出现半身不遂,口㖞,讲话不流利,左侧上、下肢不会动。立即到某西医院诊治,经15天治疗效果不明显。

刻下症:左半身不能活动,言语不利,左侧面瘫,左侧生理反射消失,病理反射可引出,眠差,纳可,二便通畅,舌质红,苔黄腻,脉弦。

查体:血压180/100mmHg。口角不对称,歪向右侧。两肺呼吸音粗糙。二尖瓣区及主动脉瓣第二听诊区可闻及二级收缩期杂音。左侧上、下肢无自主运动。病理反射可引出。

辅助检查:甘油三酯水平高。空腹血糖5.4mmol/L。头部CT示"脑血栓形成"。

【诊断依据】

1. 老年男性,年老体衰,

IV. Typical Cases

Case I Cerebral thrombosis

Li, male, 74 years old, technician, residence: Beijing.

Self-reported symptoms: Hemiplegia of the left side, with influent speaking for 15 days. Medical history: the patient was affected by cold at night 15 days ago, and hemiplegia occurred in the next morning, with wry mouth, influent speaking, immovability of left upper and lower limbs. He was sent to a western medicine hospital for treatment immediately, however the efficacy was not obvious after 15 days of treatment.

Current symptoms: Immovability of the left body, influent speaking, left facial paralysis, disappearance of left body physiological reflex while pathological reflex can be induced, poor sleep and passable appetite, smooth urination and defecation, red tongue with yellow and greasy fur, taut pulse.

Physical examination: Blood pressure 180/100 mmHg. Asymmetric mouth corners of the two sides, crooked to the right. Coarse breath sounds in both lungs. Grade 2 systolic noise at mitral valve area and second aortic valve area. No spontaneous movements of left upper and lower extremities. Pathological reflex can be induced.

Auxiliary examination: High level of triglyceride. FBG 5.4mmol/L. Head CT exam showed "cerebral thrombosis".

[Diagnostic Basis]

1. Elder male, old and feeble, Yin deficiency of liv-

肝肾阴虚，肝阳偏亢（血压180/100mmHg），高脂血症。

2. 查体：左侧半身不遂，口眼㖞斜，语言欠流利。

3. 头部CT示"脑血栓形成"。

【证治分析】

病因 肝肾阴虚，肝阳偏亢。

病机 肝肾阴虚，肝阳偏亢，值感风寒，引动内风，上扰清窍而发为本病。

证候分析 肝肾不足为酿成中风之因。肝肾之阴不足，则筋脉失养，故肢体麻木；阴虚则阳亢，故见眩晕耳鸣；风从内生，风主动，故手足拘挛；虚火内生，内扰神明，故心烦失眠。舌脉亦为阴虚内热之象。

病位 肝、肾。

病性 阴虚阳亢。

西医诊断 高血压、动脉硬化、脑血栓形成。

中医诊断 中风（中经络）、眩晕。

治法 醒脑开窍，滋补肝

er and kidney, liver Yang hyperactivity (blood pressure 180/100mmHg), hyperlipidemia.

2. Physical examination: Hemiplegia of the left side, wry eyes and mouth, influent speaking.

3. Head CT exam showed "cerebral thrombosis".

[Syndrome-treatment Analysis]

Etiology: Yin deficiency of liver and kidney, liver Yang hyperactivity.

Pathogenesis: Yin deficiency of liver and kidney, liver Yang hyperactivity, the catch of cold induced internal Wind which upwards disturbed sense organs subsequently caused this disease.

Syndrome analysis: Deficiency of liver and kidney was the cause of the stroke. Yin deficiency of liver and kidney caused nourishment loss of tendons and channels, therefore caused limb numbness; Yin deficiency was accompanied with Yang hyperactivity, therefore caused vertigo and tinnitus; Wind generated internally, and Wind governs movement, so caused contracture of hands and feet; deficiency Fire generated internally and disturbed mind and consciousness, therefore caused vexation and insomnia. Pulse condition of the tongue also indicated Yin deficiency and inner Heat.

Lesion location: Liver, kidney.

Lesion nature: Yin deficiency and Yang hyperactivity.

The diagnosis of Western Medicine: High blood pressure, arteriosclerosis, cerebral thrombosis.

The diagnosis of Traditional Chinese Medicine: Apoplexy (involving meridians and collaterals), vertigo.

Therapeutic method: Restore consciousness and

肾，疏通经络。

方法 电热针治疗。

处方 百会（DU20）、三阴交（SP6）、肾俞（BL23）、太溪（KI3）、神门（HT7）、大陵（PC7）、太冲（LR3）、极泉（HT1）、曲池（LI11）、环跳（GB30）、阳陵泉（GB34）、人中（DU26）。

方义 肾为先天之本，内藏元阴元阳，故取肾俞、太溪补肾阴而治其本；太冲是肝经原穴，可潜降上亢之风阳以治眩晕、耳鸣；用心经与心包经之原穴神门、大陵调心气，与补肾阴之穴相伍可交通心肾而治心烦失眠；三阴交既可疏通经络，又可滋肝肾之不足，为标本兼治之穴。其余穴为局部取穴，疏通经络，行气活血。

配穴 便溏纳呆者加天枢、中脘；咽干者加照海、廉泉；发声不清者加哑门；口角流涎者加颊车、四白、地仓。

induce resuscitation, nourish liver and kidney, soothe meridians and collaterals.

Method: Electrothermal acupuncture treatment.

Prescription: Baihui (DU20), Sanyinjiao (SP6), Shenshu (BL23), Taixi (KI3), Shenmen (HT7), Daling (PC7), Taichong (LR3), Jiquan (HT1), Quchi (LI11), Huantiao(GB30), Yanglingquan (GB34), Renzhong (DU26).

Mechanism of prescription: Kidney is the congenital foundation, in which stores Yuan Yin and Yuan Yang, so use Shenshu, Taixi to replenish kidney Yin so as to affect a permanent cure; Taichong is a Yuan acupoint of Liver Meridian, it can calm and descend the hyperactive Wind Yang to treat vertigo and tinnitus. Use the Yuan acupoints Shenmen, Daling of Heart Meridian and Pericardium Meridian to regulate heart Qi, and they can connect the communication between heart and kidney when being matched with acupoints effective in replenishing kidney Yin, so as to treat vexation and insomnia; Sanyinjiao can soothe meridians and collaterals as well as nourish liver and kidney to treat deficiency, is an acupoint effective in symptoms treatment as well as effecting a permanent cure. Use the method of local acupoint selecting for other acupoints, so as to soothe meridians and collaterals, activate Qi and blood circulation.

Matching acupoints: For sloppy stool and anorexia add Tianshu, Zhongwan. For dry throat add Zhaohai, Lianquan. For unclear voice add Yamen. For slobbering, add Jiache, Sibai, Dicang.

操作　选定穴位，皮肤常规消毒。电热针斜刺肾俞、太溪、三阴交、太冲、大陵、百会、阳陵泉、环跳、曲池各0.7寸，然后接通电热针仪，每穴分别给予电流量50mA，以胀而舒适为度，留针40分钟。（注：每次选3组穴给予电热针治疗，余穴用毫针治疗，每天1次。）

疗程　每日1次，留针40分钟，10次为1个疗程。疗程间可休息3～5天，再进行第2个疗程的治疗。

治疗过程　经治7次后，患者语言清楚，上肢可抬30°，下肢直腿抬高40°。配合按摩及功能训练，继续进行针灸治疗，2周后可搀扶行走，左上肢抬举过头，唯有左手握力差。30天后，四肢功能如常，言语清楚流利。继续巩固疗效，10天后痊愈出院。嘱患者坚持肢体功能锻炼，饮食要清淡，注意监测血压，心态要保持平和。随访3年，身体健康，未再发病。

Operations: Selecting the relevant acupoints, perform routine skin disinfection. Using electrothermal acupuncture needles, obliquely puncture into Shenshu, Taixi, Sanyinjiao, Taichong, Daling, Baihui, Yanglingquan, Huantiao, Quchi for 0.7" respectively, then turn on the electrothermal acupuncture equipment, apply a current of 50mA to each acupoint, and the limit is that the patient feels swelling and comfortable, leaving the needles in for 40 minutes. (Note: Select 3 pairs of acupoints for electrothermal acupuncture treatment each time, and treat the other acupoints with filiform needle, once a day.)

Therapeutic course: Once a day, leave the needles in for 40 minutes, 10 times for a course. Start the treatment for the second course after a break of 3-5 days.

Therapeutic process: After 7 treatments, the patient could speak clearly, the affected upper extremity could lift up to an angle of 30°, the affected lower extremity could lift up to an angle of 40° while keeping straight. In combination with massage and functional exercises, continued the acupuncture treatment, and the patient could walk with assistance, the left upper extremity could lift up over the head 2 weeks afterward, however the grip strength of the left hand was poor. After 30 days, the functions of extremities were recovered as normal, and the patient could speak clearly and fluently. Continue the treatment for consolidation, and the patient was cured and discharged 10 days later. Instruct the patient to adhere to limb functional exercises; diet should be light; pay attention to blood pressure monitoring; keep peaceful mind. 3 years of follow-up, the patient was healthy

【生活调摄】

1. 加强护理，卧床休息，密切观察病情的变化。

2. 清淡饮食，规律作息，防止感染和病情的进一步恶化。

3. 病情稳定后，加强语言康复和患肢的功能锻炼。

案二 脑出血

胡某，男，59岁，技术员，北京人。

主诉：右半身不遂，失语7日。病史：患者在8天前的夜晚11点左右，生气后睡觉，发现有鼾声，呼之不应，面红，叫醒后语言不清，经某医院诊治效果不显著。

刻下症：右侧肢体不利，言语不清，纳眠差，舌质红，苔黄，脉数。

查体：血压210/110mmHg。嗜睡，神志恍惚，语言不清，面红，瞳孔右略大于左。右鼻唇沟变浅，伸舌偏向右，口角不对称。颈稍僵。两肺呼吸音粗，可闻及痰鸣音，呼吸深快。二尖瓣区及主动脉瓣第二听诊区可闻及二级收缩期杂音。右侧上、下肢不能活动，病理反射可引出，生理反射健侧存在。

with no more disease attacks.

[Lifestyle Change and Health Maintenance]

1. Strengthen care, rest in bed, close observation of changes in conditions.

2. Light diet, regular life schedule, prevent infections and further deterioration of the disease.

3. After the disease is stablized, it is to improve the language rehabilitation and limb functional exercises.

Case II   Cerebral hemorrhage

Hu, male, 59 years old, technician, residence: Beijing.

Self-reported symptoms: Hemiplegia of the right side, aphasia for 7 days. Medical history: 8 days ago, around 11 o'clock at night, the patient went to bed with anger, and he was found being snoring, no response with calling, red complexion, and alalia after being waked. The effect was very little after treated by a hospital.

Current symptoms: Clumsy movements of the right side of body, alalia, poor appetite and sleep, red tongue with yellow fur, rapid pulse.

Physical examination: Blood pressure 210/110 mmHg. Drowsiness, wandering in the mind, red complexion, the right pupil slightly larger than the left one. The right nasolabial groove shallowed, the tongue crooked to the right when stretching out, the mouth corners of the two sides were asymmetric. The neck was slightly stiff. Coarse breath sounds in both lungs, wheezy phlegm could be heard, deep and rapid breath. Grade 2 systolic noise at mitral valve area and second aortic valve area. The right upper and lower extremities could not move, and pathological reflex could be induced. For the healthy

辅助检查：血脂三项指标偏高。脑脊液呈血性。头部CT示"脑出血"。

【诊断依据】

1. 中老年人，卒中体质。

2. 有高血压、高脂血症。

3. 查体见阳性体征。

4. 脑脊液呈血性。

5. 头部CT证实有出血灶。

【证治分析】

病因　恼怒所致。

病机　忧思恼怒后，以致阴阳失调，脏腑气偏，气血错乱，肌肤筋脉失去濡养，阴亏于下，肝阳暴张，肝风内动，夹痰夹火，血溢经遂所致。

证候分析　肝阳暴亢，阳升风动，气血上逆，蒙闭清窍，神不导气，故出现昏睡。风火上亢，气血逆乱，闭阻经络，故见面红、半身不遂、项强。舌脉亦为风火逆闭之象。

病位　心、肝、肾。

side psychological reflex existed.

Auxiliary examination: Three indicators for blood lipid were high. Cerebrospinal fluid was bloody. Head CT exam showed "cerebral hemorrhage".

[Diagnostic Basis]

1. Middle-aged and elderly people, with high risk of stroke.

2. Suffered from high blood pressure and hyperlipidemia.

3. Positive signs were seen in the physical examination.

4. Cerebrospinal fluid was bloody.

5. Hemorrhagic lesion was confirmed in the head CT.

[Syndrome-treatment Analysis]

Etiology: Caused by anger.

Pathogenesis: Caused by sad thoughts and anger leading to imbalance between Yin and Yang as well as between Zang Qi and Fu Qi, disorders of Qi-blood, nourishment loss of tendons and channels, Yin deficiency of lower body, over-expending of liver Yang, internal movement of liver Wind with phlegm and Fire, blood over-flooding to Jingsui.

Syndrome analysis: Hyperactivity of liver Yang, Yang ascending and Wind moving, abnormal rising of Qi-blood, obstruction and closure of sense organs, poor circulation of Qi, leading to lethargy. Hyperactivity of Wind and Fire, disorders of Qi-blood, obstruction of meridians and collaterals, therefore cause red complexion, hemiplegia, stiff neck. The pulse condition of tongue was also indicated disorder and obstruction of Wind and Fire.

Lesion location: Heart, liver, kidney.

病性 实证。

西医诊断 高血压、脑出血、高脂血症。

中医诊断 中风（中脏腑）、眩晕。

治法 开窍醒神，清肝息风。

方法 电热针治疗。

处方 人中（DU26）、十宣（EX-UE11）、内关（PC6）、太冲（LR3）、百会（DU20）、丰隆（ST40）。

方义 闭乃中风急症，故速刺十宣点刺放血，以决壅开闭，促其神智清楚。百会位于巅顶，是督脉与三阳经的交会之处，配人中以泻肝经之火，降上逆之血。泻肝经原穴太冲可镇肝降逆，清心安神。取足阳明络穴丰隆，旨在振奋脾胃气机，蠲浊化痰。诸穴合用，可达决壅开闭、镇肝潜阳、清心醒神、涤浊化痰之功效。

配穴 失语加通里、哑

Disease nature: Excess syndrome.

The diagnosis of Western Medicine: High blood pressure, cerebral hemorrhage, hyperlipidemia.

The diagnosis of Traditional Chinese Medicine: Apoplexy (involving viscera and organs), vertigo.

Therapeutic method: Induce resuscitation, clear liver and calm Wind.

Method: Electrothermal acupuncture treatment.

Prescription: Renzhong (DU26), Shixuan (EX-UE11), Neiguan (PC6), Taichong (LR3), Baihui (DU20), Fenglong (ST40).

Mechanism of prescription: Blockage syndrome is a kind of acute strokes, so quickly puncture into Shixuan for pricking blood therapy, so as to remove obstruction and facilitate opening as well as closing, to promote sanity. Baihui locates on the top, is the confluent acupoint of Du Channel and three Yang meridians. When being matched with Renzhong, it can dredge the Fire of Liver Meridian, descend upward reverse blood. Perform attenuating puncture on the Yuan acupoint Taichong from Liver Meridian can calm liver and descend adverse energy, clear heart and tranquilize mind. Use the collateral acupoint Fenglong from Yang-Ming Meridian of Foot can prosper Qi Dynamic of spleen and stomach, eliminate turbidity and phlegm. The use of combination of these acupoints can remove obstruction and facilitate opening as well as closing, calm liver and suppress Yang, clear heart and induce resuscitation, eliminate turbidity and phlegm.

Matching acupoints: For aphasia add Tongli,

门；吞咽困难加照海、天突、翳风；口角流涎加地仓、颊车、合谷；半身不遂加肩髃、曲池、外关、合谷、环跳、阳陵泉、足三里、太冲、三阴交。

操作 选定穴位，皮肤常规消毒。电热针直刺曲池、足三里、三阴交、肩髃、环跳、阳陵泉各0.7寸，分成两组，轮流交替治疗。接通电热针仪，每个穴位分别给予电流量50mA，留针40分钟，其余穴位均以毫针治疗，留针40分钟。辅以吸氧。

疗程 每日1次，留针40分钟，10次为1个疗程。疗程间可休息3～5天，再进行第2个疗程的治疗。

治疗过程 治疗后的第2天，患者神志清楚，反应迟钝，声音低微，能进食少量流质品，头痛，右侧上、下肢不能活动，舌红，苔黄腻，脉弦。除刺血针外，针刺方法同前，加廉泉、风池。连续治疗5次，头痛减轻，语言清楚，伸舌仍偏向右侧，上、下肢肌力增加，可以抬起，但右手握力差，血压150/90mmHg，舌脉同前。心志较平和，情绪

Yamen. For dysphonia, add Zhaohai, Tiantu, Yifeng. For slobbering, add Dicang, Jiache, Hegu. For hemiplegia, add Jianyu, Quchi, Waiguan, Hegu, Huantiao, Yanglingquan, Zusanli, Taichong, Sanyinjiao.

Operations: Selecting the relevant acupoints, perform routine skin disinfection. Using electrothermal acupuncture needles, vertically puncture into Quchi, Zusanli, Sanyinjiao, Jianyu, Huantiao, Yanglingquan for 0.7'' respectively, and divide these acupoints into two groups for alternate treatments. Turn on the electrothermal acupuncture equipment, apply a current of 50mA to each acupoint, leaving the needles in for 40 minutes, and treat other acupoints with filiform needles, leaving the needles in for 40 minutes. Supplemented by oxygen inhalation.

Therapeutic course: Once a day, leave the needles in for 40 minutes, 10 times for a course. Start the treatment for the second course after a break of 3-5 days.

Therapeutic process: On the second day after treatment, the patient had clear consciousness, slow response, low voice, could eat a small amount of fluid products, had headache, and the upper and lower limbs on the right side could not move, with a red tongue, yellow greasy fur, taut pulse. Remove the pricking needles, the puncture method is the same as above, add Lianquan, Fengchi. Continuously treated for 5 times, the headache was relieved, the speaking become clear, the tongue still crooked to right when stretching out, the muscle force of upper and lower extremities increased and they could be lifted up, but the grip strength of the right hand was poor,

好，能配合功能训练。经过 37 天的住院治疗，痊愈出院。出院后继续治疗，连续治疗 2 个月后，半身活动较自如，手能抬高过头，握力好，走路姿态较端正，能随意活动。

【生活调摄】

1. 加强护理，卧床休息，密切观察病情的变化。

2. 清淡饮食，规律作息，防止感染和病情的进一步恶化。

3. 病情稳定后，加强语言康复和患肢的功能锻炼。

共济失调

共济失调是一组以共济运动障碍为主要表现的中枢神经系统变性疾病。其表现为在没有肌力减退的情况下，肢体运动协调失灵，不平衡与不协调，故称共济失调。本病有遗传性倾向。根据病理损害的主要部位及程度不同，可分为脊髓型、脊髓小脑型、小脑型 3 类。共济失调多慢性起病，在疾病的发展过程中，患者可不同程度地出现行路不稳，意向

blood pressure 150/90mmHg, the tongue Channel was the same as above. Relatively peaceful mind and mood, good emotion, the patient could cooperate with functional exercises. After 37 days of hospitalization, the patient was cured and discharged. The treatment continued after discharge, and after two months of continuous treatment, the patient could relatively freely move the affected body side, the hand could rise over the head with good grip strength, the walking fashion was better and could do activities freely.

[Lifestyle Change and Health Maintenance]

1. Strengthen care, rest in bed, close observation of changes in conditions.

2. Light diet, regular life schedule, prevent infections and further deterioration of the disease.

3. After the disease is stable, strengthen the language rehabilitation and limb functional exercises.

Ataxia

Ataxia is a group of central nervous system degeneration diseases, the main presence of which is a disorder in the coordination of movements. Manifestations include failure, imbalance and dissonance of limb movements without muscle strength decreases, which is called discoordination (ataxia). The disease has a genetic tendency. It can be divided into 3 types depending on the difference in the main location and severity of pathological lesions: spinal cord type, spinocerebellar type, cerebellar type. Normally ataxia develops as a chronic disease, and during its development, patients may suffer from varying degrees of walking instability, intentional tremors and static tremors,

性和静力性震颤，头和肢体不自主动作，发育障碍或拼音困难。疾病晚期，偶可出现肌力减退，或远端肌肉萎缩等临床症状。

中医认为，本病属于"颤证""振掉"的范畴。多由气血两亏，筋脉失于濡养，或久病入络，血瘀气滞所致。

一、诊断及辨证要点

1. 脊髓型

（1）少年型脊髓型遗传共济失调（Friedreich共济失调）：此为临床最常见的一型，呈常染色体隐性遗传，多在5～13岁之间起病，最迟可致30岁，男女无差别，起病成隐性，缓慢进展。

（2）遗传性痉挛性截瘫（Strumpell病）：遗传性侧索硬化，亦是较常见的一型。遗传方式有常染色体显性遗传及隐性遗传2种。男多于女，以3～15岁之间起病者多见，起病缓慢，主要是缓慢进展的双下肢中枢性瘫痪。

（3）腓肠肌萎缩型共济失

involuntary movements of head and limbs, developmental disorders, or spelling dyslexia. In the late phase, clinical symptoms like muscle strength decease or distal amyotrophia may occasionally occur.

Traditional Chinese Medicine believes that this disease belongs to the range of "tremor syndrome" and "shakes". Most cases are caused by Qi-blood deficiency causing nourishment loss in tendons and channels, or the disease developing into collaterals causing blood stagnation and Qi stasis.

I. Key Points for Diagnosis and Syndrome Differentiation

1. Spinal cord type

(1) Juvenile hereditary spinal cord ataxia (Friedreich ataxia): This is the most clinically common type, which is an autosomal recessive inherited disease and normally develops between 5-13 years old up to 30 years old, with no difference between males and females. It is recessive when it develops and it progresses slowly.

(2) Hereditary spastic paraplegia. Also called Strumpell disease, hereditary lateral sclerosis, is a common type as well. There are two modes of inheritance: autosomal dominant inheritance and recessive inheritance. There are more male suffers than female. For most patients the disease develops from 3-15 years old, with slow disease development, and the main symptom is slowly progressing central paralysis of the lower limbs.

(3) Gastrocnemius atrophic ataxia (Roussy Levy

调（Roussy Levy 综合征）：本病多数呈常染色体显性遗传，但亦有常染色体隐性及 X 连锁遗传者，发病率约为（3～13）/10 万人口，常在 10～20 岁之间起病。肌萎缩自下肢远端开始，渐向上发展。

2. 小脑型遗传型共济失调

（1）遗传性痉挛性共济失调（Marie 型）：呈常染色体显性遗传，多在 25～55 岁起病，首先出现缓慢的步态不稳和平衡障碍，为单纯性的小脑型共济失调而无感觉型共济失调之成分。

（2）橄榄脑桥小脑萎缩（OPCA）：呈常染色体显性遗传，多在 40～50 岁发病，无性别差异，临床表现为脑功能进行性减退，开始主要表现为双下肢的小脑性行走困难及共济失调，并逐渐影响上肢。

（3）迟发性小脑皮质萎缩：呈染色体显性遗传，主要影响小脑蚓部和绒球以及橄榄体，多在 50 岁后发病，突然出刻下症状，行走和站立不稳，上肢症状相对较轻，后期出现构音轻度困难，头和躯干静止性震颤。

3. 脊髓小脑型遗传性共济

Syndrome): This disease normally is an autosomal dominant inheritance, but there are also autosomal recessive inheritances and X-linked inherited cases. The incidence rate is around (3-13)/100 thousand people, and often develops between 10-20 years old. The amyotrophy starts from the distal end of lower limbs and develops upwards gradually.

2. Hereditary cerebellar ataxia

(1) Hereditary spastic ataxia (Marie): Autosomal dominant inheritance, often develops between 25-55 years old, firstly shows slowly progressed gait instability and balance disorder; it is a simple hereditary cerebellar ataxia without elements of sensory ataxia.

(2) Olivopontocerebellar atrophy (OPCA): Autosomal dominant inheritance, often develops between 40-50 years old, with no difference between males and females; the clinical manifestation is cerebellar walking difficulties and ataxia of lower limbs, which affect upper limbs gradually.

(3) Delayed cerebellar cortical atrophy: Autosomal dominant inheritance, normally affects cerebellar vermis, floccules and olivary body, often develops after 50 years old; sudden occurrence of symptoms of instabilities of walking and standing which are relatively slighter in upper limbs, and in the late phase mild dyslexia, static tremor of head and body occur.

3. Hereditary spin cerebellar ataxia

失调

（1）棘状红细胞、血清 β 脂蛋白缺乏症：呈染色体隐性遗传，临床少见，早年发病，伴营养吸收障碍，首发症状为脂肪性腹泻，腹胀和营养障碍，多在 4～5 岁时自行减轻，其次出现动作笨拙，约在 6 岁以后出现共济失调。

（2）共济失调-毛细血管扩张症（Louis Bar 综合征）：多呈常染色体隐性遗传，为涉及多系统的一种遗传性变性疾病。婴儿期即出现小脑性共济失调，起初主要影响躯干和头，患儿等到会走路时，步态摇晃非常明显，两腿分得很宽，继而上肢出现意向性震颤。多数患儿伴舞蹈样手足徐动症，随着年龄的增长，锥体外系多动症状变得更加明显。青春期后可出现椎体受损症状，成年患者可出现肢端肌肉萎缩。3～6 岁时于眼结膜、眼睑、鼻梁和两颊部、外耳、颈项、肘窝及腋窝处经常暴露或受刺激之部位出现毛细血管扩张。成年后共济失调，有停止进展的趋势。

4. 血液生化检查

（1）血清谷氨酸脱氢酶降

(1) Deficiency of acanthocyte and serum β-lipoprotein: Autosomal recessive inheritance, clinically rare, early onset, accompanied with a disorder of nutrition absorption. The first symptoms that occur are fatty diarrhea, abdominal distension, and dystrophia, most of which relieve spontaneously at the age of 4-5 years old, followed by clumsy actions, then ataxia after 6 years old.

(2) Syndrome of ataxia-telangiectasis (Louis Bar syndrome): Normally autosomal recessive inheritance, is a hereditary degeneration disease involving multiple systems. Cerebellar ataxia occurs in the infancy stage, which mainly affects the body and head, and after the infant learned walking, the gait shaking is very obvious and the two legs are widely separated, subsequently the intentional tremor occurs. Most patients also suffer from choreoathetosis, and symptoms of the extrapyramidal system become increasingly obvious along with the age. Vertebral body damages may occur after puberty, and adult patients may suffer from amyotrophia of limb ends. At the age of 3-6 years old, telangiectasis occurs at parts that are often exposed or stimulated, like eye conjunctiva, eyelid, nose bridge and cheeks, external ears, neck, cubital fossa and armpits. After entered into the adult stage, ataxia occurs and tends to stop progressing.

4. Blood biochemical tests

(1) Reduced serum glutamate dehydrogenase level

低者为 OPCA。

（2）丙酮酸脱氢酶降低者为 Friedreich 共济失调。

（3）血清 β 脂蛋白缺乏和胆固醇降低，为棘状红细胞、β 脂蛋白缺乏症。

（4）分泌性 IgA 降低，为毛细血管扩张性共济失调。

二、治疗方法

【血虚风动证】

治法 舒筋通络，健脾养血。

处方 曲池（LI11）、阳陵泉（GB34）、足三里（ST36）、三阴交（SP6）、合谷（LI4）。

方义 本方上取手阳明经原穴合谷、合穴曲池，下取足阳明经合穴足三里，旨在疏通阳明经络，三穴合用，可使上、下肢的肌肉筋脉得到气血的正常濡养。阳陵泉为足少阳胆经之合穴，又是筋会穴，是治疗下肢痿软、步履艰难的常用穴，针之可健脾益气，助化源以生气血。舒筋通络，健脾养血是本方的主要目的。

indicates OPCA.

(2) Reduced pyruvate dehydrogenase level indicates Friedreich ataxia.

(3) Deficiency of serum β-lipoprotein and reduced cholesterol level indicated deficiency of acanthocyte and serum β-lipoprotein.

(4) Reduced secretory IgA indicates ataxia-telangiectasis.

II. Therapeutic Methods

[Syndrome of Blood Deficiency and Wind Stirring]

Therapeutic method: Relax tendons, activate collaterals, invigorate spleen, and nourish blood.

Prescription: Quchi (LI11), Yanglingquan (GB34), Zusanli (ST36), Sanyinjiao (SP6), Hegu (LI4).

Mechanism of prescription: In this prescription, use the Yuan acupoint Hegu and the He acupoint Quchi upward from Yang-Ming Meridian of Hand and the He acupoint Zusanli downward of Yang-Ming Meridian of Foot, to soothe meridians and collaterals of Yang-Ming. The combination of these three acupoints can achieve normal nourishment from Qi-blood for muscles as well as tendons and channels of upper and lower limbs. Yanglingquan is a He acupoint from Shao-Yang Gallbladder Meridian of Foot, as well as the confluent acupoint of tendons; it is a commonly used acupoint for treatment of lower limb atrophy, struggling. The acupuncture of this acupoint can invigorate spleen and tonify Qi, to facilitate source transformation so as to generate Qi and blood. The main

配穴 言语不利者加廉泉，远端肌肉萎缩者加八邪、八风，下肢抽搐者加悬钟。

方法 电热针治疗。

操作 选定穴位，皮肤常规消毒。电热针直刺曲池0.7寸，直刺合谷0.6寸，直刺阳陵泉0.7寸，直刺足三里0.8寸，直刺三阴交穴0.8寸。接通电热针仪，每个穴位分别给予50～60mA的电流量，以患者感到胀或温热舒适度，留针40分钟。

疗程 每日1次，20次为1个疗程。疗程间可休息3～5天，根据病情决定是否需要继续治疗。

三、注意事项

1. 安慰患者，使之解除思想负担，树立信心战胜疾病，更好地配合治疗。

2. 根据患者的体能，尽可能参加能做到甚至通过努力可以做到的功能训练，要帮助患者完成。

3. 本病现代医学尚无有效的治疗方法，应尽早采取中药及针灸治疗。

aim of this prescription is to relax tendons and activate collaterals, invigorate spleen and nourish blood.

Matching acupoints: For alalia add Lianquan, for distal amyotrophia add Baxie, Bafeng; for spasm of lower limbs add Xuanzhong.

Method: Electrothermal acupuncture treatment.

Operations: Selecting the relevant acupoints, perform routine skin disinfection. Using electrothermal acupuncture needles, vertically puncture into Quchi for 0.7", Hegu for 0.6", Yanglingquan for 0.7", Zusanli for 0.8", Sanyinjiao for 0.8". Turn on the electrothermal acupuncture equipment, apply a current of 50-60mA to each acupoint. The limit is that the patient feels swelling or warm and comfortable. Leave the needles in for 40 minutes.

Therapeutic course: Once a day, 20 times for a course. Rest for 3-5 days between courses, decide if continue the treatment depending on the disease conditions.

III. Precautions

1. Comfort patients and let them relieve mind burdens, establish confidence in defeating diseases and better cooperate with treatments.

2. Depending on patients' physical abilities, help them to participate in functional exercises that they can do or even can complete with efforts.

3. For this disease there is no efficient therapy in modern medicine yet, and it is therefore necessary to adopt treatments of Chinese Herb Medicine and acu-

Cerebral Agenesis

Cerebral agenesis refers to the retardation in the cerebral function development or cerebral agenesis of the infant during the embryonic period due to influence of the mother's diseases or generic factors. The main manifestations include: Dysgnosia and various symptoms of cranial nerves, among which commonly seen ones are hypophrenia, sluggish movement, normally with tetanic paralysis of lower limbs, walking with "scissors steps", inability of self-care, or accompanied with convulsion. Most are congenital diseases. However, acquired factors like birth injuries, prolong labor, intracranial infections can also cause this diseases.

Traditional Chinese Medicine believes that this disease belongs to the range of "five kinds of retardation" and the "five kinds of flaccidity". The five kinds of retardation refer to retardation in standing, walking, hair-growing, tooth eruption and speech. The five kinds of flaccidity refer to flaccidity of head top, mouth, hands, feet and muscles, most of which are caused by inadequate inherent endowment, insufficiency of Qi-blood, Yin depletion of liver and kidney.

I. Key Points for Diagnosis and Syndrome Differentiation

1. For patients with deficiencies of the liver and kidney, their sitting up, standing, walking, dentition, etc. are obviously later than those of normal children of the same age. In severe cases, patients cannot walk at the age of 4-5

而不稳者，头倾转而无力，不能抬举，少动喜卧，神倦乏力，舌质淡，舌苔薄白，指纹色淡。

2. 心血不足者，语迟发迟，智力不聪，神情呆滞，肌肤苍白，舌光无苔，指纹色淡。

3. 脾气亏损者，口软唇弛，咀嚼乏力，常有流涎，手软下垂，不能抬举，足跃迟缓，不能站立，肌肉松弛，活动无力，神情呆滞，智力迟钝，肢末不温，食欲不振，舌淡苔少，指纹色淡。

二、治疗方法

【肝肾不足证】

治法 补肾益肝，强骨健脑。

处方 百会（DU20）、四神聪（EX-HN1）、悬钟（GB39）、太溪（KI3）、肝俞（BL18）、肾俞（BL23）、志室（BL52）、命门（DU4）。

方义 头为诸阳之会，脑为髓海，取百会配四神聪，以健脑醒神；肾藏精，主骨生髓，为生长之本，而齿为骨之

years old or even at the age around 10 years old, patients cannot walk stable, with tilted and weak head, unable to lift up, less movement and preference to lying down, fatigued looks and asthenia, light tongue with thin and whitish fur, and faint fingerprints.

2. For patients with deficiency of heart blood, symptoms include retardation in speech and retardation in hair-growing, poor intelligence, sluggish look, pale skin, smooth tongue without fur, faint fingerprints.

3. For patients with depletion of spleen Qi, symptoms include soft mouth with loose lips, weakness in chewing, often with hydrostomia, soft and drooping hands unable to lift up, retardation in foot jumping, inability of standing, muscle flaccidity, weakness in movements, sluggish look, mental retardation, cold limb ends, poor appetite, light tongue with less fur, faint fingerprints.

II. Therapeutic Methods

[Liver and Kidney Deficiency]

Therapeutic method: Replenish kidney and tonify liver, strengthen bones and invigorate brain.

Prescription: Baihui (DU20), Sishencong (EX-HN1), Xuanzhong (GB39), Taixi (KI3), Ganshu (BL18), Shenshu (BL23), Zhishi (BL52), Mingmen (DU4).

Mechanism of prescription: The head is the confluent place of all Yangs and the brain is the marrow sea. Use the acupoint Baihui to match with Sishencong to invigorate the brain and awaken consciousness. Kidney

余，髓之所养，而肾俞为强肾补髓之要穴，命门为生命之门户；志室在肾俞两旁，为肾气留住之处；太溪是肾之原穴，配悬钟以培补肾气，填精益髓充脑。肝藏血主筋，手得血能握，足得血能步，因此，配肝俞以补肝肾之阴。诸穴共用，具有补肾益肝、强骨健脑之功效。

配穴 立退行迟者，加阴陵泉、足三里、三阴交、照海；齿迟者，加涌泉、通里；头软者，加天柱。

方法 电热针治疗。

操作 选定穴位，皮肤常规消毒。电热针斜刺（向中）肝俞、肾俞、志室各0.7寸，直刺命门0.7寸，平刺百会、四神聪各0.6寸，直刺悬钟0.7寸，斜刺太溪0.6寸，直刺足三里、三阴交、阴陵泉各0.7寸。（注：涌泉快速针刺，不留针；上述穴位每3～4组穴给予电热针治疗，轮流应用。）

stores essence and governs marrow generation of bones. It is the base of growth, teeth are a part of bones and nourished by marrow, while Shenshu is an important acupoint in strengthening kidney and replenishing marrow, Mingmen is the door of life. Zhishi locate on both sides of Shenshu, are the places for kidney Qi retention. Taixi is a Yuan acupoint of Kidney, when being matched with Xuanzhong, it can replenish kidney Qi, fill essence and tonify marrow and replenish brain. Liver stores blood and governs tendons; hands can grip if get blood, feet can walk if get blood, therefore, match with Ganshu to replenish Yin of liver and kidney. The use of the combination of these acupoints can replenish the kidneys and tonify the liver, strengthen bones and invigorate brain.

Matching acupoints: For standing back and retardation in walking, add Yinlingquan, Zusanli, Sanyinjiao, Zhaohai; for retardation in tooth eruption add Yongquan, Tongli; for soft head add Tianzhu.

Method: Electrothermal acupuncture treatment.

Operations: Selecting the relevant acupoints, perform routine skin disinfection. Using electrothermal acupuncture needles, obliquely puncture (with the needle tip towards spine) into Ganshu, Shenshu, Zhishi for 0.7" respectively, vertically puncture into Mingmen for 0.7", horizontally puncture into Baihui, Sishencong for 0.6" respectively, vertically puncture into Xuanzhong for 0.7", obliquely puncture into Taixi for 0.6", vertically puncture into Zusanli, Sanyinjiao, Yinlingquan for 0.7" respectively. (Note: rapidly puncture into the Yongquan, do not leave the needle in ; for the above acupoints, choose

Part II: Clinical Treatment

3-4 pairs of acupoints to apply acupuncture treatment each time, use alternatively.)

Therapeutic course: Once a day, leave the needles in for 40 minutes, 90 times for a course. Start the treatment for the second course after a break of 10-15 days. Determine the length of treatment course depending on the condition, and generally 2-6 courses are needed.

[Syndrome of Heart Blood Deficiency]

Therapeutic method: Replenish heart, nourish the blood, awaken consciousness, and induce resuscitation.

Prescription: Xinshu (BL15), Jueyinshu (BL14), Zusanli (ST36), Sanyinjiao (SP6).

Mechanism of prescription: The heart governs mind and consciousness. Therefore, use the Back-Shu acupoint Xinshu of Heart, Back-Shu acupoint Jueyinshu of Pericardium to nourish Yin and induce resuscitation. The four acupoints together can replenish heart and nourish blood, awaken consciousness and induce resuscitation.

Matching acupoints: For retardation in speech add Yamen, Lianquan, Dicang; for retardation in hair-growing add Pishu, Weishu, Ganshu.

Method: Electrothermal acupuncture treatment.

Operations: Selecting the relevant acupoints, perform routine skin disinfection. Using electrothermal acupuncture needles, obliquely puncture (with the needle tip towards spine) into the Xinshu, Jueyinshu, Ganshu, Pishu, Weishu for 0.7" respectively. Vertically puncture into the Zusanli, Sanyinjiao for 0.7" respectively. Turn

313

电流量 30～50mA，以患者感到舒适为度，留针 40 分钟。另配以毫针速刺哑门、廉泉、地仓，不留针。

疗程 每日 1 次，留针 40 分钟，90 次为 1 个疗程。疗程间可休息 7～15 天。如果需要可再进行第 2 个疗程的治疗。

【脾气亏损证】

治法 健脾益胃，补气养血。

处方 脾俞（BL20）、胃俞（BL21）、身柱（DU12）、合谷（LI4）、足三里（ST36）、三阴交（SP6）。

方义 脾为后天之本，气血生化之源，滋养肌肉、四肢、口唇，故取脾俞、胃俞，以培补后天，配足三里、三阴交以健脾益胃，补气养血，取身柱以强健筋骨，配合谷以治口面之疾及上臂之痿软。诸穴共用，有补后天、益气养血的作用。

配穴 咀嚼无力者加颊车、地仓、下关；手软下垂、

on the electrothermal acupuncture equipment, apply a current of 30-50mA to each acupoint. The limit is that the patient feels comfortable. Leave the needles in for 40 minutes. Additionally, using filiform needles, rapidly puncture into Yamen, Lianquan, Dicang, do not leave the needles in.

Therapeutic course: Once a day, leave the needles in for 40 minutes, 90 times for a course. Start the treatment for the second course after a break of 7-15 days. If necessary, start the treatment for the second course.

[Syndrome of Spleen Qi Depletion]

Therapeutic method: Invigorate spleen and tonify stomach, invigorate and nourish blood.

Prescription: Pishu(BL20), Weishu(BL21), Shenzhu (DU12), Hegu (LI4), Zusanli (ST36), Sanyinjiao (SP6).

Mechanism of prescription: The spleen is the foundation of acquired constitution, and the source of generation and transformation of Qi-blood. It nourishes muscles, limbs, the mouth and lips. Therefore, use Pishu, Weishu to replenish the acquired constitution, and match with Zusanli, Sanyinjiao to invigorate spleen and tonify the stomach, replenish Qi and nourish blood, while use Shenzhu to strengthen tendons and bones, match with Hegu to treat diseases of mouth and face as well as flaccidity of upper arms. The use of combination of these acupoints can replenish acquired constitution, tonify Qi and nourish blood.

Matching acupoints: For weakness in chewing add Jiache, Dicang, Xiaguan. For soft and drooping hands which unable to grip and lift up add Jianyu, Shousanli, Waiguan. For flaccidity of limb joints add Quchi, Yanglingquan, Xuanzhong. For mental retardation add Baihui, Sishencong, Xinshu, Shenmen and Huatuo Jiaji acupoints.

Method: Electrothermal acupuncture treatment.

Operations: Selecting the relevant acupoints, perform routine skin disinfection. Using electrothermal acupuncture needles, obliquely puncture (with the needle tip towards spine) into Pishu, Weishu for 0.7" respectively, vertically puncture into Shousanli, Waiguan, Quchi, Yanglingquan, Xuanzhong for 0.6" respectively. Turn on the electrothermal acupuncture equipment, apply a current of 30-40mA to each acupoint. The limit is that the patient feels comfortable and swollen. Leave the needles in for 40 minutes.

Therapeutic course: Once a day, leave the needles in for 40 minutes, 90 times for a course. Start the treatment for the second course after a break of 7-15 days. Generally 3-5 courses are needed.

III. Precautions

1. Do ideological work on child patients and get their cooperation, and during the needle retention after puncture, the patient must not move freely, otherwise needles cannot be left in.

2. When selecting acupoints with needle tip punctured into head, back and chest, remember that the direction and depth of needling must be appropriate to avoid injuries of large vessels, organs and brain tissues.

3. The acupoint selection must be exact, Ashi acu-

随意取阿是穴，操作要规范，一定要严格执行，避免事故。

4. 在治疗过程中，要注意肢体的功能训练，以及智力的培训和教导。如说话、走路等都要定时、有计划地教授。

5. 根据病情，必要时也应配合中、西药物治疗。

多发性神经炎

多发性神经炎又称为周围性神经炎，指运动神经与自主神经功能障碍，在四肢末端有对称性的感觉异常，在中医学的"痿证""痹证"中可以找到类似的描述。

一、诊断及辨证要点

1. 病程：急性或亚急性进行，可以在几周内到几个月内发展。

2. 感觉：初起患者肢体呈对称性感觉过敏或感觉异常，随后会出现感觉减退甚至消失。典型患者可呈手套样或袜样感觉缺失，感觉障碍可从手足末端向上伸展。

3. 运动：手足无力，进而

points mustn't be chosen freely, and the operations must comply with standards. These must be implemented strictly to avoid incidents.

4. During treatment, pay attention to limb functional exercises, as well as intelligence training and instructions. For example, regular and scheduled teaching of speaking and walking.

5. Depending on the conditions, treat in conjunction with Chinese Herb Medicine and Western Medicine therapies if necessary.

Multiple Neuritis

Multiple neuritis is also called peripheral neuritis, refers to the dysfunctions of motor nerves and automatic nerves, with symmetrical paresthesia at limb ends, and similar descriptions can be found in the "flaccidity syndrome", "arthralgia syndrome" of Traditional Chinese Medicine.

I. Key Points for Diagnosis and Syndrome Differentiation

1. Disease course: Acute or subacute, can develop in several weeks to several months.

2. Sensation: At first patients have symmetrical algesia or paresthesia, then hypoesthesia or even disappearance. Typical patients may have glove-like or sock-like anesthesia, and the sensory disturbance can radiate from limb ends upwards.

3. Movement: Weak hands and feet, subsequently

出现肌萎缩，严重时运动和感觉症状可消失。

4. 营养障碍：病变皮肤变薄，发冷，指甲变脆，出汗减少。

5. 反射：踝、膝反射及肱二头肌反射均可出现减退或消失。

6. 肺胃津伤者，病变皮肤变薄，发冷，咳嗽，发热，泄泻，口渴，小便赤，舌红苔黄，脉细数或滑数。

7. 湿热浸淫者，四肢红肿，重浊无力，或小便缺少，大便溏，舌质红，苔黄腻，脉濡数或滑数。

8. 肝肾亏虚者，四肢麻木无力，甚至瘫痪，肢冷，皮肤粗糙有裂纹，指甲干脆，头目眩晕，严重者吞咽发呛，呼吸气微，舌萎少苔，脉沉细无力。

9. 气血瘀阻者，四肢痿软无力，疼痛剧烈，发冷，皮肤有瘀斑，指甲紫暗，舌质晦黯或有瘀斑，脉细涩或沉细。

amyotrophia occurs, and in severe cases moving and sensory symptoms may disappear.

4. Dystrophia: Pathological changed skin thins, chilling, nails become brittle, sweating reduces.

5. Reflex: Reflex of ankles, knees and biceps all can degenerate or disappear.

6. For patients with lung and stomach fluid consumption, symptoms include pathological changed skin thinning, chilling, pyrexia, diarrhea, thirst, dark urine, red tongue with yellowish fur, thin and rapid or slippery and rapid pulse.

7. For patients with excessive Damp-Heat, symptoms include limb redness, heavy and turbid weakness, or lack of urine, sloppy stool, red tongue with yellow and greasy fur, soft and rapid or slippery and rapid pulse.

8. For patients with depletion and deficiency of liver and kidney, symptoms include limb numbness and weakness or even paralysis, cold limbs, rough skins with cracks, dry and brittle nails, dizziness and vertigo, in severe cases with choking when swallowing, feeble breathing, flaccid tongue with less fur, deep and thin and weak pulse.

9. For patients with stagnation of Qi-blood, symptoms include limb flaccidity, intensive pains, chilling, ecchymosis on the skin, dark purple nails, dark tongue or with ecchymosis, thin and uneven or deep and thin pulse.

二、治疗方法

【肺胃津伤证】

治法 养肺，益胃，生津。

处方 气海（RN6）、曲池（LI11）、足三里（ST36）、风府（DU16）、风池（GB20）、廉泉（RN23）、内关（PC6）。

方义 气海是强壮穴，重灸以回阳救逆，补益元气；曲池、足三里为阳明经之强壮穴，可以疏通阳明经脉，回阳救逆；风池、风府是作为治疗肺气将绝阶段之主穴，可疏通气血，以利机关，共奏益气回阳救逆之效。

配穴 痰多加丰隆、阳陵泉；多汗加复溜、阴郄。

方法 电热针治疗。

操作 选定穴位，皮肤常规消毒。电热针直刺气海0.8寸，直刺曲池0.7寸，直刺足三里0.8寸，直刺丰隆0.7寸，接通电热针仪，每个穴位分别给予电流量50～60mA，以患者感觉舒适微胀为度，留针40分钟。另配以毫针直刺廉泉0.5

II. Therapeutic Methods

[Syndrome of Lung-Stomach Fluid Consumption]

Therapeutic method: Nourishes lungs, tonifies stomach, generates fluid.

Prescription: Qihai (RN6), Quchi (LI11), Zusanli (ST36), Fengfu (DU16), Fengchi (GB20), Lianquan (RN23), Neiguan (PC6).

Mechanism of prescription: Qihai is an important tonifying acupoint, it can restore Yang and rescue collapse as well as replenish vital Qi with heavy moxibustion. Quchi and Zusanli are important tonifying acupoints of Yang-Ming Meridian, they can soothe Yang-Ming meridians and channels, restore Yang and rescue collapse. Fengchi and Fengfu are main acupoints used for treatment in the phase that lung Qi is about to run out, it can soothe Qi-blood to promote organs, and the combination of these acupoints can tonify Qi, restore Yang and rescue collapse.

Matching acupoints: For excessive phlegm add Fenglong, Yanglingquan; for hydrosis add Fuliu, Yinxi.

Method: Electrothermal acupuncture treatment.

Operations: Selecting the relevant acupoints, perform routine skin disinfection. Using electrothermal acupuncture needles, vertically puncture into Qihai for 0.8", Quchi for 0.7", Zusanli for 0.8", Fenglong for 0.7". Turn on the electrothermal acupuncture equipment, apply a current of 50-60mA to each acupoint is that the patient feels comfortable or there is slight swelling. Leave the needles in for 40 minutes. Additionally, using filiform

寸，直刺内关 0.5 寸，向下斜刺风府 0.5 寸，斜刺风池 0.5 寸，平补平泻，留针 30 分钟。

疗程 每日 1 次，90 次为 1 个疗程。疗程间可休息 7～10 天。一般治疗 1～2 个疗程即可，亦有需要治疗 3 个疗程者。

三、注意事项

1. 晚期四肢末端会出现感觉迟钝或消失。因此，必须注意保护和保温。

2. 患肢无力，或肌肉萎缩，治疗中要配合按摩，改善血液循环，减少肌萎缩。

3. 注意患肢的功能训练，保持肢体功能健全。

四、典型病例

李某，女，42 岁，职员，北京人。

主诉：四肢无力，下肢瘫痪 2 年半，加重 3 个月。病史：患者在两年半前，不明原因的四肢酸软乏力，尤其登梯走路费力，抬腿迈步困难，手提重物不能。经各医院检查始终未能明确诊断，只能对症治

needles, vertically puncture into Lianquan for 0.5", vertically puncture into Neiguan for 0.5", obliquely puncture downward into Fengfu for 0.5", obliquely puncture into Fengchi for 0.5", use the method of mild reinforcing and attenuating. Leave the needles in for 30 minutes.

Therapeutic course: Once a day, 90 times for a course. Start the treatment for the second course after a break of 7-10 days. Generally 1-2 treatment courses are needed, there are also patients that need 3 courses.

III. Precautions

1. In the late phase, dysesthesia or even sensation disappearance may occur at limb ends. Therefore must pay attention to protection and warm keeping.

2. Weakness or amyotrophia of affected limbs, the treatment should be in conjunction with massage so as to improve blood circulation and reduce amyotrophia.

3. Pay attention to functional exercises of affected limbs, keep intact limb functions.

IV. Typical Case

Li, female, 42 years old, employee, residence: Beijing.

Self-reported symptoms: Limb weakness, paralysis of lower limbs for 2 and half years, which aggravated in the recent 3 months. Medical history: 2 and a half years ago, the patient suffered from soreness and weakness of limbs due to unknown causes, in particular it was hard to climb stairs and walk, hard to lift leg and step forward, unable to hold heavy loads with hands. No clear diagno-

疗。近3个月床上翻身较困难，需要有人帮助。

刻下症：全身无力，翻身、起坐均需有人搀扶，下肢伸屈无力，全身各部尤其四肢，有不定时的蚁行感或紧绷感，或绳带捆感，有时还会出现肌肉跳动，能自然消失，倦怠乏力，饮食、睡眠时好时坏，舌质淡，有齿痕，脉细弱。

查体：二尖瓣区及主动脉瓣第二听诊区可闻及二级收缩期杂音。四肢活动不能，病理反射未引出，生理反射消失。

辅助检查：肌电图示"神经元性损害"。

【诊断依据】

1. 病变部位皮肤光滑、变薄，典型感觉减退或消失。

2. 对称性感觉障碍，弛缓性瘫痪。

3. 早期指趾麻木、刺痛，后期四肢运动无力，肌肉萎缩，出现垂腕或下垂足。

4. 腱反射消失。

【证治分析】

病因　肝肾亏虚，肺胃亏虚。

sis was obtained after examinations by several hospitals, and only symptomatic treatments could be done. In the recent 3 months, the patient was hard to turn over on the bed, which needed help from others.

Current symptoms: General weakness, turnover and sit-up both need help from others, flexion and extension weakness of lower limbs, the whole body especially limbs had formication, tension sense or sense of being bound by ropes from time to time, or in some cases even muscle jumping which disappeared naturally could occur, fatigue and asthenia, diet and sleep were sometimes good and sometimes bad, light tongue with teeth prints, thin and weak pulse.

Physical examination: Grade 2 systolic noise at mitral valve area and second aortic valve area. Inability of limb movements, failure in induction of pathological reflex, disappearance of physiological reflex.

Auxiliary examination: EMG indicated "neuronal damage".

[Diagnostic Basis]

1. Smooth and thinned skin at lesion sties, typical hypoesthesia or disappearance.

2. Symmetrical sensory disturbance, flaccid paralysis.

3. Numbness and prickling of fingers and toes in the early phase, then limb weakness in movements and amyotrophia in the late phase, with wrist drop or drop foot.

4. Disappearance of tendon reflex.

[Syndrome-treatment Analysis]

Etiology: Depletion and deficiency of liver and kidney as well as of lung and stomach.

病机 多因风寒湿外袭，淫于筋脉，经络受阻，四肢麻木、刺痛，恶寒肢凉，得温则缓，后期因足阳明络损，肢体麻木不仁，痿软无力，肌肉瘦削，瘫痪不起。

证候分析 早期因风寒阻络，出现四肢麻木，恶寒肢冷，遇温则缓，活动时加重，肤色苍白，后期阳明络损，肢体麻木不仁，痿软无力，肌肉瘦削，瘫痪不起，伴有腹胀纳呆，周身乏力，自汗，面色无华，舌淡伴有齿痕，苔薄白，脉细弱，是日久不愈之象。

病位 肝、肾、脾。

病性 虚性。

西医诊断 多发性神经炎。

中医诊断 痿证（肝肾阴虚型、脾气虚弱型）。

治法 补肝益肾，健脾益气，滋阴清热。

方法 电热针治疗、艾灸治疗。

Pathogenesis: Most are caused by external invasion of Wind, Cold and Damp, which overflood into tendons and channels, causing obstruction of meridians and collaterals, limb numbness, prickling, aversion to cold and cold limbs which relieves with warm, and in the late phase, Yang-Ming collaterals of Foot injuries, numbness of limbs and body, flaccidity, thin muscles, paralysis.

Syndrome analysis: In the early stage, due to collateral obstruction by Wind-Cold, there occur numbness of limbs, aversion to cold and cold limbs which relieves with warm and aggravates with movements, pale skins, and in the late phase, Yang-Ming collaterals injuries, numbness of limbs and body, flaccidity, thin muscles, paralysis, accompanying abdominal distension and poor appetite, general asthenia, spontaneous sweating, gloomy complexion, light tongue with tooth prints, thin and white fur, thin and weak pulse, which are signs of long-standing maladies.

Lesion location: Liver, kidney, spleen.

Disease nature: Deficiency.

The result of diagnosis of Western Medicine: Multiple neuritis.

The diagnosis of Traditional Chinese Medicine: Flaccidity syndrome (liver and kidney Yin deficiency type, spleen Qi deficiency and weakness type).

Therapeutic method: Replenish liver and tonify kidney, invigorate spleen and tonify Qi, nourish Yin and clear Heat.

Method: Electrothermal acupuncture treatment, moxa-moxibustion treatment.

（1）电热针治疗

处方 肩髃（LI15）、曲池（LI11）、合谷（LI4）、环跳（GB30）、阳陵泉（GB34）、足三里（ST36）、悬钟（GB39）、三阴交（SP6）、手三里（LI10）。

方义 依据《素问·痿论》"治痿独取阳明"之说，以取手足阳明经穴及邻近穴为主，取肩髃、曲池、手三里、足三里，以调和气血，润养经脉，配外关、环跳、阳陵泉、悬钟、三阴交等穴。其中，环跳可利枢机，疏调下肢气血；阳陵泉为筋之会，取之以调整筋脉功能；悬钟为髓会，与阳陵泉相配，用温补法能充髓壮筋骨；配三阴交以健脾化湿。诸穴共用，可奏健运脾胃，通调经络，运行气血，营养四末，濡润宗筋之功。

配穴 纳呆脘痞、便溏者，加中脘、天枢；肝肾亏损者，加肝俞、肾俞；根据病情侧重，可选用上肢的阳池、少海，

(1) Electrothermal acupuncture treatment

Prescription: Jianyu (LI15), Quchi (LI11), Hegu (LI4), Huantiao (GB30), Yanglingquan (GB34), Zusanli (ST36), Xuanzhong (GB39), Sanyinjiao (SP6), Shousanli (LI10).

Mechanism of prescription: According to the description of "use Yang-Ming alone for treatment of flaccidity" in the *Plain Questions Theory of Flaccidity*(《素问·痿论》), mainly use acupoints of Yang-Ming meridians of hand and foot as well as nearby acupoints, and choose Jianyu, Quchi, Shousanli, Zusanli to regulate Qi-blood and nourish meridians and channels, and match with acupoints like Waiguan, Huantiao, Yanglingquan, Xuanzhong and Sanyinjiao, among which Sanyinjiao can promote body essence, soothe and regulate the Qi-blood of lower limbs. Yanglingquan is a confluent acupoint of tendons, it can regulate functions of tendons and channels. Xuanzhong is a confluent acupoint of marrow, when being matched with Yanglingquan it can replenish marrow and strengthen tendons and bones with the method of warm tonifying, and when being matched with Sanyinjiao it can invigorate spleen and disperse Damp. The use of combination of these acupoints can promote transportation of spleen and stomach, soothe and regulate meridians and collaterals, activate Qi-blood circulation, nourish limb ends, and moisten convergent tendons.

Matching acupoints: For poor appetite and epigastric fullness, sloppy stool, add Zhongwan, Tianshu. For depletion and deficiency of liver and kidney add Ganshu, Shenshu. Choose acupoints of upper limbs like Yangchi,

Shaohai, of lower limbs like Fengshi, Qiuxu, as well as Bafeng, Baxie depending on the focus of disease conditions. For paralysis add Mingmen, Yaoyangguan acupoints of both sides of Bladder Meridian or Huatuo Jiaji acupoints.

Operations: Selecting the relevant acupoints, perform routine skin disinfection. Using electrothermal acupuncture needles, vertically puncture into Shousanli, Quchi, Zusanli for 0.8" respectively. Turn on the electrothermal acupuncture equipment, apply a current of 60mA to each acupoint. The limit is that the patient feels warm or swelling and comfortable. Leave the needles in for 40 minutes. Using filiform needles, vertically puncture into Jianyu, Yanglingquan, Xuanzhong for 0.7" respectively, leave the needles in for 40 minutes. (Note: Use the first acupoint group "Shousanli, Quchi, Zusanli" and the second acupoint group "Quchi, Zusanli, Sanyinjiao" alternatively.)

Therapeutic course: Once a day, 90 times for a course.

(2) Moxa-moxibustion treatment

Prescription: Quchi (LI11), Hegu (LI4), Yanglingquan (GB34), Kunlun (BL60).

Matching acupoints: For heavy upper limbs add Neiguan, Houxi; for heavy lower limbs add Sanyinjiao, Xingjian.

Operations: Perform moxibustion treatment twice a day, 15 minutes for each acupoint, use moxa-stick moxibustion, choose 2 acupoints each of upper and lower limbs and let patients perform moxibustion by themselves.

疗程 每日 1 次，90 次为 1 个疗程。疗程间可休息 7～10 天。一般治疗 1～2 个疗程即可，亦有需要治疗 3 个疗程者。

【生活调摄】

1. 本病针灸治疗有效，但疗程较长，应鼓励患者树立信心，坚持治疗。

2. 对较重患者，在治疗过程中针对病情，注意配合按摩、理疗、药物、功能训练之综合疗法。

坐骨神经痛

本病是由坐骨神经自身或其临近软组织病变所引起，属于中医"痹证"的范畴。

一、诊断及辨证要点

1. 沿坐骨神经分布区的放射性痛。神经根病变时，咳嗽、喷嚏等动作多使疼痛加重，卧床时为了减轻疼痛，膝部常有微屈。

2. 沿坐骨神经分布区有压痛点，如腰点、髂点、臀点、腘点、腓点、踝点等。

Therapeutic course: Once a day, 90 times for a course. Start the treatment for the second course after a break of 7-10 days. Generally 1-2 treatment courses are needed, there are also patients that need 3 courses.

[Lifestyle Change and Health Maintenance]

1. Acupuncture therapy is effective with this disease, but the treatment course is long. Therefore it is necessary to encourage patients to establish confidence and adhere to the treatment.

2. For patients of severe conditions, use a comprehensive therapy of massage, physical therapy, medicine, functional exercises depending on the conditions.

Sciatica

This disease is caused by pathological changes of sciatic nerves or the adjacent soft tissues, it belongs to the range of "arthralgia syndrome" in Traditional Chinese Medicine.

I. Key Points for Diagnosis and Syndrome Differentiation

1. Radiative pains along the distribution areas of sciatic nerves. For lesions of nerve roots, activities like coughing and sneezing will aggravate the pain, and when lying in the bed, knees are often slightly bended so as to relieve pains.

2. There are tenderness points along the distribution areas of sciatic nerves, such as waist point, iliac point, hip point, popliteal point, peroneal point and ankle point.

3. 坐骨神经牵拉征阳性，如 Kerning 征、Lasegue 征。

4. 坐骨神经所支配的范围内，有不同程度的运动、感觉、反射和自主神经功能障碍。常见的有患肢踇趾背屈力减弱，小腿外侧感觉迟钝，跟腱反射消失，臂部肌力降低等体征。

5. 由于发生的病因不同，尚可有其他相应的病史、体征及实验室检查所见。

6. 根据临床表现及病理特点，可进一步分为真性和假性坐骨神经痛。

（1）真性坐骨神经痛（因神经根受压所致）：①90%以上为腰椎间盘突出所致，多有因过度负重及腰部外伤病史，偶见于腰椎结核、马尾肿瘤。②起病较急，先有腰部疼痛，而后疼痛迅速沿一侧及大腿后面、小腿后外侧向下放射，直至足背外缘。咳嗽、喷嚏、行走及翻身时疼痛均加重。③站立时腰弯向患侧，患肢稍屈；第4～5腰椎、第1骶椎旁2cm处有压痛点，并且向下放射。X线诊查常可见相应椎间隙变窄或其他病变。

（2）假性坐骨神经痛（因

3. Positive in sciatic nerve stretch syndromes, such as Kerning syndrome, Lasegue syndrome.

4. Varying degrees of dysfunctions of motor, sensory, reflex and autonomic nerves in the areas governed by sciatic nerves. Most common signs include decreased dorsiflexion strength of the great toe of the affected limb, dysesthesia of the lateral lower leg, disappearance of Achilles tendon reflex, reduced muscle strength of arms.

5. Due to different disease causes, there are also other relative medical histories, physical signs, and lab findings.

6. According to clinical manifestations and pathological characteristics, it can be further divided into true sciatica and false sciatica.

(1) True sciatica (caused by injury of nerve root): ① 90% are caused by protrusion of lumbar intervertebral disc, often with a history of excessive load bearing or waist trauma, occasionally seen in lumbar tuberculosis and tumor of cauda equina. ② Acute development, at first waist pain occurs, and it radiates downwards along one side and the posterior thigh, the posterior-lateral lower leg until the outer edge of acrotarsium. Pain can aggravate when coughing, sneezing, walking and turning over the body. ③ When standing, the waist bends towards the affected side, the affected limb is bended slightly; there are tenderness points at the L 4-5 and 2cm beside the Sacral Vertebra 1, and pains radiate downwards. In the X-ray examination, relative narrowing of intervertebral space or other lesions often can be seen.

(2) False sciatica (caused by that lesions of adjacent

神经干受邻近组织病变影响所致)：①常有腰或臀部肌纤维炎、骶髂关节炎、髂关节炎、盆腔炎、梨状肌纤维炎或因臀部注射选择部位不当等病史。②一侧肢体放射性疼痛，伴有腰或臀部疼痛。③腰椎曲度正常，椎旁无压痛，直腿抬高试验阴性，肌力、跟腱反射及皮肤感觉均正常。

7. 痛痹，由寒邪偏胜所致。疼痛较剧，痛处不移，得热则痛减，遇寒则痛甚，舌质淡苔白，脉沉紧。

8. 行痹，由风邪偏胜所致。疼痛游走不定，伴有其他 2 个或更多关节游走性疼痛。屈伸不利，或见恶风、发热等症，舌苔薄白，脉浮或弦。

9. 着痹，由湿邪偏胜所致。患肢疼痛，肌肤麻木不仁，活动不便，舌苔白腻，脉濡滑。

二、治疗方法

【太阳腰腿痛（痛痹、行痹）】

治法　宣痹通络，佐以疏风。

tissues affect the nerve trunk): ① often with medical histories like myofibrositis at the waist or buttocks, sacroiliac arthritis, iliac arthritis, pelvic diseases, piriformis fibrosis or diseases caused by improper selection of injection site at buttocks. ② Radiative pains of one side limbs and body, accompanied with pains at the waist or buttocks. ③ Normal lumbar curvature, no tenderness beside lumbar vertebra, negative in the straight-leg raising test, muscle strength, Achilles tendon reflex and skin sensation are all normal.

7. Arthritis, caused by that Cold-evil toxins becoming dominant. Relatively intensive pain, the pain site does not shift, the pain is relieved with warm and aggravated with cold, light tongue with white fur, deep and tense pulse.

8. Migratory arthralgia, caused by the Wind-evil toxins becoming dominant. The pain site wanders around, accompanied with other 2 or more sites of wandering arthralgia. Inhibited bending and stretching, or symptoms like aversion to wind, pyrexia, thin and white tongue fur, floating or taut pulse.

9. Fixed arthralgia, caused by that Damp-evil toxins become dominant. Pain of affected limbs, skin numbness, difficulties in movement, white and greasy tongue fur, soft and slippery pulse.

II. Therapeutic Methods

[Tai-Yang Pain in Waist and Lower Extremities (Arthritis, Migratory Arthralgia)]

Therapeutic method: Remove stagnation and soothe collaterals, supplemented by Wind soothing.

Prescription: Shenshu (BL23), Dachangshu (BL25), Weizhong (BL40), Zhibian (BL54), Chengshan (BL57), Kunlun (BL60).

Mechanism of prescription: For pain in waist and lower extremities, respectively choose meridian acupoints of this meridian to soothe meridians and channels, activate blood and disperse stagnation, remove Wind and alleviate pains.

Matching acupoints: For waist pain and limb softness, add Fuliu, Taixi. For intensive pain and aversion to cold add Qihai, Sanyinjiao; for those caused by trauma add Xuehai, Geshu; for amyotrophia add Pishu, Zusanli.

Method: Electrothermal acupuncture treatment.

Operations: Selecting the relevant acupoints, perform routine skin disinfection. Using electrothermal acupuncture needles, vertically puncture into Shenshu for 0.6-0.8", Dachangshu for 0.6-0.8", Zhibian for 0.7-0.8". Turn on the electrothermal acupuncture equipment, apply a current of 50-80mA to each acupoint. Additionally, using filiform needles, vertically puncture into Weizhong for 0.5-0.7", Chengshan for 0.5-0.7", Kunlun for 0.4-0.5", leaving the needles in for 40 minutes.

Therapeutic course: Treat once a day, 10 times for a course, and start the treatment for the second course after a break of 3-5 days.

[Shao-Yang Pain in Waist and Lower Extremities (Arthritis, Migratory Arthralgia)]

Therapeutic method: Expel wind and disperse

处方 环跳（GB30）、风市（GB31）、阳陵泉（GB34）、悬钟（GB39）、丘墟（GB40）。

方义 选取本经经穴，可祛风散寒，活血通络。

配穴 肌肉萎缩者加足三里、丰隆；腰痛腿软者加委中、委阳；痛剧者加三阴交、太溪。

方法 电热针治疗。

操作 选定穴位，皮肤常规消毒。电热针直刺环跳0.7～0.8寸，直刺风市0.6～0.8寸，直刺阳陵泉0.6～0.7寸。然后接通电热针仪，每个穴位分别给予电流量60～80mA，以患者感到温热或胀的舒适感觉为度，留针40分钟。

疗程 每日1次，10次为1个疗程，疗程间休息3～5天，再进行第2个疗程的治疗。

【阳明腰痛】

治法 活血止痛，祛湿通络。

处方 髀关（ST31）、伏兔（ST32）、足三里（ST36）、解溪（ST41）。

方义 取本经经穴，可疏通经脉，软坚散结，活血止

cold, activate blood and soothe collaterals.

Prescription: Huantiao (GB30), Fengshi (GB31), Yanglingquan (GB34), Xuanzhong (GB39), Qiuxu (GB40).

Mechanism of prescription: Choose meridian acupoints of this meridian to expel Wind and disperse Cold, activate blood and soothe collaterals.

Matching acupoints: For amyotrophia add Zusanli, Fenglong; for waist pain and limb softness add Weizhong, Weiyang; for intensive pain add Sanyinjiao, Taixi.

Method: Electrothermal acupuncture treatment.

Operations: Selecting the relevant acupoints, perform routine skin disinfection. Using electrothermal acupuncture needles, vertically puncture into Huantiao for 0.7-0.8", Fengshi for 0.6-0.8", Yanglingquan for 0.6-0.7". Turn on the electrothermal acupuncture equipment, apply a current of 60-80mA to each acupoint. The limit is that the patient feels warmly swell and comfortable. Leave the needles in for 40 minutes.

Therapeutic course: Treat once a day, 10 times for a course, and start the treatment for the second course after a break of 3-5 days.

[Yang-Ming Waist Pain]

Therapeutic method: Activate blood and alleviate pain, expel Damp and soothe collaterals.

Prescription: Biguan (ST31), Futu (ST32), Zusanli (ST36), Jiexi (ST41).

Mechanism of prescription: Choose the meridian acupoints of this meridian to soothe meridians and chan-

痛，祛湿通络。

配穴 痛剧者加委中、委阳；外伤导致者加血海、膈俞。

方法 电热针治疗。

操作 选定穴位，皮肤常规消毒。电热针直刺髀关 0.6～0.8 寸，直刺伏兔 0.6～0.8 寸，直刺足三里 0.6～0.8 寸，接电热针仪，每个穴位给予电流量 60～80mA，以患者有舒适温热或胀感为度，留针 40 分钟。

疗程 每日 1 次，10 次为 1 个疗程，疗程间休息 3～5 天，再进行第 2 个疗程的治疗。

三、注意事项

1. 坐骨神经痛急性期，需卧床休息 1～2 周，注意腿部的保暖。

2. 积极查找病因，如为腰椎间盘突出者，可配合推拿复位（但急性期不能施术）；如为椎管肿瘤、骨结核、糖尿病等引起者，应选择治本为主，治疗坐骨神经痛为辅。

3. 针刺治疗时注意体位的安排，使患者在治疗时感到舒适，不能选勉强体位，造成患

nels, soften hardness and expel stagnation, activate blood and alleviate pain, expel Damp and soothe collaterals.

Matching acupoints: For intensive pain add Weizhong, Weiyang; for those caused by trauma add Xuehai, Geshu.

Method: Electrothermal acupuncture treatment.

Operations: Selecting the relevant acupoints, perform routine skin disinfection. Using electrothermal acupuncture needles, vertically puncture into Biguan for 0.6-0.8", Futu for 0.6-0.8", Zusanli for 0.6-0.8". Turn on the electrothermal acupuncture equipment, apply a current of 60-80mA to each acupoint, and the limit is that the patient feels warm or swelling and comfortable. Leave the needles in for 40 minutes.

Therapeutic course: Treat once a day, 10 times for a course, and start the treatment for the second course after a break of 3-5 days.

III. Precautions

1. During the acute phase of sciatica, patients should rest in bed for 1-2 weeks, pay attention to warm keeping of legs.

2. When finding the disease causes, for those caused by protrusion of lumbar intervertebral disc, treat in conjunction with massage reduction (do not perform during the acute phase). For those caused by intraspinal tumor, bone tuberculosis, diabetes, mainly focus on permanent cure, supplemented with treatment for sciatica.

3. For acupuncture treatment, pay attention to arrangement of body position to let the patient feel comfortable when receiving treatment, do not choose an

者治疗过程中的痛苦，避免过度强刺激。

4. 要针对不同病因之实情，给予合理的治疗。

臀上皮神经麻痹

臀上皮神经麻痹是外伤常见的伤筋病症，痛点多在髂后上棘的外上方，呈刺痛、酸痛或撕裂样疼痛，可向患侧下肢放射，但一般不过膝。

中医认为，本病多因局部气血运行失畅，使经络阻塞，气滞血瘀所致。

一、诊断及辨证要点

1. 检查除局部压痛外，常可触及大小不等、可移动的条索状结节，触压时患者疼痛难忍或酸胀麻木，波及下肢。

2. 体征、外观与骨科检查无异常。

3. 好发于青壮年，有时有外伤病史，多数无明显诱因。

4. 一般预后良好。

improper position which may cause pain of the patient during treatment, avoid excessive strong stimulation.

4. Perform reasonable treatment according to different diseases causes.

Superior Gluteal Cutaneous Nerve Paralysis

Superior gluteal cutaneous nerve paralysis is a tendon injury common in trauma, the pain points of which are generally located at the external superior of the posterior superior iliac spine, with prickling, aching or tearing-like pains, which can radiate downwards to the lower limb of the affected side, normally not beyond the knee.

Traditional Chinese Medicine believes that this disease is caused by inhibited local Qi-blood circulation leading to obstruction of meridians and collaterals, Qi stagnation and blood stasis.

I. Key Points for Diagnosis and Syndrome Differentiation

1. In the examination, in addition to tenderness, string-like rolling nodules with different sizes often can be touched, and the patient suffers from intolerable pain or sore and swollen as well as numb feelings when being pressed, which can involve lower limbs.

2. No abnormality found in physical sign, appearance and orthopedic examinations.

3. Most seen in young adults, sometimes patients have trauma histories. However, in most cases there are no obvious inducing causes.

4. Generally with good prognosis.

二、治疗方法

【气滞血瘀证】

治法 软坚散结，活血化瘀，消滞止痛。

处方 肾俞（BL23）、大肠俞（BL25）、委中（BL40）、阿是穴。

方义 肾俞、大肠俞、阿是穴疏通局部之经气，为局部取穴。委中特异性作用于腰背部，可加强局部活血行气之作用，属远道取穴。诸穴共用，共奏软坚散结、活血化瘀、消滞止痛之功。

方法 电热针治疗。

操作 选定穴位，皮肤常规消毒。电热针直刺肾俞 0.6～0.8 寸，直刺大肠俞 0.6～0.8 寸，直刺阿是穴 0.6～0.7 寸，接通电热针仪，每个穴位分别给予电流量 60～80mA，以患者感觉舒适为度，留针 40 分钟。另配以毫针直刺委中 0.5～0.6 寸，留针 40 分钟。

疗程 每天 1 次，10 天为 1 个疗程，疗程间可休息 7 天，

II. Therapeutic Methods

[Syndrome of Qi Stagnation and Blood Stasis]

Therapeutic method: Soften hardness and expel stagnation, activate blood circulation and remove stasis, remove stasis and alleviate pains.

Prescription: Shenshu(BL23), Dachangshu(BL25), Weizhong (BL40), Ashi acupoints.

Mechanism of prescription: Shenshu, Dachangshu, Ashi acupoints are used to soothe local meridian Qi, local acupoint selecting. Weizhong specifically effects on the waist and back area, it can strengthen the effects of local blood activation and Qi circulation, distant acupoint selecting. The use of combination of these acupoints can soften hardness and expel stagnation, activate blood circulation and remove stasis, remove stasis, and alleviate pains.

Method: Electrothermal acupuncture treatment.

Operations: Selecting the relevant acupoints, perform routine skin disinfection. Using electrothermal acupuncture needles, vertically puncture into Shenshu for 0.6-0.8", Dachangshu for 0.6-0.8", Ashi acupoints for 0.6-0.7". Turn on the electrothermal acupuncture equipment, apply a current of 60-80mA to each acupoint. The limit is that the patient feels comfortable. Leave the needles in for 40 minutes. Additionally, using filiform needles, vertically puncture into Weizhong for 0.5-0.6", leaving the needles in for 40 minutes.

Therapeutic course: Treat once a day, 10 days for a course, and start the treatment for the second course

再进行第 2 个疗程的治疗以巩固疗效。

三、注意事项

1. 急性期除治疗外，要卧床休息 2～3 周。注意局部保暖。

2. 针刺治疗中避免过度强刺激。

3. 治疗过程中，可配合活血化瘀止痛药物，以期早日恢复功能。

4. 亦可局部配合热疗。

脊髓炎

脊髓炎是脊髓灰质及白质同时受侵的非化脓性炎症，常急性起病，多数患者病因不明，部分患者可由病毒、细菌、霉菌、寄生虫等引起，亦可发生于某些发热出疹性疾病或免疫接种后。本病属于中医"痿痹""风痱"的范畴。

一、诊断及辨证要点

1. 本病好发于青壮年，起病前 1～2 周常有发烧、头痛、全身不适等上呼吸道感染症状，部分患者有肢痛、背痛、

after a break of 7 days to consolidate efficacies.

III. Precautions

1. During the acute phase, in addition to the treatment, it is necessary to rest in bed for 2-3 weeks. Pay attention to local warming.

2. Avoid excessive strong stimulation during the acupuncture treatment.

3. During treatment, drugs which can activate blood circulation and remove stasis as well as alleviate pains can be used to restore functions earlier.

4. Local thermal therapy can also be used.

Myelitis

Myelitis is a non-suppurative inflammation with simultaneous invasion into the grey matter and white matter of the spine cord, normally with acute development. For most patients the etiology remains unknown, while for some patients it can be caused by virus, bacteria, moulds, parasites, or it also may occur after certain rash and fever illness or after immunization. This disease is belongs to the ranges of "wilting and impediment", "hemiplegia" of Traditional Chinese Medicine.

I. Key Points for Diagnosis and Syndrome Differentiation

1. The disease is mostly seen in young adults, there are often symptoms of upper respiratory infections like fever, headache, systemic discomfort 1-2 weeks before onset, and some patients also have limb pain, back pain,

胸腹部束带感觉及腹泻。

2. 瘫痪症状多突然出现，数小时或 2～3 天达到高峰，但亦有缓慢进行者，数周始达高峰，症状看病变的程度和部位而异。

（1）运动障碍：病灶在颈段时产生四肢瘫痪，并可影响膈肌和肋间肌，造成呼吸肌瘫痪；病灶在胸段时则出现截瘫，病初呈迟缓性瘫痪，如无严重继发性感染及脊髓坏死，数周后可转为痉挛性瘫痪，并可出现霍纳综合征；病变位于腰骶部，下肢呈迟缓性瘫痪，可为完全性或不完全性，对称者多见。

（2）感觉障碍：感觉障碍从下向上发展，出现明显的感觉障碍平面。感觉障碍无整齐平面感者较为少见。

（3）括约肌功能障碍：脊髓休克期出现大小便潴留，继而出现失禁。

（4）自主神经功能障碍：病变水平以下常汗多或过少，瘫痪肢体水肿，皮肤苍白，干燥指（趾）甲脆弱易裂。

3. 血液：白细胞总数及多核细胞稍增加。

4. 脑脊液：蛋白或细胞数

tied-up feeling at the chest and abdomen and diarrhea.

2. The symptom of paralysis normally occurs suddenly, and reaches to a peak after several hours or 2-3 days, in some cases the progress is slow and the peak is reached after several weeks, and the symptoms vary depending on lesion degrees and lesion sites.

(1) Dyskinesia: Lesions at the neck area cause limb paralysis, and can affect diaphragm and intercostal muscles, leading to respiratory muscle paralysis. Lesions in the chest area can cause paraplegia, in the early phase it presents as flaccid paralysis, which transfers into spastic paralysis several weeks later, and Horner's syndrome may occur. Lesions at the lumbosacral portion can cause flaccid paralysis of lower limbs, complete or incomplete, most are symmetrical.

(2) Sensory disturbance: The sensory disturbance develops from bottom to top, obvious plane of sensory disturbance occurs. Patients of sensory disturbance without sensation of aligned plane are rare.

(3) Sphincter dysfunction: During the spinal cord shock period, retention of urine and stool occurs, and subsequently incontinence.

(4) Dysfunction of autonomic nerves: Normally with excessive or less sweating under the lesion level, swelling of paralytic limbs, pale skin, dry finger (toe) nails which are flimsy and easy to crack.

3. Blood: Slighted increase of total leucocytes and polykaryocytes.

4. Cerebrospinal fluid: Midly increase of or normal

轻度增高或正常，急性期有不同程度的脊髓水肿及肿胀，故可造成蛛网膜下腔一时性梗阻（要与急性感染性多发性神经炎和急性硬脊膜外脓肿鉴别）。

5. 辨证分型

（1）先驱期：外邪袭表，发热重，恶寒轻，鼻干，咳嗽，口渴，心烦，头痛，目痛，肢痛，腰酸，舌红，苔干或黄，脉浮数。

（2）瘫痪期：多为肝、肾、肺、胃受损，以补益肝肾或化瘀通督为主，临床常有如下表现：①肝肾阴亏：下肢渐渐痿软不用，腰背疼痛，肌肉麻木不仁，消瘦乏力，低热盗汗，头晕目眩，遗尿，舌红少苔，脉细数。②脾肾阴虚：腰部酸困，下肢麻木，肌肉紧胀或浮肿，行动不便，渐至瘫痪，皮肤不温，疲困倦怠，食少便溏，面色萎黄，遗尿，阳痿，舌红苔白，脉沉细。③瘀血阻滞：腰部肿胀，下肢麻木，强直或痿软无力，皮肤干燥，色紫而冷，口干目涩，食少腹胀，睡眠不宁，二便不利，舌质青紫，脉沉涩。④气血亏虚：四肢痿软不用，头目昏眩，自汗，神昏气缺，面色

protein or cell counts, during the acute period there are spinal cord edema and swelling of various degrees, therefore can cause temporary obstruction of subarachnoid space (it should be differentiated from acute inflammatory multiple neuritis and acute spinal epidural abscess).

5. Symptom differentiation and type classification

(1) Prodromal stage: Invasion of exogenous pathogenic factors to the surface, severe pyrexia and mild aversion to cold, dry noses, coughing, thirst, vexation, headache, eye pain, limb pain, waist soreness, red tongue with dry or yellow fur, floating and rapid pulse.

(2) Paralytic stage: Most are from damage of the kidneys, lungs, and stomach, focus on tonifying of liver and kidney or stasis removing or soothing Du Channel, clinical manifestations include: ① Yin depletion of liver and kidney: Gradually progressed flaccidity of lower limbs, waist and back pains, muscle numbness, emaciation and asthenia, low fever and sweating at night, dizziness and vertigo, enuresis, red tongue with less fur, thin and rapid pulse. ② Yin deficiency of spleen and kidney: Aching and tired waist, numbness of lower limbs, tension or swelling of muscles, inhibited movements which gradually develop into paralysis, cold skin, fatigue, less food intake and sloppy stool, sallow complexion, enuresis, asynodia, red tongue with white fur, deep and thin pulse. ③ Blood stasis: Swelling of waist, numbness of lower limbs, tetanus or flaccidity, dry skin, purple and cold, dry mouth and dry eyes, less food intake and abdominal distension, restless sleep, inhibited urination and defecation, cyanoze tongue, deep and uneven pulse. ④ Depletion and deficiency of Qi-blood: Limb flaccidity, dizziness

萎黄，舌质淡，苔白，脉细弱。

and vertigo, spontaneous sweating, mental fatigue and Qi lack, sallow complexion, light tongue with white fur, thin and weak pulse.

二、治疗方法

【瘫痪期】

治法 舒筋通络。

处方 百会（DU20）、内关（PC6）、曲池（LI11）、足三里（ST36）、三阴交（SP6）、太冲（LR3）、心俞（BL15）、肝俞（BL18）、肾俞（BL23）。

方义 百会为督脉腧穴，乃健脑开窍、平肝息风之要穴，内关系心包经之络穴，别走三焦经，为八脉交会阴维脉之会穴，有宁心安神之功效。曲池为手阳明经之合穴，足三里为足阳明经之合穴，阳明多为气血之腑，上下配合，可疏风清热，调和气血，强健脾胃。三阴交系肝经、脾经、肾经之交会穴，有补益脾胃，调理肝肾的作用。太冲乃肝经之原穴，可平肝通络；肝俞乃肝之背俞穴，有清肝明目之功；心俞为心之背俞穴，具有宁心安神之效；肾俞为肾之经气转输之处，可滋肾健脑，益脑明目。诸穴共用，有宁心开窍、养阴

II. Therapeutic Methods

[Paralytic stage]

Therapeutic method: Relax tendons and activate collaterals.

Prescription: Baihui (DU20), Neiguan (PC6), Quchi (LI11), Zusanli (ST36), Sanyinjiao (SP6), Taichong (LR3), Xinshu (BL15), Ganshu (BL18), Shenshu (BL23).

Mechanism of prescription: Baihui is an acupoint from Du Channel, is an important acupoint to invigorate brain and induce resuscitation, calm liver and stop Wind, Neiguan is a collateral acupoint from Pericardium Meridian and also belongs to Three-Jiao Meridian, it is one of the confluent acupoints of eight Channels, belonging to Yinwei Channel, which can soothe one's mood and calm the mind. Quchi is a He acupoint from Yang-Ming Meridian of Hand. Zusanli is a He acupoint from Yang-Ming Meridian of Foot, the most parts of Yang-Ming are the place for Qi and blood, the up and down match can disperse Wind and clear Heat, regulate Qi-blood, strengthen spleen and stomach. Sanyinjiao is the confluent acupoint of Liver Meridian, Spleen Meridian and Kidney Meridian, which can tonify spleen and stomach as well as regulate liver and kidney. Taichong is a Yuan acupoint of Liver Meridian, which can calm liver and soothe collaterals; Ganshu is a Back-shu acupoint of Liv-

通络之作用。

配穴 ①按脊髓损伤平面，颈段损伤针刺颈1～7椎；胸段损伤针刺胸1～10椎；腰骶段损伤针刺胸10～腰2椎；马尾段损伤针刺腰2～骶5椎。②按瘫痪肢体，上肢瘫痪加肩髃、曲池、外关、合谷；下肢瘫痪加环跳、八髎、承扶、委中、承山、昆仑、髀关、伏兔、风市、阴陵泉、足三里、阳陵泉、太冲、商丘、悬钟。③按中医分型，湿热重者加脾俞、阴陵泉；肝肾阴虚者加肝俞、肾俞、命门、志室、太冲、太溪；肺热重者加肺俞、大椎、尺泽。④按症状，排便障碍者加支沟、照海；排尿障碍者加肺俞、关元、三阴交、秩边、水道；兴奋易怒者加神门；痴呆者加四神聪、心俞、通里；失语者加哑门、廉泉；失明者加睛明；吞咽困难者加天突、合谷、颊车；瘫痪者加环跳、

er, which can clear liver and increase eyesight; Xinshu is a Back-shu acupoint of Heart, which can soothe one's mood and calm the mind; Shenshu is the transfer station for meridian Qi of kidney, which can nourish kidney and invigorate brain, tonify brain and increase eyesight. The combination use of these acupoints can soothe one's mood and induce resuscitation, nourish Yin and soothe collaterals.

Matching acupoints: ① As per the marrow injury levels, acupuncture of C 1-7 for cervical segment injuries; acupuncture of T 1-10 for thoracic segment injuries; acupuncture of T10-L2 for lumbosacral segment injuries; acupuncture of L2-S5 for cauda equina segment injuries. ② As per different limbs suffered from paralysis, for upper limb paralysis add Jianyu, Quchi, Waiguan, Hegu; for lower limb paralysis add Huantiao, Baliao, Chengfu, Weizhong, Chengshan, Kunlun, Biguan, Futu, Fengshi, Yinlingquan, Zusanli, Yanglingquan, Taichong, Shangqiu, Xuanzhong. ③ As per typing of Traditional Chinese Medicine, for severe Damp-Heat add Pishu, Yinlingquan; for Yin deficiency of liver and kidney add Ganshu, Shenshu, Mingmen, Zhishi, Taichong, Taixi; for severe lung Damp add Feishu, Dazhui, Chize. ④ As per symptoms for defecation disorder add Zhigou, Zhaohai; for urination disorder add Feishu, Guanyuan, Sanyinjiao, Zhibian, Shuidao; for irritability add Shenmen; for dementia add Sishencong, Xinshu, Tongli; for aphasia add Yamen, Lianquan; for blindness add Jingming; for dysphonia add Tiantu, Hegu, Jiache; for paralysis add Huantiao, Juegu, Weizhong, Taichong, Fengchi, Hegu.

绝骨、委中、太冲、风池、合谷。

方法 电热针治疗。

操作 选定穴位，皮肤常规消毒。电热针直刺曲池 0.7 寸，直刺足三里 0.7 寸，直刺三阴交 0.7 寸。接通电热针仪，每个穴位分别给予 40～60mA 的电流量，以患者有胀或温热感觉为度，留针 40 分钟。另配以毫针根据不同的症状，随症选穴，给予补法，留针 40 分钟。

疗程 每日 1 次，留针 40 分钟，90 次为 1 个疗程，疗程间可休息 10～15 天，根据病情决定是否进行第 2 个疗程的治疗。一般治疗 2～3 个疗程即可。

三、注意事项

1. 本病是一种慢性病，治疗时间长者方可取效。必须做好患者及其家属的思想工作，使之了解病情及恢复健康的可能性，因此一定要坚持配合治疗。

2. 在治疗期间，必须注重患者的功能训练，包括智能、语言及形体锻炼。

Method: Electrothermal acupuncture treatment.

Operations: Selecting the relevant acupoints, perform routine skin disinfection. Using electrothermal acupuncture needles, vertically puncture into Quchi for 0.7", Zusanli for 0.7", Sanyinjiao for 0.7". Turn on the electrothermal acupuncture equipment, apply a current of 40-60mA to each acupoint. The limit is that the patient feels swelling or warm. Leave the needles in for 40 minutes. Additionally, using filiform needles, choose acupoints depending on different symptoms and use the tonifying method, leave the needles in for 40 minutes.

Therapeutic course: Treat once a day, leave the needles in for 40 minutes, 90 times for a course, and take a break of 10-15 days after the treatment, then decide if continue the second course depending on the disease condition. Generally 2-3 courses are enough.

III. Precautions

1. This is a chronic disease, the therapy will be effective only after a long-term of treatment. Ideological work on patients and their family must let them know the disease conditions and the possibility of recovery, for which that the treatment must be adhered to.

2. During treatment, must focus on functional exercises for patients, including intelligence, language and body exercises.

强直性脊柱炎

强直性脊柱炎是一种主要累及脊柱、中轴骨骼和四肢大关节,并以椎间盘纤维环及其附近结缔组织纤维化和骨化及关节强直为病变特点的慢性炎症性疾病。此为类风湿因子血清阴性脊柱关节病的一个代表性疾病。强直性脊柱炎常见于青年男性(占90%以上),男女发病之比约在(10～14):1。一般于15岁以后发病,20～24岁多见。因发病多自骶髂关节起始,渐渐向上蔓延,故亦称"上行性脊柱炎"。

中医将本病列入"骨痹"的范畴。本病多以素体阳气虚、肝肾阳精不足为内因,风寒湿热之邪为外因。

一、诊断及辨证要点

1. 患者多为中年男性,可能有家族史,80% 左右隐匿性发病。

2. 腰背痛、脊背发僵感觉超过 3 个月以上,并经休息亦不缓解者。

Ankylosing Spondylitis

Ankylosing spondylitis is a chronic inflammatory disease that mainly affects spine, axial skeleton and major joints of limbs, while its lesion characteristics are fibrosis and ossification of intervertebral disc annulus fibrosus as well as the surrounding connective tissues and ancylosis. This is one of the representative diseases for rheumatoid factor sero-negative spondylo-arthropathy. Ankylosing spondylitis is commonly seen in young males (more than 90%), and the incidence ratio of males and females is (10-14):1. Normally the onset is after 15 years old, common seen in 20-24 years old. Since the onset normally starts from the sacroiliac joint and radiates upwards gradually, therefore it is also called "ascending spondylitis".

In Traditional Chinese Medicine this disease is included into the range of "rheumatism". For this disease, the internal cause is Yang Qi weakness of the body, Yang essence insufficiency of liver and kidney, while external factors are Wind-Cold and Damp-Heat toxins.

I. Key Points for Diagnosis and Syndrome Differentiation

1. Patients mostly are middle-aged males, may have a family history of illness, around 80% are occult onset.

2. Lumbago and backache, back stiffness for more than 3 months, which cannot be relieved by rest.

3. 触诊时在两侧骶棘肌有显著痉挛，脊柱僵硬，颈、腰、膝、髋关节活动受限，一侧或两侧骶髂关节及腰部有压痛或叩击痛。

4. 实验室检查可有轻、中度贫血，活动期可见血沉加快，"抗链球菌溶血素O"值不高，类风湿因子多呈现阴性，患者多数有HLA-B27阳性，X线表现最早改变的是骶髂关节、髂骨外硬化，关节边缘模糊不清。以后出现关节面边缘不整齐、硬化。胸、腰椎体早期出现骨质疏松，随后出现骨质增生、骨纹理增粗，之后韧带硬化，相邻椎体相互连接成竹节状。晚期常驼背畸形。

5. 本病应与类风湿性关节炎、致密髂骨炎、骨关节结核相鉴别。

二、治疗方法

【颈胸背痛者】

治法 舒筋通络，活血化瘀。

处方 以局部取穴及督脉、膀胱经、阿是穴、夹脊穴为主。

方义 以痛为输，在经络

3. During palpation, there is significant spasm of sacral spine muscles at both sides, stiff spine, limited movements of cervical, lumbar, knees and hip joints, tenderness or percussion pain of sacroiliac joints at one or two sides and of the lumbar region.

4. In the lab examinations, there can be seen mild or moderate anemia, increased erythrocyte sedimentation rate can be seen during the active period, the "ASO test" value not high, mostly RF negative, and patients mostly are HLA and B27 positive; X-ray examination indicates that the earliest occurred change is hardness of sacroiliac joints and exterior ilium, with blurred joint edges. Then edge irregularities and hardness of articular surfaces will occur. In the early phase, osteoporosis of thoracic and lumbar vertebral bodies occur, followed by osteoproliferation, enlargement of bone textures, then scleroderma, and adjacent vertebral bodies are connected to each other like bamboo joints. In the late phase often occurs kyphosis of spine.

5. This disease should be identified from rheumatoid arthritis, iliac osteitis condensans an osteoarticular tuberculosis.

II. Therapeutic Methods

[Neck, Chest and Back Pain]

Therapeutic method: Relax tendons and activate collaterals, activate blood circulation and remove stasis.

Prescription: Local acupoint selecting for acupoints of Du Channel, Bladder Meridian, Ashi acupoints, Jiaji acupoints.

Mechanism of prescription: Take pain point as

循行部位选穴，主要根据病之所在处选穴，以疏通经络、活血化瘀、温阳化湿、疏散风寒、调和气血而达到痹痛除之的目的。

配穴 大椎、腰阳关、肾俞、脾俞、大肠俞、环跳、委中、承山、足三里、三阴交、昆仑。

方法 电热针治疗。

操作 选定穴位，皮肤常规消毒。电热针直刺大椎及相应穴位各 0.7 寸，斜刺（针尖向脊柱）膀胱经背俞穴各 0.7 寸，每隔 1 个穴施 1 针，直刺肾俞、大肠俞、环跳、委中、承山、足三里、三阴交、昆仑各 0.7 寸，斜刺（针尖向脊柱）脾俞 0.7 寸，接通电热针仪，每个穴位分别给予 50mA 的电流量，以患者感到舒适为度，留针 40 分钟。

疗程 每日 1 次，留针 40 分钟，90 次为 1 个疗程，疗程间可休息 15～20 天。如果需要可进行第 2 个疗程的治疗，

acupoints, select acupoints at the parts of meridian and collateral circulation, mainly at the lesions, so as to soothe meridians and collaterals, activate blood circulation and remove stasis, warm Yang and disperse Damp, expel Wind-Cold, regulate Qi-blood to achieve the aim of removing arthralgia spasm pain.

Matching acupoints: Dazhui, Yaoyangguan, Shenshu, Pishu, Dachangshu, Huantiao, Weizhong, Chengshan, Zusanli, Sanyinjiao, Kunlun.

Method: Electrothermal acupuncture treatment.

Operations: Selecting the relevant acupoints, perform routine skin disinfection. Using electrothermal acupuncture needles, vertically puncture into Dazhui and corresponding acupoints for 0.7" respectively; obliquely puncture (with the needle tip towards spine) into the Back-Shu acupoints from Bladder Meridian for 0.7" respectively, applying one needle on an acupoint and leave the second one untreated and apply one needle on the third one, and the rest can be done in the same manner. Vertically puncture into Shenshu, Dachangshu, Huantiao, Weizhong, Chengshan, Zusanli, Sanyinjiao, Kunlun for 0.7" respectively, vertically puncture (with the needle tip towards spine) into Pishu for 0.7". Turn on the electrothermal acupuncture equipment, apply a current of 50mA to each acupoint. The limit is that the patient feels comfortable. Leave the needles in for 40 minutes.

Therapeutic course: Once a day, leave the needles in for 40 minutes, 90 times for a course. Rest for 15-20 days between courses. If necessary, start the treatment for the second course. Generally 1-2 courses are enough.

一般治疗1～2个疗程即可。

【腰骶部痛者】

治法 活血，通络，止痛。

处方 肾俞（BL23）、大肠俞（BL25）、关元俞（BL26）、阳陵泉（GB34）、委中（BL40）、阿是穴。

方义 肾俞、大肠俞、关元俞均位于腰骶，是膀胱经治腰骶疼痛之要穴，与阿是穴相配，有舒筋、镇痛之功。委中为足太阳膀胱经之合穴，又名血郄，阳陵泉为足少阳胆经之合穴，又名筋会。诸穴合用，可取其活血、通络、止痛之功效。

配穴 环跳、髀关、秩边、四髎、腰阳关、命门。

方法 电热针治疗。

操作 选定穴位，皮肤常规消毒。电热针直刺肾俞、大肠俞、关元俞、阳陵泉、委中、阿是穴各0.7寸，接通电热针仪，每个穴位分别给予60mA的电流量，以患者舒适为度，留针40分钟。

[Lumbosacral Pain]

Therapeutic method: Activate blood, activate collaterals, and alleviate pain.

Prescription: Shenshu (BL23), Dachangshu (BL25), Guanyuanshu (BL26), Yanglingquan (GB34), Weizhong (BL40), Ashi acupoints.

Mechanism of prescription: Shenshu, Dachangshu, Guanyuanshu are both at lumbosacral portion and are important acupoints for treatment of pains at lumbosacral portion, which are from Bladder Meridian, and they can relax tendons, activate blood and alleviate pain when being matched with Ashi acupoints. Weizhong is a He acupoint from Tai-Yang Bladder Meridian of Foot, also called Xuexi; Yanglingquan is a He acupoint from Shao-Yang Gallbladder Meridian of Foot, also called Jinhui. The use of combination of these acupoints can activate blood circulation, soothe collaterals and alleviate pain.

Matching acupoints: Huantiao, Biguan, Zhibian, Siliao, Yaoyangguan, Mingmen.

Method: Electrothermal acupuncture treatment.

Operations: Selecting the relevant acupoints, perform routine skin disinfection. Using electrothermal acupuncture needles, vertically puncture into Shenshu, Dachangshu, Guanyuanshu, Yanglingquan, Weizhong, Ashi acupoints for 0.7" respectively. Turn on the electrothermal acupuncture equipment, apply a current of 60mA to each acupoint. The limit is that the patient feels locally comfortable. Leave the needles in for 40 minutes.

疗程 每日 1 次，留针 40 分钟，90 次为 1 个疗程。疗程间休息 3～7 天，再进行第 2 个疗程的治疗。一般治疗 1～3 个疗程。

三、注意事项

1. 治疗后，要改善居住条件及生活习惯，注意锻炼身体，增强体质，预防感冒及上呼吸道感染，避免再发。

2. 注意保温，尤其在寒冷季节，特别是春季更应注意保温。

3. 治疗过程中，要有计划、有针对性地进行功能训练，保证正常的工作和生活能力。

进行性肌营养不良

进行性肌营养不良是一种原发于肌肉组织的遗传病，临床以假肥大型（DMD）最为常见。通常在儿童期发病，绝大多数患儿为男性。主要病变为肢体肌肉呈对称性、进行性萎缩和无力。临床表现为鸭步、跌跤、步瘘、爬坡、蹲起困难等。常早年致残或瘫痪死亡，目前现代医学尚无确定疗效的

Therapeutic course: Once a day, leave the needles in for 40 minutes, 90 times for a course. Start the treatment for the second course after a break of 3-7 days. Generally treat for 1-3 courses.

III. Precautions

1. After treatment, it is necessary to improve living conditions and living habits, pay attention to physical exercises, strengthen physique, prevent cold and infections of the upper respiratory tract, to avoid recurrence.

2. Pay attention to keeping warm, especially in the cold seasons; in particular, be aware of keeping warm in the spring.

3. During treatment, pay attention to functional exercises to cooperate with the treatment (with scheduled, targeted functional exercises), and abilities to do activities of normal work as well as daily living must be promised (sound functions).

Progressive Muscular Dystrophy (Type DMD)

Progressive muscular dystrophy is a primary hereditary disease in muscle tissues, and the most clinically common one is pseudohypertrophy (DMD). The onset normally occurs in the childhood, and most patients are male. Main pathological changes include symmetrical progressive atrophy and weakness of limb and body muscles. Clinical manifestations include waddling gait, falling over, stepping impotence, difficulties in going up slopes as well as squatting and standing up. It often causes disabilities or paralysis or even death in the early

药物和方法。

中医认为，本病属于"痿证"的范畴。病因主要为先天不足，加之后天失养。小儿禀赋根于父母，若父母精血有异，合而成形之际，遗传胚胎。出生之后，肾气不足，五脏受累，使肺不能敷布津液，脾不能主肌肉四肢，心不能主血脉，肝不能藏血主筋，肾不能藏筋主骨，皆可致痿。其中尤以脾、肾两脏关系最为密切，肾为先天之本，主骨生髓。先天不足责之于肾，肾虚则骨软髓少，筋脉随之疲软。脾为后天之本，气血生化之源，主肌肉四肢。后天失养责之于脾，脾虚则气血生化无权，不能充养四肢肌肉，故肌肉松弛，日久萎缩不用。总之，本病起于先天，失养于后天，病程中涉及五脏，而以脾肾两虚为主。

phase, and currently there have no drugs and methods which have definite efficacies yet in the Modern Medicine.

Traditional Chinese Medicine believes that this disease belongs to the range of "flaccidity syndrome". Etiology: Mainly caused by deficiency of congenital foundation, plus nourishment loss of acquired construction. The endowment of child is originated from parents, if the essence and blood of parents are abnormal, then these abnormalities will be passed on to the embryo during the formation of zoosperm. After birth, insufficiency of kidney Qi, affecting the five Zang organs, leads to that the lungs cannot distribute fluid, spleen cannot govern muscles and limbs, heart cannot govern blood and channels, liver cannot store blood and govern tendons, kidney cannot store tendons and govern bones. All of the above can cause flaccidity. Among these the connection between spleen and kidney is especially close, kidney is the congenital foundation, it governs marrow generation of bones. Deficiency of congenital foundation is attributed to kidney. Kidney deficiency causes soft bones and less marrow, therefore tendons and channels subsequently become fatigued and weak. Spleen is the foundation of acquired constitution, source of generation and transformation of Qi-blood, and it governs muscles and limbs. Nourishment loss of acquired construction is attributed to spleen. Spleen deficiency causes disorder of generation and transformation of Qi-blood impairing replenishment and nourishment of limbs and muscles, thereby causing muscular flaccidity, and subsequently leading to atrophy and uselessness. In general, this disease is caused by congenital factors and aggravated by acquired factors, the five internal organs are involved in the course of disease, among which mainly is deficiency of both spleen and kidney.

一、诊断及辨证要点

I. Key Points for Diagnosis and Syndrome Differentiation

1. 隐性起病,进行性加重之肢体肌肉对称无力,由于腰肌萎缩,呈现翼状肩、鸭步和行走登楼困难。

1. Occult onset, progressive aggravated symmetric muscle weakness of limbs, caused lumbar muscle atrophy, showed winged shoulder, waddling gait and difficulties in walking and going upstairs.

2. 多见于儿童,发病年龄为 2.5～5 岁,大部分是男性。

2. Most are seen in the children, the onset age is 2.5-5 years old, and most are male patients.

3. 具有明显的腓肠肌假性肥大,双侧对称性四肢近端肌群萎缩,萎缩起始于腰部,皮肤感觉正常。

3. Obvious gastrocnemius muscle pseudohypertrophy, bilateral symmetrical atrophy of limb proximal muscles which started from the waist portion, normal skin sensation.

4. Gower 征阳性。

4. Gower syndrome positive.

5. 肌电图检查呈肌源性损害。

5. EMG indicated myogenic damages.

6. 血清酶类(肌酸磷酸激酶、乳酸脱氢酶、谷丙转氨酶、谷草转氨酶等)显著增高。

6. Significant elevated levels of serum enzymes (creatine phosphokinase, lactic dehydrogenase, alanine aminotransferase, glutamic oxalacetic transaminase, etc.).

7. 肌肉活检可见肌纤维粗细不等、灶性坏死、脂肪组织浸润,有不同程度的肌萎缩等。

7. In the muscle biopsy, muscle fiber uneven thickness, focal necrosis, adipose tissue infiltration, amyotrophy with varying degrees, etc. can be seen.

8. 中医辨证分型:本病中医临床多参照"痿证"进行辨证论治。按照中华人民共和国

8. Symptom differentiation and type classification of Traditional Chinese Medicine: Clinically this disease is normally treated based on syndrome differentiation

行业标准——《中医病症诊断疗效标准》中关于"痿证的临床诊断原则"所确定的标准,痿证是"以肢体弛缓、软弱无力、活动不利,甚则肌肉萎缩为主要表现的病症"。另外,在中医辨证方面,因本病是先天不足和后天失调所致,故脾肾两虚始终贯穿在整个病机过程中。

(1)脾肾虚弱:患儿渐觉下肢无力,消瘦,走路易跌倒,上楼或爬坡困难,纳差,面色不华,大便溏,舌淡,苔薄白,脉细弱。

(2)肝肾阴虚:患儿肢体痿软无力,腰膝酸困,不能行走、站立,并有眩晕、耳鸣,遗尿,舌红少苔,脉细数。

(3)痰湿阻络:形体虚胖,肌肉松弛,四肢痿软,身重而活动不利,舌胖大有齿痕,苔白腻,脉沉细。

(4)肺气虚弱:频咳痰多,

according to the "flaccidity syndrome". As per the standards for "Principles of clinical diagnosis for flaccidity syndromes" defined in the Industrial Standards of the People's Republic of China—*Disease Diagnosis and Efficacy Standards for Traditional Chinese Medicine* (中华人民共和国行业标准——《中医病症诊断疗效标准》), flaccidity syndrome is a "disease that the main manifestations of which are limb and body atony, weakness, inhibited movements, or even amyotrophy". Additionally, in the respect of syndrome differentiation of Traditional Chinese Medicine, since this disease is caused by deficiency of congenital foundation and nourishment loss of acquired construction, so deficiency of both spleen and kidney exists throughout the whole process of pathogenesis.

(1) Weakness of spleen and kidney: Patients gradually feel weakness of the lower limbs, emaciation, easy to falling over during walking, difficulties in going upstairs or slopes, poor appetite, lusterless complexion, sloppy stool, light tongue with thin and white fur, thin and weak pulse.

(2) Yin deficiency of liver and kidney: Patients suffer from flaccidity and weakness of the limbs and body, soreness and tiredness of waist and knees, are unable to walk and stand, accompanying vertigo, tinnitus, enuresis, red tongue with less fur, thin and rapid pulse.

(3) Phlegm-Damp obstructing collaterals: Body puffiness, loosening muscles, flaccid limbs, heavy body and inhibited movements, fat and large tongue with teeth prints, white and greasy fur, deep and thin pulse.

(4) Weakness of lung Qi: Frequent coughing and

或易外感，纳呆懒言，大便不实，肌肉萎缩，易跌跤，舌质淡，苔薄白，脉细。

9. 周围血白细胞DNA分析发现基因变异。

二、治疗方法

【脾胃虚弱证】

治法　补脾益气。

处方　以手足阳明经穴为主。上肢取肩髃（LI15）、曲池（LI11）、手三里（LI10）、合谷（LI4），下肢取环跳（GB30）、足三里（ST36）、三阴交（SP6）、太溪（KI3）、太冲（LR3），背部取督脉穴及华佗夹脊穴。

方义　取穴以阳明经穴为主，治则来源于《内经》"治痿独取阳明"之说，但又不拘泥于此，根据患儿不同的体质、证候制订个性化的治疗方案。具体来说，取手足阳明经穴以补益后天之脾胃；肾主骨生髓，取太溪强腰壮骨充髓；肝主筋，取太冲强筋、滑利关节；取肩髃、曲池、合谷、手三里、环跳以通经接气、活血通络；足三里、三阴交是人体的主要强壮穴；督脉与华佗夹

excessive phlegm, vulnerable to exogenous infections, poor appetite and laziness to speak, non-compact stool, amyotrophy, easy to fall over, light tongue with thin and white fur, thin pulse.

9. Gene variations are found in the DNA analysis of peripheral blood leukocytes.

II. Therapeutic Methods

[Syndrome of Spleen and Stomach Weakness]

Therapeutic method: Replenish spleen and tonify Qi.

Prescription: Mainly use meridian acupoints from Yang-Ming meridians of hands and feet. For upper limbs use Jianyu (LI15), Quchi (LI11), Shousanli (LI10), Hegu (LI4), for lower limbs use Huantiao (GB30), Zusanli (ST36), Sanyinjiao (SP6), Taixi (KI3), Taichong (LR3), for back use acupoints from Du Channel and Huatuo Jia-ji acupoints.

Mechanism of prescription: Mainly use the meridian acupoints from Yang-Ming Meridian, and the therapy is originated from the Methods of Treatment "use Yang-Ming alone for treatment of flaccidity" in the *Neijing* (《内经》), while does not limited by this: Develop individual treatment schemes depending on different physical constitutions and syndromes for patients. Specifically, use acupoints from Yang-Ming meridians of hands and feet to tonify acquired foundations for spleen and stomach. Kidney governs marrow generation of bones, use Taixi to strength waist and bones and replenish marrow. Liver governs tendons, use Taichong to strengthen tendons and smooth joints; use Jianyu, Quchi, Hegu, Shousanli,

脊穴能激发、振奋全身阳经经气，有恢复肢体功能、防治肌肉萎缩之功。

配穴 中脘、上脘、梁门、滑肉门、气海、关元、肾俞、大肠俞、腰阳关、命门。

方法 电热针治疗。

操作 选定穴位，皮肤常规消毒。电热针直刺肩髃、曲池、手三里、环跳、足三里、三阴交各 0.7 寸（每次取 3 组穴，轮流交替应用）。接通电热针仪，每个穴位分别给予电流量 30～40mA，以胀而舒适为度，留针 40 分钟。其余穴位以毫针治疗，亦留针 40 分钟。

疗程 每日 1 次，30 次为 1 个疗程，中间休息 7～10 天，连续治疗 3 个疗程。

三、注意事项

1. 进针方向：督脉穴位可直刺 0.7 寸；华佗夹脊穴斜刺，针尖向脊中斜刺 0.7 寸。

Huantiao to soothe meridians and connect Qi, activate blood circulation and soothe collaterals. Zusanli and Sanyinjiao are main important tonifying acupoints for human body. Du Channel and Huatuo Jiaji acupoints can motivate and promote Yang Qi of the whole body, and can be used to recover limb and body functions, prevent and treat amyotrophia.

Matching acupoints: Zhongwan, Shangwan, Liangmen, Huaroumen, Qihai, Guanyuan, Shenshu, Dachangshu, Yaoyangguan, Mingmen.

Method: Electrothermal acupuncture treatment.

Operations: Selecting the relevant acupoints, perform routine skin disinfection. Using electrothermal acupuncture needles, vertically puncture into Jianyu, Quchi, Shousanli, Huantiao, Zusanli, Sanyinjiao for 0.7" respectively (choose 3 pairs of acupoints each time and use alternatively). Turn on the electrothermal acupuncture equipment, apply a current of 30-40mA to each acupoint. The limit is that the patient feels swelling and comfortable. Leave the needles in for 40 minutes. Treat other acupoints with filiform needles. Leave the needles in for 40 minutes as well.

Therapeutic course: Once a day, 30 times for a course. Rest for 7-10 days between courses. Continuously treat for 3 courses.

III. Precautions

1. Needling direction: For acupoints of Du Channel, vertically puncture for 0.7"; for Huatuo Jiaji acupoints use oblique puncture, obliquely puncture for 0.7" with the needle tip towards Jizhong.

2. 电热针的深度：不管采用直刺还是斜刺，必须将针尖 10 毫米能发热部位刺入穴位中，以免烫伤皮肤。

3. 电热针进针方法：刺入直达，不行捻转及捣针，因容易损伤穴位处组织，针刺入后手下有得气之沉重感（如鱼咬钩之沉重）即留针。给予 30～40mA 的电流量，患儿会感到穴位胀，不要求热感，避免烧伤。

4. 穴位按摩时，注意手法要轻（指对肌肉萎缩部位），以局部皮肤出现微红发热为宜。一般行补法，以轻揉、拿为主，以患儿愿意接受为度。

5. 中药疗法：复痿散（自拟方）。每日 1 剂，早、晚分服。组成：黄芪、全蝎、蜈蚣、明天麻、杜仲等，针对不同证型，采用配方如下：

（1）脾胃虚弱型：治宜益气健脾，活血通络，方用复痿散合参苓白术散加味。

（2）肝肾阴虚型：治宜补益肝肾，滋阴清热，活血

2. Depth of electrothermal needles: Whether for vertical puncture or oblique puncture, the 10mm of the needle tip which can radiate heat must be punctured into the acupoint so as to avoid skin burns.

3. Needling method for electrothermal needles: Puncture in and reach the target location without twirling or lifting and thrusting of needles, since these methods may injury the tissues at the acupoint locations, leave the needle in immediately once get the feeling of heaviness by Qi acquisition (like the heaviness feeling of fish biting a fishhook). Give a current of 30-40mA, the child patient will feel swelling of the acupoint site, the heat feeling is not required so as to avoid burns.

4. For acupoint massage, note that use mild manipulation (for the site of amyotrophia), and the limit is flushing and warm of local skin. The general use of the tonifying method, mainly light rolling and holding. The limit is that the patient can accept it.

5. Chinese Herb Medicine therapy: Fu Wei San (self-prescription). One dose a day, divided into two halves and take one each in the morning and in the evening respectively. Composition: Root of astragalus membranaceus, whole scorpion, rhizona gastrodiae, etc. for different syndromes use different prescriptions as followed:

(1) Spleen and stomach weakness type: Tonify Qi and invigorate spleen, activate blood circulation, soothe collaterals, so use Fu Wei San and add Shen Ling Bai Zhu San.

(2) Liver and kidney Yin deficiency type: Tonify liver and kidney, nourish Yin and clear Heat, activate

通络，方用复痿散合虎潜丸加减。

（3）痰湿阻络型：治宜健脾补肾，燥湿化痰，方用复痿散合二陈汤加减。

（4）肺气不足型：治宜培土生金，补肾强腰膝，方用复痿散合六君子汤加减。

6. 西药治疗：以营养神经的药物为主，如维生素 E、肌苷片，前者每次 20mg，每日 3 次；后者每次 0.2g，每日 3 次。能量合剂，每日 1 次静脉滴注（每个月治疗 14 天）。

7. 功能训练：根据患儿不同程度的功能不全，给予相应的训练方法，由医师指导，每天上、下午各训练 1 次。

8. 疗程：每天治疗 1 次，90 次为 1 个疗程。治疗 1 个疗程后，根据观察记录症状、体征积分，测定实验室指标，比较治疗前后之变化，再决定是否需要继续进行第 2 个疗程的治疗。一般治疗 1 个疗程后即可巩固疗效。

四、典型病例

魏某，男，7 岁，安徽人。

blood circulation and soothe collaterals, so use Fu Wei San and add Hu Qian Pills, add or remove components.

(3) Phlegm-Damp obstructing collaterals type: Invigorate spleen and replenish kidney, remove Damp and disperse phlegm, so use Fu Wei San and add Er Chen Tang, add or remove components.

(4) Lung Qi insufficiency type: Reinforce Earth to generate Metal, replenish kidney and strengthen waist and knees, so use Fu Wei San and add Liu Jun Zi Tang, add or remove components.

6. Western Medicine therapy: Mainly use drugs intended to nourish nerves, such as Vitamin E and inosine tablet, the former 20mg each time, 3 times a day; the later 0.2g each time, 3 times a day. Energy mixture, once a day by intravenous drip (14 days each month).

7. Functional exercise, provide different exercise methods depending on various degrees of incompetence, and perform once in the morning and once in the afternoon each day under physician's instruction.

8. **Therapeutic course:** Once a day, 90 times for a course. After 1 course of treatment, according to observed and recorded symptoms, integral of physical signs, measure lab indicators and compare the changes before and after the treatment, then determine if it is necessary to continue the second course. Generally the efficacies can be consolidated after 1 course.

IV. Typical Case

Wei, male, 7 years old, residence: Anhui Province.

主诉：四肢无力进行性加重2年。病史：患儿足月产，第3胎，21个月会走路，但步态不稳，跑步慢。2岁后平地走路易跌倒，行步无力，走路左右摇摆，爬坡、上楼梯逐渐费力，常需自己扶踝、再扶膝才能站起来，并发现小腿肌肉逐渐增粗变硬。曾到各大医院检查，诊断为"进行性肌营养不良DMD型"，经用药、ATP等治疗不见好转。

刻下症：患儿饮食正常，二便通调，舌质淡红，苔薄白，脉弦细无力。

查体：面色萎黄，体型瘦小。四肢近端肌肉、腰部肌肉明显萎缩，肌容积变小，双侧下肢腓肠肌假性肥大，四肢肌力0～2级。Gower征（＋），膝反射减弱，病理征（－）。

辅助检查：CPK 3936U/L，LDH 1356U/L，GPT 541U，GOT 67.6U，积分值为62分。肌电图示"肌源性损害"。

【诊断依据】

1. 儿童，男性，发病年龄为2岁。

2. 隐性起病，进行性加重

Self-reported symptoms: Progressive aggravated limb weakness for 2 years. Medical history: Full-term birthed child, the third child of his mother, learned to walk at the age of 21 months, however suffered from gait instability and ran slowly. After 2 years old, the child was easy to fall down during walking on the flat ground, weakness in taking steps, vacillated to the left and right when walking, and he felt harder and harder to go up slopes and stairs, often needed to hold against ankles or knees to stand up, and his calf muscles were found thickening and hardening. He had undergone examinations at several hospitals and was diagnosed as "progressive muscular dystrophy, Type DMD", and the condition was not improved after medication and ATP therapies.

Current symptoms: The patient had normal diet as well as urination and defecation, light-red tongue with thin and white fur, taut, thin and weak pulse.

Physical examination: Sallow complexion, lean and small body. Obvious atrophy of limb proximal muscles and lumbar muscles, reduced muscle volume, gastrocnemius muscle pseudohypertrophy of bilateral lower limbs, the muscle strength of four limbs: Grade 0-2. Gower syndrome (+), weakened knee reflex, pathological sign (-).

Auxiliary examination: CPK 3936U/L, LDH 1356U/L, GPT 541U, GOT 67.6U, 62 points of the scale. EMG indicated "myogenic damages".

[Diagnostic Basis]

1. Child, male, disease onset at the age of 2 years old.

2. Occult onset, progressive aggravated symmetric

之肢体肌肉对称无力，由于腰肌萎缩，呈现翼状肩、鸭步和行走登楼困难。

3. 具有明显的腓肠肌假性肥大，双侧对称性四肢近端肌群萎缩，萎缩起始于腰部，皮肤感觉正常。

4. Gower 征（+）。

5. 肌电图检查呈肌源性损害。

6. 血清酶类（肌酸磷酸激酶、乳酸脱氢酶、谷丙转氨酶、谷草转氨酶等）显著增高。

【证治分析】

病因 肝肾亏虚，脾气虚弱。

病机 肝肾亏虚，髓枯筋痿，患儿素体肾虚，阴精亏损，筋脉失养，脾气虚弱，精微不布，素体脾气虚弱，中焦受纳、运化、输布功能失常，气血津液生化不足，从而筋脉失养，关节不利，肌肉瘦削，导致肢体痿弱不用。

证候分析 肝肾精血亏虚，不能濡养筋骨经脉，而渐成痿

muscle weakness of limbs, caused lumbar muscle atrophy, showed winged shoulder, waddling gait and difficulties in walking and going upstairs.

3. Obvious gastrocnemius muscle pseudohypertrophy, bilateral symmetrical atrophy of limb proximal muscles which started from the waist portion, normal skin sensation.

4. Gower syndrome (+).

5. EMG indicated myogenic damages.

6. Significant elevated levels of serum enzymes (creatine phosphokinase, lactic dehydrogenase, alanine aminotransferase, glutamic oxalacetic transaminase, etc.).

[Syndrome-treatment Analysis]

Etiology: Depletion and deficiency of liver and kidney, weakness of spleen Qi.

Pathogenesis: Depletion and deficiency of liver and kidney, marrow exhaustion and tendon flaccidity. The patient had kidney deficiency, depletion of Yin essence, nourishment loss of tendons and channels, weakness of spleen Qi. Food essence was unable to be distributed, spleen Qi weakness of the body, Middle Jiao dysfunctions of food intake, transportation and transformation, transfer and distribution, insufficiency of generation and transformation of Qi-blood and fluid. This caused nourishment loss of tendons and channels, inhabited joint movements, thin muscles, leading to flaccidity and uselessness of limbs and body.

Syndrome analysis: Essence and blood depletion and deficiency of liver and kidney caused that tendons

证；腰为肾之府，肾虚则腰膝酸软；脾气虚弱，气血化源不足，筋脉失养，故肢体痿软无力，逐渐加重；脾不健运，中气不足，则食少便溏，面色不华；舌淡苔白，脉细为肝肾亏损，脾气虚弱之象。

病位 肝、肾、脾、胃。

病性 属虚。

西医诊断 进行性肌营养不良症 DMD 型。

中医诊断 痿证。

治法 补肝肾，益脾气，化痰湿。

方法 电热针治疗、中药治疗、西药治疗、穴位按摩、功能训练。

（1）电热针治疗

处方 肩髃（LI15）、曲池（LI11）、合谷（LI4）、髀关（ST31）、梁丘（ST34）、足三里（ST36）、解溪（ST41）、阳陵泉（GB34）、悬钟（GB39）、督脉穴及华佗夹脊穴。

方义 痿证以取阳明经

and bones as well as meridians and channels cannot be nourished, therefore flaccidity syndrome develops gradually; waist is the place where kidneys locate, kidney deficiency causes soreness and weakness of waist and knees; weakness of spleen Qi, insufficient transportation source of Qi-blood, nourishment loss of tendons and channels, cause flaccidity of limbs which worsens gradually; loss of normal transportation of spleen, insufficiency of Middle-Jiao Qi, lead to less food intake and sloppy stool, lusterless complexion; light tongue with white fur, thin pulses are signs of depletion and deficiency of liver and kidney, weakness of spleen Qi.

Lesion location: Liver, kidney, spleen and stomach.

Disease nature: Deficiency.

The diagnosis of Western Medicine: Progressive muscular dystrophy, Type DMD.

The diagnosis of Traditional Chinese Medicine: Flaccidity syndrome.

Therapeutic method: Replenish liver and kidney, tonify spleen Qi, disperse phlegm-Damp.

Method: Electrothermal acupuncture treatment, Chinese Herb Medicine treatment, Western Medicine treatment, acupoint massage, functional exercises.

(1) Electrothermal acupuncture treatment

Prescription: Jianyu (LI15), Quchi (LI11), Hegu (LI4), Biguan (ST31), Liangqiu (ST34), Zusanli (ST36), Jiexi (ST41), Yanglingquan (GB34), Xuanzhong (GB39), acupoints of Du Channel and Huatuo Jiaji acupoints.

Mechanism of prescription: For treatment of flac-

穴为主,取手阳明经肩髃、曲池、合谷;取足阳明经髀关、足三里、梁丘、解溪,以健运脾胃、益气养血、濡养宗筋;阳陵泉为筋之会,悬钟为髓之会,与阳陵泉相伍,用补法,能充骨髓、益筋脉。诸穴共用,可收健脾益胃、补气养血、强健筋骨之功效。华佗夹脊穴是局部取穴,可治胸、腰部及下肢疼痛和无力。

配穴 肾俞、中脘、天枢、气海、关元、腰阳关、命门。

操作 选定穴位,皮肤常规消毒。电热针直刺肩髃、曲池、合谷、足三里、三阴交各0.6寸,斜刺(针尖向脊柱)华佗夹脊穴各0.6寸,直刺督脉穴0.6寸,余者用毫针治疗。(注:每次选3组穴用电热针治疗,分组轮流交替运用。)

疗程 90次为1个疗程,每日1次,留针40分钟。疗程间根据病情可休息10～15天,再进行第2个疗程的治疗。一

cidity syndrome, mainly use the acupoints from Yang-Ming Meridian. Therefore use Jianyu, Quchi, Hegu from Yang-Ming Meridian of Hand. Use Biguan, Zusanli, Liangqiu, Jiexi from Yang-Ming Meridian of Foot to promote transportation of spleen and stomach, tonify Qi and nourish blood, tonify convergent tendon. Yanglingquan is a confluent acupoint of tendons, Xuanzhong is a confluent acupoint of marrow, when being matched with Yanglingquan it can replenish bone marrow and tonify tendons and channels. The use of combination of these acupoints can invigorate spleen and tonify stomach, replenish Qi and nourish blood, strengthen tendons and bones. Huatuo Jiaji acupoints are used with the method of local acupoint selecting, they can treat pain and weakness of chest, waist portions and lower limbs.

Matching acupoints: Shenshu, Zhongwan, Tianshu, Qihai, Guanyuan, Yaoyangguan, Mingmen.

Operations: Selecting the relevant acupoints, perform routine skin disinfection. Using electrothermal acupuncture needles, vertically puncture into Jianyu, Quchi, Hegu, Zusanli, Sanyinjiao for 0.6" respectively, obliquely puncture (with the needle tip towards spine) into Huatuo Jiaji acupoints for 0.6" respectively, vertically puncture into acupoints of Du Channel for 0.6", and for the other acupoints use filiform needles to treat. (Note: Choose 3 pairs of acupoints to apply acupuncture treatment each time, divide the acupoints into groups and use alternatively.)

Therapeutic course: 90 times for a course, once a day, leave the needles in for 40 minutes. Start the treatment for the second course depending on the condition after a break of 10-15 days. Generally treat for 1-2

般治疗 1～2 个疗程。

（2）中药治疗

复痿散加减，每日 1 剂，早、晚分服。

（3）西药治疗

维生素 E 100mg，每日 3 次；肌苷片 0.1g，每日 3 次；能量合剂，每日 1 次静脉滴注（每个月治疗 14 天）。

（4）穴位按摩

家长在医师的指导下，每日给患儿治疗 1 次。

（5）功能训练

根据每位患儿的个体差异，制订不同的训练方案，每日做 2 次，上、下午各做 1 次。

治疗过程 患儿经过上述综合治疗 5 个月后，症状、体征明显好转，走路跌倒明显减少，上楼虽然费力，但不用扶栏杆。蹲站较自如，不用扶膝站起，可连续做 35 次，积分 34 分，较治疗前明显改善，舌质淡红，苔薄白，脉细。理化检查：CPK 801.4U/L，LDH 312U/L，GPT 44U，GOT 41U。综合治疗后，指标明显下降，疗效明显，继续巩固治疗效果，定期复查。随访，患儿已治疗 5 年

courses.

(2) Chinese Herb Medicine treatment

Fu Wei San, add or remove components, one dose a day, divided into two halves and take one each in the morning and in the evening respectively.

(3) Western Medicine treatment

Vitamin E 100mg, three times a day; inosine tablet 0.1g, three times a day; energy mixture, once a day by intravenous drip (14 days each month).

(4) Acupoint massage

Under physician's instruction, the parents perform once a day for the patient.

(5) Functional exercises

Develop different exercise schemes as per individual differences of each child patient, and let them do the exercises twice a day, one in the morning and one in the afternoon.

Therapeutic process: After 5-month treatment by the above comprehensive therapy, the child patient had obvious improvements in symptoms and physical signs, and the falling times during walking reduced obviously, though it needed big efforts to go upstairs the patient could go without leaning against the handrail. Relative free squatting and standing up for 35 times continuously, no need to stand up by holding on the knees, 34 points of score which reduced significantly compared to that before treatment, light red tongue with thin and white fur, thin pulse. Physical and chemical examination: CPK 801.4U/L, LDH 312U/L, GPT 44U, GOT 41U. After treatment of the comprehensive therapy, indicators

4个月，现在体质较好，行动自如，能上学读书。

【生活调摄】

1. 治疗过程中为配合治疗，注意功能训练要有计划、有针对性的功能训练，必须能保证正常的工作和生活能力的功能健全。

2. 采用综合治疗的方法，中、西药配合治疗。

3. 规律饮食，按时作息，避免患儿过劳。

多发性硬化

多发性硬化（Multiple Sclerosis，简称MS）是一种青壮年起病的中枢神经系统脱髓鞘性疾病。因视神经、脊髓和脑内有散在多灶的脱髓鞘硬化斑块而得名。病情有缓解和复发的倾向，病因未明。女性的发病率高于男性。目前认为MS的发病与以下因素有关：①与易感的遗传素质有关，10%的患者有家族史，MS患者的亲属中有MS的发病率比一般群

reduced significantly, and obvious efficacies had been achieved; continued the treatment to consolidate the efficacies; regular reexaminations. Follow-up, the child patient has being treated for 5 years plus 4 months, now he has a relatively good physique, can move freely and go to school.

[Lifestyle Change and Health Maintenance]

1. During treatment, pay attention to functional exercises to cooperate with the treatment with scheduled, targeted functional exercises, and abilities to do activities of normal work as well as daily living must be promised.

2. Use a comprehensive therapy, to treat with the supplement of Chinese Herb Medicine treatment as well as Western Medicine treatment.

3. Have a regular diet and live a regular routine, avoid overstrain of the child patient.

Multiple Sclerosis

Multiple sclerosis (referred to MS) is a demyelinating disease of the central nervous system which is seen in the young adults. It is so named because there are multifocal demyelinating sclerotic plaques scattered in the optic nerves, spine cord and brain. The condition has a tendency to be relieved and recur, while the etiology remains unknown. The incidence of females is higher than that of males. At present, the incidence of MS is considered being related to the following factors: ① related to the genetic predisposition of susceptibility, and 10% patients have a family history of MS, while the incidence of relatives of MS patients is 5-10 times higher than that

体高 5～10 倍。单卵双胎的同胞兄弟中患病概率高达 50%。② MS 是一种自身免疫性疾病。③ 病毒感染。④ 特殊地理环境，离赤道越远发病率愈高。

中医认为，本病属于"痿证"的范畴。病变涉及脾胃，脾胃为后天之本，气血生化之源。如素体脾胃虚弱，或因外邪侵袭，情志刺激而致虚，脾胃受纳运化功能失常，气血生化不足，肌肉筋脉失养而致痿；若原有痿证经久不愈，导致脾胃虚弱，甚至久病及肝肾受损，又可使痿证加重。其病虚多实少、热多寒少。主要病机为湿热浸淫、脾胃虚弱、肝肾亏损、痰瘀阻络等，病程缓慢。

一、诊断及辨证要点

1. 年轻人临床表现为中枢神经系统白质多灶损害症状与体征（10～55 岁起病）。

of normal population. The incidence in the monozygotic twinning siblings is up to 50%. ② MS is an autoimmune disease. ③ Virus infections. ④ Special geographic environment, the farther the place from the equator, the higher the incidence in that region.

Traditional Chinese Medicine believes that this disease belongs to the category of "flaccidity syndrome". The lesions involve spleen and stomach, while spleen and stomach are foundation of acquired constitution, source of generation and transformation of Qi-blood. For example, weakness of spleen and stomach, or invasion of exogenous toxins, emotional stimulation cause deficiency, dysfunction of food reception as well as transportation and transformation of spleen and stomach, insufficient of generation and transformation of Qi-blood, nourishment loss of muscles as well as tendons and channels, leading to flaccidity; if previous flaccidity syndrome is not cured after long-term treatment and causes weakness of spleen and stomach, or even causes aeipathia and damages of liver and kidney, then the flaccidity syndrome can be aggravated. For this disease, more deficiency cases than excess ones, more Heat cases than Cold ones. Main pathogenesis: excessive Damp-Heat, spleen and stomach weakness, depletion and deficiency of liver and kidney, phlegm stasis obstructing collaterals, etc.; slow disease progress.

I. Key Points for Diagnosis and Syndrome Differentiation

1. The clinical manifestations of young adults include symptoms and physical signs for multifocal damages of CNS white matter (onset at the age of 10-55

2. 以缓解和复发交替发生的病程，缓解期在 1 个月以上。

3. 脑脊液中 IgG 增高以及 IgG 克隆带出现。

4. 头部 CT 和 MRI 检查：发现脑室周围中央白质内散在低密度阴影。急性期损害可为造影剂增强，提示脑屏障破坏。MRI 能发现较 CT 更多的损害，特别是脑干和小脑的病灶。

5. 脑脊液检查：可见以 T 淋巴细胞为主的细胞数增高，也有蛋白轻度增高。较特殊的发现为脑脊液 IgG 增高。但这些变化也可见于其他中枢神经系统疾病中。

6. 电生理检查：有关白质通路的病变、视觉、听觉或躯体感觉诱发电位的检查可发现传导速度减慢。

7. 中医辨证

（1）湿热浸淫：四肢痿软，身体困重、麻木，胸脘痞闷，小便赤涩，舌红体胖，苔薄黄腻，脉沉细数。

（2）脾胃亏虚：肢体痿软

2. During the disease course, relief and recurrence occur alternatively, and the relief period is longer than 1 month.

3. Increased IgG and IgG clone bands occur in the cerebrospinal fluid (CSF).

4. Cranial CT and MRI examinations: Scattered low-density shadows were found in the center white matter around the cerebral ventricle. In the acute period, damages can be enhanced by contrast agents, indicating destruction of brain barriers. MRI examination can find more damages compared to CT, especially lesions of brainstem and cerebellum.

5. CSF examination: Increased cell count, mainly increased T lymphocyte count can be found, as well as mild protein increase. The special finding can be increased IgG level in the CSF. However these changes also may be seen in other CNS diseases.

6. Eletrophysiological examination: Reduced conduction velocity can be found in the examinations related to lesions of white matter pathways, visual, auditory, or somatic sensory evoked potentials.

7. Syndrome differentiation of Traditional Chinese Medicine

(1) Excessive Damp-Heat: Limb flaccid, heavy and tired and numb body, fullness and distress in chest and abdomen, dark urine and inhibited urination, red tongue and fat body, thin and yellow and greasy tongue fur, deep and thin and rapid pulse.

(2) Depletion and deficiency of spleen and stomach:

无力日重，食少纳呆，腹胀，便溏，神疲乏力，气短，舌淡，苔薄白，脉沉细。

（3）肝肾亏损：发病缓慢，视物不清，复视，肢体痿软无力，腰脊酸软，不能久立，伴眩晕、耳鸣或月经不调，甚至步履全废，腿胫大肉渐脱，舌红苔少，脉沉细。

（4）痰瘀阻络：起病缓慢，视物不清，复视，肢体逐渐软弱无力，皮肤枯燥、干涩，小便短赤，大便秘结，舌暗红，苔白腻，脉弦。

二、治疗方法

【脾胃亏虚证】

治法 健脾培土，补益气血，舒筋活络。

方法 电热针治疗、中药治疗、西药治疗、功能训练、手法治疗。

（1）电热针治疗

处方 中脘（RN12）、血海（SP10）、三阴交（SP6）、足三里（ST36）、气海（RN6）。

方义 中脘调胃理气，足三里健运脾胃，是强壮要穴，

Gradually worsened flaccid and weak limbs, less food intake and poor appetite, abdominal distension, sloppy stool, fatigue look and asthenia, shortness of breath, light tongue with thin and white fur, deep and thin pulse.

(3) Depletion of liver and kidney: Slow onset, blurred vision, diplopia, flaccid and weak limbs, soreness and weakness of spinal column, inability to stand for a long time, accompanying vertigo, tinnitus or menoxenia, or even complete voiding stepping, gradually getting off of large femorotibial muscles, red tongue with less fur, deep and thin pulse.

(4) Phlegm stasis obstructing collaterals: Slow onset, blurred vision, diplopia, gradually weakening of limbs, dull and dry skin, short and dark urine, constipation, dark red tongue with white and greasy fur, taut pulse.

II. Therapeutic Methods

[Syndrome of Spleen and Stomach Deficiency]

Therapeutic method: Invigorate spleen and replenish Earth, tonify Qi and blood, relax tendons and activate collaterals.

Method: Electrothermal acupuncture treatment, Chinese Herb Medicine treatment, acupoint massage, functional exercises, manipulation therapy.

(1) Electrothermal acupuncture treatment

Prescription: Zhongwan (RN12), Xuehai (SP10), Sanyinjiao (SP6), Zusanli (ST36), Qihai (RN6).

Mechanism of prescription: Zhongwan can tonify stomach and regulate Qi; Zusanli can promote transpor-

三阴交健脾化湿、疏肝益胃，血海有清热和营、活血化瘀之作用，气海补益中气，再配合上、下肢局部穴位，可奏健脾培土、补益气血、舒筋活络之功。

配穴 上肢痿软加肩髃、曲池、合谷；下肢痿软加髀关、梁丘、足三里、解溪；湿热浸淫者，加阴陵泉、脾俞；脾胃虚弱者，加脾俞、胃俞；肝肾亏虚者，加肝俞、肾俞、悬钟；痰瘀阻络者，加丰隆、血海。

操作 选定穴位，皮肤常规消毒。电热针直刺曲池、足三里、三阴交各0.7寸，接通电热针仪，每个穴位分别给予电流量40～50mA，以患者感到胀而舒适为度。另配以毫针治疗，每次选6～8组穴，轮番应用，留针40分钟。

疗程 每日1次，90次为1个疗程，疗程间可休息10～15天，再进行第2个疗程的治疗。

（2）中药治疗

复痿散（自拟方）加味。

tation of spleen and stomach, is an important tonifying acupoint; Sanyinjiao can invigorate spleen and dispel Damp, soothe liver and tonify stomach; Xuehai can clear Heat and regulate Ying, activate blood circulation and remove stasis; Qihai can replenish Middle-Jiao Qi, plussing local acupoints of upper and lower limbs. They can invigorate spleen and replenish Earth, tonify Qi and blood, relax tendons and activate collaterals.

Matching acupoints: For upper limb flaccidity add Jianyu, Quchi, Hegu. For lower limb flaccidity add Biguan, Liangqiu, Zusanli, Jiexi. For excessive Damp-Heat add Yinlingquan, Pishu. For weakness of spleen and stomach add Pishu, Weishu. For depletion and deficiency of liver and kidney add Ganshu, Shenshu, Xuanzhong. For phlegm stasis obstructing collaterals add Fenglong, Xuehai.

Operations: Selecting the relevant acupoints, perform routine skin disinfection. Using electrothermal acupuncture needles, vertically puncture into Quchi, Zusanli, Sanyinjiao for 0.7" respectively. Turn on the electrothermal acupuncture equipment, apply a current of 40-50mA to each acupoint, and the limit is that the patient feels swelling and comfortable. Additionally, using filiform needles, select 6-8 pairs of acupoints each time and use alternatively, leaving the needles in for 40 minutes.

Therapeutic course: Treat once a day, 90 times for a course, and start the treatment for the second course after a break of 10-15 days.

(2) Chinese Herb Medicine treatment

Chinese Herb Medicine therapy: Fu Wei San

每日 1 剂，早、晚各 1 次。组成：黄芪、全蝎、蜈蚣、明天麻、白术、杜仲、山药等。针对不同证型，配方如下：①湿热浸淫型：治宜健脾利湿，活血通络，方用复痿散。②脾胃虚弱型：治宜健脾益胃，活血通络，方用复痿散合参苓白术散加味。③肝肾亏虚型：治宜补益肝肾，滋阴清热，活血通络，方用复痿散合虎潜丸加减。④痰湿阻络型：治宜健脾补肾，燥湿化痰，方用复痿散合二陈汤加味。

（3）西药治疗

以营养神经的药物为主，如维生素 B1 20mg，每日 3 次；维生素 B12 500U，每日 3 次；能量合剂，每日 1 次静脉滴注（每个月治疗 14 天）。

（4）功能训练

根据患者的具体状况，给予针对性的功能训练，由医师指导，每日上、下午各锻炼 2 小时。

(self-prescription), add or remove components. One dose a day, divided into two halves and take one each in the morning and in the evening respectively. Composition: Root of astragalus membranaceus, whole scorpion, centipede, rhizona gastrodiae, bighead atractylodes rhizome, bark of eucommia, Chinese yam, etc. For different syndromes use different prescriptions as followed: ① Excessive Damp-Heat type: Invigorate spleen and dispel Damp, activate blood and soothe collaterals, so use Fu Wei San. ② Spleen and stomach weakness type: Invigorate spleen and tonify stomach, activate blood circulation, soothe collaterals, so use Fu Wei San and add Shen Ling Bai Zhu San. ③ Depletion and deficiency of liver and kidney type: Tonify liver and kidney, nourish Yin and clear Heat, activate blood circulation and soothe collaterals, so use Fu Wei San and add Hu Qian Pills, add or remove components. ④ Phlegm-Damp obstructing collaterals type: Invigorate spleen and replenish kidney, remove Damp and disperse phlegm, so use Fu Wei San and add Er Chen Tang.

(3) Western Medicine treatment

Mainly use drugs intended to nourish nerves, such as Vitamin B1 20mg, three times a day; Vitamin B12 500U, three times a day; energy mixture, once a day by intravenous drip (14 days each month).

(4) Functional exercises

Depending on specific conditions of individual patients, perform targeted functional exercises under physician's instruction, 2 hours both in the morning and in the afternoon everyday.

Part II: Clinical Treatment

（5）手法治疗

有条件者，可给予按摩，针对无力的肢体，每日治疗1小时。

以上采取的综合疗法，治疗效果较明显。在治疗过程中，要注意患者的心理治疗，树立治病的信心与决心，配合治疗。

三、注意事项

1. 治疗后，要改善居住条件及生活习惯，注意锻炼身体，增强体质，预防感冒及上呼吸道感染。

2. 注意保温，尤其在寒冷季节，特别是春季更应注意保温。

3. 治疗过程中，要有计划、有针对性地进行功能训练，保证正常的工作和生活能力。

四、典型病例

王某，女，38岁，职员，北京人。

主诉：复视，双下肢无力5年，近日加重。病史：患者于2003年11月15日无明显诱因出现视物模糊伴复

(5) Manipulation therapy

If possible, patients can take massage for flaccid limbs, 1 hour a day.

The comprehensive therapy above has relatively significant efficacies. During treatment, attention should be paid to patient's psychological treatment, to let them be confident, determinate and cooperative during the treatment.

III. Precautions

1. After treatment, it is necessary to improve living conditions and living habits, pay attention to physical exercises, strengthen physique, prevent cold and infections of the upper respiratory tract.

2. Pay attention to warm keeping, especially in the cold seasons; in particular, be aware of keeping warm in the spring.

3. During treatment, pay attention to functional exercises to cooperate with the treatment (with scheduled, targeted functional exercises), and abilities to do activities of normal work as well as daily living must be promised (sound functions).

IV. Typical Case

Wang, female, 38 years old, employee, residence: Beijing.

Self-reported symptoms: Diplopia, limb weakness for 5 years, which was aggravated recently. Medical history: On the 15th, November, 2003, the patient developed blurred vision with diplopia without induced causes, and

视，1个月后慢慢缓解，但视力下降。自2003年12月至2004年5月，患者先出现右侧上、下肢端麻木，逐渐发展至肢体无力，进而行走困难，小便不利，大便失禁及脐以下感觉消失。经美国当地医院住院治疗，头部CT、MRI及脊髓液检查后，诊断为"多发性硬化"。经治疗稍缓解，患者可扶物行走500m。2004年7月16日，患者突发左上肢颤抖，左下肢运动障碍，颈、腰部软弱无力，不能坐立，再次住院治疗，给予激素、维生素类药物以及化疗、康复治疗，但症状无缓解，故回国就医。

刻下症：自觉躯干及四肢麻木，右侧为著，行动受限，可扶物行走，复视，纳差，饮食尚可，舌淡苔白，脉细。

查体：复视，视物模糊。小腹右侧压痛，未触及包块。左侧肱二头肌腱反射消失，右侧肱二头肌腱反射减弱，膝腱反射存在，病理反射未引出。

辅助检查：头部CT示"大脑顶叶脑室旁多发性新鲜及少量陈旧脑白质坏死病灶"。脊

it got relieved 1 month later, but the patient's eyesight declined. From December 2003 to May 2004, the patient first developed numbness of right upper and lower limb ends, which gradually developed into weakness of body and limbs, then subsequently difficulty in walking, inhibited urination, faecal incontinence and sensation disappearance of parts below the umbilicus. The patient received inpatient treatment at a local US hospital, and after examinations of cranial CT, MRI and CSF, the patient was diagnosed as "multiple sclerosis". The patient achieved relief after treatment, and could walk for 500 m with support. July 16th, 2004, the patient suddenly suffered from trembling of the left upper limb, dyskinesia of the left lower limb, weakness and feebleness of the neck and waist area, and could not sit or stand, so was sent to the hospital for inpatient treatment again. The symptoms didn't got relieved after administration of hormone and vitamin drugs. So the patient went back to China for treatment.

Current symptoms: Self-felt numbness of body and limbs, especially the right side, limited movements, walking with support, diplopia, poor appetite, fair diet, light tongue with white fur, thin pulse.

Physical examination: Diplopia, blurred vision. Tenderness at right side of the lower abdomen, no lump palpated. The reflex of left biceps tendon disappeared, the reflex of right biceps tendon reduced, the reflex of knee tendon existed, no pathological reflex induced.

Auxiliary examination: Cranial CT indicated "multiple new and few old cerebral white matter necrotic lesions beside the cerebral ventricle of the parietal lobe".

髓 MRI 示"脊髓多发新鲜坏死灶"。脑脊液检查示 T 淋巴细胞为主的细胞数增多, IgG 增高及 IgG 单克隆带出现。

【诊断依据】

1. 患者女性, 38 岁。

2. 头部 CT 示"大脑顶叶侧脑室旁多发新鲜与少量陈旧脑白质坏死灶"。脊髓 MRI 示"脊髓多发新鲜坏死灶"。

3. 症状: 四肢无力, 以右侧为甚; 双眼视物模糊, 复视; 左侧胸腹部刺痛伴紧束（捆）感。

4. 体征: 左侧肱二头肌腱反射消失, 右侧肱二头肌腱反射减弱, 左侧踝阵挛及巴宾斯基征（+）, 左跟、膝、胫试验不协调。

5. 脑脊液检查: 可见 T 淋巴细胞为主的细胞数增多, 蛋白质轻度增高, IgG 增高。

【证治分析】

病因 肝肾不足, 痰湿阻络。

证候分析 患者素体虚亏, 又劳倦过度, 耗伤精血, 精血同源, 由肝肾生成而收藏。肝主筋, 开窍于目; 肾主骨, 腰为肾之府。精血亏虚, 精血不能上荣于目, 故视物不清; 经

Spinal MRI indicated "multiple new necrotic lesions of the spinal cord". CSF examination indicated increased cell count, mainly increased T lymphocyte count, and occurrence of increased IgG and IgG clone bands.

[Diagnostic Basis]

1. Female patient, 38 years old.

2. Cranial CT indicated "multiple new and few old cerebral white matter necrotic lesions beside the cerebral ventricle of the parietal lobe". Spinal MRI indicated "multiple new necrotic lesions of spinal cord".

3. Symptoms: Limb weakness, especially right-side limbs; blurred vision, diplopia; prickling and tightly tied (bound) feeling of the left thorax and abdomen area.

4. Physical signs: The reflex of left biceps tendon disappeared, the reflex of right biceps tendon reduced, left ankle clonus and Babinski's sign (+), incoordination of left heel, knee and shin in the test.

5. CSF examination: Increased cell count, mainly increased T lymphocyte count can be found, mild protein increase, IgG increase.

[Syndrome-treatment Analysis]

Etiology: Deficiency of liver and kidney, phlegm-Damp obstructing collaterals.

Syndrome analysis: The patient suffered from body deficiency and depletion, plus overfatigue, therefore consumed essence and blood, while the essence and blood are from the same source, which are generated and stored by liver and kidney. Liver governs tendons, and opens at eyes; kidney governs bones, and waist is the

脉失养，故肢体震颤麻木。

病位 脑、脊髓。

病性 虚实夹杂，以虚为主。

预后 70%以上的患者首次发作后经过几天或几个月的治疗有所好转，有的可完全恢复正常。但多数患者随病程的进展，每次发作后恢复得不完全。急起的感觉，视神经症状发展较缓慢，涉及运动或小脑的症状预后较好。确诊 MS 的患者，25 年后大约 3/4 者尚存活，其中 2/3 者尚可行动，1/3 者可从事工作。临床上可见纯粹复发缓解型比进展基础上重叠复发缓解型为好，持续进展型的预后最差。

西医诊断 多发性硬化。

中医诊断 痿证（肝肾不足型、痰湿阻络型）。

治法 治痿独取阳明。

方法 电热针治疗、中药

place where kidneys locate. Essence and blood depletion and deficiency causes that essence and blood can not go up to eyes, therefore leads to blurred vision; nourishment loss of tendons and channels, therefore causes tremor and numbness of limbs and body.

Lesion location: Brain, spine cord.

Disease nature: Intermingled deficiency and excess, while the deficiency dominates.

Prognosis: After the first onset, more than 70% patients can get improvement after several days or months of treatment, and some even can recover completely. However most patients, along with the progressing of disease course, the recovery after each attack is not complete. The attack is sudden, while the symptoms of optic nerves develop relatively slowly, and symptoms involving movements or cerebellum have better prognosis. For patients diagnosed as MS, around 3/4 still survive after 25 years, among which 2/3 still can move, and 1/3 still can work. Pure recurrence can be seen clinically. Relapsing-remitting type can have overlapping recurrences based on the progressive type. The prognosis of relapsing-remitting type is better, and that of continuous progressive type is worst.

The diagnosis of Western Medicine: Multiple sclerosis.

The diagnosis of Traditional Chinese Medicine: Flaccidity syndrome (liver and kidney deficiency type, phlegm-Damp obstructing collaterals type).

Therapeutic method: Use Yang-Ming alone for treatment of flaccidity.

Method: Electrothermal acupuncture treatment,

下篇 临床论治　Part II: Clinical Treatment

治疗、穴位按摩、功能训练。

（1）电热针治疗

处方　肩髃（LI15）、曲池（LI11）、合谷（LI4）、阳溪（LI5）、髀关（ST31）、梁丘（ST34）、足三里（ST36）、解溪（ST41）。

方义　根据《素问·痿论》"治痿独取阳明"的治则，痿证以取阳明经为主，取手阳明经的肩髃、曲池、合谷、阳溪，取足阳明经的髀关、梁丘、足三里、解溪，以健运脾胃，益气养血，濡养宗筋；阳陵泉为筋之会，用以调整筋脉之功，悬钟为髓之会，与阳陵泉配伍，能充骨髓、益筋脉。诸穴共用，可奏补脾益胃、强健筋骨之功效。

配穴　肝肾阴亏加肝俞、肾俞；瘫痪不起加大椎、腰阳关、命门、两侧华佗夹脊穴。

操作　选定穴位，皮肤常规消毒。电热针直刺肩髃、曲池、足三里、髀关、阳陵泉、

Chinese Herb Medicine treatment, acupoint massage, functional exercises.

(1) Electrothermal acupuncture treatment

Prescription: Jianyu (LI15), Quchi (LI11), Hegu (LI4), Yangxi (LI5), Biguan (ST31), Liangqiu (ST34), Zusanli (ST36), Jiexi (ST41).

Mechanism of prescription: According to the description of "use Yang-Ming alone for treatment of flaccidity" in the *Plain Questions—Theory of Flaccidity* (《素问·痿论》) for treatment of flaccidity syndrome, mainly use the acupoints from Yang-Ming Meridian. Therefore use Jianyu, Quchi, Hegu, Yangxi from Yang-Ming Meridian of Hand. Use Biguan, Liangqiu, Zusanli, Jiexi from Yang-Ming Meridian of Foot to promote transportation of spleen and stomach, tonify Qi and nourish blood, tonify convergent tendon. Yanglingquan is a confluent acupoint of tendons, which is used to regulate tendons and channels, Xuanzhong is a confluent acupoint of marrow, when being matched with Yanglingquan it can replenish bone marrow and tonify tendons and channels. The use of combination of these acupoints can invigorate spleen and tonify stomach, strengthen tendons and bones.

Matching acupoints: For Yin depletion of liver and kidney add Ganshu, Shenshu. For paralysis add Dazhui, Yaoyangguan, Mingmen, Huatuo Jiayu acupoints on both sides.

Operations: Selecting the relevant acupoints, perform routine skin disinfection. Using electrothermal acupuncture needles, vertically puncture into Jianyu,

· 365 ·

梁丘各 0.7 寸，接通电热针仪，每个穴位分别给予电流量 40～50mA（分为两组，每组 3 组穴，轮流交替应用），留针 40 分钟。余穴用毫针治疗。

疗程 每日 1 次，90 次为 1 个疗程，疗程间休息 10～15 天，根据病情需要再进行第 2 个疗程的治疗。一般治疗 1～2 个疗程即可。

（2）中药治疗

补肝肾强筋骨，化痰活血通络。组成：胆南星 10g，全蝎 5g，明天麻 10g，蜈蚣 1 条，黄芪 30g，杜仲 10g，鸡血藤 15g，当归 15g，川芎 10g，桃仁 10g，赤芍 10g，灵芝 15g，焦白术 15g，川续断 10g，山药 15g，山萸肉 15g，菊花 10g，枸杞子 15g。每日 1 剂，水煎服，早、晚分服。

（3）穴位按摩

在医师的指导下自行按摩，每日 1 次，每次 30～60 分钟。

Quchi, Zusanli, Bigua, Yanglingquan, Liangqiu for 0.7" respectively. Turn on the electrothermal acupuncture equipment, apply a current of 40-50mA to each acupoint (divide the acupoints into two groups, 3 for each, and use alternatively), leaving the needles in for 40 minutes. Treat the other acupoints with filiform needles.

Therapeutic course: Treat once a day, 90 times for a course, and start the treatment for the second course depending on the conditions after a break of 10-15 days. Generally 1-2 courses are enough.

(2) Chinese Herb Medicine treatment

Replenish liver and kidney, strengthen tendons and bones, disperse phlegm, activate blood circulation and soothe collaterals. Composition: bile arisaema 10g, whole scorpion 5g, rhizona gastrodiae 10g, one centipede, root of astragalus membranaceus 30g, bark of eucommia 10g, suberect spatholobus stem 15g, Chinese angelica 15g, Ligusticum wallichii 10g, peach kernel 10g, root of common peony 10g, lucid ganoderma 15g, deep-fried atractylodes macrocephala koidz 15g, teasel 10g, Chinese yam 15g, pulp of dogwood fruit 15g, chrysanthemum 10g, the fruit of Chinese wolfberry 15g. One dose a day, decocted in water for oral dose, divided into two halves and take one each in the morning and in the evening respectively.

(3) Acupoint massage

Do self-massage under physician's instruction, once a day, 30-60 minutes each time.

（4）功能训练

根据患者的具体病情制订合理、切合实际的训练方案，在医师的指导下进行，每日2次，上、下午各做1次。

治疗过程　以上针灸、中药、按摩、功能训练之综合疗法，治疗6个月。治疗3个月后，患者可自由行动，达到生活自理，能外出步行1500m。随访，患者病情有反复，还要继续巩固治疗，方法同上。

【生活调摄】

1. 令患者注意情绪控制，要有一个平和乐观的心态，多与人交往，改善生活兴趣。

2. 注意预防感冒，适当保温，改善居住环境，居住地方应明亮、温暖并充满阳光。

3. 饮食合理，应清淡又富有营养。

4. 加强功能训练，保持各关节的正常功能，努力健身以增强体质。

脊髓空洞症

脊髓空洞症是脊髓的慢性进行性变性疾病。其病理特征为脊髓中央部的空洞形成。临床特点是肌肉萎缩和节段性分离性感觉障碍。空洞位于脊髓

(4) Functional exercises

Develop reasonable, practicable exercise schemes depending on the patients' conditions, and let them do the exercises under physician's instruction, twice a day, one in the morning and one in the afternoon.

Therapeutic process: Use the comprehensive therapy of acupuncture, Chinese Herb Medicine, massage, functional exercises to treat for 6 months. After 3 months of treatment, the patient can move freely, care herself and can walk outside for 1500m. Follow-up, there are relapses, she need to continue the consolidation treatment, the method is the same as above.

[Lifestyle Change and Health Maintenance]

1. Let the patients pay attention to emotional control, have a peaceful and optimistic attitude, more socialize themselves and enjoy life.

2. Prevent cold and keep warm appropriately, improve living environment, and the living place should be bright, warm and full of sunlight.

3. Proper diet, light and full of nutrition.

4. Increase functional exercises, keep normal functions of all joints, make efforts to enhance physical fitness.

Syringomyelia

Syringomyelia is a chronic progressive degenerative disease of the spine cord. Its pathologic characteristic is porosis in the central part of spinal cord. The clinical characteristics are amyotrophia and segmental dissociated sensory disturbances. Porosis is most common at the

颈段者最常见，可向下延伸至胸髓、腰髓，少数患者向上延伸到延髓。空洞常开始于中央灰质，不规则地向周围扩展，可能与中央管相通。洞壁由胶质细胞等覆盖，内含无色液体。延髓空洞多呈裂隙状，位于延髓被盖外侧部。

一、诊断及辨证要点

1. 多见于 25～40 岁，起病隐袭，进展缓慢。

2. 临床表现取决于空洞所存在的部位及破坏脊髓的范围。

3. 感觉障碍：不少患者因手无痛性伤害而意外发现痛、温觉缺失而触觉及深感觉正常。这种分离性感觉缺失的分布呈"半马甲型"或"马甲型"痛，温觉障碍区内可出现自发性剧痛。空洞进一步扩大侵犯后束，出现病灶同侧深感觉障碍。若侵及脊上束则对侧病变水平以下出现痛、温觉障碍。

4. 运动障碍：有些患者因手部肌肉萎缩而就诊，可影响整个上肢。如果累及脊椎体

cervical segment of spine, which can expand downwards to the thoracic segment and lumbar segment. In a few cases the porosis can expand upwards to the medulla oblongata. The porosis normally starts from the center of the gray matter and expand irregularly to the surrounding area. It may connect to the central canal. The cavity wall is covered by substance like colloid cells containing colorless liquid. Medulla cavities mostly are crack-like, located at the exterior medulla tegmentum.

I. Key Points for Diagnosis and Syndrome Differentiation

1. Most are seen among people aged 25-40 years, insidious onset, slow progress.

2. The clinical manifestations depend on the location of cavities and the range of damaged spine cord.

3. Sensory disturbance: Many patients found analgesia and athalposis due to painless injuries of hand, while touch sensation and deep sensation are normal. The distribution of this dissociated sensory disturbance presents as "half-vest shape" or "vest shape" pain area, and spontaneous intensive pain may occur in the area of athalposis. The cavity further expends and invades the posterior cord, then deep sensory disturbance on the same side as the lesion will occur. If the superior cord is involved, then dysalgia and temperature sensory disturbance below the contralateral lesion level.

4. Dyskinesia: Some patients make visits due to amyotrophia of hand, which can affect the whole upper limb. If the vertebral body bundle is involved, then spas-

束，则下肢出现痉挛性瘫痪。

5. 神经营养障碍：在病变分布区域出现出汗异常，皮肤发绀，破溃后易产生无痛性溃疡。指骨吸收，甚至指尖自动脱落（Morvan's 综合征）。20%的患者伴 Charcot 关节；如病变侵及颈 7 或胸 1 侧角，可有 Horner 征；晚期患者可有括约肌功能障碍。

6. 延髓空洞症较少见，多由脊髓空洞向上延伸而成，亦可单独出现。大多为单侧性，表现为周边部分痛、温觉缺失，声带、软腭瘫痪，舌肌萎缩、纤颤，眼球震颤。

7. 一般根据临床症状可作出诊断。

8. MRI 检查可见相应节段的脊髓增粗，呈半球状，中央有低信号的积水区。

9. 风寒者，症见项强，颈及肩臂疼痛，活动不利，尤以上肢为甚，手无力，伸屈不灵，伴肢体麻木，面色不华，头昏眼花，心悸，失眠，四肢不温，日久肢体肌肉萎缩，舌淡苔薄，脉细弱。

10. 气滞血瘀者，症见头颈肩背及肢体疼痛、麻木，其

tic paralysis of lower limbs will occur.

5. Dystrophia disorder: In the area of lesion distribution, there are abnormal sweating and skin cyanosis, which are easy to be developed into painless ulcers after rupture. Phalange absorption, or even automatic fall-off of finger tips (Morvan's syndrome). 20% patients have concurrent Charcot joints. If the lesion invades into the Cervical Vertebra 7 or Thoracic Vertebra 1 lateral corner, there may be Horner syndrome. In the advanced phase patients may have sphincter dysfunction.

6. Syringobulbia is less common, and in most cases it is caused by upward extension of the spine cord cavity. Also it can occur alone. Most are unilateral ones, and manifestations include pain of the surrounding area, athalposis, vocal cord paralysis, paralysis of soft palate, tongue muscle atrophy, fibrillation, nystagmus.

7. Generally the diagnosis can be made based on clinical symptoms.

8. In the MRI examination there can be seen spine cord thickening of the respective segment, with a shape of hemispherical, and there is a low-signal water accumulated area in the center.

9. For patients with Wind-Cold, symptoms include stiff neck, pain of neck, shoulder and arms, inhibited movements, weakness of hand, inhibited stretching and flexing, accompanying cold limbs, amyotrophia of limbs after long-term disease course, light tongue with thin fur, thin and weak pulse.

10. For patients with Qi stagnation and blood stasis, symptoms include pains and numbness of head, neck,

痛多为刺痛，固定不移而拒按，手部肌肉萎缩，指端麻木，指甲凹陷，无光泽，皮肤枯燥而痒，有的可有肢体无力或抽痛。尚可见头晕目眩，视物模糊，失眠健忘，烦躁，肌肤甲错，面色无华，舌紫黯或有瘀斑，脉弦细或弦涩。

11. 风寒湿痹者，症见头项肩背和四肢疼痛，痛有定处，喜热恶寒，颈僵，活动受限，上肢沉重、无力、麻木，肌肉萎缩，手指伸屈不利，指端麻木，不知痛痒，舌胖有齿痕，脉沉迟或弦。

二、治疗方法

【风寒证】

治法 祛风散寒，调和营卫。

处方 大椎（DU14）、天柱（BL10）、肩外俞（SI14）、悬钟（GB39）、后溪（SI3）。

方义 大椎是督脉经穴，又是诸阳之会，督脉为阳脉之海，天柱为足太阳膀胱经经穴，肩外俞是手太阳小肠经经穴，三穴相伍，能祛风散寒，

shoulder and limbs, and the pains mostly are prickling, fixed and unmoved, refused to be pressed; amyotrophia of hand, numbness of finger tips, depressed fingernails without luster, dry and itching skin; and in some cases there may be limb weakness or throbbing pain. As well as dizziness and vertigo, blurred vision, insomnia and amnesia, vexation, squamous and dry skin, gloomy complexion, dark and purple tongue or with ecchymosis, taut and thin or taut and uneven pulse.

11. For patients with Wind-Cold-Damp arthralgia, symptoms include pains of head, neck, shoulder and limbs, and the pain lesion is fixed; preference for warm and aversion to cold, stiff neck, limited movements, heavy-feeling, weakness, numbness of upper limbs, amyotrophia, inhibited stretching and flexing of fingers, numbness of finger tips with no feeling of pain or itching, fat tongue with teeth prints, deep and slow or taut pulse.

II. Therapeutic Methods

[Syndrome of Wind-Cold]

Therapeutic method: Dispel wind and disperse cold, tonify Ying and Wei for balance.

Prescription: Dazhui (DU14), Tianzhu (BL10), Jianwaishu (SI14), Xuanzhong (GB39), Houxi (SI3).

Mechanism of prescription: Dazhui is a meridian acupoint of Du Channel, as well as the confluent point of all Yangs. Du Channel is the sea of Yang channels. Tianzhu is a meridian acupoint of Tai-Yang Bladder Meridian of Foot, Jianwaishu is a meridian acupoint of Tai-Yang

宣通后项部及肩部经气，用于颈肌发僵或拘挛、肩背疼痛；悬钟是足少阳胆经穴、髓会，与通督脉的八脉交会穴后溪共用，可以疏通后颈项部经气，使督脉与少阳经在颈部及四肢气血得以畅通。诸穴合用，共奏祛风散寒、调和营卫之功效。

配穴 表郁明显者，加合谷、风池；表虚者，加足三里、列缺；前后不能俯仰者，加昆仑、列缺；不能回顾者，加支正、后溪；头痛者，加太阳、百会、风府。

方法 电热针治疗。

操作 选定穴位，皮肤常规消毒。电热针向下斜刺大椎 0.7 寸，直刺天柱 0.7 寸，斜刺肩外俞 0.6 寸，直刺悬钟 0.7 寸，直刺合谷、风池、太阳、昆仑各 0.6 寸，平刺列缺 0.7 寸，平刺百会 0.7 寸，直刺风府 0.7 寸，接通电热针仪，每个穴位分别给予电流量 30～50mA，以胀感舒适为度，留针 40 分钟。（注：每次

Small Intestine Meridian of Hand, the match of these three acupoints can dispel wind and disperse cold, dredge the meridian Qi of back neck and shoulder, relieve stiffness or spasm of neck muscles, shoulder and back pains. Xuanzhong is an acupoint of Shao-Yang Gallbladder Meridian of Foot, the convergent place of marrow, when being used together with the confluent acupoints of eight channels, Houxi, which is connected to Du Channel, it can dredge the meridian Qi of back neck, let Du Channel and Shao-Yang Meridian in the neck and Qi-blood of limbs be smooth. The use of combination of these acupoints can dispel Wind and disperse Cold, tonify Ying and Wei for balance.

Matching acupoints: For obvious exterior stasis, add Hegu, Fengchi. For exterior deficiency, add Zusanli, Lieque. For incapability of moving upwards and downwards, add Kunlun, Lieque. For incapability of turning back, add Zhizheng, Houxi. For headache, add Taiyang, Baihui, Fengfu.

Method: Electrothermal acupuncture treatment.

Operations: Selecting the relevant acupoints, perform routine skin disinfection. Using electrothermal acupuncture needles, obliquely puncture toward into Dazhui for 0.7", vertically puncture into Tianzhu for 0.7", obliquely puncture into Jianwaishu for 0.6", vertically puncture into Xuanzhong for 0.7", vertically puncture into Hegu, Fengchi, Taiyang, Kunlun for 0.6" respectively, horizontally puncture into Lieque for 0.7", horizontally puncture into Baihui for 0.7", vertically puncture into Fengfu for 0.7". Turn on the electrothermal acupuncture equipment, apply a current of 30-50mA to each acupoint,

选 3～4 组穴，交替使用；头部穴位给予电流量 30mA。）

疗程 每日 1 次，30 次为 1 个疗程，中间休息 7～10 天，继续进行第 2 个疗程的治疗。

【气滞血瘀证】

治法 活血化瘀，疏通经脉。

处方 大椎（DU14）、肩井（GB21）、肩髃（LI15）、养老（SI6）、条口（ST38）、膈俞（BL17），以及相应颈夹脊穴或哑穴 1～4、颈百劳（EX-HN15）。

方义 证属痹证日久，督脉受累，致血气瘀阻，故取阳经交会穴大椎及相应病变颈椎之夹脊穴、哑穴或颈百劳，以通利诸阳之经脉，调和督脉气血，使颈椎局部气滞血瘀得以消散；取肩井与经筋结聚之肩髃，使少阳、阳明经气得通；养老乃手太阳之郄穴，能舒筋通络，是历代医家治疗颈椎病之经验穴；条口为阳明经穴，阳明多气多血，二穴合用能理气活血；膈俞是血会，取之以除血分之瘀滞。诸穴合用，能活血化瘀，疏通经脉之痹阻。

and the limit is that the patient feels comfortable and swelling, leaving the needles in for 40 minutes. (Note: Select 3-4 pairs of acupoints each time, and use alternately, apply a current of 30mA to each acupoint at the head region.)

Therapeutic course: Treat once a day, 30 times for a course, and start the treatment for the second course after a break of 7-10 days.

[Syndrome of Qi Stagnation and Blood Stasis]

Therapeutic method: Activate blood circulation and remove stasis, soothe meridians and channels.

Prescription: Dazhui (DU14), Jianjing (GB21), Jianyu (LI15), Yanglao (Si6), Tiaokou (ST38), Geshu (BL17), and corresponding Jiaji acupoints of neck or Ya acupoints 1-4, Jingbailao (EX-HN15),

Mechanism of prescription: Long-term arthralgia syndrome affects Du Channel therefore leads to Qi-blood stagnation and stasis, so use the confluent acupoint Dazhui of Yang meridians and the corresponding Jiaji acupoint (lesion site of neck) or Bailao to soothe meridians and collaterals of all Yangs, regulate Qi-blood of Du Channel, so as to disperse the Qi stagnation and blood stasis of local cervical vertebra. Use Jianjing and the confluent site of meridians and tendons, Jianyu, to dredge meridian Qi of Shao-Yang and Yang-Ming meridians; Yanglao is a Xi acupoint of Tai-Yang Meridian of Hand, it can relax tendons and activate collaterals, is a historically used experienced acupoint for cervical spondylosis treatment; Tiaokou is a meridian acupoint of Yang-Ming Meridian of Foot, Yang-Ming Meridian is full of Qi and blood, so the combination of these two can regulate Qi, activate blood; Geshu is the confluent acupoint of blood, it can remove the stagnation of blood system. The use of combination of these acupoints can activate blood circulation and remove stasis, soothe retention of stagnation in the meridians and channels.

Matching acupoints: For dry skin, amyotrophia add Zusanli, Sanyinjiao and Yanglingquan to nourish blood and tendons. For dizziness and blurred sight, insomnia and amnesia, add Xinshu, Ganshu, Zusanli to nourish blood, tranquilize mind and improve eyesight.

Method: Electrothermal acupuncture treatment.

Operations: Selecting the relevant acupoints, perform routine skin disinfection. Using electrothermal acupuncture needles, obliquely puncture downwards into Dazhui for 0.7", vertically puncture into Jianjing for 0.6", puncture into Jianyu for 0.8" with the needle tip towards the arm, obliquely puncture toward the elbow into Yanglao for 0.7", vertically punture into Tiaokou for 0.8", obliquely puncture (with the needle tip towards spine) into Geshu for 0.7", vertically puncture into Zusanli, Sanyinjiao, Yanglingquan for 0.8" respectively, obliquely puncture (with the needle tip towards spine) into Xinshu, Ganshu for 0.7" respectively. Turn on the electrothermal acupuncture equipment, apply a current of 50mA to each acupoint, and the limit is that the patient feels warm or swelling and comfortable, leaving the needles in for 40 minutes. (Note: Select 3 pairs of acupoints each time, and use alternately.)

Therapeutic course: Treat once a day, 30 times for a course, and start the treatment for the second course

继续进行第 2 个疗程的治疗。

【风寒湿痹证】

治法 祛风散寒，舒筋通络除痹。

处方 大椎（DU14）、风池（GB20）、天柱（BL10）、肩井（GB21）、外关（SJ5），以及相应病变颈椎之夹脊穴或膀胱经穴、哑穴 1～4。

方义 取诸阳之会大椎及相应的颈夹脊穴、膀胱经穴或哑穴，能祛风散寒、疏通经脉，配足少阳胆经之肩井、阳维之会风池及天柱，能宣痹通络。外关是手少阳之络穴，配合上述诸穴，可奏活血通络之功。诸穴共用，可取祛风散寒、舒筋通络除痹之功效。

配穴 改善四肢与手的症状，加肩髃、曲池、手三里、阳溪、合谷、后溪、大陵（每次选 2～3 个穴）；颈部活动受限，加昆仑、列缺；胸闷纳呆加中脘。

方法 电热针治疗。

after a break of 7-10 days.

[Syndrome of Wind-Cold-Damp Arthralgia]

Therapeutic method: Dispel Wind and disperse Cold, relax tendons and activate collaterals and remove arthralgia.

Prescription: Dazhui（DU14), Fengchi (GB20), Tianzhu (BL10), Jianjing (GB21), Waiguan (SJ5), and Jiaji acupoints of the corresponding cervical vertebral lesion or acupoints of Bladder Meridian, Ya acupoints 1-4.

Mechanism of prescription: Use the confluent acupoint of all Yangs, Dazhui, and corresponding Jiaji acupoints of neck, acupoints of Bladder Meridian or Ya acupoints, to dispel wind and disperse Cold, soothe meridians and channels, and when being matched with the acupoint Jianjing of Shao-Yang Gallbladder Meridian of Foot and the confluent acupoints of Weijing Channel, Fengchi and Tianzhu, can relieve stagnation and soothe collaterals. Waiguan is a collateral acupoint of Shao-Yang Meridian of Hand, it can activate blood and soothe collaterals when being matched with the above acupoints. The use of combination of these acupoints can dispel Wind and disperse Cold, relax tendons and activate collaterals and remove arthralgia.

Matching acupoints: for improvement of symptoms at limbs as well as at hands, add Jianliao, Quchi, Shousanli, Yangxi, Hegu, Houxi, Daling (choose 2-3 acupoints each time); for limited neck movement, add Kunlun, Lieque. For chest distress and anorexia, add Zhongwan.

Method: Electrothermal acupuncture treatment.

Operations: Selecting the relevant acupoints, perform routine skin disinfection. Using electrothermal acupuncture needles, obliquely puncture toward into Dazhui for 0.7", obliquely puncture toward the contralateral eye into Fengchi for 0.6", vertically puncture into Tianzhu, Jianjing, Waiguan for 0.6" respectively, vertically puncture into Quchi, Shousanli for 0.7" respectively, obliquely puncture with the needle tip towards spine into Jiaji acupoints and meridian acupoints of Bladder Meridian for 0.6-0.7" respectively, vertically puncture into Houxi, Hegu, Yangxi, Daling for 0.6" respectively, vertically puncture into Zhongwan, Kunlun for 0.7" respectively, horizontally puncture into Lieque for 0.6". Turn on the electrothermal acupuncture equipment, apply a current of 40mA to each acupoint, leaving the needles in for 40 minutes.

Therapeutic course: Once a day, 90 times for a course. Start the treatment for the second course after a break of 10-15 days. The decision for whether carry out the second course of treatment depends on the disease conditions. Generally recovered after 2 courses.

III. Precautions

1. During treatment, for needling of acupoints at the neck and shoulder, the needling direction and depth must be controlled to avoid damage of spine cord and lungs.

2. Massage is also necessary during the acupuncture treatment, especially for limbs with amyotrophia.

3. Instruct patients to do corresponding functional exercises to ensure recovery of limb physiological func-

恢复。

4. 病情严重的患者一定要采取综合疗法，如中西药、针灸、按摩、功能训练，促进患者早日康复。

重症肌无力

重症肌无力是一种神经肌肉接头传递功能障碍的慢性疾病。主要临床表现是受累的骨骼肌极易疲劳，经休息后有一定的恢复，其中以眼睑下垂、复视等为主症的眼肌受累者最为多见，约占90%以上，严重病例可累及全身随意肌群。本病以10～35岁多见。女性发病率高于男性，感染、精神刺激、过度疲劳、分娩以及某些药物等可以促进本病发作及加重。

中医认为，本病属于"痿证""睑废"的范畴，病变主要涉及脾胃。脾胃为后天之本、气血生化之源，如素体脾胃虚弱或因病致虚，脾胃受纳运化功能失调，气血化生不足，肌肉筋脉失养，渐而成痿；若原有痿证经久不愈，导致脾胃虚弱，甚至病久及髓，肝肾受损，又可使痿证加重。

tions.

4. For severe patients a comprehensive therapy, like the combination of Chinese Herb Medicine treatment, Western Medicine treatment, massage, functional exercises, must be adopted to facilitate the early recovery.

Myasthenia Gravis

Myasthenia gravis is a chronic disease with transmission disorder of neuromuscular junctions. Main clinical manifestations include fatigue-affected skeletal muscles, and the fatigue can be relieved to a certain extent after rest. The most common is eye muscle involvement with main symptoms like ptosis and diplopia, which accounted for 90% of the cases, and in severe cases any muscle group of the body can be involved. Mostly common among people of 10-35 years old. More female patients than male patients; infections, mental stimulations, over-fatigue, deliveries and administration of certain drugs can promote the onset and aggravation of the disease.

Traditional Chinese Medicine believes that this disease belongs to the range of "flaccidity syndrome", "blepharoptosis". The lesions main involve spleen and stomach. Spleen and stomach are the foundation of acquired constitution, the source of generation and transformation of Qi-blood. For example, weakness of spleen and stomach or diseases cause deficiency, dysfunction of food reception as well as transportation and transformation of spleen and stomach, insufficient of generation and transformation of Qi-blood, nourishment loss of muscles as well as tendons and channels, gradually leading to flaccidity. If previous flaccidity syndrome is not cured after long-term treatment and causes weakness of spleen and stomach, or even the long-term disease develops into the bone cord and causes damages of liver and kidney, then the flaccidity syndrome can be aggravated.

一、诊断及辨证要点

I. Key Points for Diagnosis and Syndrome Differentiation

1. 以受累横纹肌为主症，晨轻晚重，休息后减轻，多次活动后加重，多在 10～35 岁起病，女性较多。

1. The main symptom involves with striated muscles, which is mild in the morning and severe in the evening, relieved after rest and aggravated after several times of movement. Most of onsets occur at the age of 10-35. More female patients than male ones.

2. 根据受累部位不同可分为三型，部分为混合型，其主要表现如下：

2. It can be divided into three types depending on the areas, and some are mixed type. The main manifestations are as followed:

（1）眼肌型：眼睑下垂，眼外肌麻痹而斜视、复视等。

(1) Eye muscle type: Ptosis, strabismus and diplopia due to external ophthalmoplegia.

（2）球型：声音低哑，构音不清，吞咽困难，饮水反呛；重者尚有咀嚼无力，以致进食困难，面部表情肌无力。

(2) Bulbar type: Low and hoarse voice, asophia, dysphonia, gastric reflex; in severe cases there may be weakness in chewing, leading to difficulty in feeding, weakness of facial expression muscles.

（3）全身型：全身横纹肌均有不同程度的受累，严重者因呼吸肌无力，出现呼吸、咳痰困难而危及生命。

(3) Systemic type: The striated muscles of the whole body are involved with different levels, and in severe cases the patient's life may be threatened due to difficulties in breathing and expectoration caused by weakness of respiratory muscles.

3. 临床结合试验帮助诊断。

3. Combine clinical symptoms and tests to facilitate diagnosis.

（1）疲劳试验：受累肌群做快速、重复动作后出现疲劳。

(1) Fatigue test: Fatigue occurs after rapid and repeated movement of the affected muscle group. For

例如，提上眼睑肌受累有睑下垂，嘱闭眼稍休息后，睑下垂即见改善或消失，再嘱患者两眼持续向上凝视，片刻后眼睑下垂又出现或加重。

（2）抗胆碱酯酶药物试验：肌肉注射新斯的明 0.5～1mg，半小时至 1 小时后有显著效果者，即可确诊为本病。

（3）电刺激试验：以感应电持续刺激受损肌，短时间内不发生收缩，称为肌无力。

4. 重症肌无力危象诊断要点：重症肌无力患者，病程中有两种危象可能会出现，即肌无力危象及胆碱能危象。两者都有肌无力和通气严重不足，表现为呼吸困难，吞咽困难，咳嗽及排痰无力。应严格鉴别，以免延误病情及抢救。

（1）肌无力危象：①多在感染、创伤、月经、妊娠、分娩、减药或停药后发生。②无抗胆碱酯酶药物中毒症状。③应用氯化滕喜龙静脉注射（方法：先注入 2mg，如无反应，30 秒后再注入 8mg），呼吸肌和咽部肌力有明显改善。

（2）胆碱能危象：①由于胆碱酯酶药物应用过量所

example, ptosis occurs after lifting of the upper eyelid muscle, and the ptosis is relieved or disappears after rest; then let the patient continuously peering upwards with both eyes, a moment later the ptosis occurs again or gets aggravated.

(2) Anti-cholinesterase drug test: Significant effects occur 0.5-1 hour after the muscle injection of 0.5-1mg neostigmine, then the diagnosis of this disease can be conformed.

(3) Electric stimulation test: Continuously stimulate the damaged muscle with induced electricity, and the muscle has no contraction in a short time. This is called myasthenia.

4. Key points of diagnosis for crisis of myasthenia gravis: For patients with myasthenia gravis, two types of crises may occur during the disease course: crisis of myasthenia gravis and cholinergic crisis. The two both include myasthenia and severe hypoventilation, and the manifestations include dyspnea, dysphonia, coughing and weakness in phlegm excretion. Must be strictly identified to avoid delay of the disease and rescue.

(1) Crisis of myasthenia: ① normally occurs after infections, trauma, menstruation, pregnancy, delivery, drug reduction or drug discontinuation. ② No symptom of cholinesterase drug poisoning. ③ Apply IV injection of edrophonium chloride (method: Inject 2mg first, if no response, inject another 8mg 30 seconds later), and the strength of respiratory muscles and pharyngeal muscles show obvious improvement.

(2) Cholinergic crisis: ① Caused by overdose of cholinesterase drugs. ② Often accompanied with symp-

toms of alkalosis like contraction of pupils, increase of tears, saliva, respiratory secretions, abdominal pain, diarrhea, and muscular fasciculation. ③ The condition of myasthenia is aggravated after injection of edrophonium chloride.

5. Syndrome differentiation: This disease is mainly caused by deficiency and impairment of spleen and kidney, and can be roughly divided into three types.

(1) Syndrome of spleen deficiency and Qi weakness: Common in the simple eye muscle type. Symptoms include ptosis, poor appetite, sloppy stool, fat tongue with thin fur, thin pulse.

(2) Syndrome of Qi and Yin deficiency of spleen and kidney: Common in the systemic type, bulbar type or eye muscle type accompanied with diplopia. Accompanied with asthenia, poor appetite, loosen stool, red tongue tip or dry and peeling tongue fur, thin and rapid pulse.

(3) Syndrome of spleen and kidney Yang deficiency: Seen in the systemic type or bulbar type, relatively rare. Symptoms include aversion to cold, soreness and weakness of waist and knees, soft and weak neck, general weakness, light tongue with tooth prints at the edge, thin and white fur, thin and weak pulse.

II. Therapeutic Methods

[Syndrome of Spleen Deficiency and Qi Weakness]

Therapeutic method: Invigorate spleen and replenish Earth, tonify Qi and blood, relax tendons and activate collaterals.

Prescription: Zhongwan (RN12), Xuehai (SP10),

海（SP10）、三阴交（SP6）、足三里（ST36）、气海（RN6）。

方义 中脘调胃健脾理气；足三里健运脾胃，是强壮要穴；三阴交健脾化湿，疏肝益胃；血海有清热和营，活血化瘀的作用；气海补益中气，再配合局部远端的有关穴位，可收健脾培土，补益气血，舒筋活络之功。

配穴 上眼睑下垂者加阳辅、申脉；吞咽困难者加哑门、天突、风池、廉泉；咀嚼无力者加下关、合谷；发音不清者加哑门、廉泉；抬头无力者加风池、天柱、列缺。

方法 电热针治疗。

操作 选定穴位，皮肤常规消毒。电热针直刺中脘0.8寸，直刺足三里0.7寸，直刺三阴交0.7寸。接通电热针仪，每个穴位分别给予电流量60～70mA，以患者感到胀感或温热舒适为度，留针40分钟。根据相应的兼症选择相应的配穴，用毫针给予轻刺激补法，留针40分钟。

疗程 每日1次，90次

Sanyinjiao (SP6), Zusanli (ST36), Qihai (RN6).

Mechanism of prescription: Zhongwan can tonify stomach, invigorate spleen and regulate Qi; Zusanli, an important tonifying acupoint, can promote transportation of spleen and stomach; Sanyinjiao can invigorate spleen and dispel Damp, soothe liver and tonify stomach. Xuehai can clear Heat and regulate Ying, activate blood circulation and remove stasis. Qihai can replenish Middle-Jiao Qi, plus local acupoints of distal ends, they can invigorate spleen and replenish Earth, tonify Qi and blood, relax tendons and activate collaterals.

Matching acupoints: For ptosis add Yangfu, Shenmai. For dysphonia add Yamen, Tiantu, Fengchi, Lianquan. For weakness in chewing add Xiaguan, Hegu. For asophia add Yamen, Lianquan. For weakness in head raising add Fengchi, Tianzhu, Lieque.

Method: Electrothermal acupuncture treatment.

Operations: Selecting the relevant acupoints, perform routine skin disinfection. Using electrothermal acupuncture needles, vertically puncture into Zhongwan for 0.8", Zusanli for 0.7", Sanyinjiao for 0.7". Turn on the electrothermal acupuncture equipment, apply a current of 60-70mA to each acupoint, and the limit is that the patient feels swelling or warm and comfortable, leaving the needles in for 40 minutes. Choose matching acupoints as per corresponding accompanied with symptoms, apply tonifying method with slight stimulation using filiform needles, leave the needles in for 40 minutes.

Therapeutic course: Treat once a day, 90 times for

为 1 个疗程，疗程间可休息 7～10 天，再进行第 2 个疗程的治疗。一般治疗 1～2 个疗程，病情即能控制。

三、注意事项

1. 针灸治疗重症肌无力的疗效较好，但必须帮助患者树立信心配合治疗，因为疗程较长，只要能坚持配合治疗均能获效。

2. 在针治的同时配合药物（中药）治疗能够提高疗效，缩短治疗时间。尤其对早期重症肌无力患者的疗效较好。

3. 在治疗期间要保持良好的心态，避免情绪激动，注意休息，避免过劳。

4. 对卧床患者，应保持四肢的功能体位，并不断给予变换体位，防止褥疮发生，更要防止造成胯松、足下垂、内翻等。必须注意护理，必要时用护理架及夹板托扶，勤翻身拍背。

5. 患者（严重者）一旦出现肌无力危象，应采取中西医结合的抢救措施。

a course, and start the treatment for the second course after a break of 7-10 days. Generally the condition can be controlled after 1-2 courses of treatment.

III. Precautions

1. Acupuncture therapy has a relatively good efficacy on myasthenia gravis, however due to long treatment course, it is necessary to help patients to be confident and cooperative during the treatment. And efficacies can always be achieved given that patients adhere to cooperate with the treatment.

2. Application of medication (Chinese Herb Medicine therapy) along with the acupuncture therapy can improve efficacies and shorten treatment time. The efficacy is especially good for patients of early myasthenia gravis.

3. During the treatment, patients should keep good mental state, avoid emotional excitement, get proper rest and avoid overstrain.

4. For bedbound patients, the functional positions of limbs should be kept, and continuously change their positions to prevent bed ulcers, not mention to prevent loosing of hips, foot drop and strephenopodia. Pay attention to nursing, use nursing frames and splints if necessary, perform frequent body turnover and backslap.

5. Once patients (critically ill ones) show crisis of myasthenia, the comprehensive rescue measure with Traditional Chinese Medicine and Western Medicine combined should be taken.

脑外伤后神经症

脑外伤后神经症是一种最常见的轻度原发性脑损伤，病发于脑震荡或轻度脑挫伤后数日或数年，仍有头痛；甚至有自主神经系统的体征。临床表现主要是头痛、头晕、记忆力减退、耳鸣、失眠、急躁、心悸、倦怠等。其头痛多为胀痛或悸动性疼痛，常因疲劳、噪音、震动、生活环境或习惯改变而加重，头晕常与体位变化有密切关系。本病有明显的外伤史。

中医认为，本病属于"头痛""眩晕"的范畴。因外伤后气血瘀阻，经络不畅，脑失所养，清阳阻遏所致。由于患者体质不同，发病后多表现为肝肾阴虚证、气虚痰阻证。

一、诊断及辨证要点

1. 肝肾阴虚证，症见头痛、眩晕、耳鸣、失眠、健忘、心悸、急躁、腰膝酸软、舌红瘦、苔黄、脉弦细或弦数。

Neurosis After Traumatic Brain Injury

Neurosis following traumatic brain injury is a most common mild primary brain injury. It attacks several days or several years after cerebral concussion or mild cerebral contusion, with long-lasting headaches or even physical signs of the autonomic nerve system. Main clinical manifestations include headache, dizziness, memory deterioration, tinnitus, insomnia, quick temper, palpitation, fatigue, etc. The headache is mostly distending pain or throbbing pain, often aggravated by tiredness, noise, shake, changes of living environment or habits, and the dizziness normally has close relationship with the change of body position. The onset of this disease is accompanied with a history of significant trauma.

Traditional Chinese Medicine believes that this disease belongs to the range of "headache" and "vertigo". Caused by Qi-blood stagnation and obstructed meridians and collaterals, nourishment loss of brain, repression of Qing-Yang after trauma. Due to different physiques of patients, most are syndrome of Yin deficiency of liver and kidney, syndrome of Qi deficiency and phlegm obstruction.

I. Key Points for Diagnosis and Syndrome Differentiation

1. For syndrome of Yin deficiency of liver and kidney, symptoms include headache, vertigo, tinnitus, insomnia, amnesia, palpitation, soreness and weakness of waist and knees, red and slim tongue with yellow fur, taut and thin or taut and rapid pulse.

2.气虚痰阻证,症见头痛而重、神疲倦怠、反应迟钝、纳呆、恶心、舌淡、苔白腻、脉细滑或涩。

二、治疗方法

【肝肾阴虚证】

治法 行气活血,通络止痛。

处方 风池(GB20)、百会(DU20)、合谷(LI4)、四神聪(EX-HN1)、太冲(LR3)、太溪(KI3)。

方义 风池是足少阳胆经腧穴,百会是督脉腧穴,督脉为阳脉之海,二穴均为治头痛、眩晕之要穴。四神聪是经外奇穴,善治头痛、眩晕、健忘。合谷是大肠经之原穴,长于治头痛之疾,具有行气活血之功效。肝之原穴太冲,肾之原穴太溪,二穴共用有育阴潜阳之功。诸穴合用,具有行气活血、通络止痛、育阴潜阳的作用。

配穴 失眠健忘者加神门;头痛者加太阳、后溪;耳鸣者加翳风、听宫;反胃者加

2. For syndrome of Qi deficiency and phlegm obstruction, symptoms include heavy and painful head, fatigue look, slow response, poor appetite, light tongue with white and greasy fur, thin and sloppy or uneven pulse.

II. Therapeutic Methods

[Syndrome of Yin Deficiency of Liver and Kidney]

Therapeutic method: Activate Qi and blood circulation, soothe collaterals and alleviate pain.

Prescription: Fengchi (GB20), Baihui (DU20), Hegu (LI4), Sishencong (EX-HN1), Taichong (LR3), Taixi (KI3).

Mechanism of prescription: Fengchi is an acupoint from Shao-Yang Gallbladder Meridian of Foot, Baihui is an acupoint from Du Channel, and Du Channel is the sea of Yang channels; both two are important acupoints for treatment of headache and vertigo. Sishencong is an external nerve acupoint, it is good at treatment of headache, vertigo and amnesia. Hegu is a Yuan acupoint from Large Intestine Meridian, good at treatment of headache, and it can activate Qi and blood circulation. The Yuan acupoint Taichong of Liver and the Yuan acupoint Taixi of Kidney can nourish Yin and suppress Yang if they are used together. The use of combination of these acupoints can activate Qi and blood circulation, soothe collaterals and alleviate pain, nourish Yin and suppress Yang.

Matching acupoints: For insomnia and amnesia add Shenmen. For headache add Taiyang, Houxi. For tinnitus add Yifeng, Tinggong. For gastric disorder causing

内关、足三里。

方法 电热针治疗。

操作 选定穴位,皮肤常规消毒。电热针直刺神门0.7寸,平刺百会0.7寸,向脊中斜刺风池0.7寸,直刺足三里0.8寸,平刺四神聪0.7寸,直刺太溪0.7寸。接通电热针仪,每个穴位分别给予40～50mA的电流量,使患者感到温热或胀感舒适为度,留针40分钟。另配以毫针泻太冲。

疗程 每天1次,留针40分钟,20次为1个疗程,疗程间可休息3～5天,再进行第2个疗程的治疗。一般治疗1～2个疗程即可恢复。

【气虚痰阻证】

治法 健脾和中,益气化痰。

处方 风池(GB20)、百会(DU20)、合谷(LI4)、四神聪(EX-HN1)、足三里(ST36)、三阴交(SP6)、丰隆(ST40)。

方义 风池为足少阳胆经腧穴,百会为督脉之腧穴,督脉为阳脉之海,二穴均为治头

nausea, add Neiguan, Zusanli.

Method: Electrothermal acupuncture treatment.

Operations: Selecting the relevant acupoints, perform routine skin disinfection. Using electrothermal acupuncture needles, vertically puncture into Shenmen for 0.7", horizontally puncture into Baihui for 0.7", obliquely puncture toward Jizhong into Fengchi for 0.7", vertically puncture into Zusanli for 0.8", horizontally puncture into Sishencong for 0.7", vertically puncture into Taixi for 0.7". Turn on the electrothermal acupuncture equipment, apply a current of 40-50mA to each acupoint, and the limit is that the patient feels warm or swelling and comfortable, leaving the needles in for 40 minutes. Additionally, using the filiform needles, apply the tonifying method for Taichong.

Therapeutic course: Once a day, leave the needles in for 40 minutes, 20 times for a course, and start the treatment for the second course after a break of 3-5 days. Generally recovered after 1-2 courses.

[Syndrome of Qi Deficiency and Phlegm Obstruction]

Therapeutic method: Invigorate spleen and regulate Middle Jiao, tonify Qi and disperse phlegm.

Prescription: Fengchi (GB20), Baihui (DU20), Hegu (LI4), Sishencong (EX-HN1), Zusanli(ST36), Sanyinjiao (SP6), Fenglong (ST40).

Mechanism of prescription: Fengchi is an acupoint from Shao-Yang Gallbladder Meridian of Foot, Baihui is an acupoint from Du Channel, and Du Channel

痛、眩晕之要穴。四神聪是经外奇穴，善治头痛、眩晕、健忘。大肠经之原穴合谷长于治头面之疾，具有行气活血之功。足三里是足阳明胃经之下合穴，长于益气和中。丰隆系胃经络穴，别走足太阴脾经，长于化痰。诸穴合用，可收行气活血、通络止痛、健脾和中、益气化痰之功效。

配穴 恶心者加内关；头痛者加后溪、太阳。

方法 电热针治疗。

操作 选定穴位，常规皮肤消毒。电热针向脊中斜刺风池0.7寸，平刺百会0.7寸，直刺足三里0.8寸，直刺三阴交0.7寸，直刺丰隆0.7寸。接通电热针仪，每个穴位分别给予电流量40～60mA，以温热或胀感舒适为度，留针40分钟。另配以毫针平刺四神聪0.7寸，直刺合谷0.5寸，直刺后溪0.5寸，直刺内关0.5寸，直刺太溪0.5寸，留针40分钟。

is the sea of Yang channels; both two are important acupoints fro treatment of headache and vertigo. Sishencong is an external nerve acupoint, it is good at treatment of headache, vertigo and amnesia. The Yuan acupoint from Large Intestine Meridian, Hegu, is good at treatment of head and face diseases, and it can activate Qi and blood circulation. Zusanli is a He acupoint from Yang-Ming Stomach Meridian of Foot, it is good at tonify Qi and regulate Middle Jiao. Fenglong is a collateral acupoint from Stomach Meridian, and also is connected to Tai-Yin Spleen Meridian of Foot, it is good at disperse phlegm. The use of combination of these acupoints can activate Qi and blood circulation, soothe collaterals and alleviate pain, invigorate spleen and regulate Middle Jiao, tonify Qi and disperse phlegm.

Matching acupoints: For nausea add Neiguan. For headache add Houxi, Taiyang.

Method: Electrothermal acupuncture treatment.

Operations: Selecting the relevant acupoints, perform routine skin disinfection. Using electrothermal acupuncture needles, obliquely puncture toward Jizhong into Fengchi for 0.7", horizontally puncture into Baihui for 0.7", vertically puncture into Zusanli for 0.8", Sanyinjiao for 0.7", Fenglong for 0.7". Turn on the electrothermal acupuncture equipment, apply a current of 40~60mA to each acupoint, and the limit is that the patient feels warm or swelling and comfortable, leaving the needles in for 40 minutes. Additionally, using filiform needles, horizontally puncture into Sishencong for 0.7", vertically puncture into Hegu for 0.5", vertically puncture into Houxi for 0.5", vertically puncture into Neiguan for 0.5", vertically puncture into Taixi for 0.5", leaving the needles in for 40 minutes.

Therapeutic course: Once a day, 20 times for a course, and take a break of 3-5 days after the treatment, then decide if continue the second course depending on the disease condition. Generally basically cured after 2-3 courses.

III. Precautions

1. Let patients load off their thought burdens, establish confidence in defeating diseases and make them accept and cooperate with the treatment actively.

2. Develop reasonable and appropriate functional exercise schemes for patients depending on different dysfunctions. For mental abilities related dysfunctions, special instructions are required.

3. During treatment, guide patients to have more social activities, and instruct them to do functional exercises of affected limbs, so as to facilitate functional recovery of affected limbs.

4. Chinese Herb Medicine treatment and Western Medicine treatment also can be taken if necessary, so as to improve efficacies as soon as possible and promote early recovery of patients.

Rheumatoid Arthritis

Rheumatoid arthritis is a common inflammation of connective tissues, which repeatedly attacks. Histories of acute amygdalitis or angina before onset; lesions mainly involve big joints like shoulder, knee, hip joints, etc. Multiple, wandering pains or fixed ones, or liquid aggre-

游走性疼痛，或固定不移，或关节腔有积液，并伴有不同程度的发热。躯干或四肢皮肤可出现环形红斑，在关节伸侧或四周可以触到黄豆大小的皮下结节，数周后可逐渐消退。儿童及青年发病率较高。本病的发生与寒冷、潮湿及气候急骤变化有密切关系，尤其多发在秋冬之际或早春季节。

中医认为，本病属于"痹证""历节""白虎历节""痛风"的范畴。多因素体虚弱，正气不固，或劳累、汗后当风，或淋雨、受寒或久卧湿地等，致风寒湿邪乘虚而入，闭阻经脉，气血不畅，发为风寒湿痹。其中，风邪偏胜则为行痹；寒邪偏胜为痛痹；湿邪偏胜则为着痹。

一、诊断及辨证要点

风寒湿痹，关节或肌肉酸痛，阴雨天加重，反复发作，时轻时重，为其临床共性，根据其不同的表现又可分为行痹、痛痹、着痹。

gation of joint cavity, accompanying pyrexia of different degrees. Erythema annulare may occur at body or limb skin, and subcutaneous nodules of soybean size can be palpated at the stretching side of joints or around joints, which may subside several weeks later. The incidences of children and young adults are higher. The onset of this disease is closely related to cold, damp and sharp climatic changes, especially in the autumn and winter as well as early spring.

Traditional Chinese Medicine believes that this disease belongs to the range of "arhralgia syndrome", "Lijie", "severe and migratory arhralgia", "gout". Most are caused by body deficiency, non-consolidation of vital Qi, or facing wind after overwork, sweating, or exposure to the rain, cold or long-term lying on the damp ground, leading to swooping in of Wind, Cold, Damp toxins, obstruction of meridians and channels, obstructed Qi and blood, which developing into Wind-Cold-Damp arthralgia. Among which Wind-evil toxins become dominant indicating migratory arthralgia; Cold-evil toxins become dominant indicating arthritis; Damp-evil toxins become dominant indicating fixed arthralgia.

I. Key Points for Diagnosis and Syndrome Differentiation

Wind-Cold-Damp arthralgia, soreness and pain in the joints or muscles, which get aggravated in the wet weather and attack repeated with varying severities, are the common features of this diseases. Again it can be divided into three types as per different manifestations:

1. 行痹，症见肢体关节疼痛，游走不定，关节伸屈不利，或恶风发热，舌苔薄白或略腻，脉浮或细。

2. 痛痹，症见肢体关节疼痛剧烈，痛有定处，遇寒痛增，得热痛减，局部皮肤不红，触之不热，舌苔白，脉弦紧。

3. 着痹，症见肢关节疼痛重着，或关节局部肿胀，肤色不红，痛有定处，肌肤麻木不仁，活动受限，苔白腻，脉濡或缓。

二、治疗方法

【行痹】

治法 祛风止痛。

处方 大椎（DU14）、风门（BL12）、风市（GB31）、膈俞（BL17）、血海（SP10）。

方义 大椎是手足三阳经、督脉之会，可疏风解表，又能调和诸阳经之气机。风门疏风散寒，风市祛风除湿，两穴均为祛风之要穴。膈俞、血海活血养血，取其"血行风自灭"之意。

migratory arthralgia, arthritis, fixed arthralgia.

1. Migratory arthralgia, symptoms include wandering pains in the limb joints, inhibited flexing and stretching of joints, aversion to Wind and pyrexia, thin and white or slightly greasy tongue fur, floating or thin pulse.

2. Arthritis, symptoms include fixed intensive pains in the limb joints, which get aggravated with cold and get relieved with warm; non-red of local skin, the skin is not warm when being touched; white tongue fur, taut and tight pulse.

3. Fixed arthralgia, symptoms include severe pains in the limb joints, or local joint swelling, non-red of local skin, and the pain lesion is fixed; numbness of skin, limited movements; white and greasy tongue fur, soft or slow pulse.

II. Therapeutic Methods

[Migratory Arthralgia]

Therapeutic method: Remove Wind and alleviate pains.

Prescription: Dazhui (DU14), Fengmen (BL12), Fengshi (GB31), Geshu (BL17), Xuehai (SP10).

Mechanism of prescription: Dazhui is the confluent acupoint of three Yang meridians of hand and foot as well as Du Channel, it can soothe Wind and resolve diaphoresis, and regulate Qi Dynamic of all Yang meridians. Fengmen can soothe Wind and disperse Cold, Fengshi can remove Wind and Damp, both two are important acupoints for Wind removing. Geshu, Xuehai can activate and nourish blood, the principle is "Wind will be dispersed naturally given that blood is activated".

配穴　肩关节疼痛者加肩髎、肩井、曲池、外关；肘关节疼痛者加曲池、手三里、合谷；腕关节疼痛者加阳溪、阳池、曲池、腕骨；髋关节痛者加环跳、居髎、秩边、委中、阳陵泉；膝关节痛者加梁丘、膝眼、足三里、阳陵泉、鹤顶、阴陵泉、三阴交；踝关节痛者加解溪、昆仑、悬钟；全身关节痛者加身柱、上髎、中髎、下髎、后溪、申脉、外关、足三里、曲池、合谷。

Matching acupoints: For pain of shoulder joint add Jianliao, Jianjing, Quchi, Waiguan. For pain of elbow joint add Quchi, Shousanli, Hegu. For pain of wrist joint add Yangxi, Yangchi, Quchi, Wangu; For pain of hip joint add Huantiao, Juliao, Zhibian, Weizhong, Yanglingquan. For pain of knee joint add Liangqiu, Xiyan, Zusanli, Yanglingquan, Heding, Yinlingquan, Sanyinjiao. For pain of ankle joint add Jiexi, Kunlun, Xuanzhong. For pain of joints of the whole body add Shenzhu, Shangliao, Zhongliao, Xialiao, Houxi, Shenmai, Waiguan, Zusanli, Quchi, Hegu.

方法　电热针治疗。

操作　选定穴位，皮肤常规消毒。电热针向上斜刺大椎 0.7 寸，直刺风市 0.8 寸，向脊柱方向斜刺膈俞 0.7 寸，直刺血海 0.7 寸。接通电热针仪，每个穴位分别给予电流量 50mA，以患者感到舒适为度，留针 40 分钟。

Method: Electrothermal acupuncture treatment.

Operations: Selecting the relevant acupoints, perform routine skin disinfection. Using the electrothermal acupuncture needles, obliquely puncture upward into Dazhui for 0.7", vertically puncture into Fengshi for 0.8", obliquely puncture toward spine into Geshu for 0.7", vertically puncture into Xuehai for for 0.7". Turn on the electrothermal acupuncture equipment, apply a current of 50mA to each acupoint, and the limit is that the patient feels comfortable, leaving the needles in for 40 minutes.

疗程　每日 1 次，30 次为 1 个疗程，疗程间休息 5～7 天，再继续进行第 2 个疗程的治疗，共需要治疗 3 个疗程。

Therapeutic course: Once a day, 30 times for a course, and start the treatment for the second course after a break of 5-7 days, 3 courses in total.

【痛痹】

治法　温经散寒，通经止痛。

[Arthritis]

Therapeutic method: Warm meridians and dissipate cold, dredge meridians and alleviate pain.

处方 关元（RN4）、肾俞（BL23）、大椎（DU14）、居髎（GB29）、环跳（GB30）。

方义 关元、肾俞益气温阳，驱散风寒。居髎祛风寒、通经络，擅治痛痹。环跳是少阳、太阳二脉之会穴，与大椎同用，可疏风祛湿，通络止痛。诸穴合用，以温针治之，可增强其温阳散寒、通经止痛之力。

配穴 取穴同行痹。

方法 电热针治疗。

操作 选定穴位，皮肤常规消毒。电热针直刺关元0.8寸，直刺肾俞0.7寸，向上直刺大椎0.7寸，直刺居髎1.2寸，直刺环跳1.2寸。接通电热针仪，每个穴位分别给予电流量50mA，以患者感到局部舒适为度，留针40分钟。

疗程 每日1次，30次为1个疗程，疗程间休息5～7天，再继续进行第2个疗程的治疗，共需要治疗3个疗程。

Prescription: Guanyuan (RN4), Shenshu (BL23), Dazhui (DU14), Juliao (GB29), Huantiao (GB30).

Mechanism of prescription: Guanyuan, Shenshu can tonify Qi and warm Yang, disperse Wind-Cold. Juliao can dispel Wind-Cold, dredge meridians and collaterals, it is good at treatment of arthritis. Huantiao is the confluent acupoint of Shao-Yang and Tai-Yang channels, when use Huantiao together with Dazhui, they can soothe Wind and dispel Damp, soothe collaterals and alleviate pain. The use of combination of these acupoints with the method of warm needling can strengthen the efficacies of warming Yang and dissipating cold, dredging meridians and alleviating pain.

Matching acupoints: The same as that of migratory arthralgia.

Method: Electrothermal acupuncture treatment.

Operations: Selecting the relevant acupoints, perform routine skin disinfection. Using electrothermal acupuncture needles, vertically puncture into Guanyuan for 0.8", vertically puncture into Shenshu for 0.7", vertically puncture upward into Dazhui for 0.7", vertically puncture into Juliao for 1.2", vertically puncture into Huantiao for 1.2". Turn on the electrothermal acupuncture equipment, apply a current of 50mA to each acupoint, and the limit is that the patient feels locally comfortable, leaving the needles in for 40 minutes.

Therapeutic course: Once a day, 30 times for a course, and start the treatment for the second course after a break of 5-7 days, 3 courses in total.

【着痹】

治法 健脾祛湿，疏风散寒。

处方 商丘（SP5）、漏谷（SP7）、合阳（BL55）、脾俞（BL20）、阴陵泉（SP9）、足三里（ST36）。

方义 商丘、漏谷能健脾利湿、通络止痛，均是治疗痹证的要穴。合阳可祛风湿、健腰腿，擅长治疗下肢酸痛、腰痛。脾俞、阴陵泉、足三里合用，能健运脾胃而温化寒湿。本法取穴，目的是祛湿与健脾并重，相得益彰，兼有疏风散寒之功效。

配穴 取穴同行痹。

方法 电热针治疗。

操作 选定穴位，皮肤常规消毒。采用温补法，电热针直刺商丘0.6寸，直刺漏谷0.7寸，直刺合阳0.8寸，向脊中斜刺脾俞0.7寸，直刺阴陵泉0.7寸，直刺曲池0.7寸，直刺足三里0.7寸。接通电热针仪，每穴分别给予电流量60mA，以患者感到舒适为度，留针40

[Fixed Arthralgia]

Therapeutic method: Invigorate spleen and remove Damp, soothe Wind and dispel Cold.

Prescription: Shangqiu (SP5), Lougu (SP7), Heyang (BL55), Pishu (BL20), Yinlingquan (SP9), Zusanli (ST36).

Mechanism of prescription: Shangqiu, Lougu can invigorate spleen and dispel Damp, soothe collaterals and alleviate pain, they both are important acupoints for treatment of arthralgia syndromes. Heyang can remove Wind-Damp, invigorate waist and legs, and it is good at treating soreness and pain of lower limbs, lumbago. The combination of Pishu, Yinlingquan, Zusanli can be used to promote transportation of spleen and stomach, so as to warm and disperse Cold-Damp. The use of this method for acupoint selecting is aimed to focus on Damp removing and spleen invigorating which can complement each other, as well as to soothe Wind and dispel Cold.

Matching acupoints: The same as that of migratory arthralgia.

Method: Electrothermal acupuncture treatment.

Operations: Selecting the relevant acupoints, perform routine skin disinfection. With the method of warm tonifying, Using electrothermal acupuncture needles, vertically puncture into Shangqiu for 0.6", vertically puncture into Lougu for 0.7", Heyang for 0.8", obliquely puncture toward Jizhong into Pishu for 0.7", vertically puncture into Yinlingquan for 0.7", Quchi for 0.7", and Zusanli for 0.7". Turn on the electrothermal acupuncture equipment, apply a current of 60mA to each acupoint, and the limit is that the patient feels comfortable, leaving the needles in for 40 minutes.

Therapeutic course: Treat once a day, 30 times for a course, and start the treatment for the second course after a break of 7-10 days. Generally cured after 2-3 courses.

III. Precautions

1. For joints with severe pains, the method of encircling needling for joints can be used. Puncture with 2-3 needles around the joint, however it is forbidden to puncture the needle into the joint cavity and the operator must be familiar with the local anatomical structure, perform accurate locating and control the needling direction, angle and depth. Apply a current of 60mA respectively, let the patient feel locally warm and comfortable at the joint, leaving the needles in for 40 minutes.

2. During the active stage of rheumatoid arthritis, for patients with redness and swellings of joints as well as pyrexia, the medication must be used together with acupuncture.

3. After symptom relief, the patient is required to adhere to do functional exercises of joints and appropriate physical exercises, so as to remain as well as recover normal functions of joints.

Rheumatoid Arthritis

Rheumatoid arthritis is a common chronic joint disease accompanied with general symptoms, and the lesions can involve any joint, mainly small joints, among

节，多累及小关节，以近侧指关节、掌指关节、趾关节最多见。也可累及膝、踝、腕、肩、髋关节，少数病例可累及下颌关节。一般均为多关节且两侧关节对称受累。

中医学统称"痹证"，属于"尫痹""骨痹""筋痹"的范畴。其病因及证治，早期与风湿性关节炎基本相同，故不重述。

晚期因风寒湿邪渗入筋骨，阻滞气血，或湿聚成痰，致痰瘀痹阻筋骨关节之间，或损伤肝肾精血，筋骨失荣，关节拘挛，渐致畸形难以扭转。故其证多本虚标实，本文着重介绍类风湿性关节炎晚期的证治。

一、诊断及辨证要点

1. 痰湿痹阻者，痹证日久，关节疼痛时轻时重，午夜尤甚，关节肿大如鹤膝，或呈强直、屈伸不利，舌质暗紫，或有瘀斑，苔白腻，脉细涩。

which most common are proximal knuckles, metacarpophalangeal joints, toe joints and knee joints, ankle joints, wrist joints, shoulder joints, hip joints can also be involved in, while in a few cases the mandibular joint also may be involved in. Generally multiple, symmetrical involvement of joints on both sides.

In Traditional Chinese Medicine these are collectively called "arthralgia syndrome", which belongs the range of "lame rheumatism", "bone rheumatism", "rheumatism". In the early phase, its etiology and syndromes are similar to those of rheumatoid arthritis, therefore no repeated details here.

In the advanced phase, Wind, Cold, and Damp toxins invade the tendons and bones, obstruct Qi and blood, or accumulated Damp transforms into phlegm, leading to that stagnated phlegm to accumulate within tendons, bones and joints, or impairs essence and blood of liver and kidney, leading to nourishment loss of tendons and bones, joint spasm. It gradually develops into deformation that is hard to be reversed. Therefore, most cases of this syndrome are asthenia in origin and sthenia in superficiality. This article mainly introduce the diagnosis and treatment for late rheumatoid arthritis.

I. Key Points for Diagnosis and Syndrome Differentiation

1. For patients with phlegm Damp stagnation, the arthralgia syndrome lasts for a long time, and the degree of joint pain varies from time to time, which becomes especially severe at midnight, the swollen joint is like a crane knee, or with stiffness and inhibited flexing and

stretching, dark purple tongue which may has ecchymosis, white and greasy fur, thin and uneven pulse.

2. 正虚邪恋者，久病痹痛，反复发作，顽固难愈，关节肿大，甚则畸形，或呈强直、屈伸不利，肌肉痿软，腰背酸痛，四肢消瘦，面色白，神疲乏力，舌质淡，苔薄白，或舌红少苔，脉细弱或细数。

2. For patients with lingering pathogen due to deficient vital Qi, the long-term pain due to arthralgia attacks repeats and is hard to be cured, the joint is swollen or even deformed, stiffness and inhibited flexing and stretching, muscle flaccidity, soreness and pain of waist and back, emaciation of limbs, pale complexion, fatigue look and asthenia, light tongue with thin and white fur, or red tongue with less fur, thin and weak or thin and rapid pulse.

二、治疗方法

【痰瘀痹阻证】

治法 祛湿蠲痰，通络止痛。

处方 膈俞（BL17）、血海（SP10）、脾俞（BL20）、天井（SJ10）。

方义 膈俞是血会，可活血化瘀；血海是"脾血归聚之海"，有祛瘀血、生新血之功；脾俞有健脾祛湿、通络止痛、化痰散结之作用。诸穴共用，能取祛痰蠲痰、通络止痛之功效。

配穴 掌指关节痛者，加八邪、阳溪、阳池、阳谷；趾关节痛者，加解溪、太冲、公

II. Therapeutic Methods

[Syndrome of Phlegm Stagnation]

Therapeutic method: Remove Damp and disperse phlegm, soothe collaterals and alleviate pain.

Prescription: Geshu (BL17), Xuehai (SP10), Pishu (BL20), Tianjing (SJ10).

Mechanism of prescription: Geshu is the convergent place of blood, it can activate blood circulation and remove stasis. Xuehai is "the sea for convergence of spleen blood", it can disperse static blood and generate new blood. Pishu can invigorate spleen and remove Damp, soothe collaterals and alleviate pain, disperse phlegm and eliminate stagnation. The use of combination of these acupoints can dispel and remove phlegm, soothe collaterals and alleviate pain.

Matching acupoints: For pain of metacarpophalangeal joints, add Baxie, Yangxi, Yangchi, Yanggu. For pain of toe joints add Jiexi, Taichong, Gongsun, Qiuxu.

孙、丘墟；脊柱关节痛者，加病变相应部位之夹脊穴或膀胱经的背俞穴。

方法 电热针治疗。

操作 选定穴位，皮肤常规消毒。电热针斜刺（针尖向脊柱）膈俞、脾俞各 0.7 寸，直刺血海、天井各 0.6 寸，斜刺背部膀胱经的背俞穴各 0.7 寸。接通电热针仪，每个穴位分别给予 60mA 的电流量，以患者感到局部舒适为度，留针 40 分钟。

疗程 每天 1 次，90 天为 1 个疗程。疗程间可休息 7～10 天，再根据病情决定是否进行第 2 个疗程的治疗。一般治疗 1～2 个疗程后病情基本稳定。

【正虚邪恋证】

治法 补气养血，蠲痹止痛。

处方 肝俞（BL18）、肾俞（BL23）、大杼（BL11）、阳陵泉（GB34）、足三里（ST36）、三阴交（SP6）。

方义 肝俞、肾俞补益肝肾、扶正祛邪，大杼、阳陵泉分别为骨、筋之会穴，可以强

For pain of spine joints add corresponding JiaJi acupoints of the lesion or Back-Shu acupoints from Bladder Meridian.

Method: Electrothermal acupuncture treatment.

Operations: Selecting the relevant acupoints, perform routine skin disinfection. Using electrothermal acupuncture needles, obliquely puncture (with the needle tip towards spine) into Geshu, Pishu for 0.7" respectively, vertically puncture into Xuehai, Tianjing for 0.6" respectively, obliquely puncture into Back-Shu acupoints from Bladder Meridian on the back for 0.7" respectively. Turn on the electrothermal acupuncture equipment, apply a current of 60mA to each acupoint, and the limit is that the patient feels locally comfortable, leaving the needles in for 40 minutes.

Therapeutic course: Once a day, 90 days for a course. Rest for 7-10 days between courses, then determine if perform the second course, depending on the disease conditions. Generally the condition can be basically stable after 1-2 courses.

[Syndrome of Lingering Pathogen Due to Deficient Vital Qi]

Therapeutic method: Replenish Qi and nourish blood, eliminate arthralgia and alleviate pain.

Prescription: Ganshu (BL18), Shenshu (BL23), Dazhu (BL11), Yanglingquan (GB34), Zusanli (ST36), Sanyinjiao (SP6).

Mechanism of prescription: Ganshu, Shenshu can tonify liver and kidney, strengthen vital Qi and eliminate pathogenic factors; Dazhu, Yanglingquan are the conflu-

壮筋骨、通痹止痛，足三里、三阴交健脾和胃，以助气血生化之源。诸穴共用，使精血充足，髓生骨健，筋脉关节得以营养，而达蠲痹止痛之功效。

配穴 取穴同痰湿痹阻证。

方法 电热针治疗。

操作 选定穴位，皮肤常规消毒。电热针斜刺（针尖向脊柱方向）肝俞、肾俞、大杼各 0.7 寸，直刺足三里 0.7 寸，直刺三阴交 0.6 寸。接通电热针仪，每个穴位分别给予 50mA 的电流量，以患者感到胀或温热舒适为度，留针 40 分钟。另配以毫针直刺八邪 0.3 寸，直刺阳溪、阳池、阳谷各 0.5 寸，直刺解溪、太冲、公孙、丘墟各 0.3 寸。脊椎关节痛时，若针夹脊穴，用毫针直刺 0.5 寸；若针膀胱经背俞穴时，亦可用电热针向脊中斜刺 0.7 寸，或毫针斜刺 0.7 寸，均留针 40 分钟。

ent acupoints of bones and tendons respectively, they can strengthen tendons and bones, dredge arthralgia and alleviate pain; Zusanli, Sanyinjiao can invigorate spleen and regulate stomach, so as to promote the source of generation and transformation of Qi-blood. The use of combination of these acupoints can facilitate sufficient essence blood, marrow generation and strong bones, nourishment of tendons and channels as well as joints, so as to eliminate arthralgia and alleviate pain.

Matching acupoints: The same as that of syndrome of phlegm Damp stagnation.

Method: Electrothermal acupuncture treatment.

Operations: Selecting the relevant acupoints, perform routine skin disinfection. Using electrothermal acupuncture needles, obliquely puncture (with the needle tip towards spine) into Ganshu, Shenshu, Dazhu for 0.7" respectively, vertically puncture into Zusanli for 0.7", Sanyinjiao for 0.6". Turn on the electrothermal acupuncture equipment, apply a current of 50mA to each acupoint, and the limit is that the patient feels swelling or warm and comfortable, leaving the needles in for 40 minutes. Additionally, using filiform needles, vertically puncture into Baxie for 0.3", vertically puncture into Yangxi, Yangchi, Yanggu for 0.5" respectively, vertically puncture into Jiexi, Taichong, Gongsun, Qiuxu for 0.3" respectively. For vertebral joint pain, if acupuncture is performed on Jiaji acupoints, vertically puncture for 0.5" with filiform needles. For acupuncture of Back-Shu acupoints from Bladder Meridian, the electrothermal needles can be used to obliquely puncture towards Jizhong into the acupoints for 0.7", or use filiform needles to obliquely puncture into the acupoints for 0.7"; for both methods, leave the needles in for 40 minutes.

Therapeutic course: Once a day, 90 times for a course. Start the treatment for the second course after a break of 10-15 days. Generally 2-3 courses are enough.

III. Precautions

1. Use acupuncture therapy to treat this disease, and the sooner the treatment, the better the efficacies. For patients in the active period it is better to use Chinese Herb Medicine treatment as well to improve efficacies and shorten the treatment course.

2. Along with the acupuncture treatment, patients should do functional exercises of limbs and joints, which has important effects on reducing or preventing joint deformations, remaining functions of limbs and joints.

3. This disease is hard to be cured, therefore the treatment time should be increased for longer disease courses, while patients should closely cooperate with medical personnel and adhere to the treatment. Normally the treatment will last for 3-6 months. After that the condition has improved and the symptoms have basically disappeared, consolidation treatment is still required to prevent recurrence.

4. For patients with joint deformation and inhibited limb movements, the functional exercises should be performed slowly with gradual increase, meanwhile perform massage therapy with mild manipulation.

5. Avoid accidentally falling, injuries or bone fractures.

6. For damp and cold environments, dampness-proof and cold-proof measures should be adopted depending on specific situations.

Raynaud Disease

Raynaud disease, also called "acra artery spasm", is a spastic disease of acra arterioles caused by dysfunction of vascular nerves. The main clinical features include paroxysmal, intermittent pallor, cyanossis or flushing of limb ends. Normally at finger tips, generally are symmetry; most onsets are attributed to cold or emotional excitement. Commonly seen among young females.

Traditional Chinese Medicine believes that this disease is caused by Yang deficiency of spleen and kidney, external infection of Cold toxins. Cold toxins accumulates within meridians and channels, and causes Yang Qi stagnation, therefore the Yang Qi cannot reach limb ends, leading to cold of limbs. It belongs to the range of "blood arthralgia".

I. Key Points for Diagnosis and Syndrome Differentiation

1. Commonly seen among young females with an age of 20-30 years old, slow onset.

2. Main characteristics: With cold, limb ends show intermittent pallor, flushing or cyanosis, symmetry and paroxysmal whitening.

3. Most are induced by emotional excitement and

诱发，遇热则减。

4. 辨证

（1）寒邪阻络者（缺血期）：多因素体虚弱，气血不足所致。每遇外界寒冷刺激即出现四肢末端皮肤发冷、发白、发麻或潮红、疼痛等，脉细弦或紧。

（2）气滞血瘀者（缺气期）：可见患指（趾）皮色紫红或青紫，作胀疼痛，舌紫黯，苔薄白，脉沉细。

（3）寒邪化热者（充血期）：症见患肢发冷较轻，肢端潮红或紫红而胖胀，灼热疼痛，或继发轻度溃疡，舌质红，苔黄，脉滑数。

5. 实验室检查：风湿指标正常。

6. 病理：指（趾）端动脉早期可无任何变化，后期可出现动脉内膜增生，弹力膜断裂，层纤维化，管腔狭窄闭塞和血栓形成，以及毛细血管扭曲。

二、治疗方法

【脾肾阳虚证】

治法　温阳散寒，通脉活血。

cold, and will be relieved with warm.

4. Symptom differentiation

(1) Cold toxins obstructing collaterals (blood-lacking period): Most are caused by body deficiency and weakness, insufficiency of Qi-blood. Each time with external cold stimulations there will be cold, pale color, numbness or flushing, pain at the skin of limb ends, as well as thin and taut or tight pulse.

(2) Qi stagnation and blood stasis (Qi-lacking period): Purplish red or cyanoze skin at the patient's fingers (toes) which is swelling and painful, dark purple tongue with thin and white fur, deep and thin pulse.

(3) Cold toxins transforming into Heat (congestive period): Symptoms include mild cold of affected limbs, flushing or purplish red and swelling limb ends, or burning-like pains, or secondary mild ulcers, red tongue with yellow fur, slippery and rapid pulse.

5. Lab examination: Rheumatism indicators normal.

6. Pathology: In the early phase the arteries of finger (toe) ends may have no changes, and in the advanced phase there may occur arterial intimal hyperplasia, elastic membrane fragmentation, muscular fibrosis, vascular lumen stenosis and obstruction and thrombosis, and distortion of capillaries.

II. Therapeutic Methods

[Syndrome of Yang Deficiency of Spleen and Kidney]

Therapeutic method: Warm Yang and dispel Cold, dredge channels and activate blood.

处方 缺盆（ST12）、照海（KI6）、三阴交（SP6）。

方义 缺盆位于锁骨上窝，属足阳明胃经之穴位。阳明多气多血，刺之可鼓舞阳气外达四肢，以温阳散寒，通脉活血。照海隶属于足少阳肾经，又是八脉交会穴；三阴交是足三阴经脉的交会穴，此二穴合用可引命门真火，中土脾阳外达四肢末端，以通阳散寒。

配穴 病位在上肢者加手三里、内关、小海、八邪；病位在下肢者加环跳、秩边、阳陵泉、八风；必要时可加手足十宣。

方法 电热针治疗（温补法）。

操作 选定穴位，常规皮肤消毒。电热针直刺三阴交0.7寸，直刺照海0.7寸，直刺手三里0.7寸，直刺阳陵泉0.8寸，直刺环跳0.9寸，直刺秩边0.9寸。接通电热针仪，每个穴位分别给予电流量60～70mA。另配以毫针向背后直刺缺盆0.2寸，得气后做

Prescription: Quepen (ST12), Zhaohai (KI6), Sanyinjiao (SP6).

Mechanism of prescription: Quepen is located at the supraclavicular fossa, is an acupoint from Yang-Ming Stomach Meridian of Foot. Yang-Ming Meridian is full of Qi and blood, the needling of this meridian can promote Yang Qi to reach limbs outwards, so as to warm Yang and dispel Cold, dredge channels and activate blood. Zhaohai belongs to Shao-Yang Kidney Meridian of Foot, as well as a confluent acupoint of eight channels; Sanyinjiao is the confluent acupoint of three Yin Meridians of Foot, so the combination of these two can induce true Fire of Mingmen, let spleen Yang of Middle Earth reach limb ends, so as to warm Yang and dispel Cold.

Matching acupoints: For lesions at upper limbs add Shousanli, Neiguan, Xiaohai, Baxie. For lesions at lower limbs add Huantiao, Zhibian, Yanglingquan, Bafeng; add Shoushixuan and Zushixuan if necessary.

Method: Electrothermal acupuncture treatment (warm tonifying).

Operations: Selecting the relevant acupoints, perform routine skin disinfection. Using electrothermal acupuncture needles, vertically puncture into Sanyinjiao for 0.7", Zhaohai for 0.7", Shousanli for 0.7", Yanglingquan for 0.8", Huantiao for 0.9", Zhibian for 0.9". Turn on the electrothermal acupuncture equipment, apply a current of 60-70mA to each acupoint. Additionally, using filiform needles, vertically puncture toward the back into Quepen for 0.2", after getting Qi, lift and thrust at a

小幅度雀啄法提插，不留针。

疗程 每日1次，20次为1个疗程。疗程间休息3天，再继续进行第2个疗程的治疗。

三、注意事项

1. 针刺缺盆时必须严格掌握进针方向及深度，不可向下深刺，避免刺伤肺尖，造成气胸。

2. 治疗过程中，要求患者注意患肢的保温，防止寒冷刺激。

3. 加强活动，锻炼身体，促进肢体的血液流通，以帮助康复。

4. 病情稳定后，亦要坚持巩固治疗，以求提高疗效。病情严重者可配合中、西药物综合疗法，以求康复。

多发性大动脉炎（无脉症）

多发性大动脉炎又称为"主动脉弓分支血栓闭塞性动脉炎""主动脉弓综合征""原发性动脉炎综合征"，是主动脉及其分支的慢性、进行性、闭塞性炎症，以头臂部受累者多见。

small extent using the method of bird-peck needling, do not leave the needles in.

Therapeutic course: Once a day, 20 times for a course. Start the treatment for the second course after a break of 3 days.

III. Precautions

1. For acupuncture of Quepen, the needling direction and depth must be controlled, and deeply puncture downwards is forbidden, so as to avoid impairing the lung apex leading to pneumothorax.

2. During treatment, patients are required to keep warm of the affected limb and prevent stimulations of Cold.

3. Increase movements and physical exercises, promote the blood circulation of limbs so as to facilitate recovery.

4. After the disease is stable, the consolidation treatment should be adhered to, so as to improve the efficacies. For severe patients, Chinese Herb Medicine and Western Medicine treatments should also be used to facilitate recovery.

Takayasu's Arteritis (Pulseless Disease)

Takayasu's Arteritis is also called "throbus-occlusive arteritis of aortic arch branches", "aortic arch syndrome", "primary arteritis syndrome", refers to chronic, progressive, obliterative inflammations of aortae and their branches, and the most common ones are lesions in the head and arm region.

中医学尚无相应的病名。根据其临床表现，应属于"无脉症""脉痹""臂厥（上肢）""骭厥（下肢）"的范畴。多由先天不足或后天失调，风寒湿邪侵入经脉，以致气血亏损，脉络空虚，或痰瘀凝滞，脉道不通所致。

一、诊断及辨证要点

1. 病在上肢者，主要表现为单侧或双侧桡动脉、肱动脉、腋动脉、颈动脉或颞动脉搏动减弱或消失。

2. 病在下肢者，则从股动脉开始，单侧或双侧腘动脉、足背动脉搏动减弱或消失，并有间歇性跛行。

3. 可有全身不适，肢体疼痛、麻木、肢冷无力，头晕、头痛，视力下降，心前区疼痛，遇冷则四肢末端指（趾）关节呈现白色、厥冷，遇热则缓解。

There is no corresponding name in Traditional Chinese Medicine yet. According to the clinical manifestations, it should belongs to the ranges of "pulseless disease", "vascular arthralgia", "cold arms (upper limbs)", "cold shins (lower limbs)". Most are caused by deficiency of congenital foundation or nourishment loss of acquired construction, invasion of Wind, Cold, and Damp toxins into meridians and channels, leading to Qi-blood depletion, deficiency of channels and collaterals, or retention of stagnated phlegm, obstruction of channel pathways.

I. Key Points for Diagnosis and Syndrome Differentiation

1. For lesions at upper limbs, the main manifestations include pulse weakness or disappearance of unilateral or bilateral radial arteries, brachial arteries, axillary arteries, carotid arteries or temporal arteries.

2. For lesions at lower limbs, the main manifestations include pulse weakness or disappearance of unilateral or bilateral popliteal arteries, dorsal pedal arteries which start from the femoral arteries, companied with intermittent claudication.

3. There can be general discomfort, pain and numbness of limbs, cold and weakness of limbs, dizziness, headache, reduced eyesight, pain in the precordium, and the finger (toe) joints at limb ends present pale and cold with cold, which will be relieved with heat.

II. Therapeutic Methods

[Syndrome of Cold Stagnation and Qi Stasis]

Therapeutic method: Tonify Qi and dredge channels.

Prescription: Renying (ST9), Taiyuan (LU9).

Mechanism of prescription: Renying is the place where Qi of Yang-Ming Stomach Meridian and channel of foot locates, it is the confluent acupoint of Yang-Ming and Shao-Yang. Yang-Ming Meridian is a meridian full of Qi and blood, the use of its acupoints can regulate Qi and blood, dredge meridians and channels. Taiyuan is a Shu acupoint of Lung Meridian, as well as a confluent acupoint of channels, it can tonify Qi and dredge channels. The use of the combination of these two acupoints can tonify Qi and blood, dredge meridians and channels.

Matching acupoints: For lesions at upper limbs add Neiguan, Chize, Shenmen. For lesions at lower limbs add Qichong, Chongyang. For dizziness and headache add Fengchi. For hypopsia add Cuanzhu, Jingming, Sibai. For pain of precordium add Xinshu, Zusanli, Tongli, Sanyinjiao.

Method: Electrothermal acupuncture treatment (warm tonifying).

Operations: Selecting the relevant acupoints, perform routine skin disinfection. Using electrothermal acupuncture needles, vertically puncture into Renying for 0.8", Zusanli for 0.8", Sanyinjiao for 0.7", obliquely puncture toward vertebral bodies into Xinshu for 0.8", vertically puncture into Qichong for 0.7". Turn on the electrothermal acupuncture equipment, apply a current

40分钟。另配以毫针直刺内关0.5寸，直刺尺泽0.5寸，直刺神门0.4寸，直刺太渊0.3寸，向下斜刺攒竹0.4寸，直刺睛明0.2寸，直刺四白0.4寸，留针30分钟。

疗程 每天1次，10次为1个疗程，疗程间可休息3天。

三、注意事项

1. 注意保暖避寒，避免风寒刺激。

2. 若发现因感染或结核等病继发者，要积极治疗原发病。

3. 并发心脏病者，要注意心脏病的治疗与监护。

4. 加强营养，改善饮食，清淡食物有助于康复。

5. 注意加强锻炼，但要劳逸适度。

高脂血症

高脂血症是指血浆脂质中一种或多种成分的浓度超过正常高限而言，40岁以内者胆固醇和甘油三酯含量分别在180mg/dl和110mg/dl以下者属正常；分别在220mg/

of 60-80mA to each acupoint, leaving the needles in for 40 minutes. Additionally, using filiform needles, vertically puncture into Neiguan for 0.5", vertically puncture into Chize for 0.5", Shenmen for 0.4", Taiyuan for 0.3", obliquely puncture downward into Cuanzhu for 0.4", vertically puncture into Jingming for 0.2", vertically puncture into Sibai for 0.4", leaving the needles in for 30 minutes.

Therapeutic course: Once a day, 10 times for a course. Rest for 3 days between courses.

III. Precautions

1. Pay attention to warm keeping and avoiding cold, avoid stimulations from Wind and Cold.

2. If the disease is found secondary to diseases like infections or tuberculosis, it is necessary to positively treat the primary diseases.

3. For patients with concurrent cardiac diseases, pay attention to treatment and monitoring of the cardiac diseases.

4. Strengthen nutrition, improve diet. Light diet facilitates recovery.

5. Increase physical exercise, but should have appropriate rest.

Hyperlipidemia

Hyperlipidemia refers to that the concentration of one or more components of plasma lipids exceed the normal upper limit. For people no more than 40 years old, it is normal if the contents of cholesterol and triglyceride are lower than 180mg/dl and 110mg/dl respectively; lipemia if higher than 220mg/dl and 160mg/dl respec-

dl 和 160mg/dl 以上者属血脂过高，处于两者之间者为血脂偏高。40 岁以上者则以后者为上限，超过此上限者为血脂偏高。临床可分为原发性与继发性两种。

中医认为，本病多因多食肥甘厚味，脾胃运化不及，遂滋湿生痰，留于肌肤脉络，着而不去所致。

一、诊断及辨证要点

1. 原发者病因不明，但大多数有家族史与遗传史。

2. 继发者则与动脉粥样硬化、冠心病、高血压、糖尿病、肾病综合征等有关。

3. 实验室、血脂、血液流变学检查均超标。

二、治疗方法

【脾虚湿困证】

治法　健脾和胃，调畅气机，祛湿降脂。

tively; high blood lipid if between the two limits respectively. For people more than 40 years old the later is the upper limit, and it can be considered as high blood lipid if the upper limit is exceeded. It can be divided as two types clinically: primary ones and secondary ones.

Traditional Chinese Medicine believes that this disease is caused by that excessive intake of fat and sweet and strong taste food leads to non-timely transportation and transformation of spleen and stomach, therefore produces Damp and generate phlegm which leave in the skin, channels and collaterals, accumulate there and do not go.

I. Key Points for Diagnosis and Syndrome Differentiation

1. For primary ones, the etiology remains unknown, however most are related to family histories and hereditary histories.

2. Secondary ones are associated with atherosclerosis, coronary heart diseases, high blood pressure, diabetes, nephritic syndrome, etc.

3. In the lab, blood lipid and blood rheological examinations, the indicators are all exceeded.

II. Therapeutic Methods

[Syndrome of Spleen Deficiency and Damp Retention]

Therapeutic method: Invigorate spleen and regulate stomach, regulate and soothe Qi Dynamic, remove Damp and reduce lipids.

(1) Method 1

Prescription: Neiguan (PC6).

Mechanism of prescription: Neiguan is a collateral acupoint of Jue-Yin Pericardium Meridian of Hand as well as one of the confluent acupoints of eight channels, it can promote mental concentration and ease pain, soothe liver and regulate stomach, and is used to treat angina, stomachache, palpitation, insomnia, vomiting, etc. It have confirmed by clinical studies that Neiguan can reduce plasma lipid concentration to treat hyperlipidemia.

Method: Electrothermal acupuncture treatment (mild tonifying and attenuating).

Operations: Selecting the relevant acupoints, perform routine skin disinfection. Using electrothermal acupuncture needles, vertically puncture into Neiguan for 0.7-0.8". After getting Qi, Turn on the electrothermal acupuncture equipment, apply a current of 50-60mA (depends on individual patient), leaving the needles in for 40 minutes.

Therapeutic course: Treat once a day, 10 times for a course, and start the treatment for the second course after a break of 3-5 days.

(2) Method 2

Prescription: Sanyinjiao (SP6), Ququan (LR8), Gongsun (SP4), Zhongwan (RN12).

Mechanism of prescription: Sanyinjiao and Gongsun are both meridian acupoints from Tai-Yin Spleen Meridian of Foot, they can invigorate spleen and dispel Damp, regulate stomach and tonify Middle Jiao; Zhongwan is an acupoint of Ren Channel, it can invig-

郁之功效。四穴共用，取其健脾和胃之功，气机调畅，湿去脂降。

方法 毫针治疗（泻法）。

操作 选定穴位，常规皮肤消毒。毫针直刺公孙 0.5 寸，直刺三阴交 0.8 寸，直刺曲泉、中脘各 0.7～0.8 寸，得气后提插，留针 30 分钟。

疗程 每天 1 次，10 天为 1 个疗程。疗程间休息 3 天，再继续进行第 2 个疗程的治疗。

（3）方法 3

处方 内关（PC6）、足三里（ST36）、三阴交（SP6）、太白（SP3）、丰隆（ST40）、阳陵泉（GB34）。

方义 内关有降脂之长；三阴交、太白是足太阴脾经穴，有健脾化湿、理气和胃之功；胃之合穴足三里能和胃健脾，通腑化痰，升降气机；胃经络穴丰隆可化痰宁心；胆经合穴阳陵泉有疏肝利胆之功。诸穴合用，可使脾健湿化，气

orate spleen and regulate stomach, soothe abdomen and descend Qi. Ququan is a He acupoint from Jue-Yin Liver Meridian of Foot, it can soothe liver Qi stagnation. The use of combination of these four acupoints can invigorate spleen and regulate stomach, regulate and soothe Qi Dynamic, remove Damp and reduce lipids.

Method: Filiform needle acupuncture treatment (attenuating).

Operations: Selecting the relevant acupoints, perform routine skin disinfection. Using filiform needles, vertically puncture into Gongsun for 0.5", vertically puncture into Sanyinjiao for 0.8", vertically puncture into Ququan, Zhongwan for 0.7-0.8" respectively, lift and thrust the needles after Qi acquisition, leaving the needles in for 30 minutes.

Therapeutic course: Once a day, 10 days for a course. Start the treatment for the second course after a break of 3 days.

(3) Method 3

Prescription: Neiguan (PC6), Zusanli (ST36), Sanyinjiao (SP6), Taibai (SP3), Fenglong (ST40), Yanglingquan (GB34).

Mechanism of prescription: Neiguan can reduce lipid; Sanyinjiao and Taibai are both meridian acupoints from Tai-Yin Spleen Meridian of Foot, they can invigorate spleen and dispel Damp, regulate Qi and harmonize stomach. The He acupoint of Stomach, Zusanli, can harmonize stomach and invigorate spleen, soothe internal organs and dispel phlegm, ascend and descend Qi Dynamic; the meridian acupoint Fenglong of Stomach

调浊去，血脂亦可降低。

配穴 胸闷、气短、心前区疼痛者加郄门、膻中；头晕耳鸣者加太冲、风池；头痛者加太阳、百会。

方法 毫针治疗（泻法）。

操作 选定穴位，常规皮肤消毒。毫针直刺太白 0.4 寸，直刺阳陵泉 0.8 寸，直刺内关、三阴交各 0.8 寸，直刺足三里 0.8 寸，直刺丰隆 0.8 寸，分为两组，交替轮换。提插泻法，得气后留针 30 分钟。

疗程 每天 1 次，10 天为 1 个疗程。疗程间休息 3～5 天，再进行第 2 个疗程的治疗。

三、注意事项

1. 宜吃清淡食物，少吃肥甘厚味之品。

2. 注意加强锻炼，但要劳逸适度。

Meridian can dispel phlegm and tranquilize heart; the He acupoint Yanglingquan of Gallbladder Meridian can soothe liver and reinforce gallbladder. The use of combination of these acupoints can invigorate spleen and dispel Damp, regulate Qi and disperse turbidity, as well as reduce blood lipids.

Matching acupoints: For chest distress and shortness of breath, pain in the precordium add Ximen, Danzhong. For dizziness and tinnitus add Taichong, Fengchi. For headache add Taiyang, Baihui.

Method: Filiform needle acupuncture treatment (attenuating).

Operations: Selecting the relevant acupoints, perform routine skin disinfection. Using filiform needles, vertically puncture into Taibai for 0.4", vertically puncture into Yanglingquan for 0.8", vertically puncture into Neiguan, Sanyinjiao for 0.8" respectively, vertically puncture into Zusanli for 0.8", vertically puncture into Fenglong for 0.8". Divide these acupoints into two groups and use alternatively. Use method of lifting-thrusting and attenuating, leaving the needles in for 30 minutes after getting Qi.

Therapeutic course: Once a day, 10 days for a course. Start the treatment for the second course after a break of 3-5 days.

III. Precautions

1. Have a light diet and eat less fat, sweet and strong-taste food.

2. Increase physical exercise, but should have appropriate rest.

3. 防止并发症的发生。

糖尿病

糖尿病是危害人类健康比较严重的一种常见内分泌代谢紊乱性疾病。临床表现除高血糖和尿糖外，还有典型的"三多一少"症状，即多饮、多食、多尿、消瘦。常并发酮症酸中毒、感染以及心血管病变、肾脏病变、神经病变、眼病变等，严重时亦可危及生命。

中医认为，本病属于"消渴"的范畴。多因嗜食肥甘厚味，蕴为内热，情志失调，五志化火，或肾虚精亏所致。病变的脏腑主要在肺、胃、肾。临床根据其症状分为上、中、下三消。上消属肺燥，中消属胃热，下消属肾虚。病机主要以阴虚为本，燥热为标，两者互为因果。早期多以燥热为主，中期则阴虚与燥热互见，晚期则以阴虚为主。

3. Prevent incidence of complications.

Diabetes

Diabetes is a common disease of endocrine metabolic disturbances that seriously endangers human health. In addition to hyperglycemia and glycosuria, the clinical manifestations also include the classic symptom of "three excesses and one less", namely polydipsia, hyperphagia, urorrhagia, emaciation. Often accompanied with ketoacidosis, infections, cardiovascular diseases, renal diseases, neurologic disease, eye diseases, etc., which can also be life threatening in severe cases.

Traditional Chinese Medicine believes that this disease belongs to the range of "symptom-complex of excessive eating". Most are caused by excessive intake of fat and sweet and strong taste food which accumulate as internal Heat, emotional disorders, five emotions transforming into Fire, or kidney deficiency and essence depletion. The main lesion locations are lungs, stomach and kidneys. It is clinically divided as three types: diabetes involving the Upper Jiao, diabetes involving the Middle Jiao, and diabetes involving the Lower Jiao. Diabetes involving the Upper Jiao belongs to lung Dryness, diabetes involving the Middle Jiao to stomach Heat, diabetes involving the Lower Jiao to kidney deficiency. Pathogenesis: Mainly Yin deficiency is the root cause and Dryness-Heat is symptom, and they interact as both cause and effect. In the early phase there mainly is Dryness-Heat, and in the middle phase Dryness-Heat and Yin deficiency coexist, while in the advanced phase there mainly is Yin deficiency.

I. Key Points for Diagnosis and Syndrome Differentiation

1. Domestic interim diagnostic criteria

If there are typical symptoms of diabetes, like polydipsia, urorrhagia, hyperphagia, emaciation, asthenia, FBG>126mg/dl (7mmol/L), 2-hour post-meal BG>200mg/dl (11.1mmol/L), then the patient can be diagnosed as diabetes.

In the oral glucose tolerance test (OGTT), the normal upper limits of blood glucose for various time phases are: 125mg/dl (6.9mmol/L) for 0 minute, 200mg/dl (11.1mmol/L) for 30 minutes, 190mg/dl (10.5mmol/L) for 60 minutes, 150mg/dl (8.3mmol/L) for 120 minutes, 125mg/dl (6.9mmol/L) for 180 minutes. Thereinto the glucose value at 30 minutes or 60 minutes is taken as one point, and the glucose values of other time phases are taken as one point respectively, 4 points in total.

(1) Overt diabetes: With typical symptoms of diabetes or a history of diabetic ketoacidosis. FBG>110mg/dl and/or postprandial blood glucose (PBG)>200mg/d, or there are three points of the four OGTT points over the above normal upper limits.

(2) Impaired glucose tolerance (IGT): No symptoms, among four OGTT points, values of two points reach or exceed the above normal upper limits. This

值。此组属可疑病例，须经长期随访后方可确诊或排除。

（3）隐性糖尿病：无症状，但空腹血糖及餐后 2 小时血糖或 OGTT 达到上述诊断标准。

（4）非糖尿病：无症状，血糖、OGTT 均正常。

2. 世界卫生组织（WHO）暂行诊断标准

（1）糖尿病典型症状（如多饮、多尿、多食、消瘦、乏力等），并发血糖升高，空腹血糖 >126mg/dl（7mmol/L），任何时候血糖 >200mg/dl（11.1mmol/L），可确诊为糖尿病。

（2）如结果可疑，应进行 OGTT（成人口服 75g 葡萄糖，儿童每千克体重服 1.75g，总量不超过 75g），餐后 2 小时血糖 >200mg/dl，可诊断为糖尿病。餐后 2 小时血糖 <140mg/dl 可除外糖尿病。餐后 2 小时血糖 >140mg/dl，同时 <200mg/dl，为糖耐量减低或异常（IGT）。

（3）如无糖尿病症状，除上述两项诊断标准外，尚须另加 1 个指标以辅助诊断，即 OGTT 曲线上血糖 >200mg/dl，或另一次空腹血糖 >126mg/dl。

（4）妊娠期糖尿病亦可采

group belongs to suspicious cases, and diagnosis or exclusion must be made after long-term follow-up.

(3) Latent diabetes: No symptoms, but the FBG and 2-hour post-meal BG or OGTT reach the above criteria of diagnosis.

(4) Non-diabetes: No symptoms, blood glucose and OGTT are normal.

2. Interim diagnostic criteria of the World Health Organization (WHO)

(1) If there are typical symptoms of diabetes (such as polydipsia, urorrhagia, hyperphagia, emaciation, asthenia) accompanied with increased blood glucose, FGB>126mg/dl (7mmol/L), blood glucose at any time >200mg/dl (11.1mmol/L), then the patient can be diagnosed as diabetes.

(2) If any suspicious case, then it is necessary to perform OGTT (for adults, oral administration of 75g glucose. For children, oral administration of 1.75g glucose/kg body weight, no more than 75g in total), the 2-hour post-meal BG>200mg/dl, then the patient can be diagnosed as diabetes. If the 2-hour post-meal BG<140mg/dl, then diabetes can be excluded. If the 2-hour post-meal BG>140mg/dl while <200mg/dl, it indicates reduced or impaired glucose tolerance (IGT).

(3) If there is no diabetic symptom, then except the two diagnostic criteria above, another indicator should be added for auxiliary diagnosis, namely on the OGTT curve the blood glucose>200mg/dl, or another measurement of FBG>126mg/dl.

(4) These diagnostic criteria are also applied to the

用此诊断标准。

3. 糖尿病的分型标准

（1）1型糖尿病（即胰岛素依赖型糖尿病）：①发病较急。②血浆胰岛素水平低于正常，必须依赖胰岛素治疗，如停用胰岛素则有酮症发生倾向。③典型者发病于幼年，但可于任何年龄开始有症状或被发现。④多在遗传基础上加一个外来因素（如病毒感染而发病，少数病例在第Ⅵ染色体上HLA抗原阳性率增高或减低，并伴有特异性免疫或自身免疫反应），早期胰岛素细胞抗体（ICA）阳性。

（2）2型糖尿病（即非胰岛素依赖型糖尿病）：①常无或很少出现糖尿病症状。②不依赖胰岛素治疗，无酮症发生倾向，但于感染及应激反应时可出现酮症。③饮食及口服降糖药不能控制，应激或感染发生高血糖症时也需要胰岛素治疗。④血浆胰岛素水平往往正常或稍低，甚可稍高于正常，有胰岛素耐药性者可增高。⑤多数发病于40岁以后，亦可见于幼年。⑥遗传因素较强，为常染色体显性遗传。⑦肥胖常为诱因，控制饮食及加强运动

gestational diabetes.

3. Type classification standard of diabetes

(1) Type I diabetes (namely insulin dependent diabetes): ① Acute occurrence. ② Plasma insulin level is lower than normal, and it must rely on insulin treatment, and if the administration of insulin is stopped, then there will be a tendency for incidence of ketosis. ③ Typically the onset is at infancy, however the symptoms can start or the disease can be found at any age. ④ Normally in addition to the hereditary factor there is an additional external factor (such as virus infection, in a few cases the positive rate of the HLA antigen on the Chromosome VI increases or decreases, accompanied with specific immune response or autoimmune response), islet cell antibodies (ICA) positive in the early phase.

(2) Type II diabetes (namely non-insulin dependent diabetes): ① Normally with no or few diabetic symptoms. ② Do not rely on insulin treatment, with no tendency for incidence of ketosis, however ketosis can occur due to infections or stress response. ③ Can not be controlled by diet and oral antidiabetics, and for hyperglycemia due to stress response or infections insulin treatment is also required. ④ Plasma insulin level is normal or slightly lower than normal or in severe cases, it may higher than normal, and for patients with insulin resistance it may increased. ⑤ Normally occurs after the age of 40 years old, however it also can be seen at infancy. ⑥ The hereditary factor has strong influence; autosomal dominant inheritance. ⑦ Obesity is often an inducement. When the body weight is reduced due to diet

使体重下降时,高血糖症和耐糖量异常可恢复正常。

4. 中医辨证分型

(1) 上消:烦渴多饮,日夜无度,口干舌燥,尿频、量多,舌红,苔薄黄,脉数。

(2) 中消:多食善饥,形体消瘦,口干多饮,大便秘结,小便频数,舌红,苔黄燥,脉滑有力。

(3) 下消:小便频数,浑浊如脂,五心烦热,视物模糊,腰膝酸软,舌质红,苔薄黄,脉细数。

二、治疗方法

【上消】

治法 清热润肺,生津止渴。

处方 太渊(LU9)、少府(HT8)、内庭(ST44)、肺俞(BL13)、胰俞(EX-B5)。

方义 上消肺热津伤,治宜清泻心肺。肺主治节,为水之上源,肺热则治节失调。故取手太阴、手少阴之荥穴太

control and intensive physical exercises, the hyperglycemia and IGT can be recovered to normal.

4. Symptom differentiation and type classification of Traditional Chinese Medicine

(1) Diabetes involving the Upper Jiao: Polydipsia, day and night without measure, mouth parched and tongue scorched, frequent micturition with excessive volume, red tongue with yellow and thin fur and rapid pulse.

(2) Diabetes involving the Middle Jiao: Increased eating with rapid hungering, skinny body, thirst and increased drinking, constipation, frequent urination, red tongue with yellow and dry fur, slippery and strong pulse.

(3) Diabetes involving the Lower Jiao: Frequent urination, turbid urine like lipid, dysphoria in chest with palms-soles, blurred vision, soreness and weakness of waist and knees, red tongue with thin and yellow fur, thin and rapid pulse.

II. Therapeutic Methods

[Diabetes Involving the Upper Jiao]

Therapeutic method: Clear Heat and moisten lung, engender liquid and allay thirst.

Prescription: Taiyuan (LU9), Shaofu (HT8), Neiting (ST44), Feishu (BL13), Yishu (EX-B5).

Mechanism of prescription: For diabetes involving the Upper Jiao, lung Heat and fluid impairment, the treatment should focus on that clear and dredge heart and lung. Lung governs management and regulation, is the

渊、少府，以清热润肺。配足阳明经荥穴内庭，既能清胃火，又可泻心火，有"实则泻其子"之意。再伍肺俞滋补肺阴。胰俞为治疗消渴的有效奇穴。诸穴共用，有清热泻火、生津止渴之功效。

配穴 口干舌燥者加廉泉、承浆；口渴甚者加少商、膈俞。

方法 电热针治疗。

操作 选定穴位，皮肤常规消毒。电热针斜刺（针尖向脊柱）肺俞、胰俞、膈俞各0.7寸，直刺少府、太渊各0.6寸，斜刺内庭0.7寸，接通电热针仪，每个穴位分别给予电流量40～50mA，以患者感到胀而舒适为度，留针40分钟。

疗程 3个月为1个疗程，每日1次，每次留针40分钟。疗程间可休息15～20天。根据病情再决定是否进行第2个

upper source of Water, and lung heat can cause disorders of management and regulation. Therefore use the Yuan acupoint from Tai-Yin Meridian of Hand, Taiyuan, and the Xing acupoint from Shao-Yin Meridian of Hand, Shaofu, to clear Heat and moisten lung. The match with the Xing acupoint from Yang-Ming Meridian of Foot, Neiting, can clear stomach Fire as well as dredge heart Fire, with the principle of "Treat excess with dredging its child". And match the Feishu to tonify lung Yin. Yishu is an effective extra acupoint for treatment of symptom-complex of excessive eating. The use of combination of these acupoints can clear Heat and purge Fire, engender liquid and allay thirst.

Matching acupoints: For mouth parched and tongue scorched add Lianquan and Chengjiang. For extreme thirst add Shaoshang, Geshu.

Method: Electrothermal acupuncture treatment.

Operations: Selecting the relevant acupoints, perform routine skin disinfection. Using electrothermal acupuncture needles, obliquely puncture (with the needle tip towards spine) into Feishu, Yishu, Geshu for 0.7" respectively, vertically puncture into Shaofu, Taiyuan for 0.6" respectively, obliquely puncture into Neiting for 0.7". Turn on the electrothermal acupuncture equipment, apply a current of 40-50mA to each acupoint, and the limit is that the patient feels swelling and comfortable, leaving the needles in for 40 minutes.

Therapeutic course: 3 months as a course, once a day, leave the needles in for 40 minutes each time. Start the treatment for the second course after a break of 15-20 days. The decision for whether carry out the second course of treatment depends on the disease conditions. Generally the condition can be basically controlled after 1 course of treatment.

[Diabetes Involving the Middle Jiao]

Therapeutic method: Clear stomach and dredge Fire, nourish Yin and increase fluid.

Prescription: Neiting (ST44), Sanyinjiao (SP6), Weishu (BL21), Pishu (BL20), Yishu(EX-B5).

Mechanism of prescription: For diabetes involving the Middle Jiao, stomach Heat is exuberant, the treatment should focus on that clear stomach and dredge Fire, tonify Yin and store fluid. Use the Xing acupoint from Yang-Ming Meridian of Foot, Neiting, together with Weishu to clear and dredge Dryness-Heat of Middle Jiao. Use Sanyinjiao and Pishu as well to regulate spleen and stomach so as to distribute fluid. Spleen and stomach are located in the Middle Jiao, one governs absorption and the other governs transportation, they condition and use mutually, and the match of these two acupoints can tonify acquired constitution. Yishu is an effective extra acupoint for treatment of symptom-complex of excessive eating. The use of combination of these acupoints can dredge Fire and replenish Yin, generate fluid.

Matching acupoints: For large appetite with rapid hungering add Zhongwan, Fenglong. For hidrosis add Shenshu, Fuliu. For fatigue and weakness add Zusanli. For extreme Heat accumulation of three Jiaos, add Sanjiaoshu, Yangchi.

Method: Electrothermal acupuncture treatment.

Operations: Selecting the relevant acupoints, per-

form routine skin disinfection. Using electrothermal acupuncture needles, obliquely puncture (with the needle tip towards spine) into Weishu, Yishu, Pishu, Sanjiaoshu, Shenshu for 0.7" respectively, vertically puncture into Zusanli, Sanyinjiao, Fuliu, Fenglong, Zhongwan for 0.7" respectively, obliquely puncture into Neiting for 0.6". Turn on the electrothermal acupuncture equipment, apply a current of 30-40mA to each acupoint, and the limit is that the patient feels comfortable, leaving the needles in for 40 minutes. (Note: Select 3 pairs of acupoints for electrothermal acupuncture treatment each time, and treat the other acupoints with filiform needles.)

Therapeutic course: 3 months as a course, once a day, leave the needles in for 40 minutes each time. Start the treatment for the second course after a break of 15-20 days. The decision for whether carry out the second course of treatment depends on the disease conditions. Generally the condition can be basically controlled after 1 course of treatment.

[Diabetes Involving the Lower Jiao]

Therapeutic method: Nourish Yin and replenish kidney, moisten Dryness and allay thirst.

Prescription: Taixi (KI3), Ganshu (BL18), Shenshu (BL23), Yishu(EX-B5), Taichong (LR3).

Mechanism of prescription: Kidney is the congenital foundation, it governs essence storage, marrow generation, Qi absorption and Water. For diabetes involving the Lower Jiao, there is kidney deficiency, therefore the treatment should focus on that nourish and reinforce kidney. Use the acupoint where Shao-Yin channels of foot

络属，具有益阴固肾壮元阳之功。太冲为厥阴肝经之所输，又是肝之原穴，配肝俞以平肝降火。胰俞为治消渴的经验穴。诸穴合用，有滋肾养阴生津之功。

配穴 肾阳虚加命门；视物不清加攒竹、头维、光明；头晕加上星；多尿加关元、复溜、水泉；手脚麻木、疼痛，加曲池、足三里；皮肤瘙痒，加风池、曲池、合谷、血海；腹泻加天枢、公孙。

方法 电热针治疗。

操作 选定穴位，皮肤常规消毒。电热针斜刺（针尖向脊柱）肾俞、胰俞、肝俞各0.7寸，直刺足三里、三阴交、命门、复溜、曲池、天枢、关元、大椎、血海各0.7寸，接通电热针仪，每个穴位分别给予40～50mA的电流量，以患者感到胀而舒适为度，留针40分钟。（注：每次选3组穴

infuse in, Taixi, which is also a Yuan acupoint of Kidney Meridian, to nourish Yin, clear Heat and reinforce kidney, and match it with Shenshu, since these two are external and internal acupoints corresponding to each other and the meridians and collaterals belong to each other. Therefore they can tonify Yin, reinforce kidney and strengthen Yuan Yang. Taichong is the acupoint where Jue-Yin Liver Meridian infuses in, and also a Yuan acupoint of Liver Meridian, it can calm liver and reduce Fire when being matched with Ganshu. Yishu is an experienced acupoint for treatment of symptom-complex of excessive eating. The use of combination of these acupoints can nourish kidney, replenish Yin and generate fluid.

Matching acupoints: For Yang deficiency of kidney add Mingmen. For blurred vision add Cuanzhu, Touwei, Guangming. For dizziness add Shangxing. For urorrhagia add Guanyuan, Fuliu, Shuiquan. For numbness and pain of hands and feet add Quchi, Zusanli; for skin itching add Fengchi, Quchi, Hegu, Xuehai. For diarrhea add Tianshu, Gongsun.

Method: Electrothermal acupuncture treatment.

Operations: Selecting the relevant acupoints, perform routine skin disinfection. Using electrothermal acupuncture needles, obliquely puncture (with the needle tip towards spine) into Shenshu, Yishu, Ganshu for 0.7" respectively, vertically puncture into Zusanli, Sanyinjiao Mingmen, Fuliu, Quchi, Tianshu, Guanyuan, Dazhui, Xuehai for 0.7" respectively. Turn on the electrothermal acupuncture equipment, apply a current of 40-50mA to each acupoint, and the limit is that the patient feels swelling and comfortable, leaving the needles in for 40

给予电热针治疗，余者用毫针治疗。）

疗程 3个月为1个疗程，每日1次，每次留针40分钟。疗程间可休息15～20天。根据病情再决定是否进行第2个疗程的治疗。一般治疗1个疗程可基本控制病情。

三、注意事项

1. 糖尿病患者在治疗期间要养成健康饮食的习惯，适当参加体育运动，但避免过劳，注意保温，防止感冒，注意精神调养。

2. 针灸治疗1型糖尿病效果较好，对效果差者要配合药物治疗。

3. 针刺背俞穴要注意方向、深度，还要安置合适的体位，避免造成气胸。

4. 糖尿病患者抵抗力弱，极易引起感染，故针治时必须严格消毒，针时严防发生烧、烫伤。

5. 如遇病情危重者，如出现呼吸困难、四肢厥冷的患者不宜用针灸治疗，应立即用药

minutes. (Note: Select 3 pairs of acupoints for electro-thermal acupuncture treatment each time, and treat the other acupoints with filiform needles.)

Therapeutic course: 3 months as a course, once a day, leave the needles in for 40 minutes each time. Start the treatment for the second course after a break of 15-20 days. The decision for whether carry out the second course of treatment depends on the disease conditions. Generally the condition can be basically controlled after 1 course of treatment.

III. Precautions

1. During treatment, diabetic patients should establish a habit of healthy diet, participate in physical exercises appropriately, but do not be overstrained, pay attention to warm keeping so as to prevent catching a cold, pay attention to mental care.

2. Acupuncture therapy has a relatively better efficacy on Type I diabetes, and for patients got poor efficacies, medication should be implemented as well.

3. For acupuncture of Back-Shu acupoints, attentions should be paid to the direction and depth of needling, and appropriate patient body position as well, so as to avoid pneumothorax.

4. Diabetic patients have poor autoimmunity and extremely susceptible to infections, therefore strict disinfection must be performed during the acupuncture treatment, strictly prevent burns and scalds during treatment.

5. For critically ill patients, patients with dyspnea, cold limbs are not appropriate to receive acupuncture treatment, and drugs must be used immediately for res-

物进行抢救。

四、典型病例

方某，女，32岁，工人，北京人。

主诉：患糖尿病3年多，经治疗仍有口干、多饮、多尿。

刻下症：头晕心悸，腰酸神疲，体力下降，月经量多，伴血块，苔薄，舌边有齿痕。现日服二甲双胍1.5g，配合饮食治疗，尿糖（++），空腹血糖8.4mmol/L。

查体：二尖瓣区及主动脉瓣第二听诊区闻及二级收缩期杂音。

辅助检查：尿糖（+++），空腹血糖8.6mmol/L。血脂三项偏高。

【诊断依据】

1. 中年女性，多饮多尿3年。

2. 空腹血糖8.6mmol/L，尿糖（+++）。

3. 长期服用降糖药。

4. 既往无特殊病史记载。

【证治分析】

病因　饮食不节，过食肥甘。

病机　长期过食肥甘厚

IV. Typical Case

Fang, female, 32 years old, worker, residence: Beijing.

Self-reported symptoms: Diabetes for 3 years, still had symptoms like dry mouth, excessive drinking and urination after treatment.

Current symptoms: Dizziness and palpitation, soreness of waist and fatigue look, declined physical strength, excessive menstrual blood volume accompanied with blood clots, thin tongue fur with tooth prints at the edge. Currently taking Metformin 1.5g daily together with diet therapy, urine glucose (++), FBG 8.4mmol/L.

Physical examination: Grade 2 systolic noise at mitral valve area and second aortic valve area.

Auxiliary examination: Urine glucose (+++), FBG 8.6mmol/L. Slight high levels of three blood lipid indicators.

[Diagnostic Basis]

1. Middle-aged female, symptoms of excessive drinking and urination for 3 years.

2. FBG 8.6mmol/L, urine glucose (+++).

3. Long-term use of antidiabetics.

4. No previous recorded special medical history.

[Syndrome-treatment Analysis]

Etiology: Intemperate diet, excessive intake of fat and sweet food.

Pathogenesis: Long-term excessive intake of fat

味，致脾胃运化失职，积热内蕴，化燥耗津，发为消渴。

证候分析 肺热炽盛，耗伤津液，故烦渴多饮，口干咽燥；胃火炽盛，水谷腐熟过度，故多食易饥；肺主治节，燥热伤肺，治节失职，水不化津，直趋于下，故小便量多；因肺与大肠相表里，燥热下移大肠，故见大便秘结。舌红，苔薄黄，脉数为内热炽盛之象。

病位 肺、胃。

病性 阴虚为本。

西医诊断 2型糖尿病。

中医诊断 消渴（上消）。

治法 清热泻火，生津止渴。

方法 电热针治疗。

处方 太渊（LU9）、少府（HT8）、内庭（ST44）、肺

and sweet and strong taste food leading to irregulation of transportation and transformation of spleen and stomach, internal retention of accumulated Heat, consumption of fluid for removing of Dryness, therefore caused symptom-complex of excessive eating.

Syndrome analysis: Exuberance of lung Heat consumes and impairs fluid, thereby causing polydipsia, dry mouth and throat; exuberance of stomach Fire causes excessive digestion of food, therefore leads to large appetite with rapid hungering; lung governs management and regulation, Dryness-Heat impairs lung and causes disorders of management and regulation, Water does not transform into fluid but go downwards directly, thereby leading to excessive volume of urine. Since lung and large intestines are exterior and interior organs corresponding to each other, so the Dryness-Heat goes downwards to the large intestine and causes constipation. Red tongue with yellow and thin fur and rapid pulse are signs of internal Heat exuberance.

Lesion location: Lung, stomach.

Lesion nature: Yin-oriented deficiency.

The diagnosis of Western Medicine: Type 2 diabetes.

The diagnosis of Traditional Chinese Medicine: Symptom-complex of excessive eating (diabetes involving the Upper Jiao).

Therapeutic method: Clear Heat and purge fire, engender liquid and allay thirst.

Method: Electrothermal acupuncture treatment.

Prescription: Taiyuan (LU9), Shaofu (HT8), Neiting (ST44), Feishu(BL13), Yishu(EX-B5).

俞（BL13）、胰俞（EX-B5）。

方义 上消肺热津伤，治宜清泻心肺。肺主治节，为水之上源，肺燥则治节失调，故取手太阴之原穴太渊、手少阴之荥穴少府，以清热润肺。足阳明经荥穴内庭，既能清胃火，又能泻心火，再配肺俞滋补肺阴。胰俞为治疗消渴病之有效奇穴。诸穴共用，可清热泻火，生津止渴。

配穴 多食多饥者加中脘、丰隆；多汗者加肾俞、复溜；神疲乏力者加足三里；视物不清者加光明、头维、攒竹；头晕者加上星；多尿者加关元；口干舌燥者加廉泉。

操作 选定穴位，皮肤常规消毒。电热针直刺太渊、少府、内庭各0.6寸，斜刺（针尖向脊柱）肺俞、胰俞、肾俞各0.7寸，直刺中脘、丰隆、复溜、足三里、曲池各0.8寸，接通电热针仪，每个穴位分别给予电流量40mA，以患者感

Mechanism of prescription: Diabetes involving the Upper Jiao, lung Heat and fluid impairment, the treatment should focus on clear and dredge heart and lung. Lung governs management and regulation, is the upper source of Water, and lung dryness can cause disorders of management and regulation, therefore use the Yuan acupoint from Tai-Yin Meridian of Hand, Taiyuan, and the Xing acupoint from Shao-Yin Meridian of Hand, Shaofu, to clear Heat and moisten lung. The Xing acupoint from Yang-Ming Meridian of Foot, Neiting, can clear stomach Fire as well as dredge heart Fire, and the match of Neiting and Feishu can tonify lung Yin. Yishu is an effective extra acupoint for treatment of symptom-complex of excessive eating. The use of combination of these acupoints can clear Heat and purge fire, engender liquid and allay thirst.

Matching acupoints: For frequent eating and hunger add Zhongwan, Fenglong. For hidrosis add Shenshu, Fuliu. For fatigue look and asthenia add Zusanli. For blurred vision add Guangming, Touwei, Cuanzhu. For dizziness add Shangxing. For urorrhagia add Guanyuan. For mouth parched and tongue scorched add Lianquan.

Operations: Selecting the relevant acupoints, perform routine skin disinfection. Using electrothermal acupuncture needles, vertically puncture into Taiyuan, Shaofu, Neiting for 0.6" respectively, obliquely puncture (with the needle tip towards spine) into Feishu, Yishu, Shenshu for 0.7" respectively, vertically puncture into Zhongwan, Fenglong, Fuliu, Zusanli, Quchi for 0.8" respectively. Turn on the electrothermal acupuncture equipment, apply

到胀而舒适为度，留针40分钟。（注：每次选3组穴给予电热针治疗，分组交替应用，眼区及颌下的穴位均用毫针治疗。）

疗程 每日1次，90次为1个疗程。疗程结束后症状基本控制，要配合饮食治疗。

【生活调摄】

1. 糖尿病患者自身抵抗力差，容易感染，治疗过程中要严格消毒，防止感染。

2. 针灸治疗过程中或之后要注意控制饮食，适当加强身体锻炼，但不要过劳。

3. 注意保暖，防止感冒，注意精神调养。

4. 对病情危重或酸中毒者，要配合中西药综合治疗，切忌单纯用针灸治疗。

甲状腺腺瘤

甲状腺腺瘤为常见的甲状腺良性肿瘤，病理上可分为滤泡状和乳头状囊性腺瘤两种，但前者较为多见。

中医认为，本病属于"瘿"的范畴。中医将瘿病分为气

a current of 40mA to each acupoint, and the limit is that the patient feels swelling and comfortable, leaving the needles in for 40 minutes. (Note：Select 3 pairs of acupoints for electrothermal acupuncture treatment each time, group them and use alternately, and treat the acupoints at the eye region and under chins with filiform needles.)

Therapeutic course: Once a day, 90 times for a course. After end of courses, symptoms can be basically controlled, it is necessary to perform diet therapy as well.

[Lifestyle Change and Health Maintenance]

1. Diabetic patients have poor autoimmunity and susceptible to infections, therefore strict disinfection must be performed during the treatment so as to prevent infections.

2. During or after acupuncture treatment, it is necessary to control diet and appropriately increase physical exercises, but do not overstrain.

3. Pay attention to warm keeping so as to prevent catching a cold, pay attention to mental care.

4. For critically ill patients or patients with acidosis, it is necessary to perform Chinese Herb Medicine therapy plus Western Medicine therapy as well, do not perform acupuncture therapy alone.

Thyroid Adenoma

Thyroid adenoma is a common benign thyroid tumor, and can be pathologically divided into two types, follicular and papillary cystic adenoma, while the former is more common.

Traditional Chinese Medicine believes that this disease belongs to the range of "goiter". In Traditional Chi-

瘿、肉瘿、筋瘿、石瘿等，根据临床特点，甲状腺腺瘤相当于肉瘿。多因忧思郁怒，痰浊凝结，留注于结喉，气血为之壅滞，聚而形成，发为肉瘿。

一、诊断及辨证要点

1. 本病多发于 40 岁以下的妇女，腺瘤多为单发，成圆形或椭圆形，局限在一侧腺体内。

2. 质地较周围甲状腺稍硬，表面光滑，无压痛，可随吞吐动作而上下移动，生长缓慢。

3. 一般多无明显全身状况，如果肿块增大，压迫气管，可引起呼吸困难，甚则声音嘶哑。

4. 甲状腺同位素碘 –131 扫描图显示多为温结节。

5. 约 20% 的概率引起甲状腺功能亢进，约 10% 的概率发生恶变，故应早期治疗。

二、治疗方法

【痰凝血瘀证】

治法　行气活血，化痰散结。

nese Medicine, the goiter is divided into Qi goiter, flesh goiter, tendon goiter, stone goiter, etc., and as per clinical characteristics, thyroid adenoma is equivalent to flesh goiter. Most are caused by deep sorrow and stagnated anger, retention of phlegm stagnation within adam's apple, leading to Qi-blood stagnation, therefore causing flesh goiter.

I. Key Points for Diagnosis and Syndrome Differentiation

1. Commonly seen among females with an age under 40 years old, and the adenomas are mostly single ones with a round or oval shape, confined to the gland of one side.

2. The texture of the adenoma is harder than the surrounding thyroid, and the surface is smooth without tenderness, while the adenoma will move upwards and downwards along with swallowing and spiting out, slow growing.

3. Normally no obvious systemic symptoms. If the lump enlarges and compress the air tract, it can cause dyspnea or even hoarse voice.

4. Generally thyroid scan with isotope iodine-131 indicates warm nodules.

5. A probability of 20% to cause hyperthyroidism, 10% to cause malignant transformation, therefore early treatment is necessary.

II. Therapeutic Methods

[Syndrome of Phlegm Stasis and Blood Stagnation]

Therapeutic method: Activate Qi and blood circulation, disperse phlegm and eliminate stagnation.

Prescription: Ashi acupoints, Tianrong (SI17), Tiantu (RN22), Naohui (SJ13), Qugu (RN2), Tianzhu (BL10), Dazhu(BL11), Neiguan (PC6).

Mechanism of prescription: This is mostly caused by unsmooth Qi circulation as well as phlegm stasis and blood stagnation, therefore use Ashi acupoints of the local lump and Tianrong, Tiantu to activate Qi-blood, regulate meridians and channels, disperse stagnation. Use Neiguan to soothe liver Qi stagnation; along both sides of Three-Jiao Meridians of Shao-Yang, the isthmus of thyroid gland is the circulation part for Ren Channel, therefore use Naohui and Qugu from two meridians to dredge meridians and eliminate stagnation. According to the theory "activate Yang for diseases about Yin, activate Yin for diseases about Yang" in the "Classics on Medical Problems: Sixty-seven difficulties' (《难经·六十七难》), use Tianzhu and Dazhu for "induce Yin from Yang". The prescription can activate Qi and blood circulation, disperse phlegm and eliminate stagnation.

Matching acupoints: For long-term disease add Hegu. For transformation of liver stasis into Fire add Taichong, Xingjian. For dyspnea, hoarse voice add Dingchuan, Lianquan, Jialianquan.

Method: Electrothermal acupuncture treatment.

Operations: Selecting the relevant acupoints, perform routine skin disinfection. Using electrothermal acupuncture needles, vertically puncture into Ashi acupoints for 0.7" (3-4 needles in the centre of the lump and the surrounding area), vertically puncture into Tianrong for

处方 阿是穴、天容（SI17）、天突（RN22）、臑会（SJ13）、曲骨（RN2）、天柱（BL10）、大杼（BL11）、内关（PC6）。

方义 本病多因气行不畅、痰凝血瘀所致，故选取肿块局部之阿是穴及天容、天突诸穴，以行气血、调经脉、散瘀结；取内关以疏肝解郁，于少阳三焦经循顾于两侧，甲状腺峡部为任脉循行部位，故取二经之臑会、曲骨通经散结。据《难经·六十七难》中"阴病行阳，阳病行阴"的理论，取天柱、大杼二穴为"从阴引阳"之义。全方可奏行气活血、化痰散结之功效。

配穴 发病较久者可加合谷；肝郁化火者加太冲、行间；呼吸困难、声音嘶哑者加定喘、廉泉、夹廉泉。

方法 电热针治疗。

操作 选定穴位，皮肤常规消毒。电热针直刺阿是穴0.7寸（肿块中心及周围刺3～4针），直刺天容0.8寸，直刺天鼎0.7寸，直刺臑会、曲骨各 0.8 寸。接通电热针仪，每个穴位分别给予电流量 40～60mA，以患者感觉舒服为度，留针 40 分钟。另配以毫针靠近胸骨柄面刺入 0.8 寸，直刺天柱、大杼各 0.5 寸，直刺内关 0.6 寸，平补平泻，留针 40 分钟。

0.8", vertically puncture into Tianding for 0.7", vertically puncture into Naohui, Qugu for 0.8" respectively. Turn on the electrothermal acupuncture equipment, apply a current of 40-60mA to each acupoint, and the limit is that the patient feels comfortable, leaving the needles in for 40 minutes. Additionally, using filiform needles, vertically puncture near the manubrium surface for 0.8", vertically puncture into Tianzhu, Dazhu for 0.5", vertically puncture into Neiguan for 0.6", use the method of mild reinforcing and attenuating, leaving the needles in for 40 minutes.

疗程 每天 1 次，90 次为 1 个疗程。疗程间若无不适，可继续治疗，否则可休息 5 天。

Therapeutic course: Once a day, 90 times for a course. Perform continuous treatment if no discomfort during the courses, or rest for 5 days.

三、注意事项

1. 保持心情舒畅，避免不良的精神刺激。

2. 针刺治疗时，肿块局部的针刺要注意深度和方向，以免损伤血管及喉返神经。

3. 经过 1 个疗程（90 次）治疗后，肿块缩小不明显，或伴有甲亢症状，或肿块迅速增大，质地坚硬，疑有恶变或压迫症状明显者，应及时考虑手术切除。

4. 可配合中药治疗，如海藻玉壶汤加味或四物舒郁丸加减等，以增强行气活郁之力。

III. Precautions

1. Keep good mood, avoid mental stimulation by adverse factors.

2. During acupoint treatment, pay attention to the depth and direction for needling of local lump, so as to avoid damages of vessels and the recurrent laryngeal nerve.

3. After a course of treatment (90 times), shrinking of the lump is not obvious, or with systems of hyperthyroidism, or the lump enlarges rapidly and has a hard texture. For suspicious malignant transformation or obvious compressive symptoms, prompt surgical resection should be considered.

4. Chinese Herb Medicine treatment also can be used in the meantime, such as Haizao Yuhu decoction (add or remove ingredients) or Siwu Shuyu pills (add or

remove ingredients), to enhance the effecacies of activating Qi and removing stagnation.

Hyperhidrosis

Hyperhidrosis is a symptom which can occur alone and also can be found in other diseases. Usually symmetrically appear on relatively limited parts on both sides of the body, such as sweating of hands, feet and cheek, and the sweating will be more obvious with warm, mental stress, emotional excitements or intake of stimulating food. Modern medicine believes that this disease is associated with neurological diseases, endocrine diseases and vegetative nerve functional disturbance.

Traditional Chinese Medicine believes that hyper hidrosis is caused by opening and closing disorders of the grain of skin and the texture of the subcutaneous flesh, abnormal excretion of Yin fluid, which belongs to the range of "spontaneous sweating"' and "night sweating". "Spontaneous sweating" is characterized as frequent profuse sweating which will be aggravated with movements, mostly caused by Qi deficiency and insecurity; "night sweating" is characterized as that sweat during sleep and stop upon waking up, mostly caused by Yin deficiency and internal Heat.

I. Key Points for Diagnosis and Syndrome Differentiation

1. For patients with Yang deficiency, symptoms include sweating when wake up which may be aggravated after movements, as well as cold body and limbs, fatigue

脉沉细而微。

2. 阴虚者，入睡汗出，兼见心烦，午后潮热，手足心热，口干咽燥，头晕，耳鸣，舌红少苔，脉细数。

二、治疗方法

【阳虚证】

治法 扶阳益气，护卫止汗。

处方 大椎（DU14）、膏肓（BL43）、复溜（KI7）。

方义 自汗责之脾胃，因脾胃为生化之源，肾藏真阴而寓元阳，阳不敛阴，卫外不固，则自汗出。督脉总督诸阳，故取督脉与手足三阳经之交会穴大椎，宣通诸阳经之经气，则卫外固而汗可止；复溜为足少阴肾经穴，有培补肾阳之功；佐以膏肓补益气血。三穴共用，有扶阳益气、护卫止汗之功。

配穴 形寒肢冷者加气

and weakness, shortness of breath and pale complexion, dark limps and light tongue, deep and thin and weak pulse.

2. For patients with Yin deficiency, symptoms include sweating during sleep, accompanying vexation, afternoon tidal fever, hot palms and sole centers, dry mouth and throat, dizziness, tinnitus, red tongue with less fur, thin and rapid pulse.

II. Therapeutic Methods

[Syndrome of Yang Deficiency]

Therapeutic method: Benefit Yang and tonify Qi, protect Wei and stop sweating.

Prescription: Dazhui (DU14), Gaohuang (BL43), Fuliu (KI7).

Mechanism of prescription: Spontaneous sweating is attributed to spleen and stomach, since spleen and stomach are the source of generation and transformation of Qi-blood, kidney stores real Yin and Yuan Yang, therefore the inability of Yang to restrain Yin and insecurity of external Wei can cause spontaneous sweating. Du Channel governs Yang of the whole body, therefore use the confluent acupoint Dazhui of Du Channel and three Yang meridians of hands and feet to drain meridian Qi, then external Wei can be enhanced and the sweating can be stopped. Fuliu is a meridian acupoints from Shao-Yin Kidney Meridian of Foot, it can replenish kidney Yang. In addition, use Gaohuang to tonify Qi and blood. The use of combination of these three acupoints can benefit Yang and tonify Qi, protect Wei and stop sweating.

Matching acupoints: For cold body and limbs add

海、关元；纳少者加足三里、中脘；腹胀者加三阴交、公孙；便溏者加丰隆、天枢。

方法 电热针治疗。

操作 选定穴位，皮肤常规消毒。电热针直刺大椎 0.7 寸，向脊中直刺膏肓 0.7 寸，直刺复溜 0.8 寸，接通电热针仪，每个穴位分别给予电流量 40～60mA，以患者感到胀或温热舒适为度，留针 40 分钟。余者随症配穴。

疗程 每日 1 次，10 次为 1 个疗程。疗程间可休息 3～5 天，再进行第 2 个疗程的治疗。

【阴虚证】

治法 滋阴固卫生津。

处方 肺俞（BL13）、复溜（KI7）、合谷（LI4）。

方义 阴液不能敛藏，故盗汗频作，方取肺俞泻肺火，养肺阴，为主穴；取复溜泻相火而坚阴，为辅穴；佐以合谷健脾益气，气血充则腠理密固而汗不出。

Qihai and Guanyuan. For less food intake add Zusanli, Zhongwan. For abdominal distension add Sanyinjiao, Gongsun. For sloppy stool add Fenglong, Tianshu.

Method: Electrothermal acupuncture treatment.

Operations: Selecting the relevant acupoints, perform routine skin disinfection. Using electrothermal acupuncture needles, vertically puncture into Dazhui for 0.7", vertically puncture toward Jizhong into Gaohuang for 0.7", vertically puncture into Fuliu for 0.8". Turn on the electrothermal acupuncture equipment, apply a current of 40-60mA to each acupoint, and the limit is that the patient feels warmly swelling and comfortable, leaving the needles in for 40 minutes. For others use matching acupoints depending on symptoms.

Therapeutic course: Once a day, 10 times for a course. Start the treatment for the second course after a break of 3-5 days.

[Syndrome of Yin Deficiency]

Therapeutic method: Nourish Yin, reinforce Wei and generate fluid.

Prescription: Feishu (BL13), Fuliu (KI7), Hegu (LI4).

Mechanism of prescription: Yin fluid is unable to be stored, therefore causes frequent night sweating, so in this prescription use Feishu as the main acupoint to purge lung Fire and nourish lung Yin. Use Fuliu as the main acupoint to purge Ministerial Fire and strengthen Yin. Add Hegu to invigorate spleen and tonify Qi; plentiful Qi and blood can lead to the grain of skin and the texture of the subcutaneous flesh solid, then there won't be night sweating.

Matching acupoints: For afternoon tidal fever add Dazhui. For irregular menstruation add Sanyinjiao. For nocturnal emission or spermatorrhea add Zhishi, Mingmen. For lean body add Shenshu, Zusanli.

Method: Electrothermal acupuncture treatment.

Operations: Selecting the relevant acupoints, perform routine skin disinfection. Using electrothermal acupuncture needles, obliquely puncture into Dazhui for 0.7", obliquely puncture into Fuliu for 0.7", vertically puncture into Hegu for 0.7", vertically puncture into Zusanli for 0.8", Sanyinjiao for 0.7". Turn on the electrothermal acupuncture equipment, apply a current of 50-60mA to each acupoint, and the limit is that the patient feels swelling or warm and comfortable, leaving the needles in for 40 minutes. For others use matching acupoints depending on symptoms.

Therapeutic course: Once a day, 10 times for a course. Start the treatment for the second course after a break of 3-5 days. Generally 2-3 courses are enough.

III. Precautions

1. Pay attention to needling direction for acupuncture of acupoints on the back, not to be too deep, and the direction should be towards Jizhong.

2. During treatment, smoking, alcohol drinking, intake of spicy and stimulating food as well as seafood are forbidden.

3. Patients are required to have stable emotion,

peaceful mind, do not be angry, exited, agitated, nervous, and cooperate with treatments.

4. Do not catch colds, take showers and change underwear frequently, pay attention to personal hygiene.

Esophagus Cancer

Esophagus cancer is one of common malignant tumors, ranked as 2 in the digestive system cancers in China.

Traditional Chinese Medicine believes that this disease belongs to the range of "dysphagia". Mostly are caused by impairment due to diet, emotional upset, depletion of vital Qi, leading to Qi and phlegm and Heat stasis as well as blood stagnation, long-term lump enlargement and exhaustion of fluid and blood. Esophagus cancer is a syndrome of asthenia in origin and sthenia in superficiality.

I. Key Points for Diagnosis and Syndrome Differentiation

1. Most common in patients with an age of 35-60 years old, more male patients than female ones.

2. Lesion location: Most are at middle or lower esophagus, or junction of lower esophagus and the cardia.

3. Symptoms: ① In the early phase symptoms are slight and are often neglected, patients only feels distress and fullness or feeling of food accumulation behind the sternum after eating. ② In the middle phase patients may have dysphonia which is intermittent at first, then occurs obstruction of food swallowing, accompanied with sense

常带有黏液样痰沫；③胸骨及后背部闷胀疼痛加重，食管部位出现灼热或针刺样疼痛，兼伴有干咳、声嘶、气短、形体消瘦等恶病质；④癌肿有转移时可摸到右锁骨上淋巴结肿大。

4. 食道癌的发生多与喜热饮、过食醇酒、辛辣煎烩的食物有关。情绪抑郁等精神因素也是本病的诱发因素之一。

5. 鳞状上皮细胞癌多见于食管中段，而腺癌主要发生在食管下段或贲门处。

6. 临床辨证当视患者体质强弱、病程长短、邪正消长之势而论。一般初、中期，当以标实为主，本虚次之；晚期则以本虚表现较为突出。

（1）初期

①气滞郁结者，症见情绪抑郁，情性急躁，口干，胸骨后食管部有闷胀感，或食咽时有不适感，苔薄黄，脉弦。

②痰湿伤络者，症见食咽不畅，或进食后呃逆，或饭后有泛恶吞酸，或厌食油腻，苔黄腻，脉滑数。

of vomiting, and there are often mucus foamy phlegm in the vomitus. ③ The fullness and distending pains of the sternum and back are aggravated, and burning-like or prickling-like pains occurs at the esophagus pat, accompanied with cachexia like dry cough, hoarseness, shortness of breath, body emaciation. ④ With cancer metastasis, enlargement of the supraclavicular lymph node can be palpated.

4. The occurrence of esophagus cancer is often associated with preference to hot drink, excessive intake of mellow wine, spicy, fried and stewed food. Mental factors like low spirits are also inducing factors of this disease.

5. Squamous cell carcinoma is normally seen at the middle esophagus, while adenocarcinoma often occurs at the lower esophagus or cardia.

6. The clinical syndrome differentiation should be done depending on the physical strength, duration of disease, waning and waxing tendency of vital Qi and pathogenic factors. Generally, in the early phase sthenia in superficiality dominates, followed by asthenia in origin; and in the advanced phase asthenia in origin dominates.

(1) Early phase

① For patients with Qi stagnation, symptoms include depressed emotions, quick temper, dry mouth, distress and fullness of the esophagus part behind the sternum, or uncomfortable feeling when swallowing, yellow and greasy thin tongue fur, taut pulse.

② For patients with phlegm Damp impairing collaterals, symptoms include unsmooth swallowing, or hiccup after food intake, or nausea and acid regurgitation after meals, or dislike to greasy food, yellow and greasy

（2）中期

①痰气交阻者，症见食咽不畅，进食过快则时见呃逆呕吐，咽部不适似物梗塞，胸骨后闷胀疼痛，苔薄黄腻，脉弦滑。

②痰阻互结者，症见食咽困难，纳谷呆滞，胸闷隐隐作痛，掣引背部，食后泛恶呕吐，呕吐物常多见清水或痰涎，苔白厚腻，脉滑。

③瘀热内积者，症见食咽困难，食入即吐，胸骨后疼痛，或背部疼痛，口干，大便干结，舌边瘀紫，苔黄，脉涩或弦数。

（3）晚期

①瘀毒伤阳者，症见食咽难下，食入呕吐，带有黏稠痰涎，口干欲饮，饮不慎则呛咳，五心烦热，舌质晦黯，舌下脉瘀紫而粗，苔薄腻，脉细弦数。

②气滞津少者，症见食咽难下，神疲乏力，气短，音哽，纳少形瘦，口干，且伴有低

tongue fur, slippery and rapid pulse.

(2) Middle phase

① For patients with stagnation of phlegm and Qi, symptoms include unsmooth swallowing, hiccup and vomiting upon eating too fast, uncomfortable feelings of the throat like being obstructed by something, fullness and distending pain behind the sternum, yellow and greasy thin tongue fur, taut and slippery pulse.

② For patients with phlegm obstruction and stagnation, symptoms include difficulty in swallowing, indigestion and loss of appetite, chest distress with dull pain extending to the back, nausea and vomiting after meals, clear water or sputum often seen in the vomitus, white and thick and greasy tongue fur, slippery pulse.

③ For patients with internal accumulation of stagnated Heat, symptoms include difficulty in swallowing, immediate vomiting after food intake, pain behind the sternum, or back pain, dry mouth, dry and hard stool, purple bruises at the tongue edge, yellow tongue fur, uneven or taut and rapid pulse.

(3) Advanced phase

① For patients with stagnated toxins impairing Yang, symptoms include difficulty in swallowing, vomiting after food intake with sticky sputum, dry mouth with desire to drink, bucking with careless drinking, dysphoria in chest with palms-soles, dark and gloomy tongue, stagnated purple and thick sublingual vessel, thin and greasy tongue fur, thin and taut and rapid pulse.

② For patients with Qi stagnation and less fluid, symptoms include difficulty in swallowing, fatigue look and asthenia, shortness of breath, choked voice, less food

热，舌红少苔，脉沉细。

③津液枯槁者，症见食咽难下，唯饮流质，汤水咽下过快也会返出，低热缠绵，口干口臭，饮而不能食，形容憔悴，骨瘦如柴，舌质红绛，光剥如镜，脉细数。

（4）术后、化疗、放疗后

①脾胃气虚者，症见纳谷少馨，神疲乏力，动则气短，或有自汗，颜面苍白，舌质淡，脉濡细。

②气血双亏者，症见头晕眼花，颜面无华，口唇爪甲淡白，神疲乏力，心悸怔忡，纳谷呆滞，舌质胖而有齿痕，苔瘦，脉细软。

③阴虚火旺者，症见口干呕物，干咳喑哑，心烦，夜寐不安，舌质红绛，无苔，脉细数。

二、治疗方法

【初期】

治法 开胃利膈，宽胸理气。

intake and body emaciation, dry mouth, and accompanied with lower fever, red tongue with less fur, deep and thin pulse.

③ For patients with dry-up of fluid, symptoms include difficulty in swallowing, only to eat liquid food and the liquid will also be backflowed with too fast swallowing, endless lower fever, dry mouth and ozostomia, only drink with no food intake, wan-looking, skinny body, red dark tongue, mirror-like tongue, thin and rapid pulse.

(4) Post-operation, post-chemotherapy, post-radiotherapy

① For patients with Qi deficiency of spleen and stomach, symptoms include no pleasure in eating, fatigue look and asthenia, shortness of breath with movement, or spontaneous sweating, pale complexion, light tongue, soft and thin pulse.

② For patients with deficiency of Qi and blood, symptoms include dizziness and vertigo, lusterless complexion, light and white lips and nails, fatigue look and asthenia, palpitation and cardiopalmus, indigestion and loss of appetite, fat tongue with tooth prints, thin tongue fur, thin and soft pulse.

③ For patients with Yın deficiency and extreme hyperactivity of Fire, symptoms include dry mouth and vomiting, dry cough and hoarse voice, vexation, disturbed sleep at night, red dark tongue with no fur, thin and rapid pulse.

II. Therapeutic Methods

[Early Phase]

Therapeutic method: Stimulate appetite and clear

处方 内关（PC6）、上脘（RN13）。

方义 食道癌初期虽然症状轻微，但体内已潜伏着隐患。其病因多为情绪抑郁或饮食所伤，而其病变部位主要在胸骨后食道及贲门处。取手厥阴心包经的络穴内关，有治疗胸闷、食不下之功效。上脘位于中脘之上，为任脉与足阳明、手太阳经的交会穴，有和中开胃、平逆止呕之功效，与内关相配，可开胃利膈以消食，宽胸理气以散郁。

配穴 若要扶正，加曲池、足三里；若见气滞郁结者，加膈俞、膻中；痰湿伤络者，加中脘、内庭。

方法 电热针治疗。

操作 选定穴位，皮肤常规消毒。电热针直刺内关 0.5 寸，直刺上脘 0.8 寸，直刺曲池 0.7 寸，直刺足三里 0.8 寸。接通电热针仪，每个穴位分别给予电流量 40～50mA，以患者感到温热舒适或胀感为度，

Prescription: Neiguan (PC6), Shangwan (RN13).

Mechanism of prescription: In the early phase of esophagus cancer, there have been lurking hidden dangers in the body though the symptoms are slight. Etiology: Most are cause by depressed emotions or impairment due to diet, and the main lesion locations are at the esophagus or cardia behind the sternum. Use the collateral acupoint Neiguan from Jue-Yin Pericardium Meridian of Hand to treat chest distress and food unable to flow down. Shangwan is located above Zhongwan, and is the confluent acupoint of Ren Channel and Yang-Ming Meridian of Foot as well as Tai-Yang Meridian of Hand. It can harmonize Middle Jiao and stimulate appetite, descend adverse energy and stop vomiting, and the match of this acupoint with Neiguan can stimulate appetite and clear diaphragm to help digestion, relieve chest distress and regulate Qi to disperse stasis.

Matching acupoints: For strengthen vital Qi, add Quchi, Zusanli. For Qi stagnation add Geshu, Danzhong. For phlegm Damp impairing collaterals add Zhongwan, Neiting.

Method: Electrothermal acupuncture treatment.

Operations: Select the relevant acupoints, perform routine skin disinfection. Using electrothermal acupuncture needles, vertically puncture into Neiguan for 0.5", vertically puncture into Shangwan for 0.8", vertically puncture into Quchi for 0.7", vertically puncture into Zusanli for 0.8". Turn on the electrothermal acupuncture equipment, apply a current of 40-50mA to each acupoint,

留针40分钟。

疗程 每日1次，30次为1个疗程。疗程间可休息5～7天，然后再进行第2个疗程的治疗。若患者无不适感觉亦可连续治疗。

【中期】

治法 疏膈利气，标本兼顾。

处方 膻中（RN17）、膈俞（BL17）、内关（PC6）、足三里（ST36）。

方义 食道癌中期主要症状是吞咽困难，胸背疼痛，呕吐。取膻中、膈俞为的是宽胸下气，以便梗阻之食道畅通。膻中是八会穴之一，所谓"气会膻中"，有疏调气机之功效；膈俞亦属于八会穴之一，所谓"血会膈俞"，故有疏膈利气、养血和血之功。膻中与膈俞相配，更有行气活血以消癥块之效，亦宗调和气血阴阳之理，行气止痛之功；足三里是强壮之穴，旨在和胃悦中，使中气继而化源足也。本病进入中期，每见癥块积留而正气亏损，用足三里以助胃气，乃标本兼顾之法。

and the limit is that the patient feels warmly swell and comfortable, leaving the needles in for 40 minutes.

Therapeutic course: Once a day, 30 times for a course. Start the treatment for the second course after a break of 5-7 days. If the patient have no discomfort, continuous treatment is also practicable.

[Middle Phase]

Therapeutic method: Soothe diaphragm and promote Qi circulation, treat symptoms as well as to effect a permanent cure.

Prescription: Danzhong (RN17), Geshu (BL17), Neiguan (PC6), Zusanli (ST36).

Mechanism of prescription: The main symptoms in the middle phase of esophagus cancer are dysphonia, pain of chest and back, vomiting. Use Danzhong and Geshu to relieve chest stuffiness and depress Qi, so as to unobstruct the esophagus. Danzhong is one of the eight confluent acupoints, "Qi converges at Danzhong", it can soothe and regulate the Qi dynamic. Geshu is also one of the eight confluent acupoints, "Blood converges at Geshu", it can soothe diaphragm and promote Qi circulation, nourish and regulate blood. The match of Danzhong and Geshu can activate Qi and blood circulation to subside lumps, and also can regulate the Yin-Yang balance of Qi and blood, so as to activate Qi and alleviate pains. Zusanli is an important tonifying acupoint, can harmonize stomach and pacify Middle Jiao, enable endless Middle-Jiao Qi therefore achieve sufficient transformation source. Once entering the middle phase, the lump

配穴　若见痰气交阻者加公孙，痰浊互结者加丰隆，瘀热内积者加合谷、大都。

方法　电热针治疗（温补法）。

操作　选定穴位，皮肤常规消毒。电热针直刺足三里 0.8 寸，平刺膻中 0.8 寸。接通电热针仪，每个穴位给予电流量 40～50mA，留针 40 分钟。另配以毫针直刺内关 0.6 寸，直刺合谷 0.5 寸，直刺丰隆 0.8 寸，留针 40 分钟。

疗程　每日 1 次，30 次为 1 个疗程。疗程间可休息 5～7 天，然后再进行第 2 个疗程的治疗。若患者无不适感亦可连续治疗。

【晚期】

治法　养阴清热，止呕保津。

处方　三阴交（SP6）、内关（PC6）、天突（RN22）、大都（SP2）。

方义　食道癌晚期的主要

enlarges and vital Qi depletes, so use Zusanli to promote stomach Qi. This is a method to treat symptoms as well as to effect a permanent cure.

Matching acupoints: For stagnation of phlegm and Qi add Gongsun. For stagnation of phlegm and turbidity add Fenglong. For internal accumulation of stagnated Heat add Hegu, Dadu.

Method: Electrothermal acupuncture treatment (warm tonifying).

Operations: Selecting the relevant acupoints, perform routine skin disinfection. Using electrothermal acupuncture needles, vertically puncture into Zusanli for 0.8", horizontally puncture into Danzhong for 0.8". Turn on the electrothermal acupuncture equipment, apply a current of 40-50 mA to each acupoint, leaving the needles in for 40 minutes. Additionally, using the filiform needles, vertically puncture into Neiguan for 0.6", vertically puncture into Hegu for 0.5", vertically puncture into Fenglong for 0.8", leaving the needles in for 40 minutes.

Therapeutic course: Once a day, 30 times for a course. Start the treatment for the second course after a break of 5-7 days. If the patient have no discomfort, continuous treatment is also practicable.

[Advanced Phase]

Therapeutic method: Nourish Yin and clear Heat, stop vomiting and preserve fluid.

Prescription: Sanyinjiao (SP6), Neiguan (PC6), Tiantu (RN22), Dadu (SP2).

Mechanism of prescription: The main symptoms

症状是食入即吐，只能食流质或半流质，此时癥块邪毒内积已甚，整日消耗，津液亏损，治疗当重在扶正保津，降逆止呕。取三阴交重在健脾保津，此穴是足三阴经的交会穴，能通调肝、肾、脾以护养阴津；与通于阴维的内关穴相配，既有疏通胸脘之气机，又有维系阴液以保津之义。选天突以平逆降气，使水谷入而得养，况且天突又为阳维与任脉之会，有降逆而护阳，祛邪而不伤正之义。大都是足太阳脾经的荥穴，有清脾经之邪热和运脾醒脾之功。诸穴共用，可奏养阴清热，止呕保津之功。

配穴 瘀毒伤阳者，加膈俞、血海；气虚津少者，加脾俞、气海、足三里；津液枯槁者，加肝俞、肾俞、太溪。

方法 电热针治疗（温补法）。

操作 选定穴位，皮肤

in the advanced phase of esophagus cancer is immediate vomiting after food intake, and patients can only eat fluid or semi-fluid food, at that time the internal accumulation of pathogenic toxins of the lump has been quite serious, with endless consumption and depletion of fluid. The treatment should be aimed to strengthen vital Qi and retain fluid, descend adverse energy and stop vomiting. The use of Sanyinjiao is aimed to invigorate spleen and retain fluid. This is the confluent acupoint of three Yin Meridians of Foot, and it can tonify liver, kidney and spleen to protect and nourish Yin fluid. The match of this acupoint with the acupoint Neiguan connected to Yin-Wei can soothe thoracic and epigastric Qi Dynamic, as well as maintain Yin fluid to retain fluid. Choose Tiantu to clam down adverse energy and descend Qi, to facilitate entrance of food for nourishment, and Tiantu also is the confluent acupoint of Yang-Wei and Ren Channel, it can descend adverse energy and protect Yang, expel pathogenic factors without impairment on vitality. Dadu is a Xing acupoint from Tai-Yang Spleen Meridian of Foot, it can clear Heat toxins of Spleen Meridian and activate spleen transformation and refresh mind. The use of combination of these acupoints can nourish Yin and clear Heat, stop vomiting and preserve fluid.

Matching acupoints: For stagnated toxins impairing Yang add Geshu, Xuehai. For Qi deficiency and less fluid add Pishu, Qihai, Zusanli. For dry-up of fluid add Ganshu, Shenshu, Taixi.

Method: Electrothermal acupuncture treatment (warm tonifying).

Operations: Selecting the relevant acupoints, per-

常规消毒。电热针直刺三阴交 0.7 寸,直刺足三里 0.8 寸,直刺内关 0.7 寸。接通电热针仪,每个穴位分别给予电流量 50～60mA。另配以毫针顺胸骨柄向下刺天突 0.8 寸,直刺大都 0.3 寸,留针 40 分钟。

疗程 每日 1 次,30 次为 1 个疗程。疗程间可休息 5～7 天,然后再进行第 2 个疗程的治疗。若患者无不适感亦可连续治疗。

【术后、化疗、放疗后】

(1) 脾胃气虚证
治法 健中益气。

处方 脾俞(BL20)、胃俞(BL21)、足三里(ST36)、三阴交(SP6)、合谷(LI4)、内关(PC6)。

方义 术后及放、化疗后白细胞下降者,或胃肠道反应明显者,均可选用本组穴位治疗。脾俞与胃俞相配,主要是调整其脾胃,促进胃肠的消化及吸收功能;配足三里、三阴交,旨在鼓舞中气,增加食欲,加内关、合谷可降逆止呕,诸穴共用,有健中益气之功效。

form routine skin disinfection. Using electrothermal acupuncture needles, vertically puncture into Sanyinjiao for 0.7", Zusanli for 0.8", and Neiguan for 0.7". Turn on the electrothermal acupuncture equipment, apply a current of 50-60mA to each acupoint. Additionally, using the filiform needles, vertically puncture along the manubrium surface downwards into Tiantu for 0.8", vertically puncture into Dadu for 0.3", leaving the needles in for 40 minutes.

Therapeutic course: Once a day, 30 times for a course. Start the treatment for the second course after a break of 5-7 days. If the patient have no discomfort, continuous treatment is also practicable.

[Post-operation, post-chemotherapy, post-radiotherapy]

(1) Syndrome of Qi deficiency of spleen and stomach
Therapeutic method: Invigorate Middle Jiao and tonify Qi.

Prescription: Pishu(BL20), Weishu(BL21), Zusanli (ST36), Sanyinjiao (SP6), Hegu (LI4), Neiguan (PC6).

Mechanism of prescription: This group of acupoints are appropriate to patients with reduced leukocyte count after operation or radiotherapy, chemotherapy for treatments. The match of Pishu and Weishu is to regulate spleen and stomach so as to facilitate digestion and absorption functions of the stomach and intestine. The addition of Zusanli, Sanyinjiao is to promote Middle-Jiao Qi, improve appetite, and the addition of Neiguan, Hegu can descend adverse energy and stop vomiting. The use of combination of these acupoints can invigorate Middle Jiao and tonify Qi.

配穴 瘀毒伤阳者，加膈俞、血海；气虚津少者，加气海；津液枯槁者，加太溪。

Matching acupoints: For stagnated toxins impairing Yang add Geshu, Xuehai. For Qi deficiency and less fluid add Qihai. For dry-up of fluid add Taixi.

方法 电热针治疗。

Method: Electrothermal acupuncture treatment.

操作 选定穴位，皮肤常规消毒。电热针直刺足三里、三阴交各0.8寸，斜刺（针尖向脊柱）肾俞、脾俞各0.8寸。接通电热针仪，每个穴位分别给予电流量40～50mA，以患者有温胀的舒适感觉为度。另配以毫针直刺内关0.6寸，直刺合谷0.5寸，留针40分钟。

Operations: Selecting the relevant acupoints, perform routine skin disinfection. Using electrothermal acupuncture needles, vertically puncture into Zusanli, Sanyinjiao for 0.8" respectively, obliquely (with the needle tip towards spine) into Shenshu, Pishu for 0.8" respectively. Turn on the electrothermal acupuncture equipment, apply a current of 40-50mA to each acupoint, and the limit is that the patient feels warmly swelling and comfortable. Additionally, using the filiform needles, vertically puncture into Neiguan for 0.6", vertically puncture into Hegu for 0.5", leaving the needles in for 40 minutes.

疗程 每日1次，30次为1个疗程。疗程间可休息5～7天，然后再进行第2个疗程的治疗。若患者无不适感觉亦可连续治疗。

Therapeutic course: Once a day, 30 times for a course. Start the treatment for the second course after a break of 5-7 days. If the patient have no discomfort, continuous treatment is also practicable.

（2）气血两虚证

治法 补气养血。

(2) Syndrome of Qi-blood deficiency

Therapeutic method: Replenish Qi and nourish blood.

处方 肝俞（BL18）、脾俞（BL20）、足三里（ST36）、关元（RN4）。

Prescription: Ganshu(BL18), Pishu(BL20), Zusanli (ST36), Guanyuan (RN4).

方义 肝藏血，脾统血，故肝脾二穴相配，有良好的养血生血之功。足三里是阳明经

Mechanism of prescription: Liver stores blood and spleen governs blood, therefore the match of the acupoints from Liver and Spleen have good efficacies

之合穴，合治内腑，有补益中气，助气血化源之功。取关元以培补元气。诸穴合用，可奏益气生血之功。本方对术后气血不足，或放、化疗后所致的骨髓抑制或神经系统等症状，均有较好的辅助治疗效果。

配穴 气虚者加气海、关元；血瘀者加血海；局部疼痛者加阿是穴。

方法 电热针疗法（温补法）。

操作 选定穴位，皮肤常规消毒。电热针直刺足三里0.8寸，斜刺（针尖向脊柱）肝俞、脾俞各0.8寸。接通电热针仪，每个穴位分别给予电流量40～50mA，以患者有温胀的舒适感觉为度。另配以毫针直刺太溪、太冲各0.5寸，直刺内关0.6寸，直刺合谷0.5寸，留针40分钟。

疗程 每日1次，10次为1个疗程。疗程间可休息5～7天，若无不适者可连续治疗。

of nourishing and generating blood. Zusanli is a He acupoint of Yang-Ming Meridian, He acupoints can treat internal organs, therefore this acupoint can tonify Middle-Jiao Qi, promote transportation source of Qi-blood. Use Guanyuan to replenish vital Qi. The use of combination of these acupoints can tonify Qi and generate blood. This prescription has good auxiliary effects on postoperative Qi-blood deficiency, myelosuppression or neurological symptoms after radiotherapy and chemotherapy.

Matching acupoints: For Qi deficiency add Qihai, Guanyuan. For blood stasis add Xuehai. For local pains add Ashi acupoints.

Method: Electrothermal acupuncture treatment (warm tonifying).

Operations: Selecting the relevant acupoints, perform routine skin disinfection. Using electrothermal acupuncture needles, vertically puncture into Zusanli for 0.8", obliquely (with the needle tip towards spine) into Ganshu, Pishu for 0.8" respectively. Turn on the electrothermal acupuncture equipment, apply a current of 40-50mA to each acupoint, and the limit is that the patient feels warmly swelling and comfortable. Additionally, using the filiform needles, vertically puncture into Taixi, Taichong for 0.5" respectively, vertically puncture into Neiguan for 0.6", vertically puncture into Hegu for 0.5", leaving the needles in for 40 minutes.

Therapeutic course: Once a day, 10 times for a course. Start the treatment for the second course after a break of 5-7 days, or perform continuous treatment if there is no discomfort.

（3）阴虚火旺证

治法　滋阴清热降火。

处方　脾俞（BL20）、章门（LR13）、三阴交（SP6）。

方义　在放、化疗的过程中，多出现口干舌燥、津液亏少、舌绛苔剥的征象。方中脾俞与章门相配，为俞募配穴法，旨在益脾阳而维护五脏功能，即所谓存得一分津液，就有一分生机。其与三阴交相伍，共调肝、脾、肾之功能，使阴津得养而虚火自退也。

配穴　阴虚火旺甚者加太溪；胸闷气短者加膻中。

方法　电热针疗法（温补法）。

操作　选定穴位，皮肤常规消毒。电热针向脊柱方向斜刺脾俞0.8寸，沿肋下斜刺章门0.8寸，直刺三阴交0.7寸。接通电热针仪，每个穴位分别给予电流量40～50mA，留针40分钟。

(3) Syndrome of hyperactivity of Fire and Yin deficiency

Therapeutic method: Nourish Yin and clear Heat, reduce Fire.

Prescription: Pishu (BL20), Zhangmen (LR13), Sanyinjiao (SP6).

Mechanism of prescription: During radiotherapy, chemotherapy, symptoms like dry mouth and tongue, depletion and reduction of fluid, crimson tongue with peeling fur often occur. In the prescription, the match of Pishu and Zhangmen uses the method of Shu-Mu acupoints combination, which is aimed to tonify spleen Yang so as to maintain functions of five internal organs, the so-called "there is fluid, there is a slim chance of survival". Adding Sanyinjiao, the combination of these three acupoints can regulate liver, spleen and kidney, so as to nourish Yin fluid and the deficiency Fire back down naturally.

Matching acupoints: For Yin deficiency and extreme hyperactivity of Fire add Taixi. For chest distress and shortness of breath add Danzhong.

Method: Electrothermal acupuncture treatment (warm tonifying).

Operations: Selecting the relevant acupoints, perform routine skin disinfection. Using electrothermal acupuncture needles, obliquely puncture toward spine into Pishu for 0.8", obliquely puncture along the rib downward into Zhangmen for 0.8", vertically puncture into Sanyinjiao for 0.7". Turn on the electrothermal acupuncture equipment, apply a current of 40-50mA to each acupoint, leaving the needles in for 40 minutes.

疗程　每日1次，10次为1个疗程。疗程间可休息5～7天，若无不适者可连续治疗。

三、注意事项

1. 食道癌目前首选的治疗方法是手术，其次是放、化疗，再次是中药、针灸等综合治疗。针灸临床所见的食道癌患者大多数是中晚期，或化疗、放疗后患者。实践证明，针灸对本病的辅助治疗作用是肯定的，效果很好，尤其在缓解症状，减轻患者的痛苦，减少放、化疗的毒副反应，延长肿瘤患者的生命等方面，均取得了较好的疗效。

2. 食道癌患者在针灸治疗的过程中，饮食调养很重要，不宜食粗糙、黏稠、油腻、煎炒的食物；宜食用富有营养、易吞咽、润滑的食物，如米仁粥、山药粥、糯米粥、牛奶、蛋汤、新鲜蔬菜及水果，蔬菜最好切成细末。

3. 针灸治疗期间，患者要适当参加一些体育运动。

4. 针刺天突、章门及背俞穴时，要掌握好针刺方向、深

Therapeutic course: Once a day, 10 times for a course. Start the treatment for the second course after a break of 5-7 days, or perform continuous treatment if there is no discomfort.

III. Precautions

1. The preferred therapeutic method for esophagus cancer is surgery, followed by radiotherapy, chemotherapy, then the comprehensive therapy with Chinese Herb Medicine treatment and acupuncture treatment. The clinically seen patients with esophagus cancer of acupuncture therapy mostly are patients in the middle phase or advanced phase, or patients who have received chemotherapy and radiotherapy. Practice has proved that the efficacies of acupuncture as an auxiliary therapy on this disease is definite, especially in respects like symptom relief, pain alleviating, reducing toxic and side effects from radiotherapy and chemotherapy, prolonging the life of cancer patients.

2. For patients with esophagus cancer, diet regulation is important during treatment. Do not eat rough, sticky, greasy, fried food; eat nutritious, easy to swallow, lubricative food, like rice kernel porridge, yam porridge, glutinous rice porridge, milk, egg soup, fresh vegetables and fruits, and vegetables are better to be chopped into fine particles.

3. During treatment, patients should have some physical exercises properly.

4. For acupuncture of the acupoints Tiantu, Zhangmen and Back-Shu acupoints, it is important to control

度，以免刺伤内脏器官。

四、典型病例

宋某，男，47岁，职员，天津人。

主诉：胸骨后引背部疼痛，吞咽困难50多天，近1周加重。病史：患者2个月前因与朋友聚餐，过食生冷及辛辣食品，之后食道及胃脘部不适，呃逆沉缓有力，得热则减，遇寒则甚，饮食减少，口不渴，舌淡苔润，脉迟。经中、西医对症治疗不减轻，之后经食道镜活检诊为"食道中上段癌"。因放疗食道水肿，出现梗阻、滴水不进，要求针灸配合治疗。

刻下症：进食困难，甚则滴水不进，形体消瘦，面色无华，神疲气短，纳少，二便通畅，舌淡苔润，脉迟。

查体：两肺呼吸音粗糙。二尖瓣区及主动脉瓣第二听诊区可闻及二级收缩期杂音。

辅助检查：X线示"食道中段癌"。白细胞计数：$12×10^9$/

IV. Typical Case

Song, male, 47 years old, employee, residence: Tianjin.

Self-reported symptoms: Back pain backwards extended from the sternum, dysphonia for more than 50 days, aggravated in the recent 1 week. Medical history: 2 moths ago, the patient ate excessive cold and spicy food during the dinner with friends, then he felt discomfort of espohagus and epigastrium, deep and slow and powerful hiccup which relived with warm and worsened with cold, reduced food intake, a lack of thirst, light tongue with moist fur, delay pulse. The disease was not relieved by symptomatic treatment of Traditional Chinese Medicine and Western Medicine; later "esophageal squamous cell carcinoma" was confirmed by the esophagoscopic biopsy. Esophagus edema due to chemotherapy; obstruction occurred and the patient was unable to eat or drink, matching treatment of acupuncture therapy was required.

Current symptoms: Difficulty in feeding, or even unable to eat or drink, body emaciation, gloomy complexion, fatigue look, shortness of breath, less food intake, good urination and defecation, light tongue with moist fur, delay pulse.

Physical examination: Coarse breath sounds in both lungs. Grade 2 systolic noise at mitral valve area and second aortic valve area.

Auxiliary examination: X-ray examination indicated "middle esophageal cancer". Leukocyte count $12×10^9$/L.

L。食道镜活检示"食道鳞状细胞癌"。

【诊断依据】

1. 呃逆病史2月余不减，越来越重。

2. 食欲逐渐减少，吞咽不利。

3. 食道镜活检示"黏膜细胞炎症、中度不典型增生、鳞状上皮细胞癌"。

4. 胸骨后引及背后疼痛。

5. 白细胞计数 $12×10^9$/L。

【证治分析】

病因 过食生冷、辛辣之品。

病机 多因饮食所伤，导致痰热互结，癥块日积，津血枯槁所致。

证候分析 寒邪阻遏，肺胃之气失于和降，故呃逆声沉缓有力，膈间及胃脘不适。寒邪遏热则易消散，遇寒则更增邪势，故得热则减，遇寒则甚，胃中寒冷，中阳被遏，运化迟缓，故食欲减少，口不渴。舌脉均属胃中有热之象。

病位 食道。

Esophagoscopic biopsy indicated "esophageal squamous cell carcinoma".

[Diagnostic Basis]

1. A history of hiccup for more than 2 months with no relief, increasingly worsened.

2. Gradually reducing of appetite, difficulty in swallowing.

3. Esophagoscopic biopsy indicated "inflammation of mucous cells, moderate atypical hyperplasia, squamous cell carcinoma".

4. Retrosternal and back pain.

5. Leukocyte count $12×10^9$/L.

[Syndrome-treatment Analysis]

Etiology: Excessive intake of cold and spicy food.

Pathogenesis: Most are caused by impairment due to diet, leading to stagnation of phlegm and Heat, long-term lump enlargement and exhaustion of fluid and blood.

Syndrome analysis: Cold toxins obstruction, disorders of regulation and descending of lung and stomach Qi, lead to deep, slow and powerful sound of hiccup, transdiaphragmatic and epigastric discomfort. Cold toxins suppress Heat, therefore it is easy to dissipate, and the power of toxins increases with Cold, therefore the symptom gets relieved with Warm and aggravated with Cold. The stomach is cold inside and the Middle Yang is suppressed, slow transportation and transformation, therefore lead to reduced appetite, a lack of thirst. The signs of tongue pulse are all those for the symptom of Heat inside stomach.

Lesion location: Esophagus.

病性 虚实夹杂。

西医诊断 食道癌、慢性食道炎。

中医诊断 噎膈、呃逆。

治法 温中散寒,降逆止呃。

方法 电热针治疗。

处方 天突（RN22）、膻中（RN17）、膈俞（BL17）、胃俞（BL21）、脾俞（BL20）、内关（PC6）、足三里（ST36）、中脘（RN12）、章门（LR13）、关元（RN4）。

方义 天突为任脉和阴维脉之会，能和中降逆，中脘为胃之募穴，章门为脾之募穴，分别与胃俞、脾俞相伍，乃俞募配穴，调理脾胃气机，关元补元气，以助温中散寒之力，膻中为八会穴之一，所谓"气会膻中"，有疏调气机之功。

配穴 呕吐酸水、清水，加梁门；滴水不进，加合谷。

操作 选定穴位，皮肤常规消毒。电热针直刺足三里、关元、内关、中脘各 0.7 寸,

Disease nature: intermingled deficiency and excess.

The diagnosis of Western Medicine: Esophagus cancer, chronic esophagitis.

The diagnosis of Traditional Chinese Medicine: Dysphagia, hiccup.

Therapeutic method: Warm Middle Jiao and disperse Cold, descend adverse energy and stop belching.

Method: Electrothermal acupuncture treatment.

Prescription: Tiantu (RN22), Danzhong (RN17), Geshu (BL17), Weishu(BL21), Pishu(BL20), Neiguan (PC6), Zusanli(ST36), Zhongwan (RN12), Zhangmen (LR13), Guanyuan (RN4).

Mechanism of prescription: Tiantu is the confluent acupoint of Ren Channel and Yinwei Channel, it can regulate Middle Jiao and descend adverse energy; Zhongwan is a Mu acupoint of Stomach, Zhangmeng is a Mu acupoint of Spleen, and the match of Zhongwan and Weishu as well as Zhangmen and Pishu complies with the method of Shu-Mu acupoints combination, they can tonify Qi Dynamic of spleen and stomach; Guanyuan can replenish vitality Qi to promote the efficacy of warm Middle Jiao and disperse Cold; Danzhong is one of the eight confluent acupoints, "Qi converges at Danzhong", it can soothe and regulate Qi Dynamic.

Matching acupoints: For vomiting of acid water and clear water add Liangmen. For unable to eat or drink add Hegu.

Operations: Selecting the relevant acupoints, perform routine skin disinfection. Using electrothermal acupuncture needles, vertically puncture into Zusanli,

沿胸骨柄向下直刺天突 0.7 寸，斜刺膈俞、脾俞、胃俞各 0.8 寸，平刺章门 0.8 寸，接通电热针仪，每个穴位分别给予电流量 50mA，以患者感到温热舒适为度，留针 40 分钟。另配以毫针泻合谷（提插），不留针。

疗程 每日 1 次，10 天为 1 个疗程，若无不适可连续治疗。

治疗过程 该患者治疗过程顺利，经针治 3 次后呃逆消失，针 1 次后即可进流食。1 个月后基本可进普食。为巩固疗效又配合中药治疗。治疗中配合放疗共同完成疗程，随访 5 年未复发。

【生活调摄】

1. 饮食调养很重要，不宜食粗糙、黏稠、油腻、煎炒的食物；宜食富有营养、易吞咽、润滑的食物，如米仁粥、山药粥、糯米粥、牛奶、蛋汤、新鲜蔬菜及水果，蔬菜最好切成细末。

2. 患者要适当参加一些体育运动。

Guanyuan, Neiguan, Zhongwan for 0.7" respectively, vertically puncture along the manubtium surface downwards into Tiantu for 0.7", obliquely puncture into Geshu, Pishu, Weishu for 0.8" respectively, horizontally puncture into Zhangmen for 0.8". Turn on the electrothermal acupuncture equipment, apply a current of 50mA to each acupoint, and the limit is that the patient feels warm and comfortable, leaving the needles in for 40 minutes. Additionally, using the filiform needles, attenuate Hegu (lifting-thrusting), do not leave the needles in.

Therapeutic course: Once a day, 10 days for a course, or perform continuous treatment if there is no discomfort.

Therapeutic process: The treatment for the patient was successful. After 3 times of acupuncture, the hiccup disappeared and the patient could eat fluid food after 1 time of acupuncture. After 1 month of treatment the patient basically could eat normal food. To consolidate the efficacies, Chinese Herb Medicine therapy was used as well. During treatment, chemotherapy was used too. 5-year follow-up, no recurrence.

[Lifestyle Change and Health Maintenance]

1. Diet regulation is important. Do not eat rough, sticky, greasy, fried food; eat nutritious, easy to swallow, lubricative food, like rice kernel porridge, yam porridge, glutinous rice porridge, milk, egg soup, fresh vegetables and fruits, and vegetables are better to be chopped into fine particles.

2. Patients should have some physical exercises properly.

肺癌 / Lung Cancer

肺癌是呼吸系统常见的肿瘤之一，多因吸烟、工业废气、化学性及放射性物质、粉尘等长期吸入和刺激，造成肺部慢性炎症，机体免疫功能低下，从而导致气管上皮细胞恶变而发生。吸烟与肺癌关系密切。

中医认为，本病属于"肺积""咳嗽""痞癖"等范畴。多因风、痰、热、瘀等邪毒乘虚而犯肺，肺失清肃之令，气道受阻，邪毒内结，日久形成肿块，癥块日大，正气亏损，肺之气阴耗竭所致。本病临床多见正虚邪实的表现，故早期多以实证为主，中期则以虚实夹杂证为主，晚期则多以虚证为主。

一、诊断及辨证要点

1. 初期

（1）风寒恋肺者，咳嗽反复发作，咳稍止则又作，缠绵难愈，常咳泡沫黏痰，咳痰不

Lung cancer is one of the common tumors of the respiratory system, mostly caused by smoking, long-term inhalation and stimulation of industrial waste gas, chemical and radioactive substances, and dust, which cause chronic pulmonary inflammations and impaired body immune functions, and lead to malignant transformation of tracheal epithelial cells. Smoking is closely associated to lung cancer.

Traditional Chinese Medicine believes that this disease belongs to the ranges of "lung accumulation", "cough", "lump aggregation", etc. Most are caused by that pathogenic toxins like Wind, Phlegm, Heat, Stasis invade lung when it is weak, leading to loss of strict pulmonary order, air tract obstruction, internal stagnation of pathogenic toxins, formation of lumps after a long time, long-term lump enlargement, vital Qi depletion, consumption of lung Qi Yin. Most of the clinically seen manifestations present as body resistance weakened while pathogenic factors prevailing, therefore in the early phase most are excess syndromes, in the middle phase most are syndromes of intermingled deficiency and excess, and in the advanced phase most are deficiency syndromes.

I. Key Points for Diagnosis and Syndrome Differentiation

1. Early phase

(1) For patients with Wind-Cold retention in the lung, symptoms include repeated onset of cough, which attacks again after slight relief and is hard to be cured,

净，胸闷且痛，痛引脊背，伴有咽痒，气短，舌质晦暗，苔白腻，脉浮滑。

（2）肝火犯肺者，呛咳反复不愈，甚则咳吐鲜红，胸闷痛而挚引两肺，痰少而黏，性情急躁，心烦易怒，舌质红，苔黄。

（3）痰热壅肺者，咳嗽痰多，经治难愈，肺积初成，胸痛气短，痰多黄稠，常反复发热，口干咽痛，小便黄赤，舌肿色暗，苔黄厚腻，脉弦滑。

2. 中期

（1）气滞血瘀者，肺积咳嗽，痰少，胸痛，痛有定处，咳则疼痛加剧，甚则咳嗽胸痛，汗出气短，胸腹胀满，纳食呆滞，舌质黯，舌边有瘀斑或瘀点，苔灰腻，脉弦紧而涩。

（2）肺热痰饮者，肺积咳嗽，胸胁闷痛，咳唾引痛，气短气促，颜面虚肿，纳呆心烦，心下悬饮，身重且有胸腔积

frequent occurrence of foamy sticky phlegm during coughing, endless expectoration, chest distress and pain which extending to the back, accompanied with throat itching, shortness of breath, dark and gloomy tongue with white and greasy fur, floating and slippery pulse.

(2) For patients with liver Fire invading lung, symptoms include non-cure repeated bucking with bright red vomitus, chest distending pain extending to the lungs, less and sticky phlegm, quick temper, vexation and irritability, red tongue with yellow fur.

(3) For patients with phlegm and Heat obstructing lung, excessive phlegm upon coughing, hard to be cured by treatments, initial formation of lung accumulation, chest pain and shortness of breath, excessive yellow and thick phlegm, frequent repeated pyrexia, dry mouth and painful throat, yellow dark urine, swollen tongue with dark color, yellow and thick and greasy tongue fur, taut and slippery pulse.

2. Middle phase

(1) For patients with Qi stagnation and blood stasis, lung accumulation and cough, less phlegm, chest pain with fixed pain lesions, increased pain upon coughing, or even coughing leading to chest pain, sweating and shortness of sweating, thoracico-abdominal distress and fullness, indigestion and loss of appetite, dark tongue, ecchymosis or petechia on the tongue edge, gray and greasy tongue fur, taut and tight and uneven pulse.

(2) For patients with lung Heat, phlegm and retained fluid, symptoms include lung accumulation and cough, chest and hypochondrium oppressive pain, pain caused by coughing saliva, shortness of breath, face puff-

液，舌质暗红，苔黄腻，脉滑弦数。

（3）肺阴虚者，肺积咳嗽，痰中带血，低热时起，久稽不退，午后颧红，夜热早凉，心烦口干，形体消瘦，舌红苔少，脉细数。

3. 晚期

（1）肺脾气阴两虚者，肺积咳嗽，咳声低微，咳痰少，痰中带血，咳则气短，常见自汗或盗汗，神疲倦怠，面色萎黄，口干纳少，形体消瘦，舌质嫩红或胖，苔薄或少苔，脉细弱。

（2）肺肾阴阳两虚者，肺积咳嗽，气急，胸痛痰黏，腰腿酸软，头晕耳鸣，形瘦微寒，四肢不温，舌质淡胖，苔白腻，脉沉细无力。

4. 术后、放疗、化疗后

（1）肺脾气血两虚者，咳嗽气短，神疲乏力，面色白，头晕心悸，语声低微，虚热自

iness, indigestion and loss of appetite, vexation, pleural effusion under heart, heavy body with water inside chest, dark red tongue with yellow and greasy fur, slippery and taut and rapid pulse.

(3) For patients with lung Yin deficiency, symptoms include lung accumulation and cough, blood within phlegm, frequent onset of lower fever which lingering for a long time, red cheeks in the afternoon, warm body at night and cold body in the morning, vexation and dry mouth, body emaciation, red tongue with less fur, thin and rapid pulse.

3. Advanced phase

(1) For patients with Qi and Yin deficiency of lung and spleen, symptoms include lung accumulation and cough with low coughing sound, less cough phlegm, blood within phlegm, shortness of breath upon coughing, frequent spontaneous sweating or night sweating, fatigue look and tiredness, sallow complexion, dry mouth and less food intake, body emaciation, tender and red or fat tongue with thin fur or less fur, thin and weak pulse.

(2) For patients with Yin and Yang deficiency of lung and kidney, symptoms include lung accumulation and cough, tachypnea, chest pain and sticky phlegm, aching lumbus and limp legs, dizziness and tinnitus, skinny and slightly cold body, cold limbs, light and fat tongue with white and greasy fur, deep and thin and weak pulse.

4. Post-operation, post-radiotherapy, post-chemotherapy

(1) For patients with Qi and blood deficiency of lung and spleen, symptoms include cough and shortness of breath, fatigue look and asthenia, pale complexion,

汗，食少消瘦，舌淡质胖，苔薄，脉微弱，按之无力。

（2）肺肾阴虚者，咳嗽少气，咳声低哑，咽痛，口干舌燥，腰酸腿软，午后潮热，五心烦热，动则气短，舌质红绛，苔少或剥，脉细数，按之无力。

二、治疗方法

【初期】

治法 宣肺透邪，降逆止咳。

处方 风门（BL12）、肺俞（BL13）、太渊（LU9）。

方义 肺癌初期，临床症状主要是咳嗽，反复难愈，咳痰时少时多，以外邪乘虚犯肺，或风痰热毒瘀结于肺的征象比较突出，故常表现为实证。治疗当以祛邪散结为主，辅以补益肺气。肺俞可助风门宣肺透邪，同时可疏导肺脏之气，止咳逆。

dizziness and palpitation, low speaking volume, deficiency-Heat and spontaneous sweating, less food intake and emaciation, light and fat tongue with thin fur, weak pulse which is weak when being pressed.

(2) For patients with Yin deficiency of lung and kidney, symptoms include cough and shortness of breath, low and hoarse coughing sound, throat pain, dry mouth and tongue, aching lumbus and limp legs, afternoon tidal fever, dysphoria in chest with palms-soles, shortness of breath upon moving, red dark tongue with less or peeling fur, thin and rapid pulse which is weak when being pressed.

II. Therapeutic Methods

[Early Phase]

Therapeutic method: Facilitate lung and expel pathogenic factors, descend adverse energy and stop coughing.

Prescription: Fengmen (BL12), Feishu (BL13), Taiyuan (LU9).

Mechanism of prescription: The main clinical symptom is coughing that attack repeatedly and is hard to be healed, the amount of phlegm upon coughing varies from time to time, and normally the relatively prominent signs are invasion of external pathogenic factors into the lung when it is weak, or stagnation of Wind, Phlegm, Heat, Stasis toxins within the lung, therefore normally it is excess syndrome. The treatment should focus on eliminating pathogenic Qi and stagnation, supplemented with tonifying lung Qi. Feishu can help Fengmen to facilitate lung and expel pathogenic factors, while to soothe Qi of lungs and stop coughing and dyspnea.

配穴 若见风痰恋肺者，加尺泽、列缺；若见肝火犯肺者，加行间、足临泣；若见热痰壅肺者，加丰隆、少商。

Matching acupoints: For Wind and phlegm retention in the lung add Chize, Lieque. For vexation and irritability add Xingjian, Zulinqi. For Heat and phlegm obstructing lung add Fenglong, Shaoshang.

方法 电热针治疗。

Method: Electrothermal acupuncture treatment.

操作 选定穴位，皮肤常规消毒。电热针向脊柱斜刺风门、肺俞各0.7寸，直刺太渊0.6寸。接通电热针仪，每个穴位分别给予电流量40～60mA，以患者略感舒适为度，留针40分钟。

Operations: Selecting the relevant acupoints, perform routine skin disinfection. Using electrothermal acupuncture needles, obliquely puncture toward spine into Fengmen, Feishu for 0.7" respectively, vertically puncture into Taiyuan for 0.6". Turn on the electrothermal acupuncture equipment, apply a current of 40-60mA to each acupoint, and the limit is that the patient feels slightly comfortable, leaving the needles in for 40 minutes.

疗程 每日1次，10次为1个疗程。疗程间可休息5～7天，若无不适者可连续治疗。

Therapeutic course: Once a day, 10 times for a course. Start the treatment for the second course after a break of 5-7 days, or perform continuous treatment if there is no discomfort.

【中期】

[Middle Phase]

治法 培土生金，降逆祛邪。

Therapeutic method: Reinforce Earth to generate Metal, descend adverse energy and remove pathogenic factors.

处方 肺俞（BL13）、中府（LU1）、尺泽（LU5）、支沟（SJ6）、足三里（ST36）。

Prescription: Feishu (BL13), Zhongfu(LU1), Chize (LU5), Zhigou (SJ6), Zusanli (ST36).

方义 肺癌中期，邪毒日积，癥块日大，此时咳嗽、胸痛、咯血等症俱见，癥块在肺，元气亏损，津液耗伤，故在临床多见虚实夹杂证，治疗要扶正祛邪兼顾。本方以肺俞

Mechanism of prescription: In the middle phase of lung cancer, the pathogenic factors accumulate over time and the lump enlarges over time, at that time symptoms like cough, chest pain, hemoptysis all occur, and the lump is within the lung, with Yuan Qi depletion, consumption of fluid, therefore syndromes of intermingled

配中府,取俞募配穴法,重在转输肺脏之气,以行宣肃之令,肺气宣则风痰邪毒无结滞之地,肺气肃则痰热瘀毒无稽留之害;配肺经之合穴尺泽,以宣泄肺经邪气;选手少阳三焦经之支沟穴,旨在疏通三焦气机,使三焦之气得以开泄,以祛除肺之痰热瘀积;取足阳明经合穴足三里培本补气,培土生金,中焦脾胃化源不竭,则肺金得养。诸穴合用,共奏扶正祛邪之功效。

deficiency and excess are most common clinically. The treatment should focus on both strengthening vital Qi and eliminating pathogenic factors. This prescription match Feishu with Zhongfu, using the method of Shu-Mu acupoints combination, aims to transport lung Qi to regulate strict orders of lung, and smooth lung Qi can eliminate places for stagnation of Wind and phlegm pathogenic toxins, orderly lung Qi can eliminate the harm of retention of Wind, Phlegm, Heat, Stasis. Match with the He acupoint Chize of Lung Meridian to disperse pathogenic Qi of Lung Meridian. Choose the acupoint Zhigou from Shao-Yang Three-Jiao Meridian of Hand to soothe Qi Dynamic of three Jiaos, so as to facilitate opening-dispersing Qi of three Jiaos, remove the stagnation of phlegm and Heat in the lung. Use the He acupoint Zusanli from Yang-Ming Meridian of Foot to foster foundation and replenish Qi, reinforce Earth to generate Metal, the lung Metal can be nourished as long as that the transformation source of spleen and stomach of Middle Jiao does not exhausted. The use of combination of these acupoints can strengthen vital Qi and eliminate pathogenic factors.

配穴 若肺气滞血瘀者,加行间、曲泉;若肺痰饮停,偏热者加列缺、丰隆,偏寒者加膈俞、通里;若肺阴虚者,可加三阴交、太白。

Matching acupoints: For lung Qi stagnation and blood stasis add Xingjian, Ququan. For phlegm-fluid retention of lung, add Lieque and Fenglong for excessive Heat, Geshu and Tongli for excessive Cold. For lung Yin deficiency add Sanyinjiao, Taibai.

方法 电热针治疗。

Method: Electrothermal acupuncture treatment.

操作 选定穴位,皮肤常规消毒。电热针向外斜刺肺俞0.7寸,直刺尺泽0.8寸,直刺支沟0.8寸,直刺足三里0.8寸。

Operations: Selecting the relevant acupoints, perform routine skin disinfection. Using electrothermal acupuncture needles, obliquely puncture outward into Feishu for 0.7", vertically puncture into Chize for 0.8",

接通电热针仪，每个穴位分别给予电流量 40～60mA，以患者感到舒适或温热为度，留针 40 分钟。

疗程 每日 1 次，10 次为 1 个疗程。疗程间可休息 3～5 天，若无不适可连续治疗。

【晚期】

治法 扶本培元,补肺降气。

处方 肺俞（BL13）、中府（LU1）、太渊（LU9）、膏肓（BL43）、神门（HT7）、脾俞（BL20）、肾俞（BL23）。

方义 肺癌晚期，多是气阴俱损或阴阳两虚之表现，此时虽然病位在肺，但常累及肾，因此，"肺脾同治，肺肾同调，扶本培元"是治疗肺癌晚期的常用治则。本方仍采用俞募配穴法，肺俞配中府以转输肺脏之气；配肺之原穴太渊，以补肺气，助肺脏经气之转输；取膏肓是因癥积日久，邪毒深陷，针膏肓以除邪散结，驱邪外出；用气海以壮阳气，具有补肺降气之功，使肺气得以升降出入；合心经之原穴神门，以宁心安神，心肺同

vertically puncture into Zhigou for 0.8", vertically puncture into Zusanli for 0.8". Turn on the electrothermal acupuncture equipment, apply a current of 40-60mA to each acupoint, and the limit is that the patient feels comfortable or warm, leaving the needles in for 40 minutes.

Therapeutic course: Once a day, 10 times for a course. Start the treatment for the second course after a break of 3-5 days, or perform continuous treatment if there is no discomfort.

[Advanced Phase]

Therapeutic method: Strengthen foundation and reinforce vital essence, replenish lung and descend Qi.

Prescription: Feishu(BL13), Zhongfu (LU1), Taiyuan (LU9), Gaohuang (BL43), Shenmen (HT7), Pishu (BL20), Shenshu (BL23).

Mechanism of prescription: In the advanced phase of lung cancer, most manifestations belong to depletion of both Qi and Yin or deficiency of both Yin and Yang. At that time though the lesion site is lung, however the kidneys are generally involved in, therefore "treat lung and spleen together, tonify lung and kidney together, strengthen foundation and reinforce vital essence" is the commonly used rule of treatment for advanced lung cancer. This prescription still use the method of Shu-Mu acupoints combination, match Feishu with Zhongfu to transport lung Qi. Match the Yuan acupoint Taiyuan of Lung to replenish lung Qi and facilitate the circulation of lung meridian Qi. The reason for use of Gaohuang is that the lump has been enlarging for a long time and pathogenic toxins are deeply accumulated, therefore puncture

居上焦，又为宗气之所聚，其司呼吸而贯心脉，若神安而心脉充，则有利于肺气之开合及上焦的宣通；选肾俞，以温肾益气，有助于固先天之本。

配穴 若肺脾气阴两虚，可加内关、三阴交、足三里；若肺肾阴阳两虚，加太溪、关元。

方法 电热针治疗。

操作 选定穴位，皮肤常规消毒。电热针向脊柱方向斜刺肺俞、膏肓、脾俞、肾俞、中府各0.7寸，接通电热针仪，每个穴位分别给予电流量40～60mA，以患者有温热胀感而舒服为度，留针40分钟。另配以毫针直刺神门、太渊各0.5寸，留针30分钟，气海可予以艾条灸10～20分钟。

疗程 每日1次，10次为1个疗程。疗程间可休息3～5天，若无不适可连续治疗。

Gaohuang to remove pathogenic toxins and disperse stagnation, expel pathogenic toxins out. Use Qihai to strengthen Yang Qi, and this acupoint can replenish lung and descend Qi, to facilitate ascending and descending as well as coming in and going out of lung Qi. Match the Yuan acupoint Shenmen from Heart Meridian to pacify mood and tranquillize mind; heart and lungs are both located within Upper Jiao, heart channels will be plentiful with tranquillized mind, and is good to opening and closing of Hui Qi and ventilating of Upper Jiao. Choose Shenshu to warm kidney and tonify Qi, and facilities to reinforce the congenital foundation.

Matching acupoints: For Qi and Yin deficiency of lung and spleen, add Neiguan, Sanyinjiao, Zusanli. For Yin and Yang deficiency of lung and kidney, add Taixi, Guanyuan.

Method: Electrothermal acupuncture treatment.

Operations: Selecting the relevant acupoints, perform routine skin disinfection. Using electrothermal acupuncture needles, obliquely puncture towards spine into Feishu, Gaohuang, Pishu, Shenshu, Zhongfu for 0.7" respectively. Turn on the electrothermal acupuncture equipment, apply a current of 40-60mA to each acupoint, and the limit is that the patient feels warm or swell and comfortable. Additionally, using filiform needles, vertically puncture into Shenmen, Taiyuan for 0.5" respectively, leaving the needles in for 30 minutes, and perform moxa stick moxibustion on Qihai for 10-20 minutes.

Therapeutic course: Once a day, 10 times for a course. Start the treatment for the second course after a break of 3-5 days, or perform continuous treatment if

【术后、放疗、化疗后】

治法 补益肺气,滋养肺阴。

处方 肺俞（BL13）、气海（RN6）、足三里（ST36）、三阴交（SP6）。

方义 肺癌术后、放疗、化疗的副反应,临床主要表现是肺之气阴不足。因此,补益肺气,滋养肺阴是其治疗原则。本方取肺俞为主穴,用以和调肺脏之气;选气海以益气培本,收敛气补肺之功;用足三里以培补真气,养胃生津。胃乃五脏六腑之海,主润宗筋,主束骨而利关节,胃又为后天之本,胃气不绝,则药后能发挥作用,肺气得充,生机不息也。故本组穴为肺癌术后、放疗、化疗时扶正培本的必选穴位。

配穴 若肺脾气血双虚,加脾俞、肝俞;若胃肾阴虚,热毒烧灼,加肾俞、太溪、行间、尺泽。

方法 电热针疗法（温

there is no discomfort.

[Post-operation, post-radiotherapy, post-chemotherapy]

Therapeutic method: Replenish and tonify lung Qi, nourish lung Yin.

Prescription: Feishu(BL13), Qihai (RN6), Zusanli (ST36), Sanyinjiao (SP6).

Mechanism of prescription: Side reactions after operation, radiotherapy and chemotherapy for lung cancer, and the main clinical manifestation is insufficiency of lung Qi Yin. Therefore its treatment principle is to replenish and tonify lung Qi, nourish lung Yin. This prescription use Feishu as the main acupoint to regulate lung Qi; choose Qihai to tonify Qi and foster foundation, so as to retain Qi and replenish lung. Use Zusanli to replenish genuine Qi, tonify stomach and generate fluid. Stomach is the sea of internal organs, and it governs moistening of convergent tendons, as well as governs bundling bones to facilitate joints, while stomach is the foundation of acquired constitution, the medicines can exert therapeutic effects given that stomach Qi is not exhausted, and the vitality will be on and on so long as that lung Qi is plentiful. So this group of acupoints are required to strengthen vital Qi and reinforce foundation after operation, radiotherapy and chemotherapy for lung cancers.

Matching acupoints: For Qi and blood deficiency of lung and spleen add Pishu, Ganshu. For Yin deficiency of stomach and kidney, burning of Heat toxins, add Shenshu, Taixi, Xingjian, Chize.

Method: Electrothermal acupuncture treatment

补法)。

操作 选定穴位,皮肤常规消毒。电热针向脊柱方向斜刺肺俞、脾俞、肝俞各 0.7 寸,直刺足三里 0.8 寸,直刺三阴交 0.7 寸。接通电热针仪,每个穴位分别给予电流量 40～60mA。另配以毫针直刺太溪 0.5 寸,直刺尺泽、行间各 0.6 寸,留针 40 分钟。

疗程 每日 1 次,10 次为 1 个疗程。疗程间休息 3～5 天,再进行第 2 个疗程的治疗。

三、注意事项

1. 针刺背俞穴及中府时,要特别注意针刺方向和深度,防止刺伤肺脏,引起气胸、血胸等不良反应。

2. 肺癌患者要严格掌握饮食禁忌,禁烟、酒和辛辣刺激食品,饮食宜清淡,以新鲜蔬菜、水果为好。可多食香菇、木耳、河鱼等,少食油腻厚味及不易消化的食品。

3. 患者生活要规律,早睡早起,可到户外呼吸新鲜空气,适当参加体育活动,如太极拳、气功、散步等。应保持

(warm tonifying).

Operations: Selecting the relevant acupoints, perform routine skin disinfection. Using electrothermal acupuncture needles, obliquely puncture toward spine into Feishu, Pishu, Ganshu for 0.7" respectively, vertically puncture into Zusanli for 0.8", vertically puncture into Sanyinjiao for 0.7". Turn on the electrothermal acupuncture equipment, apply a current of 40-60mA to each acupoint. Additionally, using the filiform needles, vertically puncture into Taixi for 0.5", vertically puncture into Chize, Xingjian for 0.6" respectively, leaving the needles in for 40 minutes.

Therapeutic course: Once a day, 10 times for a course. Start the treatment for the second course after a break of 3-5 days.

III. Precautions

1. For acupuncture of Back-Shu acupoints and Zhongfu, special attention should be paid to needling direction and depth to avoid puncture into the lung, causing adverse effects like pneumothorax and hemothorax.

2. Patients with lung cancers should strictly control dietetic contraindications, do not smoke, drink, eat spicy and stimulating food, better to have light diet, such as fresh vegetables and fruits. Eat more shii-take mushrooms, agaric, river fishes, etc., eat less greasy and thick taste food and food not easy to be digested.

3. Patients should have regular life, sleep early and get up early, go outside to breath fresh air, have appropriate physical exercises such as Taiji, Qigong, walking. Patients should keep happy mood and avoid mental stim-

精神愉快，避免精神刺激。

4. 针灸治疗肺癌仍是辅助治疗，治疗原则为：①早期以手术为主；②中期主要是综合治疗，控制肿瘤发展，创造有利于手术的条件；③晚期在运用化疗、放疗的同时配合针灸及中药，以辅助治疗。针灸对改善肺癌各期的症状和提高患者的免疫功能有着良好的功效。

四、典型病例

张某，男，42岁，职员，北京人。

主诉：咳嗽，痰少黏白，带血丝已10天。病史：患者10天前无原因胸痛、咳嗽，时有痰中带血丝，低热，经胸片及右锁骨上浅淋巴穿刺，诊为"原发性右周围型肺癌中期"，给予化疗后，出现恶心、不思饮食、全身困倦无力、头晕，经药物治疗症状不减，频发呕吐，需要针灸配合治疗。

刻下症：面色白，形体消瘦，神疲乏力，纳差，二便

4. For lung treatment the acupuncture therapy is still an auxiliary therapy, the treatment principles of which are: ① The main therapy in the early phase is operation. ② In the middle phase the main therapy is to use comprehensive for control of tumor development, so as to create conditions in favor of operations. ③ In the advanced phase, use acupuncture therapy and Chinese Herb Medicine therapies as auxiliary therapies along with chemotherapy and radiotherapy. Acupuncture treatment has good efficacies on improvement of symptoms in all phases of lung cancers as well as on improving immunologic functions of patients.

IV. Typical Case

Zhang, male, 42 years old, employee, residence: Beijing.

Self-reported symptoms: Cough, sticky and white, less phlegm with blood streaks for 10 days. Medical history: 10 days ago, the patient had chest pain, coughing with blood streaks inside phlegm from time to time, lower fever, reasons unknown. After chest radiography and right supraclavicular shallow lymph node biopsy, the patient was diagnosed as "primary right peripheral lung cancer, middle phase". After chemotherapy, the patient developed symptoms like nausea, apathy to food, systemic weakness, dizziness, which had no relief after mediation, and the patient had frequent vomiting, acupuncture therapy required.

Current symptoms: Pale complexion, body emaciation, fatigue look and asthenia, poor appetite, good uri-

通畅，咳嗽痰少，质黏，色白，带血丝，舌淡，苔白，脉沉细。

查体：锁骨上浅表淋巴结肿大，如枣核大小，可活动。两肺呼吸音粗。体温 37.3～37.5℃。

辅助检查：胸片示"原发性右周围型肺癌中期"。淋巴结穿刺示"肺癌淋巴转移"。痰中找到癌细胞。

【诊断依据】

1. 中年男性，无原因之胸痛，咳嗽，痰中带血丝，低热，体温 37.3～37.5℃。

2. 胸片证实为"原发性右周围型肺癌中期"。

3. 吸烟 25 年。

4. 淋巴结穿刺证实为转移癌。

5. 痰中找到癌细胞。

【证治分析】

病因 外邪浸入肺脏，正气不足。

病机 正气不足，体质虚弱，劳倦过度，耗伤气血和阳精，正气受损，抗邪能力下降，致肺气先伤，卫外减弱，外邪乘机侵入肺部，进而邪毒内结，日久形成肿块。

nation and defecation, coughing with less and sticky and white phlegm with blood streaks, light tongue with white fur, deep and thin pulse.

Physical examination: Enlargement of the supraclavicular superficial lymph node, with a size like jujube kernel, movable. Coarse breath sounds in both lungs. Body temperature: 37.3 - 37.5℃.

Auxiliary examination: Chest radiography indicated primary right peripheral lung cancer, middle phase. Lymph node puncture indicated "lymphatic metastasis of lung cancer". Cancer cells were found in the phlegm.

[Diagnostic Basis]

1. Middle-aged male, chest pain, coughing with blood streaks inside phlegm, lower fever, body temperature 37.3 - 37.5℃; reasons unknown.

2. Chest radiography confirmed "primary right peripheral lung cancer, middle phase".

3. A smoking history of 25 years.

4. Lymph node puncture confirmed metastatic cancer.

5. Cancer cells were found in the phlegm.

[Syndrome-treatment Analysis]

Etiology: Invasion of exogenous pathogenic factors into the lung, insufficiency of vital Qi.

Pathogenesis: Insufficiency of vital Qi, weakness of body, overfatigue, over-consuming Qi-blood and Yang essence, leading to impairment of vital Qi, decreased ability of anti-evil, therefore causing impairment of lung Qi, weakening of external defense, and the exogenous pathogenic factors invade into lung, then causes internal stagnation of pathogenic toxins, formation of lumps after

证候分析 阴虚肺燥，肺失滋润，故干咳少痰，胸闷隐痛，肺损络伤则痰中时夹血丝，舌脉亦为肺气阴亏之象。

病位 肺。

病性 正虚邪实。

西医诊断 肺癌、化疗后毒副反应。

中医诊断 肺积。

治法 扶正祛邪。

方法 电热针治疗。

处方 肺俞（BL13）、中府（LU1）、尺泽（LU5）、支沟（SJ6）、足三里（ST36）、太渊（LU9）、膏肓（BL43）、三阴交（SP6）、太溪（KI3）。

方义 肺俞配中府，取俞募配穴法，重在转输肺脏之气，以外宣肃之令，肺宣则风痰邪毒无结滞之地，肺气宣则痰热瘀毒无稽留之害。配肺经合穴尺泽，以宣泄肺经邪气；取三焦经之支沟，旨在疏通三焦之气机，使三焦之气得以开泄，以祛除肺之痰热瘀积；取

a long time.

Syndrome analysis: Yin deficiency and lung dryness, loss of lung nourishment, therefore cause dry coughing with less phlegm, chest distress and dull pain, and the phlegm often contains blood streaks if lung is impaired and collaterals are injured, and the pulse condition of tongue also indicates Yin deficiency of lung Qi.

Lesion location: Lung.

Disease nature: Body resistance weakened while pathogenic factors prevailing.

The diagnosis of Western Medicine: Lung cancer, toxic and side effects after chemotherapy.

The diagnosis of Traditional Chinese Medicine: Lung accumulation.

Therapeutic method: Strengthen vital Qi and eliminate pathogenic factors.

Method: Electrothermal acupuncture treatment.

Prescription: Feishu (BL13), Zhongfu (LU1), Chize (LU5), Zhigou (SJ6), Zusanli (ST36), Taiyuan (LU9), Gaohuang (BL43), Sanyinjiao (SP6), Taixi (KI3).

Mechanism of prescription: This prescription match Feishu with Zhongfu, using the method of Shu-Mu acupoints combination, aims to transport lung Qi, subsequently to regulate strict orders of lung outside, and smooth lung Qi can eliminate places for stagnation of Wind, phlegm and pathogenic toxins, orderly lung Qi can eliminate the harm of retention of phlegm, Heat, stasis and toxins. Match with the He acupoint Chize of Lung Meridian to disperse pathogenic Qi of Lung

阳明经合穴足三里，可培本补气，培土生金，中焦脾胃化源不竭，则肺金得养；配太渊及主治诸虚百损之要穴膏肓，滋阴润肺；取太溪补肾阳、滋水润肺；足三里、三阴交健运中洲，扶正祛邪。

配穴 咯血加孔最；咳嗽痰多加尺泽；肺阴虚加三阴交、太白。

操作 选定穴位，皮肤常规消毒。电热针直刺足三里、三阴交、支沟各0.7寸，斜刺（向中）肺俞、膏肓、中府各0.8寸（每次3个穴，两组交替应用）。接通电热针仪，每穴分别给予电流量40mA，留针40分钟，余穴用毫针治疗。

疗程 每日1次，10次为1个疗程。疗程间休息3～5天，

Meridian; choose the acupoint Zhigou from Three-Jiao Meridian to soothe Qi Dynamic of three Jiaos, so as to facilitate opening-dispersing Qi of three Jiaos, remove the stagnation of phlegm and Heat in the lung. Use the He acupoint Zusanli from Yang-Ming Meridian of Foot to foster foundation and replenish Qi, reinforce Earth to generate Metal, the lung Metal can be nourished as long as that the transformation source of spleen and stomach of Middle Jiao does not exhausted. Match with the acupoint Taiyuan and the acupoint Gaohuang which is an important acupoint for treatment of various deficiencies and damages, to nourish Yin and moist lung. Use Taixi to replenish kidney Yang, nourish Water and moist lung. Use Zusanli, Sanyinjiao to promote transportation of spleen and stomach, strengthen vital Qi and eliminate pathogenic factors.

Matching acupoints: For hemoptysis add Kongzui. For cough with excessive phlegm add Chize. For Yin deficiency of lung add Sanyinjiao, Taibai.

Operations: Selecting the relevant acupoints, perform routine skin disinfection. Using electrothermal acupuncture needles, vertically puncture into Zusanli, Sanyinjiao, Zhigou for 0.7" respectively, obliquely puncture (with the needle tip towards spine) into Feishu, Gaohuang, Zhongfu for 0.8" respectively (use 3 acupoints each time, use the two groups alternatively). Turn on the electrothermal acupuncture equipment, apply a current of 40mA to each acupoint, leaving the needles in for 40 minutes, and treat the other acupoints with filiform needles.

Therapeutic course: Once a day, 10 times for a course. Start the treatment for the second course after a

再进行第 2 个疗程的治疗。

治疗过程 每日 1 次，第 3 天恶心、欲吐、咳嗽均减轻，能进饮食，继续治疗，配合服中草药，每日 1 剂，治疗顺利，疗效显著（继续化疗中），患者的精神、体力均明显好转，食欲增强，咳吐血痰已消失。在化疗、中药配合下继续电热针治疗，转移淋巴结已不能触及，肿块已消失。前后共治疗 8 个月。复查胸片，肺脏肿块消退，停化疗后电热针隔日治疗 1 次（临床治愈），患者精力充沛，但始终要求继续电热针保健，观察 5 年健在，工作、生活均如常人。（注：在治疗过程中，患者配合较好，始终是中西医综合治疗。）

【生活调摄】

1. 严格掌握饮食禁忌，禁烟、酒和辛辣刺激性食品，饮食物宜清淡，以新鲜蔬菜、水果为好。可多食香菇、木耳、河鱼等，少食油腻厚味及不易

break of 3-5 days.

Therapeutic process: Once a day, and at the third day the symptoms of nausea, sense of vomiting and cough were all relived, the patient could take food; continued the treatment supplemented with Chinese Herb Medicine therapy, one dose a day. The treatment was successful with significant efficacies (continuous chemotherapy), and the mental and physical conditions of the patient all had significant improvements with increased appetite, and the symptom of coughing with bloody phlegm disappeared. Continued the electrothermal acupuncture treatment supplemented by chemotherapy and Chinese Herb Medicine therapy, the metastatic lymph node could not be touched any more, and the lump had disappeared. 8 months of treatment in total. Reexamed with chest radiography, and the lump in the lung had subsided, performed the electrothermal acupuncture treatment once every two days after termination of chemotherapy (clinically cured). The patient was full of energy but still asked to continue the electrothermal acupuncture treatment for health care. The patient is still alive after 5-year observation, with normal working and daily life. (Note: During the treatment, the patient showed good cooperation and accepted the comprehensive therapy with Traditional Chinese Medicine and Western Medicine treatments.)

[Lifestyle Change and Health Maintenance]

1. Strictly control dietetic contraindications, do not smoke, drink, eat spicy and stimulating food, better to have light diet, such as fresh vegetables and fruits. Eat more shiitake mushrooms, agaric, river fishes, etc., eat less greasy and thick foods and food not easy to be di-

消化的食品。

2.生活要规律，早睡早起，可到户外呼吸新鲜空气，适当参加体育活动，如太极拳、气功、散步等。

3.应保持精神愉快，避免精神刺激。

胃癌

胃癌是临床常见的消化道恶性肿瘤，病位主要在胃部，尤其幽门前区、胃窦、胃体小弯侧最易发病。多与饮食、环境、遗传、免疫、癌前病变等因素有关。如胃溃疡、胃息肉、慢性萎缩性胃炎伴胃黏膜肠腺化生或不典型增生等病变而被忽略；或经治无效，逐渐发展而恶变，导致本病的发生。

中医认为，本病属于"反胃""胃脘痛""积聚"等范畴。多因饮食不节，饥饱失常，过食醇酒辛辣煎炒食品；或情志所伤；或胃病久治不愈，以致胃府受损，正气亏虚，邪毒痰气瘀结，癥块日大，后天乏源，气血阴阳衰竭所致。

gested.

2. Have regular life, sleep early and get up early, go outside to breath fresh air, have appropriate physical exercises such as Taiji, Qigong and walking.

3. Keep happy mood and avoid mental stimulations.

Stomach Cancer

Stomach cancer is a clinically common malignant tumor of digestive tract, and the main lesion location is stomach, especially the proparea of pylorus, gastric antrum and the side of small curvature of stomach. Most are associated with dietary, environmental, hereditary, immunological factors and precancerous lesions. The disease may be caused by neglect of lesions like gastric ulcer, gastric polyps, chronic atrophic gastritis accompanied with gastric mucosal gland metaplasia or atypical hyperplasia. Or caused by ineffective treatment leading to gradually development of malignant transformation.

Traditional Chinese Medicine believes that this disease belongs to the ranges of "regurgitation","epigastric pain", "stomach accumulation". Most are caused by intemperate diet, irregular eating, excessive intake of mellow wine, spicy, fried and stewed food; or caused by emotional upset; or the stomach illness cannot be cured after long-term treatment, therefore cause impairment of the stomach organ, depletion and deficiency of vital Qi, stasis accumulation of pathogenic toxins and phlegm Qi, long-term lump enlargement, lack of source for acquired constitution, exhaustion of Qi-blood and Yin-Yang, leading to the cancer.

一、诊断及辨证要点

I. Key Points for Diagnosis and Syndrome Differentiation

临床属正虚邪实证。早期多为气分证候,以实证为主;中期多为邪毒瘀结,正气亏损,以虚实夹杂证为主;晚期多为癥块日积,气血津液亏损,以虚证为主。

It clinically belongs to the syndrome of body resistance weakened while pathogenic factors prevailing. In the early phase, most are Qi-Fen syndromes, and the excess syndrome dominates; in the middle phase most are syndromes of intermingled deficiency and excess, with stagnation of pathogenic toxins, depletion of vital Qi. In the advanced phase, most are deficiency syndromes, with long-term lump enlargement, depletion of Qi-blood and fluid.

1. 初期

(1) 肝气犯胃者,胃脘胀满,隐隐作痛,或痛引两胁,纳食少馨,嗳气,口干且苦,舌质红,苔薄黄,脉弦数。

(2) 脾胃虚寒者,胃脘隐痛,按之则舒,常喜热饮,神疲乏力,面色白,四肢不温,易于感冒,纳谷不振,大便溏薄,舌质暗,苔薄白滑,脉细无力。

2. 中期

(1) 痰气凝滞者,胃脘部胀满疼痛,时有泛恶吐涎,胃胀,食纳呆滞,胸闷身重,嗳气,喉间似物梗,有痰,舌暗

1. Early phase

(1) For patients with liver Qi invading stomach, symptoms include epigastric distress and dull pain, or pain extending to both sides of the chest, no pleasure in eating, blenching, dry mouth and bitter taste, red tongue with thin and yellow fur, taut and rapid pulse.

(2) For patients with deficiency and cold of spleen and stomach, symptoms include epigastric dull pain which gets relived with pressing, preference to hot drink, fatigue look and asthenia, pale complexion, cold limbs, easy to catch cold, poor appetite, sloppy and thin stool, dark tongue with thin and white and slippery fur, thin and weak pulse.

2. Middle phase

(1) For patients with cognation and stasis of phlegm and Qi, symptoms include epigastric distension and fullness as well as pain, frequent nausea and ptysis, stomach distension, indigestion and loss of appetite, chest distress

红，苔黄腻，脉弦滑。

（2）热毒内结者，胃脘疼痛，泛恶呕吐，食后常反胃，口气秽臭，口干舌燥，大便干结，小便黄赤，舌红苔黄，脉弦数。

（3）气结血瘀者，胃脘疼痛，部位固定。常呈锐痛或针刺样痛，且有灼热感，饮食少进，时见黑粪，舌质晦黯，舌边瘀紫，苔白腻，脉弦滑或细涩。

3. 晚期

胃阴不足者，胃脘隐痛，干呕不食，形体消瘦，口干咽燥，且有低热缠绵不去，午后或傍晚颧红，形体瘦削，舌绛且干，苔剥或萎黄，或灰滞，脉弦细数，按之无力。

4. 术后、化疗、放疗后

（1）胃虚气逆者，胃胀满不适，嗳气频发，甚则反胃呕吐或吐清涎，苔白腻，脉弦滑。

and heavy body, blenching, uncomfortable feelings of the throat like being obstructed by something, phlegm, dark red tongue with yellow and greasy fur, taut and slippery pulse.

(2) For patients with internal stagnation of Heat toxins, symptoms include epigastric pain, nausea and vomiting, frequent regurgitation after eating, ozostomia, dry mouth and tongue, dry and hard stool, yellow dark urine, red tongue with yellow fur, taut and rapid pulse.

(3) For patients with Qi stagnation and blood stasis, symptoms include epigastric pain with fixed lesion sites. Often are sharpen pain or prickling-like pains with burning-like feelings, less food intake, frequent dark stool, dark and gloomy tongue with purple bruises at the tongue edge, white and greasy fur, taut and slippery or thin and uneven pulse.

3. Advanced phase

For patients with insufficiency of stomach Yin, symptoms include epigastric dull pain, dry vomiting without food intake, body emaciation, dry mouth and throat, accompanied with endless lower fever, flushing cheeks in the afternoon or in the evening, skinny body, crimson and dry tongue with peeling or sallow or gray fur, taut and thin and rapid pulse which is weak when being pressed.

4. Post-operation, post-chemotherapy, post-radiotherapy

(1) For patients with stomach deficiency and reversed flow of Qi, symptoms include stomach distress and fullness, frequent blenching, or even nausea and vomiting or vomiting with clear saliva, white and greasy

（2）脾肾气阴两虚者，胃脘隐痛，癥块不化，面色苍白，精神倦怠，纳谷不馨，形疲气短，头晕眼花，口干，腰酸腿软，舌质淡，苔少或剥，脉细数。

二、治疗方法

【初期】

治法 疏肝解郁，调畅气机。

处方 中脘（RN12）、胃俞（BL21）、气海（RN6）、足三里（ST36）、三阴交（SP6）、曲池（LI11）、内关（PC6）、合谷（LI4）。

方义 胃癌初期常因情志抑郁，饮食不节而致肝失疏泄，胃失和降，出现气机郁滞不畅的表现；又可因饮食生冷、脾胃受损而导致胃不能腐谷，脾不能健运，出现中焦虚寒的表现。本方用腑会中脘，重在和调胃腑，疏理阳明气机，使胃气和降，纳腐有权，则痰气邪毒无稽留积滞之害；配阳明合穴足三里"合治内腑"，更能使中焦健运，胃气顺降，且有扶正祛邪之功；选内

tongue fur, taut and slippery pulse.

(2) For patients with Qi and Yin deficiency of lung and spleen, symptoms include epigastric dull pain, non-removed lumps, pale complexion, spiritual burn-out, no pleasure in eating, body fatigue and shortness of breath, dizziness and vertigo, dry mouth, aching lumbus and limp legs, light tongue with less or peeling fur, thin and rapid pulse.

II. Therapeutic Methods

[Early Phase]

Therapeutic method: Soothe liver Qi stagnation, regulate Qi Dynamic.

Prescription: Zhongwan (RN12), Weishu (BL21), Qihai (RN6), Zusanli (ST36), Sanyinjiao (SP6), Quchi (LI11), Neiguan (ST44), Hegu (LI4).

Mechanism of prescription: In the early phase of stomach cancer, emotional depression and intemperate diet often cause loss of liver soothing and dredging, stomach Qi rising, subsequently leading to Qi Dynamic stagnation. Meanwhile intake of raw and cold drink and food, impairment of spleen and stomach cause dysfunctions of stomach and spleen, subsequently leading to deficiency-Cold of Middle Jiao. This prescription uses the confluent acupoint of organs, Zhongwan, to regulate the stomach organ, soothe Qi Dynamic of Yang-Ming Meridian, so as to facilitate orderly stomach Qi descending and food digestion, then there won't be harm of retention and stagnation of phlegm, Qi and pathogenic toxins.

关可宽胸畅中以和调气机；配少阳胆经之合穴阳陵泉，在于疏泄胆气，使肝胆得以舒畅，则无害中焦脾胃气机升降之枢要。故此方对于胃脘积聚初起者十分相宜。

配方 若肝气犯胃，加太冲、期门；若脾胃虚寒，加内庭、气海、天枢。

方法 电热针治疗。

操作 选定穴位，皮肤常规消毒。电热针直刺中脘 0.7 寸，直刺内关 0.6 寸，直刺足三里 0.8 寸，直刺阳陵泉 0.8 寸。接通电热针仪，每个穴位分别给予电流量 40～60mA，以患者感到舒适为度。另配以毫针直刺太冲 0.6 寸，斜刺期门 0.7 寸，留针 40 分钟。

疗程 每日 1 次，10 次为 1 个疗程。疗程间休息 3～5 天，再进行第 2 个疗程的治疗。

Match with the He acupoint Zusanli from Yang-Ming Meridian, "He acupoints can treat internal organs", so this acupoint can enable normal functions of Middle Jiao and descending of stomach Qi, as well as strengthen vital Qi and eliminate pathogenic factors; choose Neiguan to relieve chest stuffiness and soothe Middle Jiao, therefore regulate Qi Dynamic. Match with the He acupoint Yanglingquan from Shao-Yang Gallbladder Meridian to dredge gallbladder Qi and unobstruct liver and gallbladder, so as to avoid impairment of the key place for ascending and descending of spleen and stomach Qi Dynamic within Middle Jiao. Therefore this prescription is very appropriate to patients with early accumulation of stomach.

Matching acupoints: For liver Qi invading stomach add Taichong, Qimen. For deficiency and cold of spleen and stomach add Neiting, Qihai, Tianshu.

Method: Electrothermal acupuncture treatment.

Operations: Selecting the relevant acupoints, perform routine skin disinfection. Using electrothermal acupuncture needles, vertically puncture into Zhongwan for 0.7", vertically puncture into Neiguan for 0.6", vertically puncture into Zusanli for 0.8", vertically puncture into Yanglingquan for 0.8". Turn on the electrothermal acupuncture equipment, apply a current of 40-60mA to each acupoint, and the limit is that the patient feels comfortable. Additionally, using the filiform needles, vertically puncture into Taichong for 0.6", obliquely puncture into Qimen for 0.7", leaving the needles in for 40 minutes.

Therapeutic course: Once a day, 10 times for a course. Start the treatment for the second course after a break of 3-5 days.

【中期】

治法 调胃护中，疏理气机，消积止呕。

处方 中脘（RN12）、足三里（ST36）、内关（PC6）、三阴交（SP6）、曲池（LI11）、胃俞（BL21）、三焦俞（BL22）。

方义 胃癌中期，邪毒痰气瘀结明显，胃脘胀满疼痛，呕吐反胃，黑便，消瘦等症状突出，此时虚实夹杂，应在祛邪的同时兼顾正气。本方重点是采用俞募配穴法。取中脘与胃俞相配，共调胃之阴阳气血，使脏腑之气转输，则邪毒痰气瘀结自除。《针灸大成·诸般积聚门》曰："心下如杯：中脘、百会。"今取中脘、胃俞以转运胃气，助其生化。合足三里以强胃气，助纳运，维护后天之本。选阴维内关以宽胸和胃，降逆止呕。取三焦俞者，旨在疏调气机，消除积滞。《针灸大成·治病要穴》认为："三焦俞，主胀满积块。"诸穴相伍，有调胃护中，疏理气机，消积止呕之功。

[Middle Phase]

Therapeutic method: Tonify stomach and protect Middle Jiao, soothe Qi Dynamic, eliminate accumulation and stop vomiting.

Prescription: Zhongwan (RN12), Zusanli (ST36), Neiguan (PC6), Sanyinjiao (SP6), Quchi (LI11), Weishu (BL21), Sanjiaoshu (BL22).

Mechanism of prescription: In the middle phase of stomach cancer, the stasis and accumulation of pathogenic toxins and phlegm Qi is obvious, with significant symptoms like epigastric distension and fullness as well as pain, vomiting and nausea, dark stools, emaciation, at this time the syndrome is the intermingled deficiency and excess one, so it is necessary to strengthen vital Qi together with removing of pathogenic toxins. The focus of this prescription is the use of the method of Shu-Mu acupoints combination. Match Weishu with Zhongwan to tonify Yin, Yang, Qi, Blood of stomach, so as to enable the Qi circulation of internal organs, then the stasis and accumulation of pathogenic toxins and phlegm Qi can be eliminated naturally. It is said in the *Compendium of Acupuncture and Moxibustion* that "for acupuncture under heart: Zhongwan, Baihui". Use Zhongwan and Weishu to promote transportation of stomach Qi and facilitate its generation and transformation. Match with Zusanli to strengthen stomach Qi, promote digestion and transportation, so as to protect the foundation of acquired constitution. Use Neiguan from Yin-Wei Channel to relieve chest stuffiness and regulate stomach, descend adverse energy and stop vomiting. Use Sanjiaoshu to dredge and regulate Qi Dynamic, remove accumulation. *Compendium of Acupuncture and Moxibustion* (《针灸大成·治病要穴》) believes that "Sanjiaoshu mainly can treat distention and lumps". The match of these acupoints can tonify stomach and protect Middle Jiao, soothe Qi Dynamic, eliminate accumulation and stop vomiting.

Matching acupoints: For congealment and stasis of phlegm and Qi, add Chize, Fenglong. For internal stagnation of Heat toxins add Dazhui, Quchi. For Qi stagnation and blood stasis add Geshu, Xuehai.

Method: Electrothermal acupuncture treatment.

Operations: Selecting the relevant acupoints, perform routine skin disinfection. Using electrothermal acupuncture needles, vertically puncture into Zusanli for 0.8", vertically puncture into Zhongwan for 0.7", vertically puncture into Neiguan for 0.6", obliquely puncture with the needle tip towards spine into Weishu, Sanjiaoshu for 0.7" respectively. Turn on the electrothermal acupuncture equipment, apply a current of 40-60mA to each acupoint, leaving the needles in for 40 minutes.

Therapeutic course: Once a day, 10 times for a course. Start the treatment for the second course after a break of 3-5 days.

[Advanced Phase]

Therapeutic method: Regulate liver, spleen and stomach, protect Yin and tonify stomach.

Prescription: Zhongwan (RN12), Weishu (BL21), Zhangmen (LR13), Pishu (BL20), Sanyinjiao (SP6).

Mechanism of prescription: In the advanced

积，正气已虚，纳食少进，化源匮乏，胃气有将绝之势，此时当扶脾胃，以维持生机。本方重在调理脾胃脏腑之功能，着重采用俞募配穴法。中脘配胃俞，以助胃气之纳腐；章门配脾俞，以助脾气之运化，因中脘为八会穴之腑会、章门是八会穴之脏会，两穴相配，有调脏腑阴阳气血之功，使脾胃和，纳运健，化源不竭，生机不息；配三阴交以调肝、脾、肾之经气，用以护阴津以养胃，使阳得阴助而生机不绝。

配穴 若胃阴不足者，加上脘、阴郄、地机；若正虚瘀结者，加气海、足三里。

方法 电热针治疗。

操作 选定穴位，皮肤常规消毒。电热针直刺中脘 0.7 寸，针尖向脊柱方向斜刺胃俞、脾俞各 0.7 寸，平刺章门 0.6 寸，直刺三阴交 0.8 寸。接

phase of stomach cancer, the lump enlarges over time, the vital Qi has weakened, food intake reduces, with lack of transformation sources, and the stomach Qi is about to exhaust, so at this time the treatment should be to strengthen spleen and stomach to maintain vitality. This prescription focuses on the tonifying of spleen and stomach functions, and mainly use the method of Shu-Mu acupoints combination. The match of Zhongwan and Weishu can promote stomach Qi to take and digest food. The match of Zhangmen and Pishu can promote the transport and transformation of spleen Qi, and Zhongwan is the Fu confluent acupoint of organs of the eight confluent acupoints, Zhangmen is the Zang confluent acupoint of organs of the eight confluent acupoints, the match of these two can tonify the Yin, Yang, Qi, blood of organs to facilitate harmony of spleen and stomach, normal intake and transportation, and the vitality will be on and on so long as that transportation source is not exhausted. Match Sanyinjiao to tonify meridian Qi of liver, spleen and kidney, and protect Yin fluid to nourish stomach, so as to promote support of Yang from Yin, then the vitality will be on and on.

Matching acupoints: For insufficiency of stomach Yin add Shangwan, Yinxi, Diji. For vital Qi deficiency and stagnation add Qihai, Zusanli.

Method: Electrothermal acupuncture treatment.

Operations: Selecting the relevant acupoints, perform routine skin disinfection. Using electrothermal acupuncture needles, vertically puncture into Zhongwan for 0.7", obliquely puncture toward spine into Weishu, Pishu for 0.7" respectively, horizontally puncture into

通电热针仪，每穴分别给予电流量40～60mA，以患者有舒适胀感为度，留针40分钟。

疗程 每日1次，10次为1个疗程。疗程间休息3～5天，再进行第2个疗程的治疗。

【术后、放疗、化疗后】

治法 补元气，壮胃气，生气血。

处方 中脘（RN12）、胃俞（BL21）、气海（RN6）、足三里（ST36）。

方义 针灸配合胃癌手术后放疗、化疗的应用，在综合治疗中有着良好的作用，其治疗原则主要在于提高机体的免疫功能，促进胃肠的消化吸收，减轻放疗、化疗的毒副反应。因此，益气和胃，助其化源是根本。方中中脘配胃俞是取俞募配穴法，以促进胃肠的消化吸收。选用足三里以强壮胃气，足阳明胃经多气多血，胃气壮则气血生。取任脉之气海，以培补元气。诸穴共用，确有补元气、壮胃气、生气血之功。

Zhangmen for 0.6", vertically puncture into Sanyinjiao for 0.8". Turn on the electrothermal acupuncture equipment, apply a current of 40-60mA to each acupoint, and the limit is that the patient feels comfortable and swelling, leaving the needles in for 40 minutes.

Therapeutic course: Once a day, 10 times for a course. Start the treatment for the second course after a break of 3-5 days.

[Post-operation, post-radiotherapy, post-chemotherapy]

Therapeutic method: Replenish vitality Qi, strengthen stomach Qi, generate Qi and blood.

Prescription: Zhongwan(RN12), Weishu(BL21), Qihai (RN6), Zusanli (ST36).

Mechanism of prescription: The combination of acupuncture therapy with radiotherapy and chemotherapy after surgery, as a comprehensive therapy, has good efficacies, and the core of its treatment principles is to improve immunological functions, promote gastrointestinal digestion and absorption functions and reduce toxic and side effects of radiotherapy and chemotherapy. Therefore, the key point is to tonify Qi and regulate stomach, promote source transportation. In this prescription, the match of Zhongwan and Weishu is based on the method of Shu-Mu acupoints combination to facilitate gastrointestinal digestion and absorption. Choose Zusanli to strength stomach Qi; Yang-Ming Stomach Meridian is full of Qi and blood, and Qi blood will be generated given that stomach Qi is strong. Use the acupoint Qihai from Ren Channel to replenish vitality Qi. The use of combination of these acupoints can replenish vital Qi, strengthen stomach Qi, generate Qi and blood.

配穴 若有胃虚气逆者，加内关、膈俞、上脘、公孙；若有脾胃气阴两虚者，加膈俞、章门、三阴交、三焦俞、关元。

Matching acupoints: For stomach deficiency and reversed flow of Qi add Neiguan, Geshu, Shangwan, Gongsun. For Qi and Yin deficiency of spleen and stomach, add Geshu, Zhangmen, Sanyinjiao, Sanjiaoshu, Guanyuan.

方法 电热针治疗。

Method: Electrothermal acupuncture treatment.

操作 选定穴位，皮肤常规消毒。电热针直刺中脘0.7寸，直刺足三里0.8寸，直刺气海0.6寸。接通电热针仪，每穴分别给予电流量40～60mA，以患者感到胀而舒适为度，留针30分钟。起针后用毫针刺胃俞，针尖向脊柱方向斜刺0.7寸，留针5分钟。

Operations: Selecting the relevant acupoints, perform routine skin disinfection. Using electrothermal acupuncture needles, vertically puncture into Zhongwan for 0.7", vertically puncture into Zusanli for 0.8", vertically puncture into Qihai for 0.6". Turn on the electrothermal acupuncture equipment, apply a current of 40-60mA to each acupoint, and the limit is that the patient feels comfortable, leaving the needles in for 30 minutes. After needle removing, using filiform needles, puncture into Weishu with the needle tip towards spine into 0.7", leaving the needle in for 5 minutes.

疗程 每日1次，10次为1个疗程。疗程间休息3～5天，再进行第2个疗程的治疗。

Therapeutic course: Once a day, 10 times for a course. Start the treatment for the second course after a break of 3-5 days.

三、注意事项

III. Precautions

1. 早期胃癌应以手术为主，中期胃癌在争取手术的前提下，积极使用放疗、化疗，同时辅以针灸及中药疗法，在综合治疗中充分发挥针灸的优势。

1. For early stomach cancer the main therapy should be surgeries. For middle stomach cancer, in the premise of fight for surgery, together with proactive use of radiotherapy and chemotherapy, use acupuncture therapy and Chinese Herb Medicine therapy as supplemented treatments, and the advantages of acupuncture therapy can be fully used in the comprehensive therapy.

2. For acupuncture of Zhagnmen and Back-shu acupoints, special attentions should be paid to the needling direction and depth so as to prevent piercing of internal organs.

3. In the advanced phase of stomach cancer, the patient is skinny, so it is important to control the needling depth, better shallow puncturing.

4. Patients with stomach cancer must keep optimistic and cheerful mood, establish confidence in conquering diseases, while participate in some appropriate physical exercises such as Taiji and Qigong.

5. The clinical treatment determination based on syndrome differentiation for stomach cancers is very important and must be mastered. Early confirmation of precancerous lesions for stomach cancer like gastric ulcer and atrophic gastritis can enable exact efficacies of acupuncture therapy, so as to achieve the aim of preventing stomach cancer. Therefore proactive treatment for precancerous lesions of stomach cancer is necessary to prevent cancerization.

6. For patients with stomach cancer, dietetic care is important, and the food and beverages should be fine, soft, thin with less amount, and patients should have diet at fixed time and with fixed amount, have more meals a day but less food at each. Eat more vegetables and fruits, do not eat spicy and stimulating or greasy food.

IV. Typical Case

Wu, female, 56 years old, retired, residence: Tangshan.

下篇 临床论治　Part II: Clinical Treatment

主诉：胃脘部隐隐作痛，常喜热饮，按之则舒，神疲乏力，纳谷不振，四肢不温已半年之久。病史：患者胃痛十余年之久，因工作繁忙，饮食不节，饥饱失常，又喜辛辣煎炒食物，久而久之患上胃病。之前喜欢冷饮，近半年不能进食凉之食物，否则胃痛，遇热痛减。

刻下症：形体消瘦，纳差，神疲乏力，胃脘部隐隐作痛，遇寒则痛，得温则减，大便偏干，小便黄，舌红苔黄，脉细数。

查体：两肺呼吸音粗，可闻及中、小水泡音。二尖瓣区及主动脉瓣第二听诊区闻及二级收缩期杂音。

辅助检查：胃镜示"胃癌"。活检示"重度不典型增生、炎性浸润"。

【诊断依据】

1. 胃痛十余年，经治不愈，患者有过食辛辣煎炒食物的习惯。

2. 胃镜确诊为胃癌。

3. 形体消瘦，纳呆，神疲乏力，面色白。

4. 胃脘隐隐作痛，大便

Self-reported symptoms: Epigastric dull pain which gets relived with pressing, preference to hot drink, fatigue look and asthenia, poor appetite, cold limbs for a half year. Medical history: The patient had being suffered from stomach pain for more than 10 years, and the stomach disease developed due to long-term busy work, intemperate diet, irregular eating, preference to spicy, fried food. The patient liked cold drinks before, however in the recent half year, she could not take cold food or beverages, or stomach pain would occur, which got relieved with warm.

Current symptoms: Body emaciation, poor appetite, fatigue look and asthenia, epigastric dull pain which got aggravated with cold and relieved with warm, dry stool, yellow urine, red tongue with yellow fur, thin and rapid pulse.

Physical examination: Coarse breath sounds in both lungs, audible fine and medium bubbling rales. Grade 2 systolic noise at mitral valve area and second aortic valve area.

Auxiliary examination: Gastroscopy indicated "stomach cancer". Biopsy indicated "severe atypical hyperplasia, inflammatory infiltuation".

[Diagnostic Basis]

1. Stomach pain for more than 10 years, which could not be cured. The patient had a habit to eat excessive spicy and fried food.

2. Gastroscopy indicated "stomach cancer".

3. Body emaciation, indigestion, fatigue look and asthenia, pale complexion.

4. Epigastric dull pain, sloppy stool, cold limbs.

溏，四肢不温。

【证治分析】

病因 饮食不节，饥饱失常，过食辛辣煎炒食物。

病机 胃痛久治不愈，以致胃府受损，正气亏虚，邪毒痰气瘀结，癥块日生，后天乏源，导致气血阴阳衰弱。

证候分析 脾胃虚寒，属正虚，故胃脘部隐隐作痛，以空腹为甚，得食后缓；寒得温而散，气得按而行，故喜温喜按；脾虚中寒水不运化而上逆，故泛吐清水；中阳不振，故神疲乏力及手足不温；脾虚生湿下渗肠间，故大便溏。舌淡，脉沉细，皆为脾胃虚弱、中阳不足之象。

病位 胃。

病性 正虚邪实。

西医诊断 胃癌。

[Syndrome-treatment Analysis]

Etiology: Intemperate diet, irregular eating, excessive intake of mellow wine, spicy, fried food.

Pathogenesis: The stomach pain cannot be cured after long-term treatment, therefore cause impairment of the stomach organ, depletion and deficiency of vital Qi, stasis accumulation of pathogenic toxins and phlegm Qi, long-term lump enlargement, lack of source for acquired constitution, leading to weakness of Qi-blood and Yin-Yang.

Syndrome analysis: Deficiency-Cold of spleen and stomach, the disease belongs to the range of weakened body resistance, therefore causes epigastric dull pain, which gets aggravated with empty stomach and gets relieved after food intake; Cold will disperse with warm, Qi will moves after pressing, therefore the patient prefers to warm and pressing; deficiency-Cold of spleen and stomach, Water cannot be transported and transformed and goes up reversely, therefore vomit clear water. Weakness of Middle Yang causes fatigue look and asthenia and cold limbs; spleen deficiency causes the generation of Damp flowing downwards to the intestine, thereby leading to sloppy stool. Light tongue, deep and thin pulse, both are symptoms of spleen and stomach weakness, insufficiency of Middle Yang.

Lesion location: Stomach.

Disease nature: Body resistance is weakened while pathogenic factors prevailing.

The diagnosis of Western Medicine: Stomach cancer.

中医诊断 脾胃虚寒型胃脘痛。

治法 温中散寒,开郁止痛。

方法 电热针治疗(温补法)。

处方 中脘(RN12)、内关(PC6)、足三里(ST36)、阳陵泉(GB34)、公孙(SP4)。

方义 胃癌初期常因情志抑郁,饮食不节而导致肝失疏泄,胃失和降,出现气机郁滞不畅之症。方用腑会中脘,重在和调胃腑,疏理阳明气机,使胃气和降,纳腐有权,则痰气邪毒无稽留之害;配阳明合穴足三里,"合治内腑",更有助中焦健运,胃气顺降,且有扶正祛邪之功;选内关可宽胸畅中以和调气机;配少阳胆经之合穴阳陵泉,在于疏泄胆气,使肝胆得以舒畅,则无害中焦脾胃气机升降之枢要;又取公孙、内关是八脉交会穴相配,能宽胸理气,开郁止痛。

The diagnosis of Traditional Chinese Medicine: Epigastric pain due to deficiency and Cold of stomach.

Therapeutic method: Warm Middle Jiao and disperse Cold, relieve stasis and alleviate pains.

Method: Electrothermal acupuncture treatment (warm tonifying).

Prescription: Zhongwan (RN12), Neiguan (PC6), Zusanli (ST36), Yanglingquan (GB34), Gongsun (SP4).

Mechanism of prescription: In the early phase of stomach cancer, emotional depression and intemperate diet often cause loss of liver soothing and dredging, stomach Qi rising, subsequently leading to Qi Dynamic stagnation. This prescription uses the confluent acupoint of organs, Zhongwan, to regulate the stomach organ, soothe Qi Dynamic of Yang-Ming Meridian, so as to facilitate orderly stomach Qi descending and food digestion, then there won't be harm of retention and stagnation of phlegm, Qi and pathogenic toxins. Match with the He acupoint Zusanli from Yang-Ming Meridian, "He acupoints can treat internal organs", so this acupoint can enable normal functions of Middle Jiao and descending of stomach Qi, as well as strengthen vital Qi and eliminate pathogenic factors; choose Neiguan to relieve chest stuffiness and soothe Middle Jiao, therefore regulate Qi Dynamic. Match with the He acupoint Yanglingquan from Shao-Yang Gallbladder Meridian to dredge gallbladder Qi and unobstruct liver and gallbladder, so as to avoid impairment of the key place for ascending and descending of spleen and stomach Qi Dynamic within Middle Jiao; and match Gongsun with one of the confluent

配穴 肝气犯胃者加太冲、期门；脾胃虚寒者加内庭、气海、天枢；嗳气者加内关、膻中、三阴交。

操作 选定穴位，皮肤常规消毒。电热针直刺中脘、建里、阳陵泉、足三里各 0.7 寸，接通电热针仪，每个穴位分别给予电流量 40mA，以患者感到温胀为度，留针 40 分钟，余者用毫针治疗。毫针直刺内关、太冲、内庭、气海、天枢、三阴交各 0.7 寸，平刺膻中 0.6 寸，直刺公孙 0.5 寸，留针 40 分钟。（注：每日选 6 穴给予电热针治疗，交替运用，余者用毫针治疗。）

疗程 每日 1 次，90 次为 1 个疗程。同时配合中草药治疗。5 个月后复查胃镜、活检，以明确疗效。

治疗过程 该患者疗效较好，治疗过程顺利，症状随治疗而递减，1 个月后症状消失，5 个月后胃镜、活检证实病变消失，黏膜基本恢复正常，呈

acupoints of eight Channels, Neiguan, to relieve chest distress and regulate Qi, relieve stasis and alleviate pains.

Matching acupoints: For liver Qi impairing stomach add Taichong, Qimen. For deficiency and Cold of spleen and stomach add Neiting, Qihai, Tianshu. For blenching add Neiguan, Danzhong, Sanyinjiao.

Operations: Selecting the relevant acupoints, perform routine skin disinfection. Using electrothermal acupuncture needles, vertically puncture into Zhongwan, Jianli, Yanglingquan, Zusanli for 0.7" respectively. Turn on the electrothermal acupuncture equipment, apply a current of 40mA to each acupoint, and the limit is that the patient feels warm and swelling, leaving the needles in for 40 minutes, and treat the other acupoints with filiform needles. Using filiform needles, vertically puncture into Neiguan, Taichong, Neiting, Qihai, Tianshu, Sanyinjiao for 0.7" respectively, horizontally puncture into Danzhong for 0.6", vertically puncture into Gongsun for 0.5", leaving the needles in for 40 minutes. (Note: Select 6 pairs of acupoints for electrothermal acupuncture treatment each time and use alternatively, and treat the other acupoints with filiform needles.)

Therapeutic course: Once a day, 90 times for a course. Use Chinese Herb Medicine therapy as well. Re-exam with gastroscopy and biopsy 5 months later to confirm efficacies.

Therapeutic process: The efficacies for this patient were good, and the treatment was successful. The symptoms were being relieved gradually along with the treatment and disappeared 1 month later. Five months later, the results of gastroscopy and biopsy confirmed that the

现浅表性胃炎。休息 30 天后又巩固治疗 30 天，追踪至今健在。

【生活调摄】

1. 令患者在治疗过程中注意饮食，禁食辛辣煎炒食物，多进清淡、软食、易消化的食品，少食多餐。

2. 针治时注意进针的深度、方向，避免发生意外。电热针每次选 6 个穴位，多为扶正祛邪之穴，保证体力的恢复。

3. 令患者有好的心态，有战胜病魔的信心，坚持治疗；医者更要坚定信心，选择有效的措施，提高疗效，缩短疗程。

肝癌

肝癌是消化系统最常见的恶性肿瘤之一，有原发性和继发性之分。前者指肝细胞或肝内胆管细胞发生一种恶性较高的癌变，后者可因其他部位之癌瘤通过淋巴、血液和癌瘤直接蔓延侵犯肝脏而发生。究其因，多为患者机体免疫功能低

lesions had disappeared and the mucous membrane had basically recovered, and indicated the presence of superficial gastritis. After a break of 30 days, performed consolidation treatment for another 30 days. Follow up till now, and the patient is still alive.

[Lifestyle Change and Health Maintenance]

1. During the treatment, ask patients pay attention to diet, do not eat spicy and fired food, eat more light, soft food and food that easy to be digested, have more meals a day but less food at each.

2. During the acupuncture, pay attention to needling depth and direction, to avoid accidents. For electrothermal acupuncture treatment, choose 6 acupoints each time, most of which are acupoints effective in strengthening vital Qi and eliminating pathogenic factors, so as to ensure the recovery of physical strength.

3. Let patients keep good mental status and establish confidence in conquering diseases, adhere to the treatment; and medical practitioners should be more confident, choose effective measures to improve efficacies and shorten the course of treatment.

Liver Cancer

Liver cancer is one of the most common malignant tumors of the digestive system, which is divided into primary ones and secondary ones. The former refers to a kind of severe cancers of liver cells or bile duct cells in the liver, and the later refers to cancers caused by direct spreading of tumors at other sites through lymphs, blood and tumors invading the liver. And the root reasons are impaired body immune functions, or development of

下，或有肝炎、肝硬化、乙型肝炎，或进食含有黄曲霉素、亚硝基化合物之大米、玉米、花生等导致肝细胞恶变而发。肝癌的临床早期症状不明显，仅有右上腹胀满疼痛明显，或肝可触及质硬，且有结节，纳呆、形体消瘦、面色萎黄。

中医认为，本病属于"胁痛""癥积""黄疸"等范畴。多因情志抑郁，饮食不节，嗜酒过度，邪毒乘虚而犯肝，造成肝失疏泄，气机不畅，气血瘀滞，脾虚湿聚，热毒内蕴，湿痰热毒瘀结于肝所致。其临床特点为本虚标实。

一、诊断及辨证要点

1. 临床检查

（1）CT、MRI检查：可见大小不等、多发的局灶性密度减低或增高区，边缘可较清楚，也可模糊。

（2）肝穿活检或手术病理检查证实者。

（3）B超检查：可见肝脏内有形状不规则、分布不均匀

hepatitis, cirrhosis, hepatitis B, or liver cell malignant transformation due to intake of rices, corns and peanuts containing aflatoxin and thiamine compounds. The early clinical symptoms of liver cancer are not obvious, with only obvious distension and pain of right upper abdomen, or palpated hard lump of liver, accompanied with nodules, indigestion, body emaciation, sallow complexion.

Traditional Chinese Medicine believes that this disease belongs to the ranges of "hypochondriac pain", "lump accumulation", "icteric", etc. Most are caused by emotional depression and intemperate diet, excessive drinking, invasion of pathogenic toxins into lung when it is weak, causing loss of liver soothing and dredging, unsmooth Qi Dynamic, Qi and blood stagnation, spleen deficiency and Damp accumulation, internal stagnation of Heat toxins, stagnation of Damp, phlegm, Heat toxins within the liver. The clinical characteristic is asthenia in origin and sthenia in superficiality.

I. Key Points for Diagnosis and Syndrome Differentiation

1.Clinical examination

(1) CT and MRI examinations: Multiple focal density-reduced or density-increased areas of different sizes, with clear or blur edges.

(2) Confirmed by liver puncture biopsy or operative pathological examination.

(3) B-ultrasonography: Irregular-shaped and uneven distributed light spots and masses with scattered tiny

的光点光团，周围有散在细小光点。A型超声检查：可见丛状波、束状波、迟钝复波、弥漫波或出波衰减。

（4）甲胎蛋白对流免疫电泳阳性。

（5）血清5核苷酸、磷酸二酯酶、γ-谷氨酰转肽酶、铁蛋白、醛缩酶、同工酶A等含量增加。

2. 中医辨证分型

（1）初期

①肝气郁滞者，情绪郁闷，右胁部作胀不适，胁下癥块按之质硬，胸闷，脘胀痛，口苦，纳谷减少，舌质红，苔薄黄，脉弦细。

②肝郁痰结者，口苦胀痛，癥块质硬，或有结节，胸闷纳少，厌食油腻，喉间有痰，苔黄厚腻，脉弦细。

（2）中期

①肝经湿热壅盛者，右胁胀痛，触及癥块，巩膜黄染，皮肤发黄如橘子色，身重懒言，小便黄赤，大便秘结，舌红，苔黄腻，脉弦有力。

light spots around can be seen within the liver. A-ultrasonography: Plexiform wave, bundle wave, slow complex wave, diffuse wave or wave attenuation can be seen.

(4) Positive in the counter immunoelectrophoresis of α-fetoprotein.

(5) Increased serum levels of nucleotide, phosphodiesterase, γ-glutamyl transpeptidase, ferroprotein, aldolase, isoenzyme.

2. Symptom differentiation and type classification of Traditional Chinese Medicine

(1) Early phase

① For patients with liver Qi stagnation and retention, symptoms include depressed mood, fullness and comfort of the the right hypochondrium, hard lump under the hypochondrium, chest distress, distending pain of gastral cavity, bitter taste, reduced food intake, red tongue with yellow and thin fur, taut and thin pulse.

② For patients with liver stagnation and phlegm accumulation, symptoms include bitter taste and distending pain, hard lump, or with nodules, chest distress and less food intake, dislike to greasy food, phlegm within the throat, yellow and thick and greasy fur, taut and thin pulse.

(2) Middle phase

① For patients with excessive Damp-Heat of Liver Meridian, symptoms include distending pain of the right hypochondrium with palpated lump, yellow sclera, yellow skin like the color of oranges, heavy body and laziness to speaking, yellow and dark urine, constipation, red

②肝经热毒内结者，右胁疼痛，癥块质硬，发热，口苦，目黄，齿衄，口臭，小便黄赤量少，舌红苔黄，脉弦数。

③肝经气滞血瘀者，右胁胀满，胁下疼痛，癥块坚硬，痛如针刺，胸闷脘胀，纳差，口干而不欲饮，舌黯红，舌边有瘀斑，苔薄腻，脉弦紧。

④肝经痰血瘀结者，右胁胀痛，痛处固定，形体消瘦，纳少气短，喉间痰黏，面色灰黑，舌质紫黯，苔白腻，脉细无力。

⑤肝脾血瘀者，右胁胀痛，癥块坚硬，面色萎黄或灰黄，纳呆气短，腹壁静脉显露，腹膨而胀，腹水，黑便，舌边有明显的条纹，呈块状的青紫色，苔黄腻，脉细数。

（3）晚期

①肝肾阴虚者，右胁癥块

tongue with yellow and greasy fur, taut and strong pulse.

② For patients with internal stagnation of Heat toxins within Liver Meridian, symptoms include pain of the right hypochondrium, hard lump, pyrexia, bitter taste, yellow eyes, gingival hemorrhage, ozostomia, yellow and dark and less urine, red tongue with yellow fur, taut and rapid pulse.

③ For patients with Qi stagnation and blood stasis of Liver Meridian, symptoms include fullness of the right hypochondrium, pain under the hypochondrium, hard lump, pricking, chest distress and fullness of gastral cavity, poor food intake, dry mouth and unable to drink, dark red tongue, ecchymosis on the tongue edge, thin and greasy fur, taut and tight pulse.

④ For patients with stagnation of phlegm and blood within Liver Meridian, symptoms include distending pain of the right hypochondrium with fixed pain lesions, emaciation of body, less food intake and shortness of breath, sticky phlegm within the throat, dark gray complexion, dark purple tongue with white and greasy fur, thin and weak pulse.

⑤ For patients with blood stagnation of liver and spleen, symptoms include distending pain of the right hypochondrium, hard lump, sallow or gray yellow complexion, poor appetite and shortness of breath, abdominal wall vein revealed, abdominal swell, ascites, tarry stool, obvious strips at the tongue edge which are cyan purple blocks, yellow and greasy tongue fur, thin and rapid pulse.

(3) Advanced phase

① For patients with Yin deficiency of liver and

胀痛，形体消瘦，低热缠绵，口干咽痛，颧红潮热，腰酸盗汗，五心烦热，舌红绛，苔黄腻，脉细数。

②热毒伤阴者，右胁癥块坚硬疼痛，呕血便血，发热神昏，谵语狂躁，小便黄赤，舌绛，镜面舌，脉细数。

（4）术后、放疗、化疗后

①脾胃气虚者，纳谷呆滞，神疲乏力，动则气短，脘腹时胀，四肢不温，舌淡苔薄，脉细弱。

②肝脾气血两虚者，头晕眼花，纳谷减少，口干，心悸，四肢无力，失眠，面色白，舌淡而胖，苔少，脉细少力。

二、治疗方法

【电热针治疗】

（1）初期

治法　疏肝理气，消癥散结。

处方　肝俞（BL18）、内关（PC6）、阳陵泉（GB34）、

kidney, symptoms include distending pain of lump at the right hypochondrium, body emaciation, repeated lower fever, dry mouth and painful throat, flushed cheeks and tidal fever, sourness of waist and night sweating, dysphoria in chest with palms-soles, crimson tongue with yellow and greasy fur, thin and rapid pulse.

② For patients with Heat toxins impairing Yin, symptoms include hard and painful lump at the right hypochondrium, haematemesis and hemafecia, pyrexia and coma, delirium and mania, yellow dark urine, crimson tongue, mirror-like tongue, thin and rapid pulse.

(4) Post-operation, post-radiotherapy, post-chemotherapy

① For patients with Qi deficiency of spleen and stomach, symptoms include indigestion and loss of appetite, fatigue look and asthenia, shortness of breath when moving, frequent abdominal distension, cold limbs, light tongue with thin fur, thin and weak pulse.

② For patients with Qi-blood deficiency of liver and spleen, symptoms include dizziness and blurred vision, reduced food intake, dry mouth, palpitation, limb weakness, insomnia, pale complexion, light and fat tongue with less fur, thin and weak pulse.

II. Therapeutic Methods

[Electrothermal Acupuncture Treatment]

(1) Early phase

Therapeutic method: Soothe liver and regulate Qi, remove cumulation and disperse stasis.

Prescription: Ganshu (BL18), Neiguan (PC6), Yanglingquan (GB34), Zusanli (ST36), Sanyinjiao (SP6),

足三里（ST36）、三阴交（SP6）、痞根（EX-B4）。

方义 肝癌早期，癥块初结，常见气机郁滞，治当疏肝理气、消癥散结，取肝俞以疏调肝脏经气，收背俞治脏之功；配手厥阴经穴内关，以疏通阴维，宽胸下气，助肝俞以调胸胁之气机；合足少阳胆经之阳陵泉，以疏利肝胆，行气散结；选足阳明胃经穴足三里、足太阴脾经穴三阴交，以维护脾胃中土之后天之本，取扶正祛邪之义；取痞根以消癥散结。诸穴共用，可奏疏调肝经瘀结之功效。

配穴 若肝气郁滞者，加太冲、外关，以疏肝解郁；若肝郁痰结者加行间、丰隆，以疏肝理气，化痰散结。

操作 选定穴位，皮肤常规消毒。电热针斜刺（向脊柱

Pigen (EX-B4).

Mechanism of prescription: In the early phase of liver cancer, the lump is just formed, and Qi Dynamic stagnation is common, therefore the treatment should be aimed to soothe liver and regulate Qi, remove cumulation and disperse stasis, so use Ganshu to soothe and regulate meridian Qi of liver, so as to obtain the efficacies of organ treatment of Back-Shu acupoints. Match the meridian acupoint Neiguan from Jue-Yin Meridian of Hand to soothe Yin-Wei, relieve chest stuffiness and depress Qi, so as to help Ganshu to regulate Qi Dynamic of chest and hypochondrium. Add Yanglingquan from Shao-Yang Gallbladder Meridian of Foot to soothe liver and gallbladder, activate Qi and disperse stasis. Choose the meridian acupoint Zusanli from Yang-Ming Stomach Meridian of Foot and the meridian acupoint Sanyinjiao from Tai-Yin Spleen Meridian of Foot to protect the foundation of acquired constitution for Middle Earth of spleen and stomach, so as to strengthen vital Qi and eliminate pathogenic factors. Use Pigen to remove cumulation and disperse stasis. The use of combination of these acupoints can soothe and regulate stagnation within Liver Meridian.

Matching acupoints: For stagnation of liver Qi, add Taichong, Waiguan to soothe liver Qi stagnation. For liver stagnation and phlegm accumulation, add Xingjian, Fenglong to soothe liver and regulate Qi, disperse phlegm and eliminate stagnation.

Operations: Selecting the relevant acupoints, perform routine skin disinfection. Using electrothermal

方向）肝俞 0.8 寸，直刺足三里、三阴交、内关、阳陵泉、丰隆、外关各 0.7 寸，斜刺痞根（针尖向脊柱）0.8 寸，平刺太冲、行间各 0.7 寸。接通电热针仪，每个穴位分别给予 40～50mA 的电流量，以患者感到胀而舒适为度，留针 40 分钟。

疗程 每日 1 次，30 天为 1 个疗程。疗程间可休息 5～7 天，再进入第 2 个疗程的治疗，一般治疗 2～3 个疗程即可。

（2）中期

治法 疏肝利胆，散结消痞。

处方 肝俞（BL18）、期门（LR14）、阳陵泉（GB34）、痞根（EX-B4）、足三里（ST36）、三阴交（SP6）。

方义 肝癌中期，癥块坚硬，脏腑受损，气血瘀阻，火热痰浊，稽留不去。临床可见胁痛、发热、黄疸、腹水、出血等。治当以和调脏腑、消癥散结为主。本方肝俞配期门，取之俞募配穴法，重在转输脏腑之气血，以和调肝胆之结滞；合足少阳胆经之合穴阳陵泉，合治内腑，用以疏导肝胆

acupuncture needles, obliquely puncture (toward spine) into Ganshu for 0.8", vertically puncture into Zusanli, Sanyinjiao, Neiguan, Yanglingquan, Fenglong, Waiguan for 0.7" respectively, obliquely puncture (with the needle tip towards spine) into Pigen for 0.8", horizontally puncture into Taichong, Xingjian for 0.7" respectively. Turn on the electrothermal acupuncture equipment, apply a current of 40-50mA to each acupoint, and the limit is that the patient feels swell and comfortable, leaving the needles in for 40 minutes.

Therapeutic course: Once a day, 30 days for a course. Start the treatment for the second course after a break of 5-7 days. Generally 2-3 courses are enough.

(2) Middle phase

Therapeutic method: Soothe liver and reinforce gallbladder, disperse stagnation and subside lumps.

Prescription: Ganshu (BL18), Qimen (LR14), Yanglingquan (GB34), Pigen (EX-B4), Zusanli (ST36), Sanyinjiao (SP6).

Mechanism of prescription: In the middle phase of liver cancer, the lump is hard, organs are damaged, with Qi and blood stagnation; Fire, Heat, phlegm and turbidity are accumulated. Hypochondriac pain, pyrexia, icteric, ascites, bleeding are also can be seen clinically. The treatment should be focus on regulating organs, removing cumulation and dispersing stasis. This prescription matches Ganshu with Qimen, uses the method of Shu-Mu acupoints combination, and is aimed to transport Qi and blood of organs so as to regulate stagnation

经气，解郁散结，清泻邪毒；选痞根穴，旨在疏散肝脾痞结之气，使经气周流则邪无碍滞之害；合足三里、三阴交以维护脾胃中土之后天之本，扶正祛邪之义。诸穴共用，可奏和调肝胆经气，散消痞结，清泻邪毒之功效。

of liver and gallbladder. Match the Yanglingquan from Shao-Yang Gallbladder Meridian of Foot to care organs, so as to soothe liver and gallbladder Qi, remove stasis and disperse stagnation, dredge pathogenic toxins; choose Pigen to soothe stagnated Qi of liver and spleen, so as to soothe the meridian Qi circulation, then the harm of pathogenic toxins can be eliminated. Add Zusanli, Sanyinjiao to protect the foundation of acquired constitution for Middle Earth of spleen and stomach, so as to strengthen vital Qi and eliminate pathogenic factors. The use of combination of these acupoints can regulate meridian Qi of liver and gallbladder, disperse lump and stagnation, dredge pathogenic toxins.

配穴 肝经湿热壅滞者，可加膈俞、中脘、至阳、阳纲，以清肝利胆而退黄，宽中和胃而化湿；若肝经热毒内结者，加膈俞、大椎、曲池，以清泻肝经之火热；若肝经气滞血瘀者，加膈俞、太冲、外关，以疏泄气机，气行则血行；若肝经痰血瘀结者，可加膈俞、丰隆、支沟，以行气化痰，活血散结；若肝脾血瘀者，可加膈俞、脾俞、气海、水分、阴陵泉，以益气健脾，活血化瘀，散结行水。

Matching acupoints: For excessive Damp-Heat of Liver Meridian, add Geshu, Zhongwan, Zhiyang, Yanggang to clear liver and reinforce gallbladder therefore eliminate jaundice, loosen Middle Jiao and harmonize stomach therefore remove Damp. For internal stagnation of Heat toxins within Liver Meridian, add Geshu, Dazhui, Quchi to purge Fire and Heat of Liver Meridian. For Qi stagnation and blood stasis of Liver Meridian, add Geshu, Taichong, Waiguan to soothe Qi Dynamic, and activated Qi can facilitate blood circulation. For stagnation of phlegm and blood within Liver Meridian, add Geshu, Fenglong, Zhigou to activate Qi and disperse phlegm, activate blood and disperse stagnation. For blood stagnation of liver and spleen, add Geshu, Pishu, Qihai, Shuifen, Yinlingquan to tonify Qi and invigorate spleen, activate blood circulation and remove stasis, disperse stagnation and activate Water.

方法 电热针治疗。

Method: Electrothermal acupuncture treatment.

下篇 临床论治 Part II: Clinical Treatment

操作 选定穴位，皮肤常规消毒。电热针斜刺（针尖向脊柱）肝俞 0.8 寸，向下平刺期门 0.8 寸，直刺阳陵泉 0.7 寸，直刺痞根 0.8 寸。接通电热针仪，每个穴位分别给予电流量 40～50mA，以患者感到胀而舒适为度，留针 40 分钟。

疗程 每日 1 次，30 天为 1 个疗程。疗程间可休息 5～7 天，再进入第 2 个疗程的治疗，一般治疗 2～3 个疗程即可。

（3）晚期

治法 和中养肝，和调肝脏气血。

处方 肝俞（BL18）、期门（LR14）、脾俞（BL20）、足三里（ST36）。

方义 晚期肝癌，癥块日积，正气耗散，津液亏损，治当扶肝健脾，以维系生机。本方取俞募配穴法以维护肝胆脏腑之经气，故肝俞配期门，使脏腑和而气血流通，经气不绝则生机不息，合脾俞、足三里以维护脾胃中土之后天之本。《金匮要略·脏腑经络先后病》曰："见肝之病，知肝传脾，当先实脾。"故健脾运中，和调脾

Operations: Selecting the relevant acupoints, perform routine skin disinfection. Using electrothermal acupuncture needles, obliquely puncture (with the needle tip towards spine) into Ganyu for 0.8", horizontally puncture downwards into Qimen for 0.8", vertically puncture into Yanglingquan for 0.7", vertically puncture into Pigen for 0.8". Turn on the electrothermal acupuncture equipment, apply a current of 40-50mA to each acupoint, and the limit is that the patient feels swell and comfortable, leaving the needles in for 40 minutes.

Therapeutic course: Once a day, 30 days for a course. Start the treatment for the second course after a break of 5-7 days. Generally 2-3 courses are enough.

(3) Advanced phase

Therapeutic method: Regulate Middle Jiao and tonify liver, regulate liver Qi and blood.

Prescription: Ganshu (BL18), Qimen (LR14), Pishu (BL20), Zusanli (ST36).

Mechanism of prescription: In the advanced phase of liver cancer, the lump has accumulated for a long time, vital Qi is consumed and dissipated, with depletion of fluid, therefore the treatment should be aimed to strengthen liver and invigorate spleen to sustain vitality. This prescription use the method of Shu-Mu acupoints combination to protect the meridian Qi for liver and gallbladder and other organs, so match Ganshu with Qimen to facilitate organ harmony and Qi-blood circulation, the vitality will be on and on so long as meridian Qi is ceaselessly. Add Pishu and Zusanli to protect the foundation

· 485 ·

胃，是预防肝病传变向逆的重要治则，这不仅适用于肝癌之晚期，对早、中期肝癌患者亦同样适用。《素问·经脉别论》曰："食气入胃，散精于肝，淫气于筋。"由此得知，肝脏的濡养离不开脾胃后天之本。本方之组合，重在调中养肝，和调肝脏气血，正切合晚期肝癌的治疗。

of acquired constitution for Middle Earth of spleen and stomach. It is said in the *Synopsis of Prescriptions of the Golden Chamber* (《金匮要略·脏腑经络先后病》) that "liver diseases indicate that liver affects spleen functions, so it is necessary to tonify spleen first". Therefore invigorating spleen and Middle transportation, spleen and stomach regulation are important rules of treatment for prevention transfer and transformation of liver disease, which is applied to not only advanced liver cancer, but also patients with early and middle liver cancers. It is said in the *Plain Questions* (《素问·经脉别论》) that "when food and Qi enter the stomach, the essence is distributed into the liver and Qi is spread into tendons". Which shows that the nourishment of liver cannot be done without the foundation of acquired constitution for spleen and stomach. The combination in this prescription is focused on tonify Middle Jiao and nourish liver, regulate Qi and blood of liver, which just meet with the treatment for advanced liver cancer.

配穴 若肝肾阴虚，可加肾俞、太溪、三阴交，以滋水养肝；若热毒伤阴，可加三阴交、人中、十宣、涌泉，以凉血滋阴，清热解毒，开窍醒神。

方法 电热针治疗。

操作 选定穴位，皮肤常规消毒。电热针斜刺（针尖向脊柱）肝俞、脾俞各 0.7 寸，平刺期门 0.8 寸，直刺足三里 0.7 寸。接通电热针仪，每个穴

Matching acupoints: For Yin deficiency of liver and kidney, add Shenshu, Taixi, Sanyinjiao to nourish Water and tonify liver. For Heat toxins impairing Yin, add Sanyinjiao, Renzhong, Shixuan, Yongquan to cool blood and nourish Yin, clear Heat and toxins, induce resuscitation.

Method: Electrothermal acupuncture treatment.

Operations: Selecting the relevant acupoints, perform routine skin disinfection. Using electrothermal acupuncture needles, obliquely puncture (with the needle tip towards spine) into Ganshu, Pishu for 0.7" respectively, horizontally puncture into Qimen for 0.8", vertically

位分别给予 30mA 电流量，以患者感到胀而舒适为度，留针 40 分钟。

疗程 每日 1 次，30 天为 1 个疗程。疗程间可休息 5～7 天，再进入第 2 个疗程的治疗，一般治疗 2～3 个疗程即可。

（4）术后、放疗、化疗后

治法 补益气血，补脾养肝。

处方 足三里（ST36）、气海（RN6）、合谷（LI4）、脾俞（BL20）、胃俞（BL21）。

方义 肝癌放、化疗后，其副反应主要是消化系统及造血系统的反应，故气血不足是其特征。本方四穴均为强壮穴。足三里为足阳明经合穴，重在维护中气以助气血之生化；取任脉之气海，元气所聚之处，以培元固本，必使脏腑之气不衰，肝脏得其所养；合谷为手阳明经原穴，与足三里相配，有调阳明经气、补益气血之功，况且阳明为多气多血之乡，气血充则经脉得养，与脾俞相配以维护脾胃中土之后天之本。诸穴共用，共奏补益

puncture into Zusanli for 0.7". Turn on the electrothermal acupuncture equipment, apply a current of 30mA to each acupoint, and the limit is that the patient feels swell and comfortable, leaving the needles in for 40 minutes.

Therapeutic course: Once a day, 30 days for a course. Start the treatment for the second course after a break of 5-7 days. Generally 2-3 courses are enough.

(4) Post-operation, post-radiotherapy, post-chemotherapy

Therapeutic method: Tonify Qi-blood, replenish spleen and nourish liver.

Prescription: Zusanli (ST36), Qihai (RN6), Hegu (LI4), Pishu (BL20), Weishu (BL21).

Mechanism of prescription: The main side reactions after radiotherapy and chemotherapy for liver cancer are reactions of the digestive system and hematopoietic system, therefore the characteristic is deficiency of Qi and blood. The four acupoints in this prescription are all important tonifying acupoints. Zusanli is a He acupoint from Yang-Ming Meridian of Foot, it can maintain Middle-Jiao Qi to promote generation and transportation of Qi and blood. Use the acupoint Qihai from Ren Channel, the convergent place of vital Qi, to reinforce vital essence and foundation, then the organic Qi can be endless and the liver can be nourished. Hegu is a Yuan acupoint from Yang-Ming Meridian of Hand, if being matched with Zusanli it can tonify meridian Qi of Yang-Ming Meridian and tonify Qi and blood, and Yang-Ming

气血、补益脾胃之气、濡养肝脏之功。

配穴 若脾胃气虚者，可加脾俞、胃俞，以补益脾胃之气；若肝脾气血两虚者，加肝俞、脾俞、三阴交，以补益肝脾之气血。

方法 电热针治疗。

操作 选定穴位，皮肤常规消毒。电热针直刺足三里、气海、合谷各0.7寸，斜刺脾俞、胃俞各0.7寸，接通电热针仪，每个穴位分别给予40～50mA的电流量，以患者感到胀而舒适为度，留针40分钟。

疗程 每日1次，10次为1个疗程。疗程间可休息3～5天，再进行第2个疗程的治疗。一般与放、化疗同步进行。

【中药治疗】

本法是自拟方配合放疗、化疗、免疫治疗的综合疗法。在辨证用药的基础上，加入具有抗肝癌作用的药物。具体治

Meridian is full of Qi and blood, while plentiful Qi and blood can nourish meridians and channels, and the match with Pishu can protect the foundation of acquired constitution for Middle Earth of spleen and stomach. The use of combination of these acupoints can tonify Qi-blood, replenish Qi of spleen and stomach, nourish liver.

Matching acupoints: For Qi deficiency of spleen and stomach, add Pishu, Weishu to tonify Qi of spleen and stomach. For Qi-blood deficiency of liver and spleen, add Ganshu, Pishu, Sanyinjiao to tonify Qi and blood of liver and spleen.

Method: Electrothermal acupuncture treatment.

Operations: Selecting the relevant acupoints, perform routine skin disinfection. Using electrothermal acupuncture needles, vertically puncture into Zusanli, Qihai, Hegu for 0.7" respectively, obliquely puncture into Pishu, Weishu for 0.7" respectively. Turn on the electrothermal acupuncture equipment, apply a current of 40-50mA to each acupoint, and the limit is that the patient feels warm or swelling and comfortable, leaving the needles in for 40 minutes.

Therapeutic course: Once a day, 10 times for a course. Start the treatment for the second course after a break of 3-5 days. Normally perform together with radiotherapy and chemotherapy.

[Chinese Herb Medicine Treatment]

This method is a comprehensive therapy of self-prescription together with radiotherapy, chemotherapy and immunotherapy. On the basis of prescription according to the differentiation of syndromes, add herbal medicines

法有：①疏肝理气法：主要用于肝癌肝气郁结者，常用逍遥散合温胆汤或二陈汤。②化瘀消癥法：适用于肝癌血络瘀阻者，方选膈下逐瘀汤或鳖甲煎丸等。③解毒利湿法：适用于热毒炽盛、湿热内阻所致的黄疸、腹水，多用茵陈蒿汤合四苓散加味。④益肾柔肝法：适用于肝癌后期之肝肾阴虚证，方选六味地黄汤加味，伴有腹水者，加商陆、车前子、玉米须等化湿利尿药。⑤益气健脾法：适用于肝癌脾虚证，多用六君子汤加味。

以上各种治法，可以合并使用。例如，化瘀消癥合益气健脾法，解毒利湿法合益肾柔肝法。总之，临床应根据患者的病情变化灵活运用。常用的抗肝癌中药有：半枝莲、虎杖、小叶金钱草、冬凌草、土茯苓、板蓝根、喜树果、茵陈蒿、莪术、枸杞子、土鳖虫、半边莲、蜈蚣、蛇莓、白

which have efficacies of anti-hepatocarcinoma. Specific therapies include: ① Soothe liver and regulate Qi: Mainly used for liver cancer patients with liver Qi stagnation; normally use Xiao Yao San plus Wen Dan Tang or Er Chen Tang. ② Disperse blood stasis and eliminate lumps: Applicable to liver cancer patients with obstruction of blood and collaterals. Choose Ge Xia Zhu Yu Tang or Bie Jia Jian Wan for the prescription. ③ Remove toxins and eliminate Damp: Applicable to icterus and ascites caused by excessive Heat toxins and internal retention of Damp-Heat; normally use Yin Chen Gao Tang plus Si Ling San (add ingredients). ④ Tonify kidney and soften liver: Applicable to syndromes of liver and kidney Yin deficiency in the advanced phase of liver cancer. Choose Liu Wei Di Huang Tang (add ingredients), and for accompanied ascites add herb medicines like pokeberry root, plantain seed and stigma of corn which can remove Damp and facilitate urination. ⑤ Tonify Qi and invigorate spleen: Applicable to spleen deficiency syndromes of liver cancer; normally use Liu Jun Zi Tang (add ingredients).

The above therapies can be used combined. For example, use the method ② together with ⑤. In general, these therapies can be clinically used flexibly according to changes of patient conditions. Normally used anti-hepatoma herb medicines include: scutellaria barbata, giant knot weed, herba lysimachiae granules, herba rabdosiae, rhizoma smilacis glabrae, isatis root, fruit of camptotheca acuminate, artemisia capillaris, curcuma zedoary, fruit of Chinese wolfberry, ground beetle, Chinese lobelia, centipede, mock-strawberry, solanum lyratum, etc.

英等。

【化学药物治疗】

肝癌化疗的适应证：①饮食及体力状态较好。②肝肾功能及造血功能基本正常。③单纯型、硬化型Ⅰ、Ⅱ期不适于手术的患者及单纯型Ⅲ期一般状态较好的患者。

化疗常用的药物：5-氟尿嘧啶、阿霉素、顺铂、氨甲蝶呤、丝裂霉素C、长春新碱等。

【放射治疗】

肝癌放疗的适应证：①患者体质尚好，肝功能基本正常，肝硬变不严重。②肝癌肿比较局限，无远处转移。放疗时照射野面积不宜过大，一野照射在10cm²左右为宜，每日组织量75～125rad，总组织量在4000～6000rad。放疗期间，可小剂量用药，如噻潜派，每次10mg，每周1～2次，或氟尿嘧啶250～500mg，1周或10天1次，常可增加放射敏感性。放疗的同时合用电热针、中药治疗，可减轻副作用并提高临床疗效。

【免疫治疗】

在针、药治疗的同时，亦可配合免疫治疗。目前免疫治

[Chemotherapy]

Indications for chemotherapy of liver cancer: ① Relatively good diet and physical status. ② Liver and kidney functions and hematopoietic function are basically normal. ③ Patients with simple-type and sclerotic-type Phase I & II liver cancers who are not suitable for surgeries, and patients with simple-type Phase III liver cancers who have relatively good conditions.

Normally used drugs for chemotherapy: 5-fluorouracil, adriamycin, cis-platinum, amethopterin, mitomycin C, vincristine, etc.

[Radiotherapy]

Indications for radiotherapy of liver cancer: ① Patients who still have relatively good physique and basically normal liver functions, with non-serious cirrhosis. ② Limited liver tumors with no distant metastasis. The radiation field area shouldn't be too large, and normally the appropriate area is around 10cm², daily tissue amount 75-125rad, total tissue amount 4000-6000rad. During the radiotherapy treatment, mediation of a small dose which can increase radiosensitivity is allowable. For example, 10mg of Saiqianpai, 1-2 times a day; or 250-500mg of fluorouracil, once a week or once every 10 days. Use electrothermal acupuncture treatment and Chinese Herb Medicine treatment during the radiotherapy treatment can reduce side effects and improve clinical efficacies.

[Immunotherapy]

The immunotherapy also can be used together with acupuncture therapy and mediation. Current methods

疗法有自体或异体肝癌瘤苗、免疫核糖核酸、转移因子等，通过合并免疫治疗，患者一般状况都可有所改善，部分患者能延长生命，有的甚至可以临床治愈。

三、注意事项

1. 肝癌是一种恶性程度较大、发展最快、预后较差的肿瘤。早期肝癌大多在体检中发现，手术治愈率较高，中晚期肝癌以化疗、放疗、电热针、中药治疗为主，针灸作为综合治疗中的一种重要手段，有着较好的效果。尤其在减轻疼痛、改善胃肠道反应及放化疗对造血系统的影响方面，都有很好的疗效。

2. 积极治疗肝癌前期病变很重要。如乙型肝炎、肝硬化，以中医药治疗为主，辅以针灸治疗，能起到防止肝癌发生的作用。

3. 针刺背俞穴及腹部穴，应注意针刺的方向及深度，慎防刺伤内脏。

4. 肝癌患者饮食物以清淡

of immunotherapy include antilogous or allogeneic tumor vaccines of liver cancer, immune ribonucleic acid (iRNA), transfer factor (TF). Normally patients can achieve improvements by combined immunotherapy, and some patients can get life extension or even clinical cure.

III. Precautions

1. Liver cancer is a kind of tumors with high malignant degree and fastest progress as well as poor prognosis. Most cases of early liver cancer are found by physical examination, and the cure rate of surgery is relatively high. The main treatment methods for middle and advanced liver cancer are chemotherapy, radiotherapy, electrothermal acupuncture treatment and Chinese Herb Medicine therapy. As an important approach for comprehensive therapies, the acupuncture therapy has good efficacies. Especially in the respects of reliving pains, improving gastrointestinal reactions as well as impacts on the hematopoietic system due to radiotherapy and chemotherapy, it have really good efficacies.

2. Active treatment for precancerous lesions of liver cancer is important. For hepatitis B and cirrhosis, the main therapy should be Chinese Herb Medicine therapy supplemented with acupuncture therapy, which can prevent the occurrence of liver cancers.

3. For acupuncture of Back-Shu acupoints and acupoints located at the abdomen, attentions should be paid to the needling direction and depth so as to prevent piercing of internal organs.

4. Patients with liver cancer are better to have light

细软、容易消化为上，忌食辛辣油腻及粗糙的食物。

5. 要注意肝癌患者的情绪变化，以乐观豁达为好，切勿忧郁恼怒。同时要有适当的活动，增强体质。选择适合的健康运动。

四、典型病例

林某，女，33岁，职员，新加坡人。

主诉：右上腹隐痛已有3年，近日加重。病史：患者出生后发现是乙肝病毒携带者，但无明显症状。

刻下症：右上腹时有胁肋隐痛，纳谷减少，口干，心悸，头晕目眩，四肢无力，劳累后加重，失眠，面色白，舌淡而胖，苔少，脉细。

查体：二尖瓣区及主动脉瓣第二听诊区闻及二级收缩期杂音。

辅助检查：MRI检查发现肝有5cm×3cm大小的肿块。白细胞计数11×10^9/L。

【诊断依据】

1. 中年女性，自幼是乙肝病毒携带者。

2. MRI检查：肝有5cm×3cm大小的肿块，已确诊为

and soft, easily digestible food, and intake of spicy, greasy and rough food is forbidden.

5. Pay attention to emotional changes of patients with liver cancer, let patients be optimistic and open-minded, not be melancholy and indignant. Do appropriate exercises to strengthen physique. Choose proper and healthy activities.

IV. Typical Case

Lin, female, 33 years old, employee, Singaporean.

Self-reported symptoms: Dull pain of the right upper abdomen for 3 years, aggravated recently. Medical history: The patient was found as a hepatitis B virus carrier after birth, with no obvious symptoms.

Current symptoms: Frequent hypochondrium dull pain of the right upper abdomen, reduced food intake, dry mouth, palpitation, dizziness and vertigo, limb weakness, aggravated with tiredness, insomnia, pale complexion, light and fat tongue with less fur, thin pulse.

Physical examination: Grade 2 systolic noise at mitral valve area and second aortic valve area.

Auxiliary examination: One lump on the liver with a size of 5cm×3cm was found in the MRI examination. Leukocyte count 11×10^9/L.

[Diagnostic Basis]

1. Middle-aged female, a hepatitis B virus carrier since childhood.

2. MRI examination: One lump on the liver with a size of 5cm×3cm, diagnosed as "liver cancer".

"肝癌"。

3. 纳谷呆滞，形体消瘦，神疲乏力。

4. 西医给予治疗中。

【证治分析】

病因 禀赋不足，后天失养。

病机 肝脾气血双亏。

证候分析 肝血亏损，不能濡养肝络，故胁肋痛；肝胆气血亏虚，不能上荣，故头晕目眩；阴虚易生内热，故口干，心悸，失眠。舌淡苔少，脉沉细，皆为肝脾气血双亏之象。

病位 肝、脾。

病性 本虚标实。

西医诊断 肝癌、乙型肝炎。

中医诊断 肝脾双亏型胁痛。

治法 疏肝理气，消癥散结。

方法 电热针治疗（补法）。

3. Indigestion and loss of appetite, body emaciation, fatigue look and asthenia.

4. During treatment of Western Medicine therapy.

[Syndrome-treatment Analysis]

Etiology: Inadequate inherent endowment, nourishment loss of acquired construction.

Pathogenesis: Qi-blood depletion of both liver and spleen.

Syndrome analysis: Depletion of liver blood causes that liver meridians cannot be nourished, thereby leading to hypochondrium pain; depletion and deficiency of Qi-blood of liver and gallbladder causes the Qi and blood cannot go upwards, thereby leading to dizziness and vertigo; Yin deficiency is easy to cause generation of internal Heat, thereby leading to dry mouth, palpitation, and insomnia. Light tongue with less fur, deep and thin pulse, are all symptoms for Qi and blood depletion of liver and spleen.

Lesion location: Liver, spleen.

Nature of disease: Asthenia in origin and sthenia in superficiality.

The diagnosis of Western Medicine: Liver cancer, Hepatitis B.

The diagnosis of Traditional Chinese Medicine: Hypochondriac pain caused by Qi and blood depletion of liver and spleen.

Therapeutic method: Soothe liver and regulate Qi, remove cumulation and disperse stasis.

Method: Electrothermal acupuncture treatment (tonifying).

处方 肝俞（BL18）、内关（PC6）、阳陵泉（GB34）、足三里（ST36）、三阴交（SP6）。

方义 肝癌早期，癥块初结，常见气机郁滞之象，治当疏肝理气，消癥散结。取肝俞以疏肝理气，取背俞治脏之功；配手厥阴经之内关，以通阴维，宽胸下气，助肝俞以调胸胁之气机；合足少阳胆经之阳陵泉以疏利肝胆，行气散结；选痞根以消癥散结；取阳明胃经之合足三里，脾经之三阴交扶助脾胃，以资生化之源。

配穴 头晕者加百会；头痛者加头维、太阳；肝气郁滞者加太冲、外关，以疏肝解郁；胃脘痛者加中脘、梁门、天枢。

操作 选定穴位，皮肤常规消毒。电热针直刺内关、阳陵泉、足三里、三阴交各 0.7 寸，斜刺（针尖向脊柱）肝俞、脾俞、肾俞各 0.8 寸，直

Prescription: Ganshu (BL18), Neiguan (PC6), Yanglingquan (GB34), Zusanli (ST36), Sanyinjiao (SP6).

Mechanism of prescription: In the early phase of liver cancer, the lump is just formed, and Qi Dynamic stagnation is common, therefore the treatment should be aimed to soothe liver and regulate Qi, remove cumulation and disperse stasis. Use Ganshu to soothe and regulate meridian Qi of liver, so as to obtain the efficacies of organ treatment of Back-Shu acupoints. Match the meridian acupoint Neiguan from Jue-Yin Meridian of Hand to soothe Yin-Wei, relieve chest stuffiness and depress Qi, so as to help Ganshu to regulate Qi Dynamic of chest and hypochondrium. Add Yanglingquan from Shao-Yang Gallbladder Meridian of Foot to soothe liver and gallbladder, activate Qi and disperse stasis. Use Pigen to remove cumulation and disperse stasis. Use the confluent acupoint Zusanli of Yang-Ming Stomach Meridian, Sanyinjiao from Spleen Meridian to reinforce spleen and stomach, so as to facilitate the source of generation and transformation.

Matching acupoints: For dizziness, add Baihui. For headache add Touwei, Taiyang. For stagnation of liver Qi, add Taichong, Waiguan to soothe liver Qi stagnation. For epigastric pain add Zhongwan, Liangmen, Tianshu.

Operations: Selecting the relevant acupoints, perform routine skin disinfection. Using electrothermal acupuncture needles, vertically puncture into Neiguan, Yanglingquan, Zusanli, Sanyinjiao for 0.7" respectively, obliquely puncture (with the needle tip towards spine)

刺中脘、梁门、天枢各 0.7 寸，接通电热针仪，每个穴位分别给予 40mA 的电流量，以患者感到温胀为度，留针 40 分钟。（注：每次选 3 对主穴给予电热针治疗，余者用毫针治疗。）

疗程 每日 1 次，10 次为 1 个疗程。疗程间可休息 3～5 天，再进行第 2 个疗程的治疗。

治疗过程 该患者在治疗过程中，每日配合服中药 1 剂，针药结合，配合化疗之综合疗法，效果满意。治疗 3 个月后复查，MRI 检查示"肿块基本消失"，肝功能正常，病毒量减少，精力充沛，已于 2009 年 2 月结婚。随访 2 年健康。

【生活调摄】

1. 清淡饮食，忌食辛辣油腻及粗糙的食物。

2. 调畅情志，以乐观豁达为好，切勿忧郁恼怒。

3. 同时要有适当的活动，增强体质。选择适合的健康运动。

大肠癌

大肠癌包括直肠癌及结肠

into Ganshu, Pishu, Shenshu for 0.8" respectively, vertically puncture into Zhongwan, Liangmen, Tianshu for 0.7" respectively. Turn on the electrothermal acupuncture equipment, apply a current of 40mA to each acupoint, and the limit is that the patient feels warm and swelling, leaving the needles in for 40 minutes. (Note: Select 3 pairs of main acupoints for electrothermal acupuncture treatment each time, and treat the other acupoints with filiform needles.)

Therapeutic course: Once a day, 10 times for a course. Start the treatment for the second course after a break of 3-5 days.

Therapeutic process: During the treatment, the patient took one dose of Chinese Herb Medicine drugs, the effects of acupuncture and drug treatments plus chemotherapy were satisfactory. During the re-examination 3 months after the treatment, the MRI exam indicated "the lump basically disappeared", normal liver functions, reduced virus amount, and the patient was full of energy. She married in February, 2009. 2-year follow-up, healthy.

[Lifestyle Change and Health Maintenance]

1. Light diet, spicy, greasy and rough food is forbidden.

2. Regulate emotions, let patients be optimistic and open-minded, not be melancholy and indignant.

3. Do appropriate exercises to strengthen physique. Choose proper and healthy activities.

Colorectal Cancer

The colorectal cancer includes rectal cancer and co-

癌，其中以直肠癌为最多，占整个大肠癌的半数以上；其次是乙状结肠癌，约占1/8左右；其下依次为升结肠癌、盲肠癌、降结肠癌、横结肠癌以及肝曲和脾曲部位的癌肿。发病率仅次于胃癌和食道癌而居消化道肿瘤的第三位。中医认为，本病在"肠覃""脏毒""肠风""下痢""肠澼""下血"等病证中有类似的描述。

直肠癌常见脓血便、黏液血便、下坠感或里急后重感，大便形状不规则。腹痛、腹胀、排便困难、便次增多、便秘或腹泻交替出现。肛门指检能及肿块，形状不规则，并可见指套染脓血。直肠镜或乙状结肠镜检查窥见直肠肿块。钡剂灌肠检查有充盈缺损，黏膜破坏，肠腔狭窄、僵硬或局部梗阻等征象。病理检查证实诊断。

结肠癌临床常表现为腹胀，腹泻，腹部不适，大便习惯改变或腹泻与便秘交替出现，血便，黏液便，或黏液血便，可有结肠梗阻症状和体征，消瘦，贫血或体重减轻。

lon cancer, among which the rectal cancer is ranked first, accounting for more than a half, and the second one is sigmoid colon cancer accounting for 1/8 or so, followed by ascending colon cancer, cecal cancer, descending colon cancer, transverse colon cancer and cancers at hepatic flexure and splenic flexure parts. Its morbidity is only second to gastric cancer and esophagus cancer, ranked third among gastrointestinal cancers. It is believed in Traditional Chinese Medicine that there are similar descriptions in "female abdominal lump"(Chang Tan), "perianal abscess"(Zang Du), "intestinal wind"(Chang Feng), "diarrhea"(Xia Li), "intestinal afflux"(Chang Pi), "descent of blood"(Xia xue) and other diseases.

The common symptoms for colorectal cancer include bloody purulent stool, mucus bloody stool, feeling of bearing down or tenesmus, irregular shaped stool. Abdominal pain, abdominal distension, defecation difficulties, increased defecation frequency, constipation or diarrhea alternately appears. Irregular shaped lumpes can be felt during rectal palpation, as well as purulent blood seen on the fingerstall. Rectal lumpes are seen under rectoscopy or sigmoidoscopy. Filling defect, mucosal damage, intestinal stenosis, stiffness or local obstruction and other signs are observed under barium enema examination. Pathological examination confirmed the diagnosis.

The common clinical manifestations for colon cancer are abdominal distension, diarrhea, abdominal discomfort, defecation habits change or alternate occurrence of diarrhea and constipation, bloody stool, mucus stool, or mucus bloody stool, sometimes accompanied with symptoms and signs of colonic obstruction, emaciation,

腹部触及包块。乙状结肠镜与纤维结肠镜检查能见结肠有溃疡、肿块、狭窄，活体组织病理检查证实诊断。X 线钡剂灌肠可见结肠腔有充盈缺损，黏膜破坏，肠管僵硬和狭窄，肠梗阻等征象。

一、诊断及辨证要点

1. 脾虚湿热者，食欲不振，腹胀腹痛，面色萎黄，气短乏力，大便稀溏，或里急后重，便下脓血，苔薄黄腻，脉濡数或沉细滑。

2. 湿热瘀毒者，腹痛腹胀拒按，矢气胀减，腹有包块，推之不动，便下脓血黏膜，或里急后重，或便溏，或便秘，舌暗红，有瘀斑，苔薄黄，脉弦数。

3. 肝肾阴虚者，头晕耳鸣，消瘦乏力，心烦，口渴，失眠多梦，腰酸腿软，大便秘结，或有腹痛，舌红苔黄，脉细或细数。

4. 脾肾虚寒者，形寒肢冷，

anemia or weight loss. Abdomen lumpes are palpated. Ulceration, lump, stenosis in colon are observed under sigmoidoscopy and fibro-colonoscopy, and in vivo histopathological examination confirmed the diagnosis. Filling defect, mucosal damage, intestinal canal stiffness and stenosis, intestinal obstruction and other signs can be seen under X-ray barium enema examination.

I. Key Points for Diagnosis and Syndrome Differentiation

1. For patients with spleen deficiency and Damp-Heat, their symptoms include loss of appetite, abdominal distension and pain, sallow complexion, shortness of breath and tiredness, thin sloppy stool, or tenesmus, stool with purulent blood, yellow and greasy thin tongue fur, soft and rapid pulse or deep, thready, slippery pulse.

2. For patients with Damp-Heat and stasis, their symptoms include abdominal distension and pain and refusal of pressing, the distension will be reduce after flatus; abdominal lumps which cannot be moved by pushing; stool with purulent blood and mucus membranes, or tenesmus, or sloppy stool, or constipation; dark red tongue with ecchymosis, yellow thin tongue fur; taut and rapid pulse.

3. For patients with Yin deficiency of liver and kidney, their symptoms include dizziness and tinnitus, emaciation and asthenia, dysphoria, thirst, insomnia and dreaminess, aching lumbus and limp legs, constipation, or abdominal pain, red tongue and yellow tongue fur, thin pulse or thin and rapid pulse.

4. For patients with spleen and kidney deficiency

消瘦乏力，面色苍白，神倦纳差，腹胀腹痛，大便稀溏，舌淡苔白，脉沉细弱。

5. 气血两虚者，面色不华，少气乏力，口淡无味，纳少脘胀，大便稀薄，肛门有下坠感，形体消瘦，或有低热，舌质淡，苔薄白，脉沉细。

二、治疗方法

【早期】

治法　疏肝和胃。

处方　天枢（ST25）、大肠俞（BL25）。

方义　大肠癌早期，癥块瘀结，大肠腑气不通，传化失常，治疗当以疏导腑气为主。本方天枢配大肠俞，为俞募配穴法，重点在于疏导肝胃之气滞，胃气和顺，中焦气机升降出入有序，邪气则无郁结之弊。

配穴　若大肠气滞郁结

and cold, their symptoms include cold body and limbs, emaciation and asthenia, pale complexion, lassitude of the spirit and anorexia, abdominal distension and pain, thin sloppy stool, pale tongue and whitish tongue fur, deep, thin and weak pulse.

5. For patients with Qi-blood deficiency, their symptoms include lusterless complexion, weak breath and asthenia, tastelessness, less eating and gastric distension, thin sloppy stool, feeling of bearing down at anus, emaciation, or low-grade fever, pale tongue, thin and whitish tongue fur, deep and thin pulse.

II. Therapeutic Methods

[Early Phase]

Therapeutic method: Soothe the liver and the stomach.

Prescription: Tianshu (ST25), Dachangshu (BL25).

Mechanism of prescription: During the early phase of colorectal cancer, stasis accumulation of concretion lumps, Fu-Qi obstruction of large intestine, digestive disorders will occur, so the therapy should focus on soothing of Fu-Qi. In this prescription, the Tianshu is matched with Dachangshu, which is the method of Back-Shu points and Mu points combination, and the key points of this method are soothing of the Qi stagnation in liver and stomach. If the stomach-Qi is smooth, and for the Qi movement of the Middle Jiao, the ascending and descending as well as access are in order, then there won't be problem of pathogenic Qi stagnation.

Matching acupoints: For patients with Qi stagna-

者，可加中脘、行间，以疏导肝胃之气滞，胃气和顺，中焦气机升降出入有序，邪气则无郁结之弊；若大肠湿热下注者，可加下脘、曲池、上巨虚，以清泻湿热邪毒。

方法 电热针治疗。

操作 选定穴位，皮肤常规消毒。电热针直刺天枢0.8寸，直刺大肠俞0.8寸，直刺曲池0.7寸，接通电热针仪，每个穴位分别给予电流量40～60mA，以患者感到温胀舒适为度，留针40分钟。另配以毫针直刺上巨虚0.7寸，直刺行间0.5寸，直刺中脘0.7寸，给予补法，留针30分钟。

疗程 每日1次，10次为1个疗程，疗程间休息5～7天，再进行第2个疗程的治疗。

【中期】

治法 疏理胃肠，祛邪散结，益气补中。

处方 天枢（ST25）、大肠俞（BL25）、足三里（ST36）。

方义 大肠癌中期，肿块渐大，正气已虚，临床多见虚

tion in the large intestine, Zhongwan and Xingjian can be added to soothe the Qi stagnation in liver and stomach. If the stomach-Qi is smooth, and the ascending and descending as well as access of Qi Dynamic in Middle Jiao are in order, then there won't be problem of pathogenic Qi stagnation; for patients with downward flow of Damp-Heat at the large intestine, Xiawan, Quchi, Shangjuxu can be added to clear toxic dampness and heat.

Method: Electrothermal acupuncture treatment.

Operations: Selecting the relevant acupoints, perform routine skin disinfection. Using electrothermal acupuncture needles, vertically puncture into Tianshu for 0.8", Dachangshu for 0.8", Quchi for 0.7". Turn on the electrothermal acupuncture equipment, apply a current of 40-60mA to each acupoint, and the limit is that the patient feels warmly swell and comfortable, leaving the needles in for 40 minutes. Additionally, using the filiform needles, vertically puncture into Shangjuxu for 0.7", Xingjian for 0.5", Zhongwan for 0.7" as a supplementary treatment, leaving the needles in for 30 minutes.

Therapeutic course: Treat once a day, 10 times for a course, and start the treatment for the second course after a break of 5-7 days.

[Middle Phase]

Therapeutic method: Soothe the stomach and intestine, eliminate pathogenic Qi and stagnation, nourish vital energy.

Prescription: Tianshu (ST25), Dachangshu (BL25), Zusanli (ST36).

Mechanism of prescription: For middle-phase colorectal cancers, the lump is getting bigger, the healthy Qi

实相杂，治疗当于祛邪的同时，处处顾护正气。本方取俞募配穴法，以疏导大肠腑气，故天枢配大肠俞，在此基础上取足阳明胃经的合穴足三里，合治内腑，不仅有和调胃肠、疏导气机、清化湿热之功，且能补益元气，助脾胃以生化气血，从而达到扶正祛邪之目的。诸穴合用，共奏疏理胃肠、祛邪散结、益气补中之功效。

配穴 若大肠瘀毒内结者，可加膈俞、合谷、太冲，以疏理气机，散瘀消癥；若胃肠虚寒者，可加膈俞、胃俞、中脘、气海，以温中散寒，益气固涩；若脾胃气血两虚者，可加膈俞、肝俞、脾俞、三阴交、曲泉，以调肝、脾、肾，使肝藏血，脾统血，脾胃化源充足，气血得养，瘀积自消。

方法 电热针治疗。

操作 选定穴位，皮肤常

has been weak, the symptoms of intermingled deficiency and excess syndromes are generally seen clinically. The treatment should care for healthy Qi while eliminating pathogenic Qi. This prescription use the method of Back-Shu points and Mu points combination to soothe Fu-Qi of large intestine, so match Tianshu with Dachangshu, and use a He acupoint Zhusanli of the Yang-Ming Stomach Meridian of Foot to care organs on this basis. It not only can regulate intestines and stomach, soothe Qi Dynamic, clear Damp-Heat, but can replenish vitality, help the spleen and stomach to generate Qi-blood, so as to achieve the aim of strengthening vital Qi and eliminating pathogenic factors. The use of combination of these acupoints can soothe the stomach and intestine, eliminate pathogenic Qi and stagnation, nourish vital energy.

Matching acupoints: For patients with internal binding of static blood and poison in the large intestine, Geshu, Hegu, Taichong can be added to soothe Qi Dynamic and disperse blood stasis and eliminate lumps; for patients with stomach and intestine deficiency-cold, Geshu, Weishu, Zhongwan, Qihai can be added to warm spleen and stomach for dispelling cold and induce astringency; for patients with Qi-blood deficiency of the spleen and stomach, Geshu, Ganshu, Pishu, Sanyinjiao, Ququan can be added to regulate liver, spleen and kidney, so as to enable liver storing blood and spleen governing blood, as well as have sufficient change source of spleen and stomach, nourish Qi-blood, and the elimination of stasis accumulation.

Method: Electrothermal acupuncture treatment.

Operations: Selecting the relevant acupoints, per-

规消毒。电热针直刺天枢、大肠俞、足三里各 0.8 寸，向脊柱方向斜刺膈俞、肝俞、脾俞各 0.8 寸，直刺三阴交 0.6 寸，直刺曲池 0.7 寸。接通电热针仪，每个穴位分别给予电流量 40～60mA。另配以毫针直刺合谷、太冲各 0.5 寸，留针 40 分钟。

疗程 每日 1 次，10 次为 1 个疗程，疗程间休息 5～7 天，再进行第 2 个疗程的治疗。

【晚期】

治法 益气培元，和调胃肠。

处方 天枢（ST25）、大肠俞（BL25）、足三里（ST36）、气海（RN6）。

方义 大肠癌晚期，癥块渐大，正气日损，气血津液耗竭，治疗当补益元气。本方在治疗中期大肠癌的基础上加任脉之气海穴，重在培土补元。气海与足三里相配，更有补益脏腑元气之功。足三里益胃，胃乃五脏六腑之海，加上气海，则胃气充，脏腑得养也。诸穴共用，可奏益气培元、和调胃肠的功效。

form routine skin disinfection. Using electrothermal acupuncture needles, vertically puncture into Tianshu, Dachangshu, Zusanli for 0.8" respectively; and obliquely puncture into Geshu, Ganshu, Pishu towards the spine respectively for 0.8"; vertically puncture into Sanyinjiao for 0.6", Quchi for 0.7". Turn on the electrothermal acupuncture equipment, apply a current of 40-60mA to each acupoint. Additionally, using filiform needles, vertically puncture into Hegu and Taichong for 0.5" respectively, leaving the needles in for 40 minutes.

Therapeutic course: Treat once a day, 10 times for a course, and start the treatment for the second course after a break of 5-7 days.

[Advanced Phase]

Therapeutic method: Nourish Qi and reinforce vital essence, regulate intestines and stomach.

Prescription: Tianshu (ST25), Dachangshu (BL25), Zusanli (ST36), Qihai (RN6).

Mechanism of prescription: For advanced colorectal cancers, the lump is getting bigger, the healthy Qi is losing, the Qi-blood and fluid is exhausting, so the treatment should nourish vitality. This prescription adds the acupoint Qihai of Ren Channel on the basis of the therapy for middle-phase colorectal cancers, the emphasis is fostering Earth and nourishing vitality. The combination of Qihai and Zusanli has the efficacy of nourishing organ vitality. Zusanli is beneficial to the stomach. Stomach is the sea of internal organs, so the addition of Qihai can replenish stomach Qi and nourish internal organs. The use of combination of these acupoints can nourish Qi

配穴　若脾肾阳虚者，可加大椎、命门、肾俞、关元，以通阳补元，调养胃气；若有肝肾阴虚者，可加三阴交、太溪、肾俞、曲泉，以滋养阴津，调摄肝肾。

方法　电热针治疗。

操作　选定穴位，皮肤常规消毒。电热针直刺天枢、大肠俞、足三里各 0.8 寸，直刺气海 0.7 寸。接通电热针仪，每个穴位分别给予电流量 40～60mA。另配以毫针直刺合谷、太冲各 0.5 寸，留针 40 分钟。

疗程　每日 1 次，10 次为 1 个疗程，疗程间休息 5～7 天，再进行第 2 个疗程的治疗。

【术后、放疗、化疗后】

治法　补气生血，和调脏腑。

处方　足三里（ST36）、气海（RN6）、三阴交（SP6）。

方义　大肠癌术后、放疗、化疗的副反应主要反映在脾胃气虚、元气亏损上。本方 3 个穴都是强壮穴，取足阳明经合

and reinforce vital essence, regulate intestines and stomach.

Matching acupoints: For patients with Yang deficiency of spleen and kidney, Dazhui, Mingmen, Shenshu, Guanyuan can be added to activate Yang and replenish vitality, nurse stomach Qi; for patients with Ying deficiency of spleen and stomach, Sanyinjiao, Taixi, Shenshu, Ququan can be added to nourish Yin-Fluid, regulate liver and kidney.

Method: Electrothermal acupuncture treatment.

Operations: Selecting the relevant acupoints, perform routine skin disinfection. Using electrothermal acupuncture needles, vertically puncture into Tianshu, Dachangshu, Zusanli for 0.8" respectively, Qihai for 0.7". Turn on the electrothermal acupuncture equipment, apply a current of 40-60mA to each acupoint. Additionally, using filiform needles, vertically puncture into Hegu and Taichong for 0.5" respectively, leaving the needles in for 40 minutes.

Therapeutic course: Treat once a day, 10 times for a course, and start the treatment for the second course after a break of 5-7 days.

[Post-operation, post-radiotherapy, post-chemotherapy]

Therapeutic method: Replenish Qi and nourish blood, regulate internal organs.

Prescription: Zusanli (ST36), Qihai (RN6), Sanyinjiao (SP6).

Mechanism of prescription: After colorectal cancer surgeries, the side effects of radiotherapy and chemotherapy are mainly reflected on Qi defficiency of spleen and stomach as well as vitality loss. The three acupoints

穴足三里，主要在于维护中气以生气血；配气海穴，有助胃气以充元气；配合谷穴，乃取手足阳明同调之意，胃肠调和则水谷精微吸收，人体得养，正气日充也。诸穴合用，可以培土补元以生气血，和调胃肠以泽脏腑。

配穴 若术后假肛有炎症时，加曲池、外关、行间，以疏泄大肠经、三焦经、肝经之郁热，起清热解毒之功；若有阴虚津伤者，可加脾俞、三阴交、支沟，以养阴生津，润燥利肠；若见脾胃气虚者，可加上巨虚、中脘、脾俞、胃俞，以补益脾胃，摄养胃气。

方法 电热针治疗。

操作 选定穴位，皮肤常规消毒。电热针直刺足三里、上巨虚各0.8寸，直刺气海、三阴交、曲池各0.7寸，向脊柱方向斜刺脾俞、肾俞各0.7寸。接通电热针仪，每个穴位分别给予电流量50～60mA，

in this prescription are all important tonifying acupoints. He acupoint Zusanli of the Yang-Ming Meridian of Foot is used to maintain Middle-jiao Qi to nourish Qi-blood, and the use of Qihai is helpful to stomach Qi so as to replenish vitality; the use of Hegu is to achieve co-regulation for Yang-Ming Meridians of Hand and Foot, if the stomach and intestine are co-regulated, then the essence of water and food will be absorbed, the body can be nourished, as well as increasingly replenishing of healthy Qi. So the use of three acupoints combined can foster Earth and nourish vitality to nourish Qi-blood, as well as coordinate stomach and intestine to nourish internal organs.

Matching acupoints: If there is inflammation of false annal postoperatively, Quchi, Waiguan, Xingjian can be added to dredge the stasis-Heat of Large Intestine Meridian, Three-Jiao Meridian, Liver Meridian, so as to achieve heat-clearing and detoxifying; for patients with Yin deficiency and fluid impairment, Pishu, Sanyinjiao, Zhigou can be added to nourish Yin and generate fluid; for patients with Qi deficiency of spleen and stomach, Shangjuxu, Zhongwan, Pishu, Weishu can be added to replenish spleen and stomach as well as nourish stomach Qi.

Method: Electrothermal acupuncture treatment.

Operations: Selecting the relevant acupoints, perform routine skin disinfection. Using the electrothermal acupuncture needles, vertically puncture into Zusanli, Shangjuxu for 0.8" respectively, Qihai, Sanyinjiao, Quchi for 0.7" respectively; and obliquely puncture into Pishu, Shenshu towards the spine respectively for 0.7". Turn on the electrothermal acupuncture equipment, apply

· 503 ·

以患者感到温胀舒适为度，留40分钟针。另配以毫针直刺外关0.5寸，直刺行间0.5寸，留针30分钟。

疗程 每日1次，10次为1个疗程，疗程间休息5～7天，再进行第2个疗程的治疗。

三、注意事项

1. 大肠癌手术治疗效果较好，因此，"早期发现，早期诊断"是治疗大肠癌的关键，术后再采用针灸康复疗法。中晚期大肠癌，一般临床采用术后放化疗或放化疗配合中药治疗。针灸作为综合治疗的一种手段，可提高患者自身的免疫功能，减少放化疗的副反应，在止痛、减少消化系统及造血系统副反应方面起到良好的治疗作用。

2. 积极治疗大肠癌前期病变是预防肠癌的重要措施。针灸疗法对治疗癌前期病变有着较好的治愈效果。

3. 针刺背俞穴，要掌握好针刺的方向、深度；针刺关元时要求患者排空膀胱后施术，

a current of 50-60mA to each acupoint, and the limit is that the patient feels warmly swell and comfortable, leaving the needles in for 40 minutes. Additionally, using the filiform needles, vertically puncture into Waiguan for 0.5", Xingjian for 0.5", leaving the needles in for 30 minutes.

Therapeutic course: Treat once a day, 10 times for a course, and start the treatment for the second course after a break of 5-7 days.

III. Precautions

1. The efficacy of colorectal cancer surgeries is good, so "Early detection, early diagnosis" is the key point for colorectal cancer treatment, and the acupuncture is used postoperatively as a rehabilitation therapy. For middle-phase or advanced colorectal cancers, generally postoperative radiotherapy and chemotherapy, or radiotherapy and chemotherapy with Chinese Herb Medicine treatment are used. The acupuncture therapy, as a means of comprehensive treatments, can improve patient's own immune function and reduce side effects of radiotherapy and chemotherapy, as well as have good efficacies in reducing side effects on the digestive system and the hematopoietic system.

2. Active treatments for precancerous lesions of colorectal cancers is an important measure for prevention of colorectal cancers. The acpuncture therapy of Traditional Chinese Medicine have good healing effects on precancerous lesions of cancers.

3. For acupuncture of the Back-Shu acupoints, it is important to control the puncturing direction and depth; for acupuncture of the acupoint Guanyuan, the patient is

慎防刺伤内脏。

4. 注意患者的饮食卫生，不洁食物与发霉变质的食品不能食用。有文献报道，大肠癌与食入不洁及发霉食品有一定的关系。少吃油煎滋腻的食品，多吃新鲜蔬菜和水果。

5. 在康复后，适当参加体育活动，如散步、气功、太极拳等。

6. 大肠癌术后的人工肛门要严格消毒，勤洗勤换，保持清洁，以防假肛发炎。

四、典型病例

刘某，男，49岁，工人，北京人。

主诉：腹痛，肠鸣腹泻已3个月有余，近1周加重。

刻下症：患者腹泻与便秘交替而来，大便细，或下黏液大便，时有便意，食欲不振，苔薄腻，脉弦细。

查体：腹部有压痛。左下腹部压痛明显，肠鸣音活跃，无明显气过水声。

辅助检查：白细胞计数 12×10^9/L，红细胞计数 $3.5\times$

required to empty bladder before the procedure so as to prevent piercing of internal organs.

4. Pay attention to patient's food sanitation. Unclean and moldy food is not edible. There are literature reports which indicate a certain relationship between colorectal cancers and ingestion of unclean and modly food. Eat less fried or oily food and more fresh vegetables and fruits.

5. After recovery, take some sports activities appropriately, such as walking, Qigong and Taiji.

6. After the colorectal cancer surgery, the artificial annal should be strictly disinfected, washed and replaced frequently, and should be kept clean so as to prevent imflammation of the fake annal.

IV. Typical Case

Liu, male, 49 years old, worker, residence: Beijing.

Chief complaint: Abdominal pain, borborygmus and diarrhea for more than 3 months, aggravated in the past week.

Current symptoms: Diarrhea and constipation alternatively occurred, thin stools or mucus stools, frequent calls of defecation, loss of appetite, thin and greasy tongue fur, taut and thin pulse.

Physical examination: Tenderness at abdomen. Obvious tenderness at left lower abdomen, active bowel sound, no significant sound of gas through water.

Auxiliary examination: Leukocyte count 12×10^9/L, erythrocyte count 3.5×10^9/L. Positive stool occult blood.

10^9/L。大便潜血阳性。肠镜示"直肠病变"。活检示"腺癌"。

【诊断依据】

1. 肠镜及活检诊为肠癌（腺癌）。

2. 久泻与大便秘结交替出现，时有便意，大便细，或下黏液大便。

3. 多有忧思抑郁，劳倦体虚。

4. 常饮食不规律，喜食高脂肪、辛辣煎炒食品。

【证治分析】

病因 脾气亏虚。

病机 脾胃虚弱，运化受纳失调。

证候分析 脾之运化，胃之受纳，若长期饮食失调，劳倦内伤，致脾胃虚弱，运化受纳失调，久泻久痢，大便秘结，导致脾胃受损，运化失司，胃肠气滞，传化不利，湿热下注，蕴结瘀阻，邪毒浸淫肠道所致。

病位 肠。

病性 本虚标实。

Colonoscopy indicated "rectal lesions". Biopsy indicated "glandular cancer".

[Diagnostic Basis]

1. Diagnosed as colon cancer (glandular cancer) by colonoscopy and biopsy.

2. Chronic diarrhea and constipation alternatively occurred, frequent calls of defecation, thin stools, or mucus stools.

3. Frequent grief and sorrow, depression, fatigue and weak.

4. Often irregular diet, and prefer high fat, spicy fried food.

[Syndrome-treatment Analysis]

Etiology: Deficiency and weakness of spleen Qi.

Pathogenesis: Weakness of spleen and stomach, imbalance of transportation and transformation as well as reception.

Syndrome analysis: Transportation and transformation of spleen, reception of stomach. Long-term eating disorders, fatigue and internal injuries will lead to weakness of spleen and stomach, imbalance of transportation and transformation as well as reception, prolonged diarrhea and dysentery, constipation, causing impairment of spleen and stomach, irregulation of transportation and transformation, Qi stagnation in stomach and intestine, unfavourable transportation and transformation, downward flow of Damp-Heat, retention of stasis blocking, caused by pathogenic toxin spreading in intestine.

Lesion location: Intestine.

Nature of disease: Asthenia in origin and sthenia in superficiality.

西医诊断 大肠癌。

中医诊断 肠覃。

治法 疏理肠胃，祛邪散结，益气补中。

方法 电热针治疗。

处方 天枢（ST25）、大肠俞（BL25）、足三里（ST36）。

方义 大肠癌早期，癥块瘀结，大肠腑气不通，传化失常，治以疏导腑气为主，天枢配大肠俞，为俞募配穴法，重点在于疏导腑气，传化经气，使瘀结的癥块有疏散之机；另有大肠腑气得通，传化复常，癥块无日积增大之害。在此基础上，取足阳明胃经之合穴足三里，合治内腑，不仅有和调胃肠、疏理气机、清化湿热之功，且能补益元气，助脾胃以生化气血，从而达到扶正祛邪之目的。诸穴共用，可奏疏理肠胃，祛邪散结，益气补中之功效。

The diagnosis of Western Medicine: Colorectal cancer.

The diagnosis of Traditional Chinese Medicine: Female abdominal lump.

Therapeutic method: Soothe the stomach and intestine, eliminate pathogenic Qi and stagnation, nourish vital energy.

Method: Electrothermal acupuncture treatment.

Prescription: Tianshu (ST25), Dachangshu (BL25), Zusanli (ST36).

Mechanism of prescription: During the early phase of colorectal cancer, stasis accumulation of concretion lumps, Fu-Qi obstruction of large intestine, digestive disorders will occur, so the therapy should focus on soothing of Fu-Qi. The match of Tianshu and Dachangshu is a method of Back-Shu points and Mu points combination, and the key points of this method are soothing of the Qi stagnation in liver and stomach, transportation and transformation of Meridian Qi, so as to provide changes for eliminating lumps; the large intestine Fu-Qi becomes smooth, transportation and transformation recovers, and there is no harm of lump increasing day by day. On this basis, use a He acupoint Zhusanli of the Yang-Ming Stomach Meridian of Foot to care organs. It not only can regulate intestines and stomach, soothe Qi Dynamic, clear Damp-Heat, and can replenish vitality, help the spleen and stomach to generate Qi-blood, so as to achieve the aim of strengthening vital Qi and eliminating pathogenic factors. The use of combination of these acupoints can soothe the stomach and intestine, eliminate pathogenic Qi and stagnation, nourish vital energy.

配穴 大肠气滞郁结者，加膈俞、合谷、太冲，以疏理气机，散瘀消癥；胃肠虚寒者，加中脘、行间，以疏导肝胃之气滞，气机升降出入有序，邪气则无郁结之弊；大肠湿热下注者，加下脘、曲池、上巨虚，以清泻湿热邪毒；脾胃气血两虚者，加膈俞、肝俞。

操作 选定穴位，皮肤常规消毒。电热针直刺中脘、曲池、足三里、下脘各0.7寸，斜刺（针尖向脊柱）膈俞、大肠俞、肝俞、脾俞各0.8寸。接通电热针仪，每个穴位分别给予40mA的电流量，以患者感到胀而舒适为度，留针40分钟。（注：上脘、下脘、曲池、足三里每次都用电热针治疗，治疗10次后，改为电热针刺天枢、下脘、足三里、三阴交。两组穴可交替应用，其余穴位用毫针治疗。）

疗程 90次为1个疗程。根据病情决定是否进行下1个疗程的治疗。

Matching acupoints: For patients with Qi stagnation in the large intestine, Geshu, Hegu, Taichong are added to soothe Qi Dynamic, disperse blood stasis and eliminate lumps; for patients with stomach and intestine deficiency-Cold, Zhongwan and Xingjian can be added to soothe the Qi stagnation in liver and stomach. If the the ascending and descending as well as access of Qi Dynamic are in order, then there won't be problem of pathogenic Qi stagnation; for patients with downward flow of Damp-Heat in the large intestine, Xiawan, Quchi, Shangjuxu can be added to clear toxic Damp and Heat; for patients with Qi-blood dificiency of spleen and stomach, add Geshu, Ganshu.

Operations: Selecting the relevant acupoints, perform routine skin disinfection. Using the electrothermal acupuncture needles, vertically puncture into Zhongwan, Quchi, Zusanli, Xiawan for 0.7" respectively, obliquely puncture (towards Jizhong) into Geshu, Dachangshu, Ganshu, Pishu for 0.8" respectively. Turn on the electrothermal acupuncture equipment, apply a current of 40mA to each acupoint, and the limit is that the patient feels swell and comfortable, leaving the needles in for 40 minutes. (Note: Each time treat Shangwan, Xiawan, Quchi, Zusanli with electrothermal acupuncture needles, and after 10 times of treatment, switch to electrothermal acupuncture treatment for Tianshu, Xiawan, Zusanli and Sanyinjiao. The two acupoint groups can be used alternatively, and other acupoint are treated with filiform needles.)

Therapeutic course: Each course consists of 90 treatments. The decision for whether carry out the next course of treatment depends on the disease conditions.

治疗过程 该患者在治疗过程中,疗效显著,1个月后症状基本消失,治疗90次后肠镜复查,取活检证实病灶消失,体力恢复正常。除针灸治疗之外,每天配合服1剂中药。

【生活调摄】

1. 早期肠癌针灸效果较好,要早发现早治疗。积极治疗大肠癌的前期病变是预防肠癌的重要措施。

2. 肠癌与食入不洁饮食及发霉变质的食品有一定的关系,故应注意饮食卫生。

3. 为提高疗效,针灸与中药结合效果更好。

晚期癌肿

胃癌、肺癌、肝癌、宫颈癌等各种癌肿晚期,由于瘤体增大,压迫或侵犯邻近器官、神经末梢或神经干,患者均有不同程度的疼痛,如烧灼痛、隐痛或顽固、持续性剧痛,这种疼痛与肿瘤所在部位、生长方向和增长速度有关。

中医认为,晚期癌肿的疼

Treatment process: For this patient, the efficacies during treatment were significant, and the symptoms basically disappeared after 1 month. Performed colonoscopy after 90 times of treatment, and the biopsy confirmed that the lesions have disappeared and physical strength returned to be normal. In addition to acupuncture therapy, took a dose of Chinese Herb Medicine daily as supplement.

[Lifestyle Change and Health Maintenance]

1. The efficacy of acupuncture therapy on early colorectal cancers is relatively good, so early detection and early treatment is important. Active treatments for precancerous lesions of colorectal cancers is an important measure for prevention of colorectal cancers.

2. Colorectal cancers have a certain relationship with ingestion of unclean diet and moldy food, so attentions should be paid to food sanitation.

3. In order to improve efficacies, the combination of acupuncture therapy and Chinese Herb Medicine has better effects.

Advanced Cancer

For various advanced cancers such as stomach cancer, pulmonary cancer, liver cancer and cervical cancer, due to the growing of tumors, compressing or invading adjacent organs, nerve endings or nerve trunks, patients are all suffer from pain with different levels, such as burning pain, dull pain or refractory persistent sharp pain. This pain is associated with the tumor site, growth direction and growth speed.

Traditional Chinese Medicine believes that the pain

痛，多由气滞血瘀，脉络痹阻所致。病程较长，正气严重耗伤，多表现为虚实夹杂证。

of advanced cancer is mostly caused by Qi stagnation and blood stasis, as well as collaterals stagnation. Long disease course and serious consumption of healthy Qi, mostly are presented as syndrome of intermingled deficiency and excess.

一、诊断及辨证要点

1. 气血不足者，症见头晕乏力，面色白，心悸失眠，舌淡苔白，脉细无力。

2. 肝胃不和者，症见恶心呕吐，腿酸胀满，食少嗳气，舌红苔腻，脉弦滑。

3. 肝肾两亏者，症见五心烦热，食少乏力，腰酸耳鸣，舌红苔少。

4. 气滞血瘀者，症见疼痛，入夜加重或持续难忍，神疲乏力，舌紫黯，苔白，脉细涩。

二、治疗方法

【气滞血瘀证】

治法　活血止痛。

处方　足三里（ST36）、

I. Key Points for Diagnosis and Syndrome Differentiation

1. For patients with Qi-blood deficiency, the symptoms include dizziness and asthenia, pale complexion, palpitation and insomnia, thin and weak pulse.

2. For patients with syndrome of disharmony between liver and stomach, the symptoms include nausea and vomiting, leg soreness and distention, less ingestion and warm Qi, red tongue and greasy tongue fur, taut and slippery pulse.

3. For patients with liver and kidney depletion, the symptoms include dysphoria in chest with palms-soles, less ingestion and asthenia, waist soreness and tinnitus, red tongue and less tongue fur.

4. For patients with Qi stagnation and blood stasis, the symptoms include pain which will aggravate at night or persistent and hard to endure, mental fatigue and asthenia, purple and dark tongue, whitish tongue fur, thin and sluggish pulse.

II. Therapeutic Methods

[Syndrome of Qi Stagnation and Blood Stasis]

Therapeutic method: Activate blood and alleviate pain.

Prescription: Zusanli (ST36), Hegu (LI4), Ashi

合谷（LI4）、阿是穴（疼痛局部取穴）。

方义 足三里是足阳明胃经的合穴，能调理气血，补气养虚；合谷为手阳明经的原穴，可和血通络，是镇痛要穴；针刺阿是穴及疼痛局部经穴，旨在疏通经络，行气活血。诸穴合用，共奏行气活血，通络镇痛之功，寓"通则不痛"之意。

配穴 胸闷气短者加膻中；瘀血重者加血海；气滞甚者加太冲；气短乏力者加气海和关元。

方法 电热针治疗。

操作 选定穴位，皮肤常规消毒。电热针直刺足三里0.8寸，直刺合谷0.6寸，直刺阿是穴0.7～0.8寸，接通电热针仪，每个穴位分别给予电流量40～60mA，以患者感到舒适为度，留针40分钟。根据不同的部位掌握进针的深度，每日上、下午各治疗1次。

疗程 每日1次，10次为

acupoints (local acupoint selection for pain).

Mechanism of prescription: The acupoint Zusanli is a He acupoint of Yang-Ming Stomach Meridian of Foot, which can nurse Qi-blood, replenish Qi and nourish deficiency; the acupoint Hegu is a Yuan acupoint of Yang-Ming Meridian of Hand, which can activate blood circulation and dredge collaterals, is one of the key acupoints for pain ease; the acupuncture of Ashi acupoints and local meridian acupoints for pain is intended to dredge meridians and collaterals, activate Qi and blood circulation. The use of combination of these acupoints can activate Qi and blood circulation, dredge collaterals as well ease pain, indicating the meaning of "stagnation leading to pain".

Matching acupoints: For patients with chest distress and shortness of breath, add Danzhong; for patients with serious blood stasis, add Xuehai; For patients with Qi stagnation, add Taichong; For patients with shortness of breath and asthenia, add Qihai and Guanyuan.

Method: Electrothermal acupuncture treatment.

Operations: Preparing the selected acupoints, perform routine skin disinfection. Using electrothermal acupuncture needles, vertically puncture into Zusanli for 0.8", Hegu for 0.6", Ashiacupoint for 0.7-0.8". Turn on the electrothermal acupuncture equipment, apply a current of 40-60mA to each acupoint, and the limit is that the patient feels comfortable, leaving the needles in for 40 minutes. Control the depth of needle insertion according to different body parts, and treat once each morning and afternoon.

Therapeutic course: Treat once a day, 10 times for

1个疗程，疗程间休息3~5天，再继续进行第2个疗程的治疗。

三、注意事项

1. 清淡饮食，进食容易消化、易吸收的食物，多食蔬菜和水果。

2. 舒畅情致，保持乐观的态度。

3. 做力所能及的运动。

肿瘤放疗与化疗之副反应

放射治疗，是一种利用高能电磁辐射来杀伤癌细胞的方法；化学治疗，是一种利用具有抗癌作用的化学药物消除原发病灶及扩散的癌细胞的方法。这两种方法和手术一样，已成为治疗肿瘤的重要手段之一，对于某些恶性肿瘤的治疗和缓解有明显的作用。但由于其杀伤癌细胞的同时，或多或少伤害了人体正常的细胞或破坏人体某些正常机能，因此，肿瘤患者接受放疗或化疗后会出现一些局部或全身的不良反应。常见的副反应有：骨髓抑制而致血小板和白细胞减少；消化道反应，如恶心、呕吐、厌食、腹泻等；泌尿系统反应，

a course, and start the treatment for the second course after a break of 3-5 days.

III. Precautions

1. Light diet, eat food that easy to digest and absorb, eat more vegetables and fruits.

2. Keep happy and optimistic attitude.

3. Do exercises whatever you can.

Side Effects of Tumor Radiotherapy and Chemotherapy

Radiotherapy is a method that use high-energy electromagnetic radiation to kill cancer cells; chemotherapy is a method that use chemical drugs to eliminate primary lesions and spread cancer cells. These two methods, like surgeries, have become one of the important approaches for tumor treatment, and have significant effects in treatment and mitigation of some malignant tumors. However, since while killing cancer cells, these two therapies will damage normal human cells or impair some normal body functions more or less, so some local or systematic adverse reactions will occur after radiotherapy or chemotherapy of tumor patients. Common side effects include: Myelosuppression causing thrombocytopenia and leukocytopenia; gastrointestinal reactions, such as nausea, vomiting, anorexia, diarrhea; urinary system reactions, such as frequent micturition, urgent micturition, painful micturition, hematuria; skin reactions, such as lipsotrichia, dermatitis, ulcers, macula, desquamation; mucosal

如尿频、尿急、尿痛、血尿等；皮肤反应，如脱毛、皮炎、溃疡、斑疹、脱屑等；黏膜出现充血、水肿、溃疡、假膜、出血等；出现全身症状，如乏力、头晕、失眠、脱发等。

中医学目前虽未有与之相对应的病名，但可根据临床表现归纳为较有规律的证候，因而也可以对本病进行中医的辨证施治。

一、诊断及辨证要点

1. 气血不足者，症见头晕乏力，面色白，心悸失眠，舌淡苔白，脉细无力。

2. 肝胃不合者，症见恶心呕吐，腿酸胀满，食少嗳气，舌红苔腻，脉弦滑。

3. 肝肾两亏者，症见五心烦热，食少乏力，腰酸耳鸣，舌红苔少。

二、治疗方法

【气血不足证】

治法　补气养血。

congestion, edema, ulcers, pseudomembrane, bleeding, etc.; systematic symptoms, such as asthenia, dizziness, insomnia, alopecia.

Currently there is no corresponding disease name for these symptoms in Traditional Chinese Medicine. These can be summarized as relative regular syndromes according to clinical manifestations, so as to include this disease into the path of "Treatment determination based on syndrome differentiation" in Traditional Chinese Medicine.

I. Key Points for Diagnosis and Syndrome Differentiation

1. For patients with Qi-blood deficiency, the symptoms include dizziness and asthenia, pale complexion, palpitation and insomnia, thin and weak pulse.

2. For patients with syndrome of disharmony between liver and stomach, the symptoms include nausea and vomiting, leg soreness and distention, less ingestion and warm Qi, red tongue and greasy tongue fur, taut and slippery pulse.

3. For patients with liver and kidney depletion, the symptoms include dysphoria in chest with palms-soles, less ingestion and asthenia, waist soreness and tinitus, red tongue and less tongue fur.

II. Therapeutic Methods

[Syndrome of Qi-blood Deficiency]

Therapeutic method: Replenish Qi and nourish

blood.

Prescription: Xinshu (BL15), Geshu (BL17), Pishu (BL20), Zusanli (ST36), Sanyinjiao (SP6).

Mechanism of prescription: Heart controls bloodline, spleen is the source of engendering transformation of Qi-blood, and Geshu is the confluence of blood, so use of the combination of Xinshu, Pishu and Geshu can nourish heart and invigorate spleen, as well as replenish Qi and nourish blood. Zusanli is an important tonifying acupoint. It can invigorate spleen and tonify Qi, open the source of engendering transformation, replenish the deficiency of the five internal organs. Sanyinjiao is the confluence of the three Yin Meridians of Foot. It can nurse three Yins, tonify Qi and replenish bloodline. The use of combination of these acupoints can replenish Qi as well as nourish blood.

Matching acupoints: For patients with anorexia, nausea and vomiting, add Neiguan, Zhongwan; for patients with dizziness and insomnia, add Shenmen, Baihui, Taichong.

Method: Electrothermal acupuncture treatment.

Operations: Selecting the relevant acupoints, perform routine skin disinfection. Using electrothermal acupuncture needles, vertically puncture into Zusanli for 0.8", Sanyinjiao for 0.7", and obliquely puncture into Xinshu, Geshu, Pishu towards the spine respectively for 0.8". Turn on the electrothermal acupuncture equipment, apply a current of 40-60mA to each acupoint, and the limit is that the patient feels comfortable, leaving the needles in for 40 minutes.

疗程 每日 1 次，10 次为 1 个疗程。疗程间休息 3～5 天，再继续进行第 2 个疗程的治疗。

三、注意事项

1. 清淡饮食，进食容易消化、易吸收的食物，多食蔬菜和水果。

2. 舒畅情致，保持乐观的态度。

3. 做力所能及的运动。

Therapeutic course: Once a day, 10 times for a course. Start the treatment for the second course after a break of 3-5 days.

III. Precautions

1. Light diet, eat food that easy to digest and absorb, eat more vegetables and fruits.

2. Keep happy and optimistic attitude.

3. Do exercises whatever you can.

Gynecological diseases

Menoxenia

For abnormalities in the cycle, blood volume, color and quality of menstruation accompanied with other symptoms, this is called menoxenia. Clinical manifestations: The menstrual cycle starts more than 7 days in advance, or even appears twice a month, this is called Advanced Menstruation; the menstrual cycle starts more than 7 days delayed, or even appears each 40-50 days, this is called Delayed Menstruation; the menstruation does not come on time, it appears in advance or delayingly, this is called Irregular Menstruation. If the menstrual cycle is normal, but the menstrual blood volume is too much or too less, this is called hypermenorrhea and hypomenorrhea. This disease is caused by endocrine disorders.

Traditional Chinese Medicine believes that this disease is caused by the Cold, Heat, Damp-evil of the six exogenous evils, or caused by seven emotions stimulating, excess sexual intercourse or childbearing, causing the Meridian Qi disorder of Chong Channel and Ren Channel.

I. Key Points for Diagnosis and Syndrome Differentiation

1. Advanced Menstruation: The main symptoms

而至，量多为主症，或伴有小腹发凉，面色苍白，舌淡，脉沉细；或伴有血色红，质黏稠，舌红，脉数；或伴有血色淡，质清稀，舌淡，脉弱。

2. 月经后期：以月经延后，甚至四五十天一至，量少为主症，或伴有小腹发凉，面色苍白，舌淡，脉沉细；或伴有血色暗，胸胁乳房发胀，舌苔薄白，脉弦。

3. 月经先后不定期：以月经提前错后，量或多或少为主症，或伴有胸胁乳房作胀，经行不畅，舌苔薄白，脉弦；或伴有血色淡，质清稀，腰膝酸软，夜尿多，舌淡，脉沉细。

二、治疗方法

【月经先期】

治法 益气通经，调理冲任。

处方 中极（RN3）、气海（RN6）、三阴交（SP6）。

includes that the menstruation comes in advance with excess menstrual blood volume, or accompanied with chill of lower abdomen, pale complexion, light tongue, deep and thin pulse; or accompanied with red blood color, viscous blood quality, red tongue, rapid pulse; or accompanied with light blood color, thin quality, light tongue, weak pulse.

2. Delayed Menstruation: The main symptoms includes that the menstruation comes delayingly, sometimes even comes once each 40-50 days, with less menstrual blood volume, or accompanied with chill of lower abdomen, pale complexion, light tongue, deep and thin pulse; or accompanied with dark blood color, swell of chest and hypochondrium and breast, thin and whitish tongue fur, taut pulse.

3. Irregular menstruation: The main symptoms includes that the menstruation comes in advance or delayingly, with excess or less menstrual blood volume, or accompanied with swell of chest and hypochondrium and breast, poor menstrual blood flow, thin and whitish tongue fur, taut pulse; or accompanied with light menstrual blood color, soreness and weakness of waist and knees, frequent urination at night, light tongue, deep and thin pulse.

II. Therapeutic Methods

[Advanced Menstruation]

Therapeutic method: Tonify Qi and dredge meridians, nurse Chong Channel and Ren Channel.

Prescription: Zhongji (RN3), Qihai (RN6), Sanyinjiao (SP6).

方义 中极为任脉经穴，又是足三阴经的交会穴，有调理冲任的作用；气海同为任脉经穴，可调一身之气，气充则能统血；三阴交为足三阴经之交会穴，有补脾肾、通经络、调和气血的作用。三穴配伍，具有益气通经，调理冲任之功效。冲任得固，则经血自调。

配穴 血热配血海、行间、曲池；气虚配足三里、脾俞。

方法 电热针治疗。

操作 选定穴位，皮肤常规消毒。电热针向下斜刺中极0.8寸，直刺气海0.7寸，直刺三阴交0.7寸，得气后，每个穴位分别给予电流量60mA，以患者舒适为度，留针40分钟。另配以毫针直刺足三里0.8寸，直刺太溪、太冲各0.6寸，留针40分钟。

疗程 每日1次，10天为1个疗程，每次留针40分钟。连续观察3个月。（注：月经前

Mechanism of prescription: The acupoint Zhongji is a meridian acupoint of Ren Channel, and aslo is the confluent acupoint of the three Yin Meridians of Foot, it can nurse Chong Channel and Ren Channel; Qihai also is a meridian acupoint of Ren Channel, it can nurse the Qi of the whole body, and plentiful Qi is able to control blood; Sanyinjiao is the confluent acupoint of the three Yin Meridians of Foot, it can tonify spleen and kidney, dredge meridians and collaterals as well as regulate Qi-blood. The use of the combination of these three acupoints, can tonify Qi and dredge meridians, nurse Chong Channel and Ren Channel. The menstrual blood can be regulated naturally once the Chong Channel and Ren Channel are reinforced.

Matching acupoints: For blood-Heat patients, add Xuehai, Xingjian, Quchi; for patients with Qi deficiency, add Zusanli, Pishu.

Method: Electrothermal acupuncture treatment.

Operations: Prepare selected acupoints, perform routine skin disinfection. Using the electrothermal acupuncture needles, obliquely puncture downward into Zhongji for 0.8", vertically puncture into Qihai for 0.7", Sanyinjiao for 0.7". After getting Qi, apply a current of 60mA to each acupoint, and the limit is that the patient feels comfortable, leaving the needles in for 40 minutes. Additionally, using the filiform needles, vertically puncture into Zusanli for 0.8", Taixi and Taichong for 0.6" respectively, leaving the needles in for 40 minutes.

Therapeutic course: Treat once a day, 10 times for a course, indwell the needles for 40 minutes each time. Continuous observation for 3 months. (Note: Start treat-

10 天开始治疗，月经来潮则停针，月经过后开始针治 10 天，每个月治疗 20 天。）

【月经后期】

治法 疏通经络，益气生血，调理冲任。

处方 关元（RN4）、气海（RN6）、三阴交（SP6）。

方义 关元为足三阴经与任脉之交会穴，有补肾固本、调理冲任的作用；气海主一身之气，气行则血行，有益气生血、活血通经的功能；三阴交为足三阴经之交会穴，可疏通经络，调和气血。三穴相配，具有疏通经络，益气生血，调理冲任之功能。

配穴 血寒配命门、百会；气滞配期门、太冲。

操作 选定穴位，皮肤常规消毒。电热针直刺关元、气海、三阴交各 0.7 寸，接通电热针仪，每个穴位分别给予电流量 60mA，以患者舒适为度。再配以毫针直刺命门，平补平泻，不留针。毫针直刺百会

ment 10 days before menstruation till the coming of menstruation, and restart the treatment after the menstruation for 10 days, totally 20 days of treatment for each month.)

[Delayed Menstruation]

Therapeutic method: Dredge meridians and collaterals, tonify Qi and nourish blood, nurse Chong Channel and Ren Channel.

Prescription: Guanyuan(RN4), Qihai (RN6), Sanyinjiao (SP6).

Mechanism of prescription: The acupoint Guanyuan is the confluent acupoint of the three Yin Meridians of Foot and the Ren Channel, it can replenish kidney and reinforce the basis, nurse Chong Channel and Ren Channel. Qihai control the Qi of the whole body, and blood flows when Qi flows. It can tonify Qi and nourish blood, activate blood circulation and dredge meridians. Sanyinjiao is the confluent acupoint of the three Yin Meridians of Foot, it can dredge meridians and collaterals, regulate Qi-blood. The use of the combination of these three acupoints can dredge meridians and collaterals, tonify Qi and nourish blood, nurse Chong Channel and Ren Channel.

Matching acupoints: For patients with cold blood, add Mingmen, Baihui; for patients with Qi stagnation, add Qimen, Taichong.

Operations: Prepare selected acupoints, perform routine skin disinfection. Using electrothermal acupuncture needles, vertically puncture into Guanyuan, Qihai, Sanyinjiao for 0.7" respectively. Turn on the electrothermal acupuncture equipment, apply a current of 60mA to each acupoint, and the limit is that the patient feels comfortable. Additionally, vertically puncture Mingmen for

0.5 寸，斜刺期门 0.7 寸，直刺太冲 0.6 寸，留针 40 分钟。

mild reinforcing and attenuating, do not leave the needle in. Additionally, using filiform needles, vertically puncture into Baihui for 0.5", obliquely puncture into Qimen for 0.7", and vertically puncture into Taichong for 0.6", leaving the needles in for 40 minutes.

疗程 每日 1 次，10 次为 1 个疗程。连续观察 3 个月。（注：月经前 10 天开始治疗，月经来潮则停针，月经过后开始针治 10 天，每个月治疗 20 天。）

Therapeutic course: Once a day, 10 times for a course. Continuous observation for 3 months. (Note: Start treatment 10 days before menstruation till the coming of menstruation, and restart the treatment after the menstruation for 10 days, totally 20 days of treatment for each month.)

【月经先后不定期】

治法 疏肝解郁，调和气血。

处方 关元（RN4）、气海（RN6）、间使（PC5）。

方义 关元是足三阴经与任脉之交会穴，是治疗妇科病之主穴；气海为生元气之海。关元配气海，有行气血、调冲任的作用；间使属足厥阴肝经，有疏肝解郁、理气调经的作用。三穴配伍，可使气血调和，冲任得固，经血按时下。

配穴 肝郁加期门、太冲；肾虚加肾俞、太溪；若要扶正加曲池；气虚加足三里。

[Irregular Menstruation]

Therapeutic method: Soothe liver Qi stagnation, regulate Qi-blood.

Prescription: Guanyuan(RN4), Qihai (RN6), Jianshi (PC5).

Mechanism of prescription: The acupoint Guanyuan is the confluent acupoint of the three Yin Meridians of Foot and the Ren Channel, also a main acupoint for treatment of gynecological diseases. Qihai generates vitality. The match of Guanyuan with Qihai can promote Qi-blood flow and nurse Chong Channel and Ren Channel. Jianshi belongs to the Jue-Yin Liver Meridian of Foot, it can soothe liver Qi stagnation, regulate Qi and nurse meridians. The use of the combination of these three acupoints, can regulate Qi-blood, reinforce Chong Channel and Ren Channel and regulate menstruation to be normal.

Matching acupoints: For patients with liver stagnation, add Qimen, Taichong; for patients with kidney deficiency, add Shenshu, Taixi; for strengthening the healthy Qi, add Quchi; for patients with Qi deficiency, add Zusanli.

方法 电热针治疗。

Method: Electrothermal acupuncture treatment.

操作 选定穴位，皮肤常规消毒。电热针直刺关元、气海各0.7寸，直刺三阴交0.6寸，直刺足三里0.8寸，接通电热针仪，每个穴位分别给予电流量60mA，以患者感到舒适为度，留针40分钟。另配以毫针斜刺期门0.6寸，直刺太冲、太溪各0.5寸，直刺曲池0.7寸，留针40分钟。肾俞可在电热针治疗前给予快针。

Operations: Prepare selected acupoints, perform routine skin disinfection. Using electrothermal acupuncture needles, vertically puncture into Guanyuan and Qihai for 0.7" respectively, Sanyinjiao for 0.6", Zusanli for 0.8". Turn on the electrothermal acupuncture equipment, apply a current of 60 mA to each acupoint, and the limit is that the patient feels comfortable, leaving the needles in for 40 minutes. Additionally, using filiform needles, obliquely puncture into Qimen for 0.6", and vertically puncture into Taichong and Taixi for 0.5" respectively, Quchi for 0.7", leaving the needles in for 40 minutes. Give rapid acupuncture for the acupoint Shenshu before electrothermal acupuncture treatment.

疗程 同月经后期。

Therapeutic course: The same as that of delayed menstruation.

三、注意事项

III. Precautions

1. 治疗期间令患者保持心志平和，生活要有规律，遇到不愉快之事能安慰自己，不要过虑。

1. During treatment, patients should keep gentle mood and regular life, and comfort themselves when unhappy things happen, do not think too much.

2. 注意经期卫生，注意保暖，不要用凉水洗脚。

2. Pay attention to menstrual health and keep warm, do not wash feet with cold water.

3. 清淡饮食，做适量的活动。

3. Light diet, do appropriate amount of activities.

四、典型病例

IV. Typical Cases

案一 月经先期

Case Ⅰ. Advanced menstruation

周某，女，24岁，职员，

Zhou, female, 24 years old, employee, residence:

北京人。

主诉：月经提前7～8天，量少，已有2年多。

刻下症：月经周期不定，多提前7天左右，量少，色紫红，有血块，行经不畅，胸胁、乳房胀，脘闷不适，有时少腹痛，苔薄白，脉细弦。

查体：未见阳性体征。

辅助检查：未见异常。

【诊断依据】

1. 青年女性，月经周期不定，已有2年之久，多提前7～8天。

2. 多愁善感，苦思多虑之人。

3. 妇科诊查未见异常。

【证治分析】

病因 肝郁、肾虚。

病机 因肝郁肾虚，气血失调，导致血海蓄溢失常，月经周期提前或延后7天以上之不定期。

证候分析 郁怒伤肝，肝失疏泄，故月经先后不定期；情志不舒，气机郁滞，则经行不畅，色紫红，有血块；肝脉

Beijing.

Chief complaint: Menstruation came 7-8 days in advance, less blood volume, for more than 2 years.

Current symptoms: Irregular menstrual cycle, normally came around 7 days in advance, less blood volume, prunosus blood color, blood clots, unsmooth menstrual blood flow, swell of chest and hypochondrium and breast, abdominal tightness and discomfort, sometimes accompanied with lateral lower abdomen pain, thin and whitish tongue fur, thin and taut pulse.

Physical examination: No positive signs were seen.

Auxiliary examination: No abnormalities.

[Diagnostic Basis]

1. Young female with irregular menstrual cycle for 2 years, normally the period came 7-8 days in advance.

2. Sentimental and thoughtful person.

3. No abnormalities were observed in the gynecological examination.

[Syndrome-treatment Analysis]

Etiology: Liver stagnation and kidney deficiency.

Pathogenesis: Liver stagnation and kidney deficiency, disorder of Qi and blood, causing disorder of blood sea storage and overflow, as well as irregular menstrual cycle which generally came more than 7 days in advance or delayingly.

Syndrome analysis: Depressed anger damaged the liver, liver dysfunction caused irregular menstruation; emotional upset and Qi Dynamic stagnation caused unsmooth menstrual blood flow, prunosus blood color,

布两胁，肝气郁滞胸胁，则乳房胀痛；肝气犯胃，故脘闷不舒。病无寒热，故苔薄白，脉细弦，为肝郁气滞之象。

病位 肝、肾。

病性 虚性。

西医诊断 月经不调。

中医诊断 月经先后不定期。

治法 疏肝解郁，行血调经。

方法 电热针治疗。

处方 中极（RN3）、气海（RN6）、三阴交（SP6）、太冲（LR3）、蠡沟（LR5）、血海（SP10）、归来（ST29）。

方义 中极为任脉经穴，又是足三阴经之交会穴，有调理冲任的作用；气海为任脉经穴，可调一身之气，气充则能统血；三阴交为足三阴经之交会穴，有补脾胃、通经络、调和气血的作用；足厥阴肝经的原穴太冲与络穴蠡沟相配，能疏肝、行气、调经；足太阴经穴血海与足三阴经交会穴三阴交均为治妇科病的要穴，可行

blood clots; the liver channels were distributed at the two-side hypochondrium, and the stagnation of liver Qi at chest and hypochondrium caused breast swelling pain; the liver Qi invaded stomach, so caused abdominal tightness and discomfort. The disease had no cold and heat symptoms, so the tongue was thin and whitish, and the pulse was thin and taut, which are symptoms of liver and Qi stagnation.

Lesion location: Liver, kidney.

Disease nature: Deficiency.

The diagnosis of Western Medicine: Menoxenia.

The diagnosis of Traditional Chinese Medicine: Irregular menstruation.

Therapeutic method: Soothe liver Qi stagnation, promote blood flow and nurse meridians.

Method: Electrothermal acupuncture treatment.

Prescription: Zhongji (RN3), Qihai (RN6), Sanyinjiao (SP6), Taichong (LR3), Ligou (LR5), Xuehai (SP10), Guilai (ST29).

Mechanism of prescription: The acupoint Zhongji is a meridian acupoint of Ren Channel, and aslo is the confluent acupoint of the three Yin Meridians of Foot, it can nurse Chong Channel and Ren Channel. Qihai is a meridian acupoint of Ren Channel, it can nurse the Qi of the whole body, and plentiful Qi is able to control blood. Sanyinjiao is the confluent acupoint of the three Yin Meridians of Foot, it can replenish spleen and stomach, dredge meridians and collaterals, regulate Qi-blood. The match of the Yuan acupoint Taichong and the collateral acupoint Ligou of the Jue-Yin Liver Meridian of Foot,

血调经固冲；归来可疏通局部气血。

can dredge liver, promote Qi circulation, nurse meridians. The acupoint of the Tai-Yin Meridian of Foot, Xuehai, and the confluent acupoint of the three Yin Meridians of Foot, Sanyinjiao, are both key acupoints for treatment of gynecological diseases, and can promote blood flow and nurse meridians as well as reinforce Chong Channel. The acupoint Guilai can dredge local Qi-blood.

配穴 气虚加足三里、脾俞；气滞加太冲、期门；肾虚加太溪、肾俞。

Matching acupoints: For patients with Qi deficiency, add Zusanli, Pishu; for patients with Qi stagnation, add Taichong, Qimen; for patients with kidney deficiency, add Taixi, Shenshu.

操作 选定穴位，皮肤常规消毒。电热针直刺中极、气海、三阴交、足三里、血海、归来、蠡沟各0.7寸，斜刺（针尖向脊柱）肾俞、脾俞各0.8寸，斜刺期门0.7寸，直刺太冲、太溪各0.6寸。接通电热针仪，每个穴位分别给予电流量40mA，以胀为度，留针40分钟。（注：每次选6穴给予电热针治疗，每日1次，余穴用毫针治疗。）

Operations: Preparing the selected acupoints, perform routine skin disinfection. Using electrothermal acupuncture needles, vertically puncture into Zhongji, Qihai, Sanyinjiao, Zusanli, Xuehai, Guilai, Ligou for 0.7" respectively, obliquely puncture (towards Jizhong) into Shenshu and Pishu for 0.8" respectively, Qimen for 0.7", and vertically puncture into Taichong and Taixi for 0.6" respectively. Turn on the electrothermal acupuncture equipment, apply a current of 40mA to each acupoint, and the limit is that the patient feels swell, leaving the needles in for 40 minutes. (Note: Select 6 acupoints for electrothermal acupuncture treatment, once a day, and treat the other acupoints with filiform needles.)

疗程 每日1次，10次为1个疗程。一般连续治疗3个月，即可恢复正常。（注：月经前10天开始治疗，月经来潮则停针，月经过后开始针治10天，每个月治疗20天。）

Therapeutic course: Once a day, 10 times for a course. Generally the patient will return to normal conditions after 3 months of continuous treatment. (Note: Start treatment 10 days before menstruation till the coming of menstruation, and restart the treatment after the menstruation for 10 days, totally 20 days of treatment for each month.)

治疗过程 该患者治疗3个月后，次月月经期如时来潮，5天后结束；继续治疗2个月，效果满意。随访1年，一切正常。

【生活调摄】

1. 治疗期间令患者保持心志平和，生活要有规律，遇到不愉快之事能安慰自己，忌多虑。

2. 注意经期卫生，注意保暖，不要用凉水洗脚。

3. 针灸见效快，令人满意，但必须医患合作，坚持治疗就会收到满意的疗效。

案二 月经后期

赵某，女，20岁，学生，北京人。

主诉：月经初潮至今先后不定期，量少，常延后2～3个月或更长，已有10年。

刻下症：月经先后不定期，多延后2～3个月或更长，伴乳房发胀，小腹发凉作痛，胸胁胀满，血量少，质稀，色暗淡，面色苍白，舌淡，脉沉细。

查体：未见阳性体征。

辅助检查：未见异常。

Therapeutic process: Treated the patient for 3 months, her next menstruation came in time, and ended after 5 days. Continued the treatment for 2 months, and the effects were satisfied. Followed up for 1 year, and everything was normal.

[Lifestyle Change and Health Maintenance]

1. During treatment, patients should keep gentle mood and regular life, and comfort themselves when unhappy things happen, do not think too much.

2. Pay attention to menstrual health and keep warm, do not wash feet with cold water.

3. The acupuncture therapy has quick and satisfying effects, but the patients must cooperate with doctors. Satisfying efficacies can be achieved with long-term treatment.

Case Ⅱ. Delayed menstruation

Zhao, female, 20 years old, student, residence: Beijing.

Chief complaint: Irregular menstrual period since the menarche, less blood amount, generally came 2-3 months or more delayingly, for 10 years.

Current symptoms: Irregular menstruation, generally came 2-3 months or more delayingly, accompanied with breast swell, lower abdomen cold and pain, chest and hypochondrium swell, less blood volume, thin quality, pale color, pale complexion, light tongue, deep and thin pulse.

Physical examination: No positive signs were seen.

Auxiliary examination: No abnormalities.

【诊断依据】

1. 青年女性，月经初潮至今不定期。

2. 经前乳房胀及小腹痛，胸胁胀满，行经不畅，量少质稀，色暗淡，神疲乏力，腰膝酸痛，头晕耳鸣。

3. 舌淡，苔少，脉细尺弱。

【证治分析】

病因　肾虚。

病机　肾气不足，肾主封藏，司开阖，素体肾气不足，损伤冲任，致肾失闭藏，开阖不利，则经期不定。

证候分析　肾气不足，封藏开阖失调，冲任不调，胞宫蓄溢失常，故行经无定期。肾藏精，肾气不足，五脏精气不能上荣于面，则面色晦暗。肾阴虚则血量少，肾阳虚则经色淡、质稀。肾主骨生髓，开窍于耳，脑为髓海，肾虚髓海不足，清窍失养，故神疲乏力，头晕耳鸣。腰为肾之府，小腹为胞宫所居之地，而胞脉系于肾，肾虚则胞脉失养，故腰骶酸痛。舌淡，苔少，脉细尺弱，均为肾气不足之象。

[Diagnostic Basis]

1. Young female, irregular menstrual period since the menarche.

2. Before menstruation, breast swell and lower abdomen pain, unsmooth blood flow, less blood volume and thin quality, pale color, mental fatigue and asthenia, soreness of waist and knees, dizziness and tinnitus.

3. Pale tongue, less tongue fur, thin, and weak pulse.

[Syndrome-treatment Analysis]

Etiology: Kidney deficiency.

Pathogenesis: The kidney governs storage, control open and closure, so kidney Qi deficiency impaired Chong and Ren channels, causing storage loss of kidney, unsmooth open and closure, therefore caused irregular menstrual period.

Syndrome analysis: Kidney Qi deficiency, disorder of storage and open and closure, disharmony of Chong and Ren channels, disorder of uterus storage and overflow, causing irregular menstrual period. The kidney stores vital essence. Kidney Qi deficiency causes that the vital essence of five internal organs cannot go up to the face, leading dim complexion. For kidney Yin deficiency, the blood volume is less; for kidney Yang deficiency, the blood has light color and thin. The kidney governs marrow generation of bones, the ears are windows of kidneys, and the brain is the marrow sea. Kidney deficiency causes marrow sea deficiency, nourishment loss of clear orifices, leading to mental fatigue and asthenia, dizziness and tinnitus. Waist is where the kidneys locate, and the lower abdomen is where the uterus locates. The

Uterus Channel depends on kidney, so kidney deficiency will cause nourishment loss of Uterus Channel, causing soreness of lumbosacral parts. Pale tongue, less tongue fur, thin, and weak pulse, are all symptoms of kidney Qi deficiency.

Lesion location: Kidney.

Disease nature: Deficiency.

The diagnosis of Western Medicine: Menoxenia.

The diagnosis of Traditional Chinese Medicine: Irregular menstruation (kidney Qi deficiency).

Therapeutic method: Replenish kidney and nurse meridians, mainly focus on Ren Channel and acupoints of the Shao-Yin Kidney Meridian of Foot.

Method: Electrothermal acupuncture treatment.

Prescription: Guanyuan (RN4), Qixue (KI13), Shenshu (BL23), Taixi (KI3).

Mechanism of prescription: The Qi Acupoint is the confluent acupoint of the Shao-Yin Meridian of Foot and the Chong Channel, and Taixi is the Yuan acupoint of the Shao-Yin Meridian of Foot, so the match of these two acupoints can tonify kideny Qi, nourish essence and blood. Shenshu and Guanyuan can replenish kidney Qi and nurse Chong Channel and Ren Channel.

Matching acupoints: For patients with cold and pain at waist and knees as well as lower abdomen, add Mingmen; for patients with symptoms of dry mouth, vexation, insufficient sleep, add Yanggu, Sanyinjiao; for patients with Qi stagnation, add Qimen, Taichong.

Operations: Prepare selected acupoints, perform routine skin disinfection. Using electrothermal acu-

穴、太溪各 0.7 寸，斜刺（针尖向脊柱）肾俞 0.7 寸，直刺命门、太冲、阳谷各 0.7 寸，平刺期门 0.8 寸，接通电热针仪，每穴分别给予电流量 40mA，以胀而舒适为度，留针 40 分钟。（注：每次选 3 组穴，交替轮流使用。）

疗程　每日 1 次，10 次为 1 个疗程。一般连续治疗 3 个月，即可恢复正常。（注：月经前 10 天开始治疗，月经来潮则停针，月经过后开始针治 10 天，每个月治疗 20 天。）

治疗过程　该患者治疗后，月经周期正常，不提前也不延后，经前不适症状全部消失。

【生活调摄】

1. 针下腹部穴位时令患者排空小便，避免伤及膀胱。

2. 经期注意腹部保暖防寒，不要用冷水洗脚，忌冷凉饮食。

3. 经期不施针治，一定要在月经前 10 天开始，月经终止以后再开始治疗，避免经期针治引起月经量多。

puncture needles, vertically puncture into Guanyuan, Qi acupoint, Taixi for 0.7" respectively, obliquely puncture (towards Jizhong) into Shenshu for 0.7", vertically puncture into Mingmen, Taichong, Yanggu for 0.7" respectively, horizontally puncture into Qimen for 0.8". Turn on the electrothermal acupuncture equipment, apply a current of 40mA to each acupoint, and the limit is that the patient feels comfortable, leaving the needles in for 40 minutes. (Note: Select 3 pairs of acupoints each time, and use alternatively.)

Therapeutic course: Once a day, 10 times for a course. Generally the patient will return to normal conditions after 3 months of continuous treatment. (Note: Start treatment 10 days before menstruation till the coming of menstruation, and restart the treatment after the menstruation for 10 days, totally 20 days of treatment for each month.)

Therapeutic process: The menstrual cycle was normal, not be in advance or delayed, with all uncomfortable symptoms before menstruation disappeared.

[Lifestyle Change and Health Maintenance]

1. For acupuncture of acupoints at lower abdomen, the patient should empty urine to avoid bladder damage.

2. During the menstrual period, attentions should be paid to keeping warm and cold-resistance of abdomen do not wash feet with cold water, do not eat cold diet.

3. The acupuncture treatment is not performed during a menstrual period, and it must be started 10 days before the period, and restarted after the end of the period, so as to avoid excess blood volume caused by the acupuncture treatment.

痛经

痛经是指妇女行经前后或行经期间，出现小腹及腰部疼痛，甚至剧痛难忍，并随着月经周期而发作，亦称"行经腹痛"，为青年妇女的常见病之一。临床有原发性和继发性之分。前者是指月经初潮时即有腹痛，后者指初潮时无症状，以后逐渐发病。痛经的发生除与精神紧张等心理因素关系密切外，原发性者常见于子宫发育不良（包括前屈、后倾等位置异常和颈口狭窄等）和内分泌失调者；继发性者则多与盆腔内生殖器官病变（如盆腔内的慢性炎症、充血、子宫肌瘤、子宫内膜异位症等）有关。症状多为下腹疼痛、刺痛、胀痛，伴有腰酸腿软；重者可伴有头痛、恶心、呕吐或其他不适。疼痛可延续几个小时至几天不等，严重者会影响工作和生活。

中医认为，本病多因气血运行不畅所致，即所谓的"不通则痛"。情志不舒，肝瘀气滞，血行受阻，经血滞于胞宫；或经前受寒饮冷，坐卧湿地，

Dysmenorrhea

Dysmenorrhea refers to that before, after or during the menstrual period, the patient experiences pain at lower abdomen and waist, or even unbearable sharp pain. It occurs with the menstrual cycle, and also called "menstrual abdomen pain", which is one of the common diseases of young females. The disease is clinically divided into primary and secondary diseases. The former refers to that the abdomen pain occurs at the menarche, while the later one refers to that there is no symptom at the menarche, however gradually occurs later. The occurrence of dysmenorrhea is closely related to mental factors such as psychentonia, additionally, the primary ones are commonly seen in patients with uterine dysplasia (including positon abnormalities such as anteflexion and retroversion, as well as neck stenosis, etc.) and endocrine disorders; while the secondary ones are normally related to pelvic reproductive organ lesions (such as chronic inflammations in the pelvic cavity, congestion, myoma of uterus, endometriosis). Common symptoms include pain, prickling, swelling pain of lower abdomen, accompanied with aching lumbus and limp legs; in severe cases, headache, nausea, vomiting or other discomforts may also accompany. The pain may last for several hours to several days, and in severe cases it even can affect work and life.

Traditional Chinese Medicine believes that this disease is normally caused by unsmooth of Qi-blood circulation, namely the so-called "stagnation leading to pain". Caused by emotional upset, liver stasis and Qi stagnation, obstruction of blood circulation, the menstru-

寒湿客于胞宫，经血为寒湿所凝；或素体不足，大病、久病之后，气血两亏，行经后血海空虚，胞脉失养；或肝郁日久化火，热入营血，血热互结，血行不畅而致。

一、诊断及辨证要点

1. 实证：经前或经期小腹胀痛，行经量小，淋漓不畅，血色紫暗，有血块，伴有胸胁乳房作胀，舌质紫或有瘀点，脉沉弦。

2. 虚证：经期或经后小腹隐隐作痛，局部喜按，经水色淡，质清稀，血色少华，伴有头晕、耳鸣，腰脊酸痛，舌淡苔薄，脉细弱。

3. 寒证：经前或经期小腹冷痛，痛处拒按，连及腰脊，得热则舒，经行量少，色暗，有血块，苔薄白，脉沉紧。

al blood is stagnated in the uterus; or before menstrual period, catch a chill and drink cold things, sit and lie on the damp ground, damp and heat accumulate in the uterus, so the menstrual blood clots due to damp-heat; or body deficiency, Qi-blood deletion after server diseases or long-time disease, the blood in the blood sea is insufficient after menstruation, nourishment loss of Uterus Channel; or long-time liver stasis changes into Fire, and the Fire enters Ying-blood, the blood and heat mixes up, causing unsmooth blood flow.

I. Key Points for Diagnosis and Syndrome Differentiation

1. Excess Syndrome: Lower abdomen swelling pain before or during the menstruation period, less blood volume, dripping and unsmooth blood flow, dark and purple blood color, blood clots, accompanied with swell of chest and hypochondrium and breast, purple tongue or with petechia, deep and taut pulse.

2. Deficiency Syndrome: Lower abdomen dull pain before or during the menstruation period, locally pressure-relieved, light blood, thin quality, pale complexion, accompanied with dizziness, tinnitus, lumbar spinal soreness and pain, light tongue and thin tongue fur, thin and weak pulse.

3. Cold Syndrome: Lower abdomen cold and pain before or during the menstruation period, pressure-refused, extend to lumbar spinal parts, relieved with heat, less blood volume, dark color, blood clots, thin and whitish tongue fur, deep and tight pulse.

二、治疗方法

【实证】

治法 疏肝理气,活血化瘀。

处方 中极(RN3)、血海(SP10)、阳陵泉(GB34)、太冲(LR3)。

方义 中极属于任脉经穴,又是足三阴经与任脉之会,可通调冲任脉气,配血海行气活血;阳陵泉是胆经合穴,太冲为肝经原穴,两者同用,疏肝利胆,理气调经。诸穴共用,可收疏肝理气、活血化瘀之功。

配穴 腹痛甚者加次髎;胸胁胀痛者加期门。

方法 电热针治疗。

操作 选定穴位,皮肤常规消毒。电热针直刺中极0.8寸,直刺血海、阳陵泉各0.7寸。接通电热针,每个穴位分别给予电流量60~70mA,以患者感到舒适为度,留针40分钟。另配以毫针直刺太冲、太溪各

II. Therapeutic Methods

[Excess Syndrome]

Therapeutic method: Soothe liver and regulate Qi, activate blood circulation and remove stasis.

Prescription: Zhongji (RN3), Xuehai (SP10), Yanglingquan (GB34), Taichong (LR3).

Mechanism of prescription: Zhongji is a meridian acupoint of Ren Channel, and also is the confluent acupoint of the three Yin Meridians of Foot and the Ren Channel, it can nurse Qi of Chong Channel and Ren Channel, and activate Qi and blood circulation when matching with Xuehai; Yanglingquan is a He acupoint of Gallbladder Meridian, and Taichong is a Yuan acupoint of Liver Meridian, the use of the combination of these two can soothe liver and reinforce gallbladder, regulate Qi and nurse meridians. The use of combination of these acupoints can soothe liver and regulate Qi, activate blood circulation and remove stasis.

Matching acupoints: For patients with severe abdomen pain, add Ciliao; for patients with swelling pain of chest and hypochondrium, add Qimen.

Method: Electrothermal acupuncture treatment.

Operations: Preparing the selected acupoints, perform routine skin disinfection. Using electrothermal acupuncture needles, vertically puncture into Zhongji for 0.8", Xuehai and Yanglingquan for 0.7" respectively. Turn on the electrothermal acupuncture equipment, apply a current of 60-70mA to each acupoint, and the limit is that the patient feels comfortable, leaving the

0.5 寸，直刺足三里 0.7 寸，直刺三阴交 0.6 寸，以达滋阴潜阳、扶正祛邪之效，留针 40 分钟。

疗程 每日 1 次，20 次为 1 个疗程（月经前 10 天开始治疗，月经来潮则停针，月经过后开始针治 10 天）。连续治疗 3 个疗程，即可治愈。

【虚证】

治法 益气养血，调补冲任。

处方 气海（RN6）、足三里（ST36）、膈俞（BL17）、脾俞（BL20）。

方义 气海为任脉经穴，具有补益气血、调理冲任的作用；脾胃乃气血生化之源，故取足阳明经所入之合穴足三里、脾俞补脾胃，资生化，使气血充足，胞脉得养；膈俞乃血之会，具有调血、补血之功。诸穴合用，共奏益气养血、调补冲任之功。

配穴 头晕耳鸣加肾俞、

needles in for 40 minutes. Additionally, using the filiform needles, vertically puncture into Taichong and Taixi for 0.5" respectively, Zusanli for 0.7", Sanyinjiao for 0.6", to achieve the effects of nourishing Yin and suppressing Yang as well as strengthening body resistance and eliminating evil, leaving the needles in for 40 minutes.

Therapeutic course: Once a day, 20 times for a course (start treatment 10 days before menstruation till the coming of menstruation, and restart the treatment after the menstruation for 10 days, totally 20 days of treatment for each month). Cured after 3 continuous treatment courses.

[Deficiency Syndrome]

Therapeutic method: Tonify Qi-blood, nurse and replenish Chong Channel and Ren Channel.

Prescription: Qihai (RN6), Zusanli (ST36), Geshu (BL17), Pishu(BL20).

Mechanism of prescription: Qihai is a meridian acupoint of Ren Channel, it can tonify Qi-blood, nurse and replenish Chong Channel and Ren Channel; spleen and stomach are the source of engendering transformation of Qi-blood, so use the He acupoints Zusanli and Pishu, where the Yang-Ming Meridian of Foot enters, to replenish spleen and stomach, tonify engendering of transformation, to promote sufficient Qi-blood and nourish Uterus Channel; Geshu is the confluent acupoint of blood, it can regulate and tonify blood. The use of combination of these acupoints can tonify Qi-blood, nurse and replenish Chong Channel and Ren Channel.

Matching acupoint: For dizziness and tinnitus, add

太溪；腰背酸困加命门。

方法 电热针治疗。

操作 选定穴位，皮肤常规消毒。电热针直刺气海0.7寸，直刺足三里0.8寸，直刺三阴交0.7寸，接通电热针仪，每个穴位分别给予电流量60～70mA，以患者舒适为度，留针40分钟。另配以毫针直刺太溪0.5寸，速刺命门、膈俞，不留针。

疗程 每日1次，20次为1个疗程（月经前10天开始治疗，月经来潮则停针，月经过后开始针治10天）。连续治疗3个疗程。

【寒证】

治法 温化寒湿，通经止痛。

处方 气海（RN6）、关元（RN4）、阴陵泉（SP9）、地机（SP8）、三阴交（SP6）。

方义 气海可调气机，用电热针治疗可温暖子宫以散寒化瘀；关元可温阳散寒通胞脉；阴陵泉乃脾经合穴，能健脾利湿，温运中焦；地机乃脾经郄穴；三阴交乃调经止痛的要穴。诸穴共用，可达温化寒湿、通经止痛之效。

Shenshu and Taixi; for low back soreness, add Mingmen.

Method: Electrothermal acupuncture treatment.

Operations: Preparing the selected acupoints, perform routine skin disinfection. Using electrothermal acupuncture needles, vertically puncture into Qihai for 0.7", Zusanli for 0.8", Sanyinjiao for 0.7". Turn on the electrothermal acupuncture equipment, apply a current of 60-70mA to each acupoint, and the limit is that the patient feels comfortable, leaving the needles in for 40 minutes. Additionally, using filiform needles, vertically puncture into Taixi for 0.5", quickly puncture into Mingmen and Geshu, do not leave the needles in.

Therapeutic course: Once a day, 20 times for a course (start treatment 10 days before menstruation till the coming of menstruation, and restart the treatment after the menstruation for 10 days, totally 20 days of treatment for each month). 3 continuous treatment courses.

[Cold Syndrome]

Therapeutic method: Warm cold-dampness, dredge meridians and alleviate pain.

Prescription: Qihai (RN6), Guanyuan (RN4), Yinlingquan (SP90, Diji (SP8), Sanyinjiao (SP6).

Mechanism of prescription: Qihai can regulate Qi Dynamic, electrothermal acupuncture treatment at this acupoint can warm up the uterus to dispel cold and removing stasis; Guanyuan can warm up Yang, dispel cold and dredge Uterus Channel; Yinyangquan is a He acupoint of Spleen Meridian, it can invigorate spleen and remove dampness, warm and activate Middle Jiao, Diji is a Xi acupoint of Spleen Meridian; Sanyinjiao is a key acupoint for tonifying meridians and alleviating pain. The combination use of these acupoints can warm cold-dampness, dredge meridians and alleviate pain.

Matching acupoints: For nausea and vomiting, add Zhongwan, Neiguan.

Method: Electrothermal acupuncture treatment.

Operations: Preparing the selected acupoints, perform routine skin disinfection. Using electrothermal acupuncture needles, vertically puncture into Qihai for 0.7", Guanyuan for 0.7", Yinlingquan for 0.8", Sanyinjiao for 0.7". Turn on the electrothermal acupuncture equipment, apply a current of 60-70mA to each acupoint, and the limit is that the patient feels comfortable. Additionally, using the filiform needles, vertically puncture into Zusanli for 0.7", Taixi and Taichong for 0.5" respectively, leaving the needles in for 40 minutes.

Therapeutic course: Once a day, 20 times for a course (start treatment 10 days before menstruation till the coming of menstruation, and restart the treatment after the menstruation for 10 days, totally 20 days of treatment for each month). 3 continuous treatment courses.

III. Precautions

1. During treatment, patients should keep gentle mood and regular life, and comfort themselves when unhappy things happen, do not think too much.

2. Pay attention to menstrual health and keep warm, do not wash feet with cold water.

3. The acupuncture therapy has quick and satisfying effects, but the patients must cooperate with doctors. Sat-

会收到满意的疗效。

四、典型病例

崔某，女，18岁，学生，北京人。

主诉：经期腹痛已2年多，近期加重。病史：患者素体虚弱，13岁月经初潮，经色、经量、周期均正常。2年前因与同学争吵，情志不舒，之后行经腹痛，月经量少，色淡质稀，经中药治疗有所好转。

刻下症：小腹隐痛喜按，神疲肢倦，头昏眼花，心悸气短，舌淡，苔薄少，脉细。

查体：二尖瓣区及主动脉瓣第二听诊区可闻及二级收缩期杂音。

辅助检查：未见异常。

【诊断依据】

1. 青年女性，未婚，经期腹痛。

2. 两年前因与同学争吵，情致不畅，而致经期腹痛。行经时月经量少，色淡质稀。

3. 舌淡，苔薄少，脉细。

【证治分析】

病因　气血亏虚。

Part II: Clinical Treatment

isfying efficacies can be achieved with long-term treatment.

IV. Typical Case

Cui, female, 18 years old, student, residence: Beijing.

Chief complaint: Menstrual abdomen pain for more then 2 years, which aggregated recently. Medical history: The patient's body is weak, menarche came at 13 years old, blood color, volume and menstrual period were all normal. 2 years ago, she experienced emotional upset due to quarrel with classmates, and after that she suffered from menstrual abdomen pain, less blood volume, light color and thin quality, which became improved after Chinese Herb Medicine treatment.

Current symptoms: Lower abdomen dull pain, pressure-relieved, mental and physical fatigue, dizziness, palpitation and shortness of breath, light tongue, thin and less tongue fur, thin pulse.

Physical examination: Grade 2 systolic noise at mitral valve area and second aortic valve area.

Auxiliary examination: No abnormalities.

[Diagnostic Basis]

1. Young female, unmarried, menstrual abdomen pain.

2. 2 years ago, she experienced emotional upset due to quarrel with classmates, causing menstrual abdomen pain. Less blood volume, light color and thin quality.

3. Pale tongue, little and thin fur, thin pulse.

[Syndrome-treatment Analysis]

Etiology: Deficiency of Qi and blood.

病机 气血不足，胞宫失养，不荣则发生痛经。

证候分析 气血虚弱，血海不足，胞脉失养，故经期小腹隐痛喜按，经量少、质稀，气血不足，神疲肢倦。气血不能上荣于脑，则头昏眼花，气血不能营心，则心悸气短，舌淡，苔薄少，脉细，均为气血亏虚之象。

病位 气血。

病性 虚性。

西医诊断 继发性痛经。

中医诊断 痛经（气血不足）。

治法 补益气血，调经止痛。以任脉、足太阴脾经穴为主。

方法 电热针治疗。

处方 气海（RN6）、足三里（ST36）、脾俞（BL20）、三阴交（SP6）、子宫（EX-CA1）、膈俞（BL17）。

方义 气海为任脉经穴，具有补益气血，调理冲任之功；脾胃乃气血生化之源，故取足阳明经所入之合穴足三里，以及三阴交、脾俞以补脾

Pathogenesis: Qi-blood deficiency, nourishment loss of uterus, and the deficiency caused dysmenorrhea.

Syndrome analysis: Weak Qi-blood, blood sea deficiency, nourishment loss of Uterus Channel, leading to pressure-relieved lower abdomen dull pain before menstrual periods, less blood volume, thin quality, Qi-blood deficiency, mental and physical fatigue. Qi-blood could not go up to the brain, causing dizziness, Qi-blood unable to nourish the heart, therefore leading to palpitation and shortness of breath, light tongue, thin and less tongue fur, thin pulse, these are all symptoms of deficiency of Qi and blood.

Lesion location: Qi-blood.

Disease nature: Deficiency.

The diagnosis of Western Medicine: Secondary dysmenorrhea.

The diagnosis of Traditional Chinese Medicine: Dysmenorrhea (Qi-blood deficiency).

Therapeutic method: Tonify Qi-blood, nurse meridians and alleviate pain. Focus on meridian acupoints of Ren Channel and Tai-Yin Spleen Meridian of Foot.

Method: Electrothermal acupuncture treatment.

Prescription: Qihai (RN6), Zusanli (ST36), Pishu (BL20), Sanyinjiao (SP6), Zigong (EX-CA1), Geshu (BL17).

Mechanism of prescription: Qihai is a meridian acupoint of Ren Channel, it can tonify Qi-blood, nurse Chong Channel and Ren Channel. Spleen and stomach are the source of engendering transformation for Qi-blood, so use the He acupoints Zusanli, Sanyinjiao and

Pishu, where the Yang-Ming Meridian of Foot enters, to reinforce spleen and stomach, tonify engendering of transformation, to promote sufficient Qi-blood and nourish Uterus Channel. Geshu is the confluent acupoint of blood, it can regulate and tonify blood. The treatment method for uterus is local acupoint selection, which can nurse meridians and alleviate pain. The use of combination of these acupoints can tonify Qi-blood, nurse and replenish Chong Channel and Ren Channel.

Matching acupoint: For patients with dizziness and tinnitus, add Shenshu and Taixi; for patients with low back soreness, add Mingmen.

Operations: Preparing the selected acupoints, perform routine skin disinfection. Using electrothermal acupuncture needles, vertically puncture into Qihai, Zusanli, Sanyinjiao, Zigong for 0.8" respectively, obliquely puncture into Pishu, Geshu, Shenshu for 0.7" respectively, vertically puncture into Mingmen and Taixi for 0.6" respectively. Turn on the electrothermal acupuncture equipment, apply a current of 40mA to each acupoint, and the limit is that the patient feels comfortable, leaving the needles in for 40 minutes. (Note: Select 3 pairs of acupoints each time, and use alternatively.)

Therapeutic course: Once a day, 20 times for a course (start treatment 10 days before menstruation till the coming of menstruation, and restart the treatment after the menstruation for 10 days, totally 20 days of treatment for each month). Cured after 3 continuous treatment courses.

[Lifestyle Change and Health Maintenance]

1. Pay attention to hygiene during menstrual period,

过度疲劳及精神刺激。

2. 经期忌食生冷食品，防止受凉，注意保温，忌用冷水洗脚。

3. 针灸治疗前要排除器质性病变，避免误诊，尤其是已婚妇女。

4. 若长期痛经，必须按疗程治疗，经前治疗 10 次，经后治疗 10 次，连续治疗 3 个疗程。

闭经

凡女子年龄超过 18 岁，仍无月经来潮（暗经除外）；或已形成月经周期，复停经 3 个月以上者（妊娠哺乳期除外），均可称为闭经。前者称原发性闭经，后者称继发性闭经。月经周期是下丘脑－垂体－卵巢的神经内分泌调节以及靶器官对性激素的周期性反应。全身性疾病，如传染病、慢性贫血、精神因素（如精神创伤、恐惧、悲伤）、环境改变以及严重的营养不良等，都可以干扰月经周期而引起闭经。

一、诊断及辨证要点

1. 血枯闭经：月经超龄未

avoid over fatigue and mental stimulations.

2. During menstrual period, do not eat raw and cold food, avoid catch of cold, pay attention to keeping warm, do not wash feet with cold water.

3. Before acupuncture treatment, organic lesions should be excluded first to avoid misdiagnosis, especially for married women.

4. Long-term dysmenorrhea must be treated as per treatment courses. Treat 10 times before and after menstrual period respectively, totally 3 continuous treatment courses.

Amenorrhea

Women over the age of 18 years, still have no menses (except latent menstruation); or the menstruation is stopped for more than 3 months after the formation of menstrual cycle (except pregnancy and lactation), are both called amenorrhea. The former is called primary amenorrhea, and the later is called secondary amenorrhea. Menstrual cycle is the cyclical responsiveness of neuroendocrine regulation and target organs of hypothalamus, hypophysis and ovarian to sexual hormones. Systematic diseases, such as infective diseases, chronic anemia, mental factors (such as mental trauma, fear, sorrow), environmental changes and severe malnutrition, all can interfere menstrual cycle and lead to amenorrhea.

I. Key Points for Diagnosis and Syndrome Differentiation

1. Amenorrhea caused by blood exhaustion: The

menstruation doesn't come over the age, or the menstrual period moves later gradually, and the blood volume reduces gradually, finally causes amenorrhea. Or companied with pale complexion, emaciation, dry skin, light tongue, thin pulse; or companied with dizziness and tinnitus, soreness and weakness of waist and knees, dysphoria in chest with palms-soles, night sweat, red tongue, taut pulse; or companied with mental fatigue and shortness of breath, palpitation, anorexia and sloppy stool, sallow complexion, light tongue, thin and weak pulse.

2. Amenorrhea caused by blood stagnation: Sudden amenorrhea, or companied with irritability and depression, swell of chest and hypochondrium, pressure-refused abdomen pain, dark tongue or with ecchymosis, deep and taut pulse; or cold body and limbs, cold and pain at lower abdomen, whitish tongue, deep and slow pulse; or obesity, swell of chest and hypochondrium, mental fatigue, excess leucorrhea, greasy tongue fur, slippery pulse.

II. Therapeutic Methods

[Amenorrhea caused by Blood Depletion]

Therapeutic method: Reinforce kidney and invigorate spleen, tonify Qi and nourish blood.

Prescription: Genshu(BL17), Pishu(BL20), Shenshu(BL23), Guanyuan (RN4), Qihai (RN6), Zusanli (ST36), Sanyinjiao (SP6).

Mechanism of prescription: Blood is the basis for women, for patients with blood depletion, replenish and nourish blood. Geshu is the confluent acupoint of blood, use it to replenish Yin blood; kidney is the congenital

事应时而下，故取肾俞合任脉穴气海、关元补肾益精；脾为后天之本，气血生化之源，取脾俞、足三里、三阴交调补后天。诸穴共用，具有补肾健脾、益气养血之功。

配穴 脾胃虚弱、食少便溏者，加胃俞、中脘、天枢、大肠俞；腰腿酸软者，加命门；头晕目眩者，加百会；潮热盗汗者，加膏肓、然谷、太溪。

方法 电热针治疗。

操作 选定穴位，皮肤常规消毒。电热针向脊柱方向斜刺膈俞、脾俞、肾俞各0.7寸，接通电热针仪，每个穴位分别给予电流量60～70mA，以患者舒适为度。另配以毫针直刺足三里0.7寸，直刺三阴交0.6寸，直刺太冲、太溪各0.5寸，留针40分钟。起针后，快针直刺关元、气海各0.7寸，施以提插补法，不留针。

foundation, the Taichong Channel will be flourish if the kidney Qi is plentiful, the menstruation comes in time, so use Shenshu and the acupoints of Ren Channel, Qihai and Guanyuan to replenish kidney and tonify vital essence; spleen is the the foundation of acquired constitution, the source of engendering transformation, so use Pishu, Zusanli and Sanyinjiao to nurse and tonify acquired constitution. The use of combination of these acupoints can reinforce kidney and invigorate spleen, tonify Qi and nourish blood.

Matching acupoints: For patients with weak spleen and stomach, anorexia and sloppy stool, add Weishu, Zhongwan, Tianshu, Dachangshu; for patients with aching lumbus and limp legs, add Mingmen; for patients with the symptom of dizziness, add Baihui; for patients with tidal fever and night sweating add Gaohuang, Rangu, Taixi.

Method: Electrothermal acupuncture treatment.

Operations: Preparing the selected acupoints, perform routine skin disinfection. Using electrothermal acupuncture needles, obliquely puncture into Geshu, Pishu, Shenshu for 0.7" respectively towards spine. Turn on the electrothermal acupuncture equipment, apply a current of 60-70mA to each acupoint, and the limit is that the patient feels comfortable. Additionally, using the filiform needles, vertically puncture into Zusanli for 0.7", Sanyinjiao for 0.6", Taichong and Taixi for 0.5" respectively, leaving the needles in for 40 minutes. After needle removal, using fast acupuncture, vertically puncture Guanyuan, Qihai for 0.7" respectively, apply the method of lifting-thrusting tonifying needling, do not leave the needles in.

Therapeutic course: Once a day, 20 times for a course (10 days of treatment both before and after menstruation), continuous treatment for 3 courses, namely end after 60 times of treatment.

[Amenorrhea caused by Blood Stagnation]

Therapeutic method: Regulate Qi and activate blood circulation, disperse phlegm and dredge meridians.

Prescription: Zhongji (RN3), Xuehai (SP10), Diji (SP8), Sanyinjiao (SP6), Hegu (LI4), Taichong (LR3), Taixi (KI3), Fenglong (ST40).

Mechanism of prescription: For patients with blood stagnation, dredge and activate blood circulation. Zhongji is an acupoint of Ren Channel, it can nurse Chong Channel and Ren Channel; Xuehai is an acupoint of Tai-Yin Meridian of Foot, it is good at treatment of blood diseases, can regulate Qi-blood, and remove stasis and nurse meridians when matching with Zhongji; Xinjian is an acupoint of Jue-Yin Meridian of Foot, it can clear heat and purge fire, soothe liver and regulate Qi; Sanyinjiao is an acupoint of Spleen Meridian, it can invigorate spleen and stomach as well as remove dampness and stasis when matching with the acupoint of Yang-Ming Meridian of Foot, Fenglong. The use of combination of these acupoints can regulate Qi and activate blood circulation, disperse phlegm and dredge meridians.

Matching acupoints: For patients with serious blood stasis, add Qichong, Ququan; for patients with swell of chest and hypochondrium, add Zhigou, Qimen; for patients with lower abdomen swelling pain, add Qi-

者，加内关、照海；神疲倦怠者，加足三里；大便干燥者，加天枢、上巨虚。

操作 选定穴位，皮肤常规消毒。电热针直刺血海 0.7 寸，直刺足三里 0.8 寸，直刺三阴交 0.6 寸。接通电热针仪，每个穴位分别给予电流量 60～70mA，以患者舒适为度，留针 40 分钟。另配以毫针直刺中极、地机各 0.7 寸，直刺合谷、太冲各 0.5 寸，直刺丰隆 0.7 寸，留针 40 分钟。

疗程 每日 1 次，20 次为 1 个疗程（月经前后各治疗 10 天），连续治疗 3 个疗程，即 60 次后结束治疗。

三、注意事项

1. 平素注意卫生，避免过度疲劳及精神刺激。

2. 忌食生冷食品，防止受凉，注意保温，忌用冷水洗脚。

3. 针灸治疗前要排除器质性病变，避免误诊，尤其是已婚妇女。

4. 若长期闭经，必须按疗程治疗，经前治疗 10 次，经

hai, Shuidao, Guilai; for patients with symptoms of chest distress, nausea and vomiting, add Neiguan, Zhaohai; for patients with mental fatigue, add Zusanli; for patients with dry stools, add Tianshu, Shangjuxu.

Operations: Preparing the selected acupoints, perform routine skin disinfection. Using electrothermal acupuncture needles, vertically puncture into Xuehai for 0.7", Zusanli for 0.8", Sanyinjiao for 0.6". Turn on the electrothermal acupuncture equipment, apply a current of 60-70mA to each acupoint, and the limit is that the patient feels comfortable, leaving the needles in for 40 minutes. Additionally, using the filiform needles, vertically puncture into Zhongji, Diji for 0.7" respectively, Hegu and Taichong for 0.5" respectively, Fenglong for 0.7", leaving the needles in for 40 minutes.

Therapeutic course: Once a day, 20 times for a course (10 days of treatment both before and after menstruation), continuous treatment for 3 courses, namely end after 60 times of treatment.

III. Precautions

1. Pay attention to hygiene, avoid over fatigue and mental stimulations.

2. Do not eat raw and cold food, avoid catch of chills, pay attention to keeping warm, do not wash feet with cold water.

3. Before acupuncture treatment, organic lesions should be excluded first to avoid misdiagnosis, especially for married women.

4. Long-term amenorrhea must be treated as per treatment courses. Treat 10 times before and after men-

后治疗 10 次，连续治疗 3 个疗程。

四、典型病例

梁某，女，28 岁，职员，北京人。

主诉：经停 3 个月。病史：患者 3 个月前，正值经期过食酒及辛辣寒凉食品，致经血渐停至今。

刻下症：经期或经后小腹隐痛喜按，头晕眼花，心悸气短，少食纳呆，面色无华，神疲乏力，舌淡，苔薄少，脉细无力。

查体：未见阳性体征。

辅助检查：未见异常。

【诊断依据】

1. 青年女性，素体虚弱，饮食不节。

2. 月经已 3 个月未见来潮。

3. 形体消瘦，营养不良，脾运失调。

4. 查体未发现明显阳性体征，妇科检查正常。

【证治分析】

病因 气血亏虚。

病机 饮食劳倦，损伤脾气，化源不足，致使冲脉血少，

strual period respectively, totally 3 continuous treatment courses.

IV. Typical Case

Liang, female, 28 years old, employee, residence: Beijing.

Self-reported symptom: The menstruation stopped for 3 months. Medical history: 3 months ago, during the menstrual period, the patient over-ingest alcohol and spicy, cold food, leading to menstrual blood gradually stopping till now.

Current symptoms: Pressure-relieved lower abdomen dull pain during or after menstrual period, dizziness, palpitation and shortness of breath, anorexia, pale complexion, mental fatigue and asthenia, light tongue, thin and less tongue fur, thin and weak pulse.

Physical examination: No positive signs were seen.

Auxiliary examination: No abnormalities.

[Diagnostic Basis]

1. Young female, weak body, intemperate diet.

2. No menstruation coming for 3 months.

3. Emaciation, malnutrition, spleen transportation disorder.

4. No significant positive signs found in the physical examination, and everything was normal in the gynecological examination.

[Syndrome-treatment Analysis]

Etiology: Deficiency of Qi and blood.

Pathogenesis: Fatigue of diet, spleen Qi impairment, insufficient source of transportation, leading to in-

发为闭经。

证候分析 气血亏虚，血海不足，故经量由少渐至闭经；血虚不能上荣于头面，故面色不华，头晕目眩；气血亏虚，心失所养，故心悸气短，神疲乏力。舌淡，苔薄少，脉细无力，均为气血不足之象。

病位 气血。

病性 虚性。

西医诊断 闭经。

中医诊断 闭经（气血不足）。

治法 益气扶脾，养血调经。

方法 电热针治疗。

处方 脾俞（BL20）、膈俞（BL17）、足三里（ST36）、三阴交（SP6）、气海（RN6）、肾俞（BL23）、关元（RN4）。

方义 女子以血为本，气血不足宜补宜养。膈俞为血之会，取之以补阴血；肾为先天之本，肾气充则太冲脉盛，月事应时而下，故取肾俞合任脉之气海、关元补肾益精；脾为后天之本，气血生化之源，取脾俞、足三里、三阴交调补后天。诸穴共用，具有补肾健

sufficient blood of Chong Channel, causing amenorrhea.

Syndrome analysis: Deficiency of Qi and blood, blood sea deficiency, therefore the menstrual blood volume gradually reduced till amenorrhea; blood deficieny, the blood could not go up to the face, causing lusterless complexion, dizziness; deficiency of Qi and blood, loss of heart nourishment, causing palpitation and shortness of breath, mental fatigue and asthenia. Light tongue, thin and less tongue fur, thin pulse, these are all symptoms of deficiency of Qi and blood.

Lesion location: Qi-blood.

Disease nature: Deficiency.

The diagnosis of Western Medicine: Amenorrhea.

The diagnosis of Traditional Chinese Medicine: Amenorrhea (Qi-blood deficiency).

Therapeutic method: Tonify Qi and reinforce spleen, nourish blood and nurse meridians.

Method: Electrothermal acupuncture treatment.

Prescription: Pishu(BL20), Geshu(BL17), Zusanli (ST36), Sanyinjiao (SP6), Qihai (RN6), Shenshu (BL23), Guanyuan (RN4).

Mechanism of prescription: Blood is the basis for women, for patients with blood deficiency, replenish and nourish blood. Geshu is the confluent acupoint of blood, use it to replenish Yin blood; kidney is the congenital foundation, the Taichong Channel will be flourish if the kidney Qi is plentiful, the menstruation comes in time, so use Shenshu and the acupoints of Ren Channel, Qihai and Guanyuan to replenish kidney and tonify vital essence; spleen is the the foundation of acquired constitu-

脾、益气养血之功。

配穴 食少便溏者，加胃俞、中脘、天枢；心悸气短者，加内关、神门；头晕目眩者，加百会。

操作 选定穴位，皮肤常规消毒。电热针直刺关元、中极、中脘、足三里、三阴交、内关、神门、气海各0.7寸，斜刺（针尖向脊柱）膈俞、脾俞、胃俞、肾俞各0.8寸，平刺百会0.7寸，接通电热针仪，每个穴位分别给予电流量40mA，以患者感到胀而舒适为度，留针40分钟。（注：每次选3组穴给予电热针治疗，交替使用，余穴用毫针治疗。）

疗程 每日1次，20次为1个疗程（月经前后各治疗10天），连续治疗3个疗程，即60次后结束治疗。

治疗过程 该患者治疗7天后月经来潮，随即停针，月经结束后再治疗10天，治疗3

tion, the source of engendering transformation, so use Pishu, Zusanli and Sanyinjiao to nurse and tonify acquired constitution. The use of combination of these acupoints can reinforce kidney and invigorate spleen, tonify Qi and nourish blood.

Matching acupoints: For patients with weak spleen and stomach, anorexia and sloppy stool, add Weishu, Zhongwan, Tianshu; for patients with palpitation and shortness of breath, add Neiguan, Shenmen; for patients with the symptom of dizziness, add Baihui.

Operations: Preparing the selected acupoints, perform routine skin disinfection. Using electrothermal acupuncture needles, vertically puncture into Guanyuan, Zhongji, Zhongwan, Zusanli, Sanyinjiao, Neiguan, Shenmen, Qihai for 0.7" respectively, obliquely puncture (towards Jizhong) into Geshu, Pishu, Weishu, Shenshu for 0.8" respectively, horizontally puncture into Baihui for 0.7". Turn on the electrothermal acupuncture equipment, apply a current of 40mA to each acupoint, and the limit is that the patient feels swell and comfortable, leaving the needles in for 40 minutes. (Note: Select 3 pairs of acupoints for electrothermal acupuncture treatment each time, use alternatively, and treat the other acupoints with filiform needles.)

Therapeutic course: Once a day, 20 times for a course (10 days of treatment both before and after menstruation), continuous treatment for 3 courses, namely end after 60 times of treatment.

Treatment process: The patient's menstruation came after 7 days of treatment, so the treatment was stopped immediately, after the end of menstruation

个疗程,从此月经周期正常,饮食恢复正常,体力恢复,体重增加,精力充沛。追踪随访1年未再闭经,次年4月怀孕。

【生活调摄】

1. 针灸治疗闭经效果较好,根据患者机体状态,必要时亦可配合中药治疗。

2. 引起闭经的原因很多,如贫血、胃炎、心脏病以及结核均可继发闭经,临床注意针对病因进行必要的检查,以便采取相应的措施。

3. 切勿将早期妊娠误诊为闭经。

白带增多症

带下是指妇女阴道内流出的一种白色黏稠液体,如涕如唾,称为白带,属正常的生理现象。若带下量多,或色、质、气味异常,并伴有腰酸腿软等全身症状者,即称为白带增多症。多与长期异物刺激、生殖器感染(如阴道炎、宫颈炎、子宫内膜炎等)、肿痛或身体虚弱等因素有关。长期慢性机械性刺激与损伤是其主要诱

continued the treatment for 10 days, totally 3 treatment courses. After that the menstrual cycle became normal, diet became normal, physical strength returned normal, body weight increased, vital energy replenished. No amenorrhea occurred during the 1-year follow-up, and the patient got pregnant the next April.

[Lifestyle Change and Health Maintenance]

1. The acupuncture treatment has good efficacy on amenorrhea, if necessary, Chinese Herb Medicine treatment can be used as supplement depending on patient's body conditions.

2. There are many causes leading to amenorrhea, for example, anemia, gastritis, cardiac diseases and tuberculosis all can induce secondary amenorrhea. Causes of disease should be focused on when being checked clinically, so as to take corresponding measures.

3. Do not mistakenly diagnose the early pregnancy as amenorrhea.

Leukorrhagia

Leukorrhea refers to a white viscous liquid flowing out from woman's vagina, like snot and saliva, which is a normal physiological phenomenon. For excessive leukorrhea or leukorrhea with abnormal color, quality and smell, accompanied with systematic symptoms such as aching lumbus and limp legs, it is called leukorrhagia. It is generally related with long-term foreign body stimulation, genital infections (such as vaginitis, cervicitis, endometritis, etc.), swelling or physical weakness and other factors. Long-term chronic mechanical stimulation and injuries are main causes. It is rare among unmarried

因。未婚妇女很少见，而婚后妇女半数以上患此病。

中医认为，本病属于"带下病"，并根据带下的颜色分为"白带""黄带""赤带""青带""黑带"。临床以前3种最为常见。带下病的发生主要与脾虚肝郁、湿热下注，或肾气不足、下元亏损、带脉失约有关，多属虚证；亦因感受湿热毒邪而致者，日久易伤肾而致肾虚。

一、诊断及辨证要点

1. 脾虚：带下量多，色白或淡黄，质稠无臭，绵绵不断，伴有面色萎黄，纳少便溏，神疲肢倦，舌淡，苔白或腻，脉缓弱。

2. 肾虚：带下清冷，量多质稀，色白，淋漓不断，腰酸如折，小腹冷感，小便清长，夜间尤甚，大便溏薄，舌淡，苔薄白，脉沉迟。

3. 湿热：带下量多，色黄黏稠，或黄白如腐渣，并有臭味，胸闷纳呆，口苦咽干，小

women, while more than half of married women are sufferring from this disease.

Traditional Chinese Medicine believes that this is a kind of leukorrheal diseases, and is divided as "white leukorrhea", "yellow leukorrhea", "red leukorrhea", "green leukorrhea", "black leukorrhea" as per leukorrhea color. The first three are most common in clinical practices. The development of leukorrheal diseases mainly are related with spleen deficiency and liver stasis, downward flow of Damp-Heat, or kidney Qi deficiency, depletion of the lower origin, Dai Channel dysfunction, most are deficiency syndromes; or caused by Damp-Heat and pathogenic toxins, it may damage kidney and cause kidney deficiency for a long time.

I. Key Points for Diagnosis and Syndrome Differentiation

1. Spleen deficiency: Excessive leukorrhea, white or yellow color, thick and odorless, endless, accompanied with sallow complexion, anorexia and sloppy stool, mental and physical fatigue, light tongue, white or greasy tongue fur, moderate and weak pulse.

2. Kidney deficiency: Light and cold leukorrhea, excessive quality and thin quality, white, dripping and endless blood flow, waist soreness like breaking, cold feeling of abdomen, clear abundant urine especially at night, thin and sloppy stool, light tongue, thin and whitish tongue fur, deep and slow pulse.

3. Damp-Heat: Excessive leukorrhea, yellowish and thick, or yellowish and whitish leukorrhea like soybean curd residue, accompanied with undesirable odor, chest

便短赤,阴中瘙痒,舌红苔黄,脉数或滑。

二、治疗方法

【脾虚证】

治法 健脾除湿止带。

处方 脾俞(BL20)、气海(RN6)、带脉(GB26)、足三里(ST36)、三阴交(SP6)、阴陵泉(SP9)。

方义 脾俞为足太阳经穴,脾气输注之处,多主脾病,取之可健脾益气;气海是任脉经穴,是先天元气汇聚之处,刺之可调理任脉,健脾益气;带脉为足少阳经穴,是足少阳、带脉二经之会,可固摄经气,约束带脉而治带下病;足三里为胃经合穴,是强壮要穴之一,既可温固下元,又可健脾渗湿;三阴交为足三阴之会穴,有健脾利湿、调理肝肾之功;取足太阴经穴阴陵泉,可健脾除湿止带。诸穴共用,脾健气运,阳升湿去,则带下自止。

distress and anorexia, bitter taste and dry throat, scanty dark urine, itching of vagina, red tongue and yellowish fur, rapid or slippery pulse.

II. Therapeutic Methods

[Spleen-deficiency Syndrome]

Therapeutic method: Invigorate spleen, remove Damp and stop leukorrhea.

Prescription: Pishu(BL20), Qihai(RN6), Daimai (GB26), Zusanli (ST36), Sanyinjiao (SP6), Yinlingquan (SP9).

Mechanism of prescription: Pishu is a meridian acupoint of Tai-Yang Meridian of Foot, the infusion point of spleen Qi, mainly governs spleen diseases, it can invigorate spleen and tonify Qi; Qihai is a meridian acupoint of Ren Channel, the convergence place of congenital vitality, acupuncture of this acupoint can nurse Ren Channel, invigorate spleen and tonify Qi; Daimai is a meridian acupoint of Shao-Yang Meridian of Foot, the confluent acupoint of the Shao-Yang Meridian of Foot and the Daimai Meridian of Foot, it can secure meridian Qi, control Daimai to treat leukorrheal diseases; Zusanli is a He acupoint of Stomach Meridian, one of the important tonifying acupoints, it can warming and astringent the lower origin as well as invigorate spleen and excrete Damp; Sanyinjiao is the confluent acupoint of three Yin Meridians of Foot, it can invigorate spleen and remove Damp, nurse liver and kidney; the use of the acupoint Yinlingquan of Tai-Yin Meridian of Foot can invigorate spleen, remove Damp and stop leukorrhea. The use of combination of these acupoints can invigorate spleen and dredge Qi, increase Yang and remove Damp, and the leukorrhea will stop naturally.

Matching acupoints: For patients with endless leukorrhea, add Chongmen, Qichong. For patients with excessive leukorrhea, add Dahe, Qixue. For patients with anorexia and sloppy stool, add Zhongwan, Tianshu. For patients that lose appetite, add Zhongwan, Zhangmen.

Method: Electrothermal acupuncture treatment.

Operations: Selecting the relevant acupoints, perform routine skin disinfection. Using electrothermal acupuncture needles, obliquely puncture into Pishu (towards spine) for 0.7", vertically puncture into Zusanli for 0.7", obliquely puncture into Daimai for 0.7". Turn on the electrothermal acupuncture equipment, apply a current of 60-70mA to each acupoint. The limit is that the patient feels comfortable. Additionally, using the filiform needles, vertically puncture into Sanyinjiao for 0.6", Yinlingquan for 0.7", Taichong and Taixi for 0.5" respectively. Leave the needles in for 40 minutes.

Therapeutic course: Once a day, 10 times for a course. Start the treatment for the second course after a break of 5-7 days. Generally cured after 2-3 courses.

[Kidney Deficiency Syndrome]

Therapeutic method: Replenish kidney and reinforce vital essence, induce astringency and stop leukorrhea.

Prescription: Guanyuan (RN4), Shenshu (BL23), Ciliao (BL32), Daimai (GB26), Baihuanshu (BL30).

Mechanism of prescription: Guanyuan is the con-

足阳明经与任脉之交会穴，有强壮作用，取之以补肾经、固肾气；肾俞为足太阳经穴，可调益肾气；足太阳经穴次髎是治带下之效穴；带脉为足少阳与带脉之会，可固摄带脉经气；白环俞是足太阳膀胱经穴，可助膀胱气化，又可固肾止带。诸穴共用，取其补肾培元、固涩止带之功。

配穴 肾阳虚者加气海、足三里；肾阴虚者加中极、三阴交、太溪。

方法 电热针治疗。

操作 选定穴位，皮肤常规消毒。电热针直刺肾俞、次髎各0.7寸，斜刺带脉0.8寸，接通电热针仪，每个穴位分别给予电流量60～70mA，以患者舒适为度，留针40分钟。另配以毫针直刺足三里0.7寸，直刺三阴交0.6寸，直刺太溪0.5寸，直刺白环俞0.7寸，留针40分钟。

疗程 每天1次，10次为1

fluent acupoint of three Yin Meridians of Foot, Yang-Ming Meridian of Foot and Ren Channel, which has tonic effects. It can replenish Kidney Meridian and secure kidney Qi; Shenshu is an meridian acupoint of Tai-Yang Meridian of Foot, it can tonify kidney Qi; the acupoint Ciliao of Tai-Yang Meridian of Foot is an effecient acupoint for leukorrheal diseases treatment; Daimai is the confluent acupoint of Shao-Yang Meridian of Foot and Dai Channel, it can secrue and astringe meridian Qi of Dai Channel; Baihuanshu is an meridian acupoint of Tai-Yang Bladder Meridian of Foot, it can promote Qi transformation of bladder and astringe kidney, stop leukorrhea. The use of combination of these five acupoints can replenish kidney and reinforce vital essence, induce astringency and stop leukorrhea.

Matching acupoints: For patients with Yang deficiency of kidney, add Qihai, Zusanli; For patients with Yin deficiency of kidney, add Zhongji, Sanyinjiao, Taixi.

Method: Electrothermal acupuncture treatment.

Operations: Selecting the relevant acupoints, perform routine skin disinfection. Using electrothermal acupuncture needles, vertically puncture into Shenshu and Ciliao for 0.7" respectively, obliquely puncture into Daimai for 0.8". Turn on the electrothermal acupuncture equipment, apply a current of 60-70mA to each acupoint. The limit is that the patient feels comfortable. Leave the needles in for 40 minutes. Additionally, using the filiform needles, vertically puncture into Zusanli for 0.7", Sanyinjiao for 0.6", Taixi for 0.5", Baihuanshu for 0.7", leaving the needles in for 40 minutes.

Therapeutic course: Once a day, 10 times for a

course. Start the treatment for the second course after a break of 5-7 days. Generally cured after 2-3 courses.

[Damp-Heat Syndrome]

Therapeutic method: Clear Heat and remove Damp, relieve turbidity and stop leukorrhea.

Prescription: Daimai (GB26), Zhongji (RN3), Yinlingquan (SP9), Sanyinjiao (SP6), Xingjian (LR2).

Mechanism of prescription: Use Daimai, the confluent acupoint of Shao-Yang Meridian of Foot and Dai Channel, to regulate Dai Channel so as to stop leukorrhea. Use the important acupoint of Ren Channel, Zhongji to regulate Ren Chanel, remove Damp and resolve turbidity; Yinlingquan is a He acupoint of Spleen Meridian, can dredge downward flow of Damp-Heat. Use the acupoint Sanyinjiao of Spleen Meridian to invigorate spleen and remove Damp. Use the Ying-spring acupoint Xingjian of Liver Meridian to purge stasis-Heat of Liver Meridian. The use of combination of these acupoints can clear Heat and remove Damp, relieve turbidity and stop leukorrhea.

Matching acupoints: For patients with red leukorrhea, add Jianshi. For patients with palpitation, add Shenmen, Taixi.

Method: Electrothermal acupuncture treatment.

Operations: Selecting the relevant acupoints, perform routine skin disinfection. Using electrothermal acupuncture needles, obliquely puncture towards Qizhong into Daimai for 0.7", vertically puncture into Yinlingquan for 0.7", Sanyinjiao for 0.6". Turn on the

40~50mA，以患者感到舒适为度，留针40分钟。另配以毫针向下斜刺中极1.5寸，直刺神门0.5寸，直刺太溪0.5寸，直刺间使0.6寸，直刺行间0.5寸，留针40分钟。

疗程 每天1次，10次为1个疗程。疗程间休息5~7天，再进行第2个疗程的治疗。一般治疗2~3个疗程。

三、注意事项

1. 针灸治疗带下病疗效较好。若发现赤带时，须做妇科检查，以进一步明确诊断。

2. 多进食健脾补肾之品，如山药、银杏、新鲜蔬菜等，特别是多摄入含维生素B1的食品，对慢性白带增多的患者大有裨益。

3. 注意卫生，保持外阴清洁，避免再感染。

四、典型病例

赵某，女，32岁，职员，北京人。

主诉：白带增多半年。病史：患者平时脾胃虚弱，纳差，曾流产1次。

electrothermal acupuncture equipment, apply a current of 40-50mA to each acupoint. The limit is that the patient feels comfortable. Leave the needles in for 40 minutes. Additionally, using the filiform needles, obliquely puncture downward into Zhongji for 1.5", vertically puncture into Shenmen for 0.5", Taixi for 0.5", Jianshi for 0.6", Xingjian for 0.5", leaving the needles in for 40 minutes.

Therapeutic course: Once a day, 10 times for a course. Start the treatment for the second course after a break of 5-7 days. Generally treat for 2-3 courses.

III. Precautions

1. The efficacies of acupuncture therapy on leukorrheal diseases are good. If red leukorrhea is found, gynecological examination is required to further confirm the diagnosis.

2. Eating more foods that can invigorate spleen and replenish kidney, such as yam, ginkgo and fresh vegetables, especially eating more foods containing vitamin B1 has great benefits for patients with chronic leukorrhagia.

3. Pay attention to hygiene, keep the vulva clean, avoid re-infection.

IV. Typical Case

Zhao, female, 32 years old, employee, residence: Beijing.

Self-reported symptoms: Leukorrhagia for half a year. Medical history: The patient usually had symptoms of spleen and stomach deficiency, anorexia, and aborted

刻下症：白带增多，伴腰酸，带下清稀，神疲肢倦，舌淡胖，苔白腻，脉沉迟。

查体：两肺呼吸音粗，二尖瓣区及主动脉瓣第二听诊区可闻及二级收缩期杂音。

辅助检查：妇科检查示"盆腔炎"。

【诊断依据】

1. 中年女性，已婚，流产1次。

2. 患者素体脾胃虚弱，饮食失常，运化失调，纳少。

3. 带下白色，无臭，量多如涕。

4. 舌淡胖，苔白腻，脉沉迟。

【证治分析】

病因　脾虚失运。

病机　饮食失节，损伤脾气，运化失司，水湿内停，流注下焦，致任脉失固，带脉失约，则生带下。

证候分析　脾虚失运，水湿不化，湿邪内困，下注胞宫，故带下色白。湿邪内阻，

once.

Current symptoms: Increased leukorrhea, accompanied with waist soreness, thin leukorrhea, mental and physical fatigue, light and fat tongue, whitish and greasy tongue fur, deep and slow pulse.

Physical examination: Coarse breath sounds in both lungs, Grade 2 systolic noise at mitral valve area and second aortic valve area.

Auxiliary examination: Gynecological examination showed "pelvic inflammatory disease".

[Diagnostic Basis]

1. Middle-aged woman, married, aborted once.

2. The patient had weak spleen and stomach, irregular diet, transportation and transformation disorders, eat less.

3. White and odorless leukorrhea, excessive amount like snot.

4. Light and fat tongue, whitish and greasy tongue fur, deep and slow pulse.

[Syndrome-treatment Analysis]

Etiology: Losing transport because of spleen deficiency.

Pathogenesis: Improper diet, spleen Qi damage, irregulation of transportation and transformation, internal retention of water-Damp, downward flow to Lower Jiao, cause loss of Ren Channel astringency, Dai Channel dysfunction, so as to develop leukorrhea.

Syndrome analysis: Losing transport because of spleen deficiency, incapable of water-Damp transportation, internal obstruction of pathogenic Damp, downward

中阳不运，故纳少，身困肢倦。舌淡胖，苔白腻，脉沉迟，为脾气虚之象。

病位 脾。

病性 虚性。

西医诊断 盆腔炎。

中医诊断 带下病。

治法 健脾益气，利湿止带。以任脉、足太阴脾经穴为主。

方法 电热针治疗。

处方 气海（RN6）、带脉（GB26）、白环俞（BL30）、脾俞（BL20）、三阴交（SP6）、足三里（ST36）、阴陵泉（SP9）。

方义 脾俞为足太阳经穴，脾气输注之处，多主脾病，取之可健脾益气；气海为任脉经穴，为先天元气汇聚之处，刺之可调任脉，健脾益气；带脉为足少阳经穴，是足少阳、带脉二经之会，可固摄经气，约束带脉而治带下病；足三里为胃经之合穴，是强壮要穴之一，既可温固下元，又可健脾渗湿；三阴交为足三阴

flow to uterus, so the color of leukorrhea is whitish. Internal obstruction of pathogenic Damp, cause less food intake and tiredness of body and limbs. Light and fat tongue, whitish and greasy tongue fur, deep and slow pulse, are symptoms of spleen Qi deficiency.

Lesion location: Spleen.

Disease nature: Deficiency.

The diagnosis of Western Medicine: Pelvic inflammatory disease.

The diagnosis of Traditional Chinese Medicine: Leukorrheal disease.

Therapeutic method: Invigorate spleen and tonify Qi, remove Damp and stop leukorrhea. Focus on meridian acupoints of Ren Channel and Tai-Yin Spleen Meridian of Foot.

Method: Electrothermal acupuncture treatment.

Prescription: Qihai (RN6), Daimai (GB26), Baihuanshu (BL30), Pishu (BL20), Sanyinjiao (SP6), Zusanli (ST36), Yinlingquan (SP9).

Mechanism of prescription: Pishu is a meridian acupoint of Tai-Yang Meridian of Foot, the infusion point of spleen Qi, mainly governs spleen diseases, it can invigorate spleen and tonify Qi; Qihai is a meridian acupoint of Ren Channel, the convergence place of congenital vitality, acupuncture of this acupoint can nurse Ren Channel, invigorate spleen and tonify Qi; Daimai is a meridian acupoint of Shao-Yang Meridian of Foot, the confluent acupoint of Shao-Yang Meridian of Foot and Daimai Meridian of Foot, it can secure meridian Qi, control Daimai to treat leukorrheal diseases; Zusanli is

之交会穴，有健脾利湿、调理肝肾之功；取足太阴经穴阴陵泉，可健脾除湿止带。

配穴 纳少便溏者加中脘、天枢。

操作 选定穴位，皮肤常规消毒。电热针直刺气海、足三里、阴陵泉、三阴交、天枢、中脘各0.8寸，针尖向脐中斜刺带脉0.8寸。接通电热针仪，每个穴位分别给予电流量40mA，以患者感到胀而舒适为度，留针40分钟。

疗程 每天1次，10次为1个疗程。

治疗过程 该患者共针治20次，症状消失。后又巩固治疗10次。随访2年，未再复发。

【生活调摄】

1. 注意卫生，保持外阴清洁，避免重复感染。

2. 多吃健脾益肾的食品，对慢性白带增多的患者有益处，如山药、新鲜蔬菜，特别

a He acupoint of Stomach Meridian, one of the important tonifying acupoints, it can warming and astringent the lower origin as well as invigorate spleen and excrete Damp; Sanyinjiao is the confluent acupoint of three Yin Meridians of Foot, it can invigorate spleen and remove Damp, nurse liver and kidney; the use of the acupoint Yinlingquan of Tai-Yin Meridian of Foot can invigorate spleen, remove Damp and stop leukorrhea.

Matching acupoints: For patients with anorexia and sloppy stool, add Zhongwan, Tianshu.

Operations: Selecting the relevant acupoints, perform routine skin disinfection. Using electrothermal acupuncture needles, vertically puncture into Shenshu, Zusanli, Yinlingquan, Sanyinjiao, Tianshu, Zhongwan for 0.8" respectively, obliquely puncture into Daimai with the needle tip towards Jizhong for 0.8". Turn on the electrothermal acupuncture equipment, apply a current of 40mA to each acupoint. The limit is that the patient feels swell and comfortable. Leave the needles in for 40 minutes.

Therapeutic course: Once a day, 10 times for a course.

Treatment process: The patients received 20 times of acupuncture treatments in total during the course, and the symptoms disappeared. Later she received 10 times of consolidation treatments. 2-year follow-up, no recurrence.

[Lifestyle Change and Health Maintenance]

1. Pay attention to hygiene, keep the vulva clean, avoid repeated infection.

2. Eating more foods that can invigorate spleen and replenish kidney, such as yam, ginkgo and fresh vegetables, especially eating more foods rich in vitamin B1, has

要多吃富含维生素 B1 的食品。

3. 针灸治疗带下病有很好的疗效。若发现赤带必须及时做相关的妇科检查。

盆腔炎

盆腔炎是常见的女性生殖系统炎症之一，有急性和慢性之分。前者是盆腔的急性炎症，发病部位包括子宫、输卵管、卵巢、盆腔腹膜及盆腔结缔组织等，可在一部分或几部分同时发病，临床表现主要为发热、下腹部疼痛、白带增多及月经失调等。多由急性输卵管炎症播散或分娩、刮宫、输卵管通气、输卵管通液等无菌操作不严格，造成细菌感染所致。后者多因急性盆腔炎未能妥善、彻底治疗，或体质较差、病程迁延所致，病情较为顽固；亦有急性炎症症状不典型，发现时已为慢性盆腔炎者。临床表现多为下腹部坠胀、疼痛，腰骶部酸痛，白带增多，月经紊乱，痛经，妇科检查子宫活动受限，输卵管增粗或有囊性物，压痛等。

中医认为，本病与"腹痛"

great benefits for patients with chronic leukorrhagia.

3. The efficacies of acupuncture therapy on leukorrheal diseases are good. If red leukorrhea is found, timely related gynecological examination is required.

Pelvic Inflammatory Disease

Pelvic inflammatory disease is one of the common female reproductive system inflammations, and is divided into acute and chronic types. The former is acute inflammation of the pelvic cavity, tension sites include uterus, fallopian tubes, ovarian, pelvic peritoneum and pelvic connective tissues, etc. It can occur at one or several parts in the same time, and the clinical manifestations mainly include fever, pain of lower abdomen, increased leukorrhea and menoxenia. It's normally caused by spread of acute fallopian tube inflammation or delivery, bacterial infection due to non-strict sterile operation of uterine dilatation and curettage, fallopian tube ventilation, fallopian tube infusion, etc. The later is normally caused by improper, incomplete treatment of acute pelvic inflammatory disease, or poor physical fitness, prolonged course of disease, and the condition is stubborn; and there are also acute inflammations with atypical symptoms, which have developed into chronic pelvic inflammatory diseases when being detected. Common clinical manifestations include lower abdominal bulge and pain, soreness of lumbosacral portion, increased leukorrhea, menstrual disorder, dysmenorrhea, limited uterine actions found in gynecologic examination, fallopian tube thickening or with cystic substances, tenderness, etc.

Traditional Chinese Medicine believes that this

"带下病""痛经"及"癥瘕"等病的某些症状相似。多因分娩或人流术中病邪感染,湿热之邪侵袭胞脉,与气血相搏而发病;或经期不注意卫生或行房,湿热之邪乘虚入侵等引起。慢性盆腔炎因过度劳累,正气虚弱,外邪乘虚而入也可急性发作。

一、诊断及辨证要点

1. 急性盆腔炎

(1)有流产、分娩、宫腔内不洁操作或月经期、产褥期性交史。

(2)高烧寒战,下腹疼痛。

(3)有腹膜炎时,可出现消化系统症状,有时有泌尿系之尿道受压或受刺激症状。直肠壁受刺激可有腹泻,直肠受压时可出现排便困难。

(4)白带增多,呈脓性,有臭味。

(5)妇科检查:下腹部肌紧张,压痛或反跳痛,肠鸣音减弱或消失。阴道内有大量脓性分泌物,阴道充血,穹隆明显触痛。子宫颈充血、水肿,压痛明显。子宫体略大,有压

disease has similar symptoms with those of "abdominal pain", "leukorrheal diseases", "abdominal mass", etc. It is normally caused by pathogenic factor infection during delivery or induced abortion, the pathogenic Damp-Heat invades Uterus Channel and fight with Qi-blood; or caused by paying no attention to hygiene or sexual intercourses during menstrual period, leading to invasion of pathogenic Damp-Heat. Excessive fatigue, weakness of healthy Qi leading to invasion of external pathogenic factors can cause acute onset of chronic pelvic inflammatory diseases.

I. Key Points for Diagnosis and Syndrome Differentiation

1. Acute pelvic inflammatory disease

(1) Has a history of abortion, delivery, unsanitary intrauterine operation or sexual intercourses during menstrual periods, puerperium periods.

(2) High fever and chills, pain of lower abdomen.

(3) With peritonitis, there may occur digestive system symptoms, as well as urinary system symptoms of urethral compression or irritation. Rectal wall irritation can cause diarrhea, while rectum compression can cause defecation difficulties.

(4) Increased leukorrhea, purulent, stinky.

(5) Gynecologic examination: Lower abdominal muscle tension, tenderness or rebound tenderness, reduction or disappearance of bowel sound. Lots of purulent secretion in the vagina, vaginal congestion, obvious tenderness of fornix. Obvious congestion, edema, tenderness of cervix uterus. The uterus is slightly larger with tender-

痛，活动受限。宫旁压痛明显，有时可扪及肿物。宫旁结缔组织炎时，可扪及下腹一侧或两侧有片状增厚。如有盆腔脓肿形成，子宫直肠陷窝饱满，有触痛及波动感。

（6）体温升高，一般在39℃左右，白细胞总数及中性粒细胞增高。

（7）必要时可做后穹隆穿刺，如抽出脓液即可确诊。

2. 慢性盆腔炎

（1）病程长，下腹部隐痛及下坠，腰骶部酸痛，月经前或经期加重，白带增多。

（2）月经量多或经期延长。

（3）性交痛。

（4）有急性盆腔炎及不孕病史。

（5）妇科检查：子宫常呈后位，活动受限，或固定。如附件炎，则在子宫一侧或两侧触到增粗的输卵管，呈条索样，有压痛。如有输卵管积水，或输卵管卵巢囊肿，可在盆腔一侧或两侧触到囊性肿物。盆腔有结缔组织炎时，宫旁可有片状增厚，压痛，子宫骶骨韧带增粗、变硬。

ness and limited activities. Obvious parametrial tenderness, sometimes masses can be palpated. For parametrial connective tissue inflammation, sheet-shaped thickening can be palpated at one or both sides of the lower abdomen. If there is pelvic abscess formed, the uterus rectum lacuna is full, with tenderness and feeling of fluctuation.

(6) Increased body temperature, normally around 39℃, increased total leucocyte counts and neutrophils.

(7) If necessary, perform puncture of posterior fornix, it can be confirmed if pus is aspirated out.

2. Chrome pelvic inflammatory disease

(1) Long course of disease, dull pain and feeling of bearing down of the lower abdomen, soreness of lumbosacral portion, worsened before or during menstrual periods, increased leukorrhea.

(2) Increased menstrual blood volume or prolonged menstrual period.

(3) Dyspareunia.

(4) History of acute pelvic inflammatory diseases or infertilitas feminis.

(5) Gynecologic examination: Uterine often is presented as a posterior location, with limited activities or fixed uterine. For appendagitis, thickened fallopian tubes can be touched at one or two side of the uterus, strip-like, with tenderness. For hydrosalpinx, or tubo-ovarian cyst, cystic masses can be touched at one or two side of the pelvic cavity. If there is connective tissue inflammation within the pelvic cavity, there will be sheet-shaped thickening and tenderness beside the uterus, with thickening and hardening of the utero-sacral ligament.

3. 结核性盆腔炎

（1）有不孕、盆腔以外结核病或慢性盆腔炎久治不愈之病史。

（2）病程较久者可有月经量逐渐减少。

（3）妇科检查：由于病程、范围大小及受累部位不同，可表现为外阴溃疡、宫颈乳头糜烂或菜花样增长，子宫正常或稍小，子宫角处触及突起，输卵管粗大质硬，表面结节状，盆腔有不规则质硬块。

（4）血液检查：淋巴细胞增高，血沉加快。

（5）X线：子宫输卵管碘酒造影，可见输卵管呈念珠状，或有灌注缺陷，子宫腔重度狭窄或变形，边缘呈锯齿状。腹部平片可见盆腔钙化点。

（6）将经血或子宫内膜做结合菌培养或动物接种可证实诊断。

（7）子宫内膜病理检查可找到典型的结核结节。

4. 辨证

（1）急性盆腔炎

①邪毒内扰：高烧，恶寒，无汗，下腹部疼痛拒按，带下量多，脓性，臭味，伴口干，

3. Tuberculous pelvic inflammatory disease

(1) History of infertilitas feminis, tuberculosis outside the pelvic cavity or permanently chronic pelvic inflammatory diseases.

(2) For patients with longer course of disease, the menstrual blood volume may decrease gradually.

(3) Gynecologic examination: Due to differences of course of disease, range and affected sites, the symptoms can be vulva ulceration, cervical nipple erosion or cauliflower-like growth, normal size or smaller uterus, palpated protuberance at cornua uteri, thick and big, hard fallopian tubes with nodular surface, irregular hard lumps in the pelvic cavity.

(4) Blood examination: Increased lymphocytes, increased erythrocyte sedimentation rate.

(5) X-ray examination: It can be found in the iodine hysterosalpingography that fallopian tubes are bead-like or have perfusion defect, the uterine cavity has serious stenosis or deformation, while the edge is jagged. Pelvic calcification points can be seen in the plain abdominal radiograph.

(6) The diagnosis can be confirmed if use the menstrual blood or endometrium to do bacterial culture or animal inoculation.

(7) Typical tuberculous nodules can be found with pathologic examination of endometrium.

4. Symptom differentiation

(1) Acute pelvic inflammatory disease

① Internal disturbance of pathogenic toxin: high fever, aversion to cold, adiapneustia, abdominal pain and refusal of pressing, excessive leukorrhea, purulent and

小便赤，大便秘结，舌红，苔黄腻，脉弦数或滑数。

②湿热内蕴：低热，汗出不畅，下腹坠痛，或刺痛拒按，带下量多，色黄，伴小便赤，舌红，苔黄腻，脉滑数。

（2）慢性盆腔炎

①气滞血瘀：少腹刺痛或胀，痛引骶部，带下量多，色黄，月经不调，舌黯或有瘀点，苔薄白，脉弦或弦细。

②肝肾不足：下腹部绵绵作痛，带下量多，色黄质稀，腥臭，伴腰腿酸软，头晕，舌红少苔，脉沉细。

③脾肾阳虚：下腹隐痛，坠胀，带下量多，质清稀，伴面肿，腰酸膝软，畏寒，舌淡体胖，苔薄白，脉沉细。

（3）结核性盆腔炎

①阴虚内热：月经稀少，后期甚者闭经，少腹隐痛，伴五心烦热，午后潮热，颧赤盗汗，口渴少饮，舌红少苔，脉细数。

stinky, accompanied with dry mouth, dark urine, constipation, red tongue, yellowish and greasy tongue fur, taut and rapid or taut and slippery pulse.

② Internal retention of Damp-Heat: Low fever, inhibited sweating, bearing-down pain of lower abdomen or prickling and refusal of pressing, excessive leukorrhea, yellow, accompanied with dark urine, red tongue, yellowish and greasy tongue fur, taut and slippery pulse.

(2) Chrome pelvic inflammatory disease

① Qi stagnation and blood stasis: Prickling or swelling of lateral lower abdomen, with pain spreading to pars sacralis, excessive leukorrhea, yellow, menoxenia, dark tongue or with petechia, thin and whitish tongue fur, taut or taut and thin pulse.

② Liver and kidney deficiency: Continuous pain of lower abdomen, excessive leukorrhea, yellow and thin, stench, accompanied with aching lumbus and limp legs, dizziness, red tongue and less tongue fur, deep and thin pulse.

③ Yang deficiency of spleen and kidney: Dull pain and bearing-down as well as swell feeling of lower abdomen, excessive leukorrhea, light and thin, accompanied with face swelling, aching lumbus and limp knees, intolerance of cold, light tongue and fat figure, thin and whitish tongue fur, deep and thin pulse.

(3) Tuberculous pelvic inflammatory disease

① Yin deficiency and internal Heat: Thin and less menstrual blood, even amenorrhea at the later period, dull pain of lateral lower abdomen, accompanies with dysphoria in chest with palms-soles, afternoon tidal fever, flushing of zygomatic region and night sweating,

②气血两亏：行经后期，量少色淡，少腹隐痛，面色萎黄，倦怠乏力，纳呆，舌淡，苔薄白，脉细无力。

二、治疗方法

【湿热内蕴，气滞血瘀】

治法 调理冲任，清热利湿，疏通经络，化瘀止痛。

处方 中极（RN3）、归来（ST29）、足三里（ST36）、三阴交（SP6）。

方义 中极系膀胱之募穴，亦系足三阴经与任脉之交会穴，具有调理冲任、清利湿热、化瘀止痛之功效；配胃经的归来穴，治疗妇科炎症疗效显著；足三里为胃经之合穴，三阴交为肝、脾、肾三经之交会穴，二穴相伍，有清热利湿、疏通经络之功。诸穴相伍，具有调理冲任、清热利湿、疏通经络、化瘀止痛的作用。

thirsty and less drinking, red tongue and less tongue fur, thin and rapid pulse.

② Depletion of Qi-blood: delayed menstruation, less volume and light color, dull pain of lateral lower abdomen, sallow complexion, tiredness and asthenia, anorexia, light tongue, thin and whitish tongue fur, thin and weak pulse.

II. Therapeutic Methods

[Internal Retention of Damp-Heat, Qi Stagnation and Blood Stasis]

Therapeutic method: Nurse Chong Channel and Ren Channel, clear Heat and remove Damp, dredge meridians and collaterals, remove stasis and alleviate pain.

Prescription: Zhongji (RN3), Guilai (ST29), Zusanli (ST36), Sanyinjiao (SP6).

Mechanism of prescription: Zhongji is a Mu acupoint of Bladder, the confluent acupoint of three Yin Meridians of Foot and Ren Channel, it can nurse Chong Channel and Ren Channel, clear Heat and remove Damp, remove stasis and alleviate pain; it has significant efficacies on treatment of gynecological inflammations matching the acupoint Guilai of Stomach Meridian; Zusanli is a He acupoint of Stomach Meridian, and Sanyinjiao is the confluent acupoint of Liver Meridian, Spleen Meridian and Kidney Meridian, the combination of these two acupoints can clear Heat and remove Damp, dredge meridians and collaterals. The combination of these four acupoints can nurse Chong Channel and Ren Channel, clear Heat and remove Damp, dredge meridians and col-

配穴 急性盆腔炎发热者，加大椎、曲池；腰骶痛甚者，加肾俞、次髎；尿频者，加阴陵泉；带下多者，加带脉；慢性盆腔炎，加肾俞、气海。

方法 电热针治疗。

操作 选定穴位，皮肤常规消毒。电热针直刺归来0.7寸，直刺足三里0.7寸，直刺三阴交0.6寸。接通电热针仪，每个穴位分别给予电流量60～70mA，留针40分钟。另配以毫针直刺曲池0.6寸，直刺中极0.7寸，直刺阴陵泉0.7寸，斜刺带脉0.7寸，留针40分钟。

疗程 每天1次，10次为1个疗程。疗程间可休息5～7天，再继续进行第2个疗程的治疗。一般治疗2～3个疗程即可痊愈。

三、注意事项

1. 针治下腹部穴位前，令患者排空小便。

2. 急性盆腔炎严重者，要配合中药或西药综合治疗，以提高疗效，避免转为慢性。

laterals, remove stasis and alleviate pain.

Matching acupoints: For patients with acute pelvic inflammatory disease accompanying fever, add Dazhui, Quchi. For patients with severe lumbosacral pain, add Shenshu, Ciliao. For patients with frequent micturition, add Yinlingquan. For patients with excessive leukorrhea, add Daimai. For chronic pelvic inflammatory diseases, add Shenshu, Qihai.

Method: Electrothermal acupuncture treatment.

Operations: Selecting the relevant acupoints, perform routine skin disinfection. Using electrothermal acupuncture needles, vertically puncture into Guilai for 0.7", Zusanli for 0.7", Sanyinjiao for 0.6". Turn on the electrothermal acupuncture equipment, apply a current of 60-70mA to each acupoint. Leave the needles in for 40 minutes. Additionally, using the filiform needles, vertically puncture into Quchi for 0.6", Zhongji and Yinlingquan for 0.7" respectively, obliquely puncture into Daimai for 0.7", leaving the needles in for 40 minutes.

Therapeutic course: Once a day, 10 times for a course. Start the treatment for the second course after a break of 5-7 days. Generally cured after 2-3 courses.

III. Precautions

1. Instruct patients to empty urine before acupuncture of acupoints at lower abdomen.

2. For patients with serious acute pelvic inflammatory diseases, it is necessary to combine with Chinese Herb Medicine treatment and comprehensive Western

3. 注意卫生，尤其是外阴部的清洁，避免重复感染。

外阴瘙痒

外阴瘙痒是妇科常见病之一。瘙痒最常发生的部位是阴蒂及小阴唇区域，严重者可波及整个外阴部，甚则波及肛门和大腿内侧。各种年龄的女子均可发生，但绝大多数患者是更年期的妇女。轻者为间断性、阵发性瘙痒，重者可持续存在。瘙痒长期折磨患者，可使其变得衰弱、憔悴、急躁和高度神经质，患处皮肤及黏膜由于长期反复刺激及搔抓损伤，可引起继发病变，皮肤常有苔藓样硬化及肥厚。外阴瘙痒除某些疾病（如妇科外阴炎、阴道炎）的分泌物刺激外阴引起外，外阴周围寄生虫感染、糖尿病、外阴皮肤病等均可引起外阴瘙痒。

中医认为，本病属于"阴痒"的范畴。由于脾虚湿盛或肝郁化热下注阴户所致，也可由素体虚弱、精血不足、血虚生风化燥、外阴失濡或滴虫侵袭引起。

Medicine treatment to improve efficacy and avoid the disease transfer into chronic one.

3. Pay attention to hygiene, especially the cleaning of vulva, avoid repeated infection.

Pruritus Vulvae

Pruritus vulvae is one of the common gynecological disease. The most common affected sites of pruritus vulvae are clitoris and labium minus areas, in serious cases it can spread to the whole vulva or even spread to the anus and inner sides of legs. It can occur on women of various ages, however most patients are menopausal women. In mild cases it may be intermittent, paroxysmal pruritus, while in serious cases it may be persistent one. Pruritus tortures patients for long times, can make them become weak, haggard, irritable and highly neurotic, and due to long-term repeated irritation and scratching damage, the skin and mucous membrane at affected sites may cause secondary lesions, often with skin lichenification and pachynsis. In addition to vulva irritation caused by secretions of some diseases (such as gynecological vulvitis, vaginitis), parasitic infections around the vulva, diabetes, vulval skin diseases all can cause pruritus vulvae.

Traditional Chinese Medicine believes that this disease belongs to the range of "vulval itching". It can be caused by spleen deficiency with overabundance of Damp or liver stasis transforming into Heat flowing downward to the pussy, and also can be cause by weak body, insufficiency of blood and essence, as well as that

一、诊断及辨证要点

1. 辨病

（1）白带增多，多为黄水状，感染严重时白带可呈脓性，有臭味，阴道黏膜有表浅溃疡时，分泌物可为血性；或有点滴出血伴外阴瘙痒，灼热感。炎症波及前庭或尿道口周围黏膜，可出现尿急、尿频、尿痛或尿失禁等症状。

（2）妇科检查：可见外阴黏膜呈老年性改变，上皮菲薄，光滑，潮红，常有散在性小出血点，或片状出血斑，严重时上皮脱落，形成浅表溃疡，宫颈也常充血，并有散在性小出血点。经久不愈者，黏膜下结缔组织纤维化，阴道弹性消失，更为狭窄。慢性炎症或溃疡还可引起阴道粘连。

（3）根据临床表现，有时有必要取分泌物做镜下检查，以鉴别滴虫性或霉菌性阴道炎。

blood deficiency generates Wind then transform into Dryness, loss of moistening of vulva or trichomonad invasion.

I. Key Points for Diagnosis and Syndrome Differentiation

1. Disease differentiation

(1) Increased leukorrhea, most is yellowish water-like, and the leukorrhea may be purulent and stinky, while the secretions can be bloody if there are superficial ulcers of the vaginal mucosa. Or there is drop-like bleeding accompanied with pruritus vulvae, feeling of burning heat. If the inflammation spread to the vestibule or mucosa around the urethral orifice, there may occur symptoms like urgent urination, frequent micturition, odynuria or uroclepsia.

(2) Gynecologic examination: Senile changes of vulva mucosa can be seen, thin epithelium, smooth and flushing, often some scattered small bleeding points or sheet-shaped bleeding spots, in severe cases there may be epithelial shedding which form superficial ulcers, and the cervix is also often congested with scattered small bleeding points. For prolonged unhealed patients, they may have submucosal connective tissue fibrosis and the vaginal elasticity disappears, becomes more narrow. Chronic inflammations or ulcers also may cause vaginal adhesions.

(3) According to clinical manifestations, sometimes it is necessary to take secretions for microscopic examinations, so as to identify trichomonas or mycotic vaginitis.

2. 辨证

（1）肝肾阴虚：带下量多，呈黄色，质黏稠，甚者如血样，阴部干涩，灼热瘙痒，五心烦热，头晕目眩，时有烘热汗出，口干不欲饮，耳鸣腰酸，舌红少苔，脉细数无力。

（2）肝经湿热：带下量多，或赤白相间，或色黄如脓，有臭味，阴部瘙痒，甚则疼痛，或尿频，尿痛，尿急，心烦少寐，口苦，胸闷不适，纳谷不香，苔黄腻，脉弦数。

二、治疗方法

【湿热内蕴证】

治法 调冲任，清湿热，通络息风。

处方 中极（RN3）、会阴（RN1）、阴廉（LR11）、三阴交（SP6）。

方义 中极系足三阴经与任脉之交会穴，具有调冲任、清利湿热、化瘀息风之功效；会阴乃任脉之络穴，阴廉为肝经之穴，二穴为近外阴部穴位，合用有清湿热、息肝风、治阴痒的作用。三阴交为肝、肾、

2. Symptom differentiation

(1) Yin deficiency of liver and kidney: Excessive leukorrhea, yellowish, thick and sticky, even blood-like, vaginal dryness, burning and itching, dysphoria in chest with palms-soles, dizziness, sometimes Heat and sweating, dry mouth without desire of drinking, tinnitus and waist soreness, red tongue and less tongue fur, thin and taut and weak pulse.

(2) Damp-Heat of Liver Channel: Excessive leukorrhea, or red and whitish, or color of yellow like pus, stinky, vaginal pruritus or even pain, or frequent micturition, painful micturition, urgent micturition, vexation and insufficient sleep, bitter taste, chest distress and discomfort, poor appetite, yellowish and greasy tongue fur, taut and rapid pulse.

II. Therapeutic Methods

[Sydrome of Internal Retention of Damp-Heat]

Therapeutic method: Nurse Chong Channel and Ren Channel, clear Damp-Heat, dredge collaterals and claim Wind.

Prescription: Zhongji (RN3), Huiyin (RN1), Yinlian (LR11), Sanyinjiao (SP6).

Mechanism of prescription: Zhongji is the confluent acupoint of three Yin Meridians of Foot and Ren Channel, it can nurse Chong Channel and Ren Channel, clear Damp-Heat, remove stasis and claim Wind. Huiyin is a collateral acupoint of Ren Channel, Yinlian is an acupoint of Liver Meridian, these two are acupoints near the vulva, the combination of them can remove Damp-Heat,

脾三经之交会穴，是主治妇科疾病及泌尿系统疾患的要穴，有疏通经络、清热利湿的作用。诸穴合用，共奏调冲任、清湿热、通络息风、治阴痒之功。

配穴 带下多、外阴潮湿者，加阴陵泉、蠡沟；胃肠积热者，加气冲；肝火盛者，加太冲；外阴营养不良者，加照海；若要扶正，加曲池、足三里。

方法 电热针治疗。

操作 选定穴位，皮肤常规消毒。电热针直刺中极0.7寸，直刺会阴0.7寸，直刺阴廉0.7寸，直刺三阴交0.6寸。接通电热针仪，每穴分别给予电流量60～70mA，留针40分钟。另配以毫针直刺足三里0.8寸，直刺阳陵泉0.7寸，直刺曲池0.7寸，直刺照海0.5寸，留针40分钟。

疗程 每日1次，10次为1个疗程。疗程间休息5～7天，再进行第2个疗程的治疗。连续治疗3～4个疗程即

claim liver Wind, and treat vaginal pruritus. Sanyinjiao is the confluent acupoint of Liver Meridian, Spleen Meridian and Kidney Meridian, an important acupoint which mainly used to treat gynecological diseases and diseases of urinary system, it can dredge meridians and collaterals, clear Heat and remove Damp. The use of combination of these four acupoints can nurse Chong Channel and Ren Channel, clear Damp-Heat, dredge collaterals and claim Wind.

Matching acupoints: For patients with excessive leukorrhea and Damp vulva, add Yinlingquan, Ligou. For patients with accumulated Heat in stomach and intestine, add Qichong; For patients with liver-fire hyperactivity, add Taichong, for patients with vulva dystrophy, add Zhaohai. For strengthening the healthy Qi, add Quchi, Zusanli.

Method: Electrothermal acupuncture treatment.

Operations: Selecting the relevant acupoints, perform routine skin disinfection. Using electrothermal acupuncture needles, vertically puncture into Zhongji, Huiyin and Yinlian for 0.7" respectively, Sanyinjiao for 0.6". Turn on the electrothermal acupuncture equipment, apply a current of 60-70mA to each acupoint. Leave the needles in for 40 minutes. Additionally, using the filiform needles, vertically puncture into Zusanli for 0.8", Yanglingquan and Quchi for 0.7", Zhaohai for 0.5", leaving the needles in for 40 minutes.

Therapeutic course: Once a day, 10 times for a course. Start the treatment for the second course after a break of 5-7 days. Cured after 3-4 continuous treatment courses.

可痊愈。

三、注意事项

1. 施针前令患者排空尿液，再针刺下腹部穴位，如中极、曲骨、会阴等穴。

2. 保持外阴部清洁干燥，注意经期卫生。

3. 如因全身疾病原因（如糖尿病）引起继发性外阴瘙痒者，应积极治疗原发病。

女阴白色病变

女阴白色病变是妇科常见病之一，又称外阴白斑或阴道白斑。本病可发生于各种年龄，但以中青年居多。

自 1885 年 Breisky 报道女阴白色病变以来，一直认为本病具有一定的恶性潜能，属于癌前病变。过去国内外多采取手术治疗，然而术后复发率高达 50%。近年来，研究人员从临床、病理方面对本病开展了深入的研究，认为本病具有上皮非典型增生者方属癌前期病变，治疗上已趋于保守疗法。

中医古代文献虽无与女阴白色病变相符的病名，但有很

III. Precautions

1. Instruct patients to empty urine before acupuncture, then puncture into acupoints at lower abdomen with needles, such as Zhongji, Qugu, Huiyin.

2. Keep vulva clean and dry, pay attention to hygiene during menstrual periods.

3. Patients with secondary pruritus vulvae caused by systemic diseases (such as diabete) should actively treat the primary disease.

Vulva White Lesion

Vulvae white lesion is one of the common gynecological diseases, which is also called leukoplakia vulvae or leukoplakia of vagina. This disease may occur on women of various ages, however it is more often found among young and middle-aged women.

Since Breisky reported the vulvae white lesion in 1885, this disease has always been considered having certain potential for malignancy, is a precancerous lesion. In the past normally surgical therapy was taken for this disease, however, the postoperative recurrence rate was as high as 50%. In recent years, researchers have carried out in-deep studies from the clinical, pathological aspects, and believe that the disease will only be considered as precancerous lesion when atypical epithelial hyperplasia occurs, and the treatment has tended to conservative therapies.

Although there is no disease name that matches with vulvae white lesion in ancient literatures of Tradi-

多对"阴痒"的描述与本病十分相似,现代中医文献《中国医学百科全书》《中医症状鉴别诊断学》等亦将本病归入阴痒门,类似的病名还有"阴肿""阴疮""阴痛""阴蠹""阴蚀"等。

一、诊断及辨证要点

1. 湿热下注

(1)全身症状:胸闷不适,口苦纳差,心烦不寐,舌质红,苔黄腻,脉弦数或滑数。

(2)局部症状:外阴瘙痒,疼痛或外阴肥厚,带下色黄,黏稠有味。

2. 肝肾不足

(1)全身症状:头晕目眩,两目干涩,腰膝酸软,舌质红,少苔,脉沉细或弦细无力。

(2)局部症状:外阴瘙痒,夜间尤甚,外阴皮肤干燥,甚则萎缩、皲裂,月经量少,白带不多。

3. 肝肾不足兼湿热下注

(1)全身症状:头晕目眩,口苦黏腻,腰脊酸困无力,舌

tional Chinese Medicine, many descriptions about "vulval itching" are very similar with this diseases. Modern Traditional Chinese Medicine literatures, such as Chinese Medical Encyclopedia, Syndrome Differentiation Diagnosis of Traditional Chinese Medicine, also classify this disease into "vulval itching", and similar disease names include "vulval swelling", "sore of vulva", "vaginal pain", "yinli", "erosion of vulva", etc.

I. Key Points for Diagnosis and Syndrome Differentiation

1. Downward flow of Damp-Heat

(1) Systemic syndromes: Chest distress and discomfort, bitter taste and poor appetite, vexation and sleeplessness, red tongue, yellowish and greasy tongue fur, taut and rapid or taut and slippery pulse.

(2) Local syndromes: Pruritus vulvae, pain or vulval hypertrophy, yellow leukorrhea, thick and stinky.

2. Liver and kidney deficiency

(1) Systemic syndromes: Dizziness, dry eyes, soreness and weakness of waist and knees, red tongue, less tongue fur, deep and thin or taut, thin and weak pulse.

(2) Local syndromes: Pruritus vulvae, especially at night, dry or even shrinking, chapped vulval skins, less menstrual blood volume, less leukorrhea.

3. Liver and kidney deficiency accompanied with downward flow of Damp-Heat

(1) Systemic syndromes: Dizziness, bitter taste and sticky, soreness and weakness of spinal column, red

质红，苔少或黄腻，脉弦细或沉细。

（2）局部症状：外阴瘙痒，或灼痛，外阴萎缩，带下量多，色黄有味。

二、治疗方法

【湿热下注证】

治法 健脾利湿,通经活络。

处方 脾俞（BL20）、阴陵泉（SP9）、三阴交（SP6）、中极（RN3）、阿是穴。

方义 脾俞为背俞穴，是脾脏之气输注于背部的腧穴，针刺脾俞可以调节脾脏功能，有健脾化湿之功；阴陵泉为足太阴脾经之合穴，可健脾化湿，通利三焦；三阴交为足太阴、足厥阴、足少阴之会，可调节三阴经经气，助脾运化，通经活络；中极为任脉经穴，可利膀胱，埋下注，治阴部疾患；丰隆为足阳明胃经之络穴，可利湿化痰，与脾俞、阴陵泉相配，可加强利湿之功。

配穴 湿热下注加丰隆；热重于湿加曲池；心烦不寐加太冲。

tongue, less or yellowish and greasy tongue fur, taut and thin or deep and thin pulse.

(2) Local syndromes: Pruritus vulvae, or vulval burning pain, vulva atrophy, excessive leukorrhea, yellowish and stinky.

II. Therapeutic Methods

[Syndrome of downward flow of Damp-Heat]

Therapeutic method: Invigorate spleen and remove Damp, dredge meridians and collaterals.

Prescription: Pishu (BL20), Yinlingquan (SP9), Sanyinjiao (SP6), Zhongji (RN3), Ashi.

Mechanism of prescription: Pishu is a Back-Shu acupoint, the acupoint where the spleen Qi infuse in. Acupuncture of Pishu can regulate spleen functions, invigorate spleen and remove Damp, dredge the three Jiaos; Sanyinjiao is the confluent acupoint of Tai-Yin Meridian of Foot, Jue-Yin Meridian of Foot and Shao-Yin Meridian of Foot, it can regulate meridian Qi of three Yin meridians, help transportation and transformation of spleen, dredge meridians and collaterals; Zhongji is an meridian acupoint of three Yin meridians, it can unblock bladder, govern downward flows, treat vulval diseases; Fenglong is a collateral acupoint of Yang-Ming Stomach Meridian of Foot, it can remove Damp and disperse phlegm, and can enhance the effect of Damp removing when being matched with Pishu and Yinlingquan.

Matching acupoints: For patients with downward flow of Damp-Heat, add Fenglong. For patients of Damp-Heat syndrome with predominant Heat, add Quchi. For patients with vexation and sleeplessness, add Taichong.

Method: Electrothermal acupuncture treatment.

Operations: Selecting the relevant acupoints, perform routine skin disinfection. Using electrothermal acupuncture needles, vertically puncture into Yinlingquan for 0.7", Sanyinjiao for 0.6", locally horizontally puncture or obliquely puncture into Ashi for 0.6". Turn on the electrothermal acupuncture equipment, apply a current of 60-70mA to each acupoint. The limit is that the patient feels partial warm and comfortable. Leave the needles in for 40 minutes. Additionally, using the filiform needles, vertically puncture into Zhongji for 0.6", Fenglong for 0.7", Taichong and Quchi for 0.6" respectively. Leave the needles in for 40 minutes.

Therapeutic course: Treat once a day, 30 times for a course. Start the treatment for the second course after a break of 7-10 days. Generally cured after 2-3 courses.

[Liver and Kidney Deficiency]

Therapeutic method: Reinforce vital essence and replenish Qi, tonify liver and kidney.

Prescriptions: Taichong (LR3), Taixi (KI3), Sanyinjiao (SP6), Guanyuan (RN4), Shenshu (BL23).

Mechanism of prescription: Taichong is a Yuan acupoint of Jue-Yin Liver Meridian of Foot, it can tonify Qi-blood of Liver Meridian; Taixi is a Yuan acupoint of Shao-Yin Kidney Meridian of Foot, it can regulate and replenish kidney Qi; Sanyinjiao is the confluent acupoint of three Yin Meridians of Foot, it can enhance Qi of me-

可培补元气，通调冲任；肾俞为背俞穴，具有补益肾气的作用。

配穴 腰膝酸痛加足三里；两目干涩加蠡沟。

方法 电热针治疗。

操作 选定穴位，皮肤常规消毒。电热针直刺足三里 0.7 寸，直刺三阴交 0.6 寸，平刺阿是穴 0.6 寸。接通电热针仪，每个穴位分别给予电流量 60～70mA，以局部温热为度。另配以毫针直刺太冲 0.5 寸，直刺太溪 0.5 寸，直刺关元 0.7 寸，留针 40 分钟。

疗程 每日 1 次，30 次为 1 个疗程。疗程间可休息 7～10 天，再进行第 2 个疗程的治疗。一般治疗 2～3 个疗程即可痊愈。

【肝肾不足兼湿热下注证】

治法 补肝益肾，清热利湿。

处方 太冲（LR3）、太溪（KI3）、阴陵泉（SP9）、三阴交（SP6）、中极（RN3）、阿是穴。

方义 太冲、太溪分别为

ridians and channels; Guanyuan is a meridian acupoint of Ren Channel located at the pubic region, it can replenish vitality, nurse Chong Channel and Ren Channel; Shenshu is a Back-Shu acupoint, it can replenish kidney Qi.

Matching acupoints: For soreness of waist and knees add Zusanli. For dry eyes add Ligou.

Method: Electrothermal acupuncture treatment.

Operations: Selecting the relevant acupoints, perform routine skin disinfection. Using electrothermal acupuncture needles, vertically puncture into Zusanli for 0.7", Sanyinjiao for 0.6", horizontally puncture into Ashi for 0.6". Turn on the electrothermal acupuncture equipment, apply a current of 60-70mA to each acupoint. The limit is that the patient feels partially warm. Additionally, using filiform needles, vertically puncture into Taichong and Taixi for 0.5" respectively, Guanyuan for 0.7", leaving the needles in for 40 minutes.

Therapeutic course: Treat once a day, 30 times for a course. Start the treatment for the second course after a break of 7-10 days. Generally cured after 2-3 courses.

[Liver and Kidney Deficiency Accompanied with Downward Flow of Damp-Heat]

Therapeutic method: Replenish liver and tonify kidney, clear Heat and remove Damp.

Prescription: Taichong (LR3), Taixi (KI3), Yinlingquan (SP9), Sanyinjiao (SP6), Zhongji (RN3), Ashi.

Mechanism of prescription: Taichong and Taixi

足厥阴肝经、足少阴肾经之原穴，可调肝肾；三阴交可交通三阴经，既可健脾利湿，又能益肾补肝；中极可泻下焦湿热；酌情选配脾俞、肾俞、会阴。

配穴 湿热下注加丰隆；热重于湿加曲池；心烦不寐加太冲；腰膝酸软加肾俞。

方法 电热针治疗。

操作 选定穴位，皮肤常规消毒。电热针直刺阴陵泉 0.7 寸，直刺三阴交 0.6 寸，平刺阿是穴 0.7 寸。接通电热针仪，每个穴位分别给予电流量 60～70mA，以局部温热舒适为度，留针 40 分钟。另配以毫针直刺太冲 0.6 寸，直刺太溪 0.5 寸，直刺中极 0.7 寸，直刺会阴 0.6 寸，留针 40 分钟。起针后，快针直刺脾俞 0.6 寸，直刺肾俞 0.6 寸，不留针。

疗程 每日 1 次，30 次为 1 个疗程。疗程间休息 7～10 天，再进行第 2 个疗程的治疗。一般治疗 2～3 个疗程即

are Yuan acupoints of Jue-Yin Liver Meridian of Foot and Shao-Yin Kidney Meridian of Foot respectively, they can tonify liver and kidney; Sanyinjiao enables connection and communication of three Yin Meridians, it can invigorate spleen and remove Damp as well as tonify kidney and liver; Zhongji can purge Damp-Heat of Lower Jiao; match with Pishu, Shenshu or Huiyin if necessary.

Matching acupoints: For patients with downward flow of Damp-Heat, add Fenglong. For patients of Damp-Heat syndrome with predominant Heat, add Quchi. For patients with vexation and sleeplessness, add Taichong. For patients with soreness and weakness of waist and knees, add Shenshu.

Method: Electrothermal acupuncture treatment.

Operations: Selecting the relevant acupoints, perform routine skin disinfection. Using electrothermal acupuncture needles, vertically puncture into Yinlingquan for 0.7", Sanyinjiao for 0.6", horizontally puncture into Ashi for 0.7". Turn on the electrothermal acupuncture equipment, apply a current of 60-70mA to each acupoint. The limit is that the patient feels partially warm and comfortable. Leave the needles in for 40 minutes. Additionally, using filiform needles, vertically puncture into Taichong for 0.6", Taixi for 0.5", Zhongji for 0.7", Huiyin for 0.6", leaving the needles in for 40 minutes. After withdrawal of needles, vertically puncture into Pishu rapidly for 0.6", Shenshu for 0.6", do not leave the needles in.

Therapeutic course: Treat once a day, 30 times for a course. Start the treatment for the second course after a break of 7-10 days. Generally cured after 2-3 courses.

可痊愈。

三、注意事项

1. 针刺会阴时注意消毒及针刺体位，避免针后不舒适感。针刺中极前令患者排空尿液。

2. 注意外阴部卫生，避免重复感染。

3. 针刺阿是穴（阴唇部位）时注意起针后的局部止血，因为黏膜部位易出血，出针后要用棉球压迫2分钟。

4. 多进食健脾补肾之品，如山药、银杏、新鲜蔬菜等，特别是要多摄入含维生素B1的食物。

功能性子宫出血

功能性子宫出血指经妇科检查未发现生殖器官器质性病变，而因内分泌失调所引起的子宫内膜异常出血，简称"宫血"。有无排卵型宫血和排卵型宫血之分。前者系排卵功能发生障碍，好发于青春期和更年期；后者系黄体功能失调，多见于育龄期妇女，临床主要表现为月经周期紊乱，经量增多，出血时间延长，淋漓不尽

III. Precautions

1. Pay attention to sterilization and body position for acupuncture of Huiyin, to avoid discomfort after puncture. Instruct patients to empty urine before acupuncture of Zhongji.

2. Pay attention to hygiene of vulva, avoid repeated infections.

3. For acupuncture of Ashi (labium area), note that after withdrawal of needles local stanching is required due to that mucosal part is easy to bleed, so the wound should be compressed with a cotton ball after needle withdrawal for 2 minutes.

4. Eat more foods that can invigorate spleen and replenish kidney, such as yam, ginkgo and fresh vegetables, especially more foods containing vitamin B1.

Functional Uterine Hemorrhage

Functional uterine hemorrhage refers to that endometrial abnormal bleeding due to endocrine dyscrasia while there is no organic lesion of genitals found in gynecological examinations, and it is called "uterine hemorrhage" for short. It is divided into anovulatory uterine hemorrhage and ovulatory uterine hemorrhage. The former refers to ovaulation dysfunction, normally occurs in adolescence and menopause; the later refers to corpus luteum disorders, normally occurs in women of childbearing age, main clinical manifestations include irregular menstrual periods, increased blood volume, prolonged

等。长期出血可伴有面色苍白、心慌无力等贫血症状。主要是由于下丘脑－垂体－卵巢这一性腺轴功能失调所致。任何因素影响这一系统的正常功能，均可造成子宫内膜的异常出血。

中医认为，本病属于"崩漏"的范畴。多因素体阳盛，七情过极，思虑过度，饮食劳倦，以及素体肾气不足及房劳多育所致，与肝、脾、肾三脏功能失调密切相关。

一、诊断及辨证要点

1. 辨病

（1）子宫不规则出血，月经量多，经期延长，经血淋漓不断，月经先期，先后无定期，经间出血等，连续发病3个月经周期以上。

（2）排除生殖器官器质性病变和妊娠并发症或全身性及血液系统疾病。

（3）卵巢功能检查

1）无排卵型宫血：经前宫内膜活检呈增殖期或各种类型的增生，少数可见萎缩性病变，阴道涂片多受雌激素高度

bleeding time and endless bleeding. The long-time bleeding may be accompanied with anemia symptoms such as pale complexion, palpitation and weakness. It is mainly caused by dysfunction of the gonadal axis composed of hypothalamus-pituitary-ovarian. Any factor affecting the normal function of this system can cause abnormal bleeding in the endometrium.

Traditional Chinese Medicine believes that this disease belongs to the range of "metrorrhagia and metrostaxis". It is caused by multi-factor Yang hyperactivity, extreme seven emotions, worry beyond measure, improper diet and fatigue, as well as insufficient kidney Qi and excess childbearing, and it is closely related with dysfunctions of liver, spleen and kidney.

I. Key Points for Diagnosis and Syndrome Differentiation

1. Disease differentiation

(1) Irregular uterine bleeding, increased blood volume, prolonged bleeding time and endless bleeding, advanced menstruation, irregular menstrual periods, intermenstrual bleeding, etc. Continuous onset for more than 3 menstrual periods.

(2) Exclude organic lesion of genitals and pregnancy complications or systemic and hematological system diseases.

(3) Ovarian function examination

1) Anovulatory uterine hemorrhage: Premenstrual endometrial biopsy shows proliferative or various types of hyperplasia, and atrophic lesions may be found in a few cases. Most vaginal smears results are greatly af-

影响，亦有低中度者，经前宫颈黏液呈半齿状结晶，基础体温为单向型。

2）排卵型宫血：①黄体不健：经前子宫内膜分泌功能不良，阴道涂片有时可见角化细胞指数偏高，细胞堆积，皱褶不佳；基础体温双相型，黄体期缩短，在10天以下，或梯形上升或下降，亦可为14天左右，但在月经前期，体温未下降时即有少量出血。②黄体萎缩不全：经前第5天子宫内膜呈内分泌期改变；基础体温呈不典型双相型，下降延迟或逐渐下降。

2. 辨证

（1）虚热证：经血非时突然而下，量多势急或量少淋漓，或经来先期，或周期正常，月经过多或经期延长，血色鲜红而质稠，心烦潮热，头昏耳鸣，小便黄，大便秘结，舌红，苔薄黄，脉细数。

（2）实热证：经血非时忽然大下，或淋漓日久，或经来先期，或周期正常，月经过多，血色深红质稠，口渴烦热，或有发热，小便黄，大便干结，舌红，苔黄腻，脉洪数。

fected by estrogens, and in some cases of low-moderate levels, the premenstrual cervix mucosa present as half-toothy crystals, the basal body temperature (BBT) is monophasic type.

2) Ovulatory uterine hemorrhage: ① Luteal phase defect: Premenstrual endometrial secretion dysfunction, sometimes high keratinocyte index, cell accumulation and poor winkles may be seen in vaginal smears; diphasic BBT, shorten luteal phase which less than 10 days, or adder-shaped decline or rise, or around 14 days, however during pre-menstrual period before the body temperature decline there also is small-volume bleeding. ② Corpus luteum atrophy: The endometrium presents secretory-phase changes 5 days before menstruation; the BBT represents as atypital diphasic type, with delayed decline or graduate decline.

2. Symptom differentiation

(1) Syndrome of deficiency-Heat: Irregular sudden menstruation, excessive and quick or less and endless, or advanced menstruation, or normal period, excessive volume or prolonged periods, red and thick menstrual blood, vexation and hot flash, dizziness and tinnıtus, yellow urine, constipation, red tongue, yellow and thin tongue fur, thin and rapid pulse.

(2) Syndrome of excess-Heat: Irregular sudden menstruation with large volume, or long-time endless menstruation, or advanced menstruation, or normal period, excessive volume or prolonged periods, dark and thick menstrual blood, thirsty and dysphoria with smothery sensation, or fever, dry stool and constipation,

（3）肾虚证：①偏肾阳虚者：经来无期，出血量多或淋漓不止，血色淡、质清，畏寒肢冷，面色晦暗，腰膝酸软，小便清长，舌质淡，苔薄白，脉沉细。②偏肾阴虚者：经乱无期，出血淋漓不尽或量多，血色鲜红，质稍稠，头晕目眩，腰膝酸软，或心烦，舌质偏红，苔少，脉细数。

（4）脾虚证：经血非时而下，崩中继而淋漓，或月经先期，或周期正常，月经过多，血色淡而质薄，气短神疲，面色白，或面浮肢肿，手足不温，或饮食不佳，舌质淡嫩，苔薄白，脉弱或沉弱。

（5）血瘀证：经血非时而下，时下时止，或淋漓不尽，或停闭日久又突然崩中下血，继而淋漓不断，血色紫黑有块，小腹疼痛或胀痛，块下痛减，舌质紫黯或舌边有瘀点，苔薄白，脉涩。

red tongue, yellow and greasy tongue fur, full and rapid pulse.

(3) Syndrome of kidney deficiency: ① Yang deficiency of kidney: Irregular menstruation with excessive or dripping and endless blood flow, light color and thin blood, intolerance of cold and extreme chilliness, gloomy complexion, soreness and weakness of waist and knees, clear abundant urine, pale tongue, thin and whitish tongue fur, deep and thin pulse. ② Yin deficiency of kidney: Irregular menstruation with excessive or dripping and endless blood flow, bright red and slight thick blood, dizziness, soreness and weakness of waist and knees, or vexation, reddish tongue and less tongue fur, thin and rapid pulse.

(4) Syndrome of spleen deficiency: Irregular menstruation, metrorrhagia followed by dripping blood, or advanced menstruation, or normal period, thin blood with light color, shortness of breath and mental fatigue, pale complexion, light and tender tongue, thin and whitish tongue, weak or deep and weak pulse.

(5) Syndrome of blood stasis: Irregular menstruation, intermittent or dripping and endless blood flow, or sudden bleeding of metrorrhagia after long-time cessation of menstruation followed by dripping and endless blood flow, dark purple blood with clots, pain or swelling of lower abdomen, pain relief with clots discharge, dark purple tongue or ecchymosis at tongue edge, thin and whitish tongue, uneven pulse.

二、治疗方法

【冲任不固证】

治法 调补冲任，统经固摄。

处方 关元（RN4）、三阴交（SP6）、太冲（LR3）、隐白（SP1）。

方义 关元为足三阴、冲脉、任脉之会，可以调补冲任，加强固摄，制约经血妄行；三阴交为足三阴经之交会穴，有补脾统血之功；太冲系肝经原穴，有疏肝理气、通络活血之功；隐白为脾经井穴，是治疗妇科出血的常用效穴。诸穴共用，可调肝、脾、肾三经，收到疏肝理气、统血固摄的效果。

配穴 血热加血海、水泉；脾虚加脾俞、足三里；血崩欲脱加百会、人中。

方法 电热针治疗。

II. Therapeutic Methods

[Syndrome of Unconsolidation of Chong Channel and Ren Channel]

Therapeutic method: Nurse and replenish Chong Channel and Ren Channel, govern meridians and secure astringency.

Prescription: Guanyuan (RN4), Sanyinjiao (SP6), Taichong (LR3), Yinbai (SP1).

Mechanism of prescription: Guanyuan is the confluent acupoint of the three Yin Meridians of Foot, Chong Channel and the Ren Channel, which can nurse and replenish Chong Channel and Ren Channel, strengthen astringency, restrict frenetic movement of Qi-blood; Sanyinjiao is the confluent acupoint of the three Yin Meridians of Foot, which can tonify spleen and regulate blood; Taichong is a Yuan acupoint of Liver Meridian, which can soothe liver and regulate Qi, dredge collaterals and activate blood circulation; Yinbai is a Jing acupoint of Spleen Meridian, which is a commonly used effective acupoint for treatment of gynecological hemorrhage. The use of combination of these acupoints can tonify Liver Meridian, Spleen Meridian and Kidney Meridian to achieve the effects of soothing liver and regulating Qi, governing blood and securing astringency.

Matching acupoints: For blood-Heat patients, add Xuehai, Shuiquan. For patients with spleen deficiency, add Pishu, Zusanli. For metrorrhagia nearing dislocation add Baihui, Renzhong.

Method: Electrothermal acupuncture treatment.

操作 选定穴位，皮肤常规消毒。电热针直刺关元0.7寸，直刺三阴交0.7寸，直刺足三里0.7寸。接通电热针仪，每个穴位分别给予电流量60～70mA，以舒适胀感为度，留针40分钟。另配以毫针直刺太冲0.5寸，直刺隐白0.3寸，直刺血海0.6寸，留针40分钟。起针后，快针斜刺脾俞，不留针。

疗程 每天1次，10次为1个疗程。疗程间可休息3～5天，再进行第2个疗程的治疗。一般治疗3～4个疗程。

三、注意事项

1. 更年期妇女如反复出血不断，需做妇科检查以明确诊断。

2. 遇大量出血而出现虚脱时，如用针灸效果欠佳，应立即采取止血、抗休克等综合处理，以免贻误治疗时机。

3. 阴道出血期间，下腹部及腰骶部穴位不宜强刺激，以免发生出血过多。亦要及时查找出血原因，予以合理处理。

Operations: Selecting the relevant acupoints, perform routine skin disinfection. Using electrothermal acupuncture needles, vertically puncture into Guanyuan, Sanyinjiao and Zusanli for 0.7" respectively. Turn on the electrothermal acupuncture equipment, apply a current of 60-70mA to each acupoint. The limit is that the patient feels comfortable and swelling. Leave the needles in for 40 minutes. Additionally, using filiform needles, vertically puncture into Taichong for 0.5", Yinbai for 0.3", Xuehai for 0.6", leaving the needles in for 40 minutes. After withdrawal of needles, obliquely and quickly puncture into Pishu, do not leave the needles in the body.

Therapeutic course: Once a day, 10 times for a course. Start the treatment for the second course after a break of 3-5 days. Generally treat for 3-4 courses.

III. Precautions

1. For menopause women with constantly repeated bleeding, gynecological examination is required to further confirm the diagnosis.

2. For collapse due to excessive bleeding, if the effect of acupuncture treatment is poor, comprehensive treatments such as hemostasis and antishock should be taken immediately to avoid losing the treatment opportunity because of a delay.

3. During vaginal bleeding, strong stimulation of acupoints at lower abdomen and lumbosacral portion should be avoid to prevent excessive bleeding. It is also necessary to find out the cause of bleeding and properly treat it.

Uterine Prolapse

Uterine prolapse refers to that the uterus moves down along the vagina to a level below the ischial spine or even out of the vaginal orifice. Uterine prolapse is a displacement diseases of female genital organs, which mainly occurs in married, delivered women and laboring women. The occurrence of this disease is related to delivery injuries, thin and weak pelvic support tissues, reduced tension, increased intra-abdominal pressure, effects of delivery position and change of pelvic tilt. It often recurs due to excessive fatigue, sharp cough, defecation straining. Non-timely treatment will cause delayed healing.

Traditional Chinese Medicine believes that uterine prolapse belongs to the range of "prolapse of the uterus", "uterine protruding", "eggplant-like vagina", "uterine procidentia", "vaginal bacteria", "uterine ptosis", etc. It is also called "non-withdrawal of birth canal" or "non-withdrawal of childbirth canal" due to that it normally occurs after delivery. It mostly caused by weak body, Middle-Jiao Qi deficiency or excessive deliveries, depletion and deficiency of kidney Qi, along with excessive efforts during delivery or too early physical labor after delivery, leading to Middle-Jiao Qi collapse, non-consolidation of kidney Qi, Dai Channel dysfunction, so in most cases this disease is a deficiency syndrome.

I. Key Points for Diagnosis and Syndrome Differentiation

1. Middle-Jiao Qi collapse: Uterine prolapse, bear-

小腹下坠，劳动后加重，神疲肢倦，面色少华，带下量多，舌淡苔白，脉细无力。

2. 肾气不固：子宫脱垂，小腹下坠，腰酸腿软，小便频数，夜间尤甚，头晕耳鸣，舌淡苔白，脉沉无力。

二、治疗方法

【中气下陷证】

治法　补气升阳，提摄子宫。

处方　百会（DU20）、维道（GB28）、三阴交（SP6）、足三里（ST36）、子宫（EX-CA1）、维胞（EX-CA）。

方义　百会为督脉穴，督脉总督一身之阳气，取之有升阳举陷之功；维道属足少阳、带脉之会穴，有收摄胞宫的作用；三阴交、足三里可健脾益气，培补中气；子宫、维胞为经外奇穴，有提摄子宫之效，是治疗子宫脱垂之效穴。诸穴共用，可收补气升阳、提摄子宫之功。

配穴　小腹下坠重者加中脘、脾俞。

ing-down feeling of lower abdomen, aggravated after physical labor, mental and physical fatigue, pale complexion, excessive leukorrhea, light tongue with whitish fur, thin and weak pulse.

2. Non-consolidation of kidney Qi: Uterine prolapse, bearing-down feeling of lower abdomen, aching lumbus and limp legs, frequent urination especially at night, dizziness and tinnitus, light tongue with whitish fur, deep and weak pulse.

II. Therapeutic Methods

[Syndrome of Middle-Jiao Qi Collapse]

Therapeutic method: Tonify Qi and ascend up Yang, raise uterus.

Prescription: Baihui (DU20), Weidao (GB28), Sanyinjiao (SP6), Zusanli (ST36), Zigong (EX-CA1), Weibao(EX-CA).

Mechanism of prescription: Baihui is an acupoint of Du Channel, and Du Channel governs systemic Yang Qi, use this acupoint can ascend up Yang and collapse; Weidao is the confluent acupoint of Shao-Yang Meridian of Foot and Dai Channel, which can control uterus; Sanyinjiao and Zusanli can invigorate spleen and tonify Qi, reinforce Middle-Jiao Qi; Zigong and Baowei are external nerve acupoints, can raise uterus, and have extremely good efficacies on uterine prolapse. The use of combination of these acupoints can tonify Qi and ascend up Yang, raise uterus.

Matching acupoints: For patients with severe bearing-down feeling of abdomen, add Zhongwan, Pishu.

Method: Electrothermal acupuncture treatment.

Operations: Selecting the relevant acupoints, perform routine skin disinfection. Using electrothermal acupuncture needles, horizontally puncture forward along the skin into Baihui for 0.7", obliquely puncture along the groin with the needle tip towards inner inferior into Weidao for 0.8", to let the patient has a feeling of twitching, vertically puncture into Sanyinjiao for 0.7", Zusanli for 0.8", Zigong for 0.7", obliquely puncture into Weibao with downward needle tip for 0.7". Turn on the electrothermal acupuncture equipment, apply a current of 60-70mA to each acupoint. The limit is that the patient feels comfortable and swelling. Leave the needles in for 40 minutes.

Therapeutic course: Once a day, 10 times for a course. Start the treatment for the second course after a break of 3-5 days, or perform continuous treatment. Generally the treatment can be ended after 3-6 courses.

[Syndrome of Non-consolidation of Kidney Qi]

Therapeutic method: Replenish kidney and enforce Chong, elevate uterus.

Prescription: Guanyuan (RN4), Dahe (KI12), Zhaohai (9KI6), Zigong (EX-CAI), Weibao(EX-CA).

Mechanism of prescription: Guanyuan is an acupoint of Ren Channel as well as a Mu acupoint of Tai-Yang Small Intestine Meridian of Hand, it has the effect of strengthening, and can replenish kidney Qi and reinforce Chong Channel when being matched with the acupoints Dahe and Zhaohai of Shao-Yin Meridian of Foot;

穴，对子宫脱垂有奇效。诸穴共用，有补肾固冲、升提胞宫之效。

配穴 脾肾阳虚者，加百会、气海、三阴交；腰膝酸软者，加肾俞、曲泉。

方法 电热针治疗。

操作 选定穴位，皮肤常规消毒。电热针向前阴部斜刺关元2寸，直刺大赫0.8寸，直刺照海0.7寸，直刺子宫0.7寸，针尖朝下斜刺维胞0.5寸。接通电热针仪，每个穴位分别给予电流量60～70mA，以患者舒适为度，留针40分钟。

疗程 每天1次，10次为1个疗程。疗程间休息3～5天，再进行第2个疗程的治疗。一般治疗3～6个疗程即可达到临床治愈。

三、注意事项

1. 针刺时，须将脱出于阴边外的子宫推入会阴后再进行针刺，同时还要垫高臀部。

2. 针刺腹部穴位时，要让针感达到会阴部或使前阴部有

Dahe is used to enforce lower origin, and Zhaohai is used to tonify kidney Qi; Zigong and Baowei are external nerve acupoints, have extremely good efficacies on uterine prolapse. The use of combination of these acupoints can replenish kidney and reinforce Chong, elevate uterus.

Matching acupoints: For Yang deficiency of spleen and kidney add Baihui, Qihai, Sanyinjiao. For aching lumbus and limp knees add Shenshu, Ququan.

Method: Electrothermal acupuncture treatment.

Operations: Selecting the relevant acupoints, perform routine skin disinfection. Using electrothermal acupuncture needles, obliquely puncture towards external genitalia into Guanyuan for 2", vertically puncture into Dahe for 0.8", Zhaohai and Zigong for 0.7" respectively, obliquely puncture into Weibao with downward needle tip for 0.5". Turn on the electrothermal acupuncture equipment, apply a current of 60-70mA to each acupoint. The limit is that the patient feels comfortable. Leave the needles in for 40 minutes.

Therapeutic course: Once a day, 10 times for a course. Start the treatment for the second course after a break of 3-5 days. Generally clinically cured after 3-6 courses.

III. Precautions

1. During acupuncture, the uterus out of vagina edge should be pushed into vagina edge before acupuncture, while the buttock should be elevated.

2. When puncturing acupoints at abdomen, the feeling of needle puncturing should be spread to perineum or

收缩感，效果会更好。

3. 治疗期间不宜参加较重的体力劳动，停止房事。

4. 应注意会阴部卫生，防止继发感染。

5. 每次电热针治疗后，患者应配合膝胸卧位30分钟；病情严重的患者，在电热针治疗的同时可加用放置子托；并指导患者做提肛运动锻炼，具体方法为一收一放，每次15～20分钟，每日1次。

不孕症

凡婚后夫妇同居3年以上未避孕而不受孕者，称原发性不孕；婚后曾有过妊娠（流产、分娩）、相距3年以上未避孕而不再受孕者，称继发性不孕。女性因素引起的不孕症，主要因卵巢分泌及卵子生成障碍、生殖道畸形等造成精子、卵子结合障碍，或孕卵着床困难所致。

中医称本病为"无子""绝产"等，其发病主要与肝肾和冲任二脉有关。肾主藏精，为先天之本，主生殖；冲为血海，任主胞胎，所以肾精亏

let the external genitalia has a feeling of shrinking, then the effect will be better.

3. During treatment, participating in heavy physical labour is improper, and sexual intercouses should be stopped.

4. Attentions should be paid to perineum hygiene, so as to avoid secondary infections.

5. Each time after electrothermal acupuncture treatment, the patient should lay in chest-knee position for 30 minutes. For patients with serious conditions, placing tray can be used; and instruct patients to do contracting anus exercises, the method is one time of contracting and one time of releasing, 15-20 minutes each time, once a day.

Infertilitas Feminis

For infertilitas feminis that patients have more than 3-year cohabitation without contraception, called primary infertility. For infertilitas feminis that patients have pregnancy history (abortion, delivery) after getting married, then have no pregnancy for more than 3 years without contraception, called secondary infertility. Infertilitas feminis due to females is mainly caused by ovarian secretion dysfunction or oogenesis dysfunction, reproductive tract malformation leading to egg-sperm binding dysfunction, or fertilized egg bedding difficulties.

In Traditional Chinese Medicine this disease is called "childless", "sterilization", etc. Its onset is mainly associated with liver, kidney and Chong Channel, Ren Channel. Kidney governs storage of essence, is the congenital foundation, and governs reproduction; Chong

损，肝郁气滞，痰湿阻胞，血瘀寒凝等，均可致肾虚不养，冲任失调而致不孕。病因肾者多为虚证不孕；病因气、血、痰湿者多为实证不孕。

Channel is the sea of blood, Ren Channel governs fetus, so depletion of kidney essence, liver stasis and Qi stagnation, phlegm Damp obstruting fetus, blood stasis and cold coagulation, all can cause kidney depletion without nourishment, disorder of Chong Channel and Ren Channel, leading to infertilitas feminis. Most infertilitas feminis caused by kidney problems are deficiency syndrome; most infertilitas feminis caused by Qi, blood, phlegm Damp are the excess syndrome.

一、诊断及辨证要点

I. Key Points for Diagnosis and Syndrome Differentiation

1. 肾虚：婚久不孕，腰膝酸软，或经行后期，量少色淡，性欲减退，便溏，舌淡，苔白，脉沉细；或经行先期，量少色赤，形体消瘦，心悸失眠，头晕耳鸣，舌红少苔，脉细数。

1. Kidney deficiency: Long-time marriage with infertility, soreness and weakness of waist and knees, or delayed menstruation, less menstrual blood volume and light color, hyposexuality, sloppy stool, light tongue with whitish fur, deep and thin pulse; or advanced menstruation, less volume and red color, emaciation, palpitation and insomnia, dizziness and tinnitus, red tongue with less fur, thin and rapid pulse.

2. 肝郁：多年不孕，经行先后不定，量少色暗或有血块，经前乳房胀痛，精神抑郁，烦躁易怒，舌红，苔薄白，脉弦。

2. Liver stagnation: Infertility for several years, irregular menstruation, less volume and dark color or with blood clots, premenstrual breast distending pain, mental depression, irritability, red tongue, thin and whitish tongue fur, taut pulse.

3. 痰湿：婚后久不受孕，形体肥胖，经行后期，带下量多、质黏，心悸头晕，胸闷呕恶，舌淡胖嫩，边有齿痕，苔白厚腻，脉滑。

3. Phlegm Damp: Long-time marriage with infertility, obesity, delayed menstruation, excessive and thick leukorrhea, palpitation and dizziness, chest distress, nausea and vomiting, light and fat and tender tongue with teeth prints at edge, thick and greasy whitish tongue fur, slippery pulse.

4. 血瘀：婚后久不孕育，经行后期，量少色黑并有血块，经行腹痛，舌黯有瘀斑，脉弦。

二、治疗方法

【肾虚证】

治法 益肾补经，调养冲任。

处方 肾俞（BL23）、关元（RN4）、三阴交（SP6）、足三里（ST36）、内关（PC6）、然谷（KI2）、气穴（KI13）、子宫（EX-CA1）。

方义 肾俞是足太阳经穴，取之补益肾气；任脉穴关元调补冲任二经；取足阳明经穴足三里培补后天；合足太阴脾经穴三阴交助后天以养先天；手厥阴经穴内关为八脉交会之一，合足少阴经穴然谷益肾固经；气穴为肾经穴，子宫为经外奇穴，取之可调养胞宫，为治不孕之效穴。诸穴共用，可收益肾补经、调养冲任之功。

4. Blood stasis: Long-time marriage with infertility, delayed menstruation, less volume and dark color with blood clots, abdominal pain during menstruation, dark tongue with ecchymosis, taut pulse.

II. Therapeutic Methods

[Kidney Deficiency Syndrome]

Therapeutic method: Tonify kidney and nourish meridians, nurse Chong Channel and Ren Channel.

Prescription: Shenshu (BL23), Guanyuan (RN4), Sanyinjiao (SP6), Zusanli (ST36), Neiguan (PC6), Rangu (KI2), Qixue (KI13), Zigong (EX-CA1).

Mechanism of prescription: Shenshu is an acupoint of Tai-Yang Meridian of Foot, it can replenish and tonify kidney Qi; the acupoint Guanyuan of Ren Channel can nurse Chong Meridian and Ren Meridian. Use the acupoint Zusanli of Yang-Ming Meridian of Foot to reinforce acquired construction, and match it with the acupoint Sanyinjiao of Tai-Yin Spleen Meridian of Foot to facilitate acquired construction so as to nourish congenital construction; the acupoint Neiguan of Jue-Yin Meridian of Hand is one of the confluent acupoints of eight Channels, which can tonify kidney and secure meridians when being matched with the acupoint Rangu of Shao-Yin Meridian of Foot; Qixue is an acupoint of Kidney Meridian, Zigong is an extra nerve point, they can tonify uterus and are effective acupoints for treatment of infertilitas feminis. The use of combination of these acupoints can tonify kidney and nourish meridians, nurse Chong

方法 电热针治疗。

操作 选定穴位，皮肤常规消毒。电热针直刺关元 0.8 寸，直刺足三里 0.7 寸，直刺子宫 0.8 寸，直刺三阴交 0.7 寸。接通电热针仪，每个穴位分别给予电流量 60～70mA，以患者舒适为度。另配以毫针直刺内关 0.6 寸，直刺气穴 0.8 寸，直刺照海 0.5 寸，直刺然谷 0.6 寸，留针 40 分钟。起针后，向脊柱方向斜刺肾俞 0.7 寸，提插后不留针。

疗程 每天 1 次，10 次为 1 个疗程。疗程间休息 3～5 天，再进行第 2 个疗程的治疗。一般治疗 3～4 个疗程。

【肝郁证】

治法 疏肝理气，养血调经。

处方 中极（RN3）、四满（KI14）、太冲（LR3）、气穴（KI13）、阳陵泉（GB34）、三阴交（SP6）。

方义 中极为任脉要穴，可疏通冲任；四满是肾经穴，与中极相配能理气通经；太冲是足厥阴经的原穴，可舒筋解郁；阳陵泉可加强太冲调肝之功；气穴为足少阴经穴，能益

Channel and Ren Channel.

Method: Electrothermal acupuncture treatment.

Operations: Selecting the relevant acupoints, perform routine skin disinfection. Using electrothermal acupuncture needles, vertically puncture into Guanyuan for 0.8", Zusanli for 0.7", Zigong for 0.8", Sanyinjiao for 0.7". Turn on the electrothermal acupuncture equipment, apply a current of 60-70mA to each acupoint. The limit is that the patient feels comfortable. Additionally, using filiform needles, vertically puncture into Neiguan for 0.6", Qixue for 0.8", Zhaohai for 0.5", Rangu for 0.6", leaving the needles in for 40 minutes. After withdrawal of needles, obliquely puncture towards spine into Shenshu for 0.7", do not leave the needles in after lifting and thrusting.

Therapeutic course: Once a day, 10 times for a course. Start the treatment for the second course after a break of 3-5 days. Generally treat for 3-4 courses.

[Syndrome of Liver Stasis]

Therapeutic method: Soothe liver and regulate Qi, nourish blood and tonify meridians.

Prescription: Zhongji (RN3), Siman (KI14), Taichong (LR3), Qixue (KI13), Yanglingquan (GB34), Sanyinjiao (SP6).

Mechanism of prescription: Zhongji is an important acupoint of Ren Channel, it can dredge Chong Channel and Ren Channel; Siman is an acupoint of Kidney Meridian, which can regulate Qi and dredge meridians; Taichong is a Yuan acupoint of Jue-Yin Meridian of Foot, which can soothe channels and resolve stagnation; Yan-

冲任，调二阴，是治疗不孕之经验穴；足太阴脾经穴三阴交可调经养血。诸穴共用，具有疏肝理气、养血调经之功。

配穴 培补后天取足阳明经穴足三里，合足太阴脾经穴三阴交，助后天以养先天。

方法 电热针治疗。

操作 选定穴位，皮肤常规消毒。电热针向曲骨方向斜刺中极0.8寸，使感觉传至会阴部为佳，直刺四满0.8寸，直刺气穴0.8寸，直刺三阴交0.6寸。接通电热针仪，每个穴位分别给予50～60mA的电流量，以患者舒适为度，留针40分钟。

疗程 每日1次，30次为1个疗程。疗程间可休息3～5天，再进行第2个疗程的治疗。一般治疗3～4个疗程即可基本治愈。

【痰湿证】

治法 理气化痰，调经种子。

gingquan can enhance the effect of liver regulating by Taichong; Qixue is an acupoint of Shao-Yin Meridian of Foot, it can tonify Chong Channel and Ren Channel, regulate two Yins, is an experienced acupoint for treatment of infertilitas feminis; the acupoint Sanyinjiao of Tai-Yin Spleen Meridian of Foot can tonify meridians and nourish blood. The use of combination of these acupoints can soothe liver and regulate Qi, nourish blood and tonify meridians.

Matching acupoints: For reinforcing of acquired construction, use the acupoint Zusanli of Yang-Ming Meridian of Foot combined with the acupoint Sanyinjiao of Tai-Yin Spleen Meridian of Foot to facilitate acquired construction so as to nourish congenital construction.

Method: Electrothermal acupuncture treatment.

Operations: Selecting the relevant acupoints, perform routine skin disinfection. Using electrothermal acupuncture needles, obliquely puncture towards Qugu into Zhongji for 0.8", better the feeling spreading to the perineum, vertically puncture into Siman and Qixue for 0.8" respectively, Sanyinjiao for 0.6". Turn on the electrothermal acupuncture equipment, apply a current of 50-60mA to each acupoint. The limit is that the patient feels comfortable. Leave the needles in for 40 minutes.

Therapeutic course: Treat once a day, 30 times for a course. Start the treatment for the second course after a break of 3-5 days. Generally basically cured after 3-4 courses.

[Phlegm-Damp Syndrome]

Therapeutic method: Regulate Qi and disperse

处方 中极（RN3）、气冲（ST30）、丰隆（ST40）、三阴交（SP6）、阴陵泉（SP9）。

方义 中极为任脉经穴，气冲为足阳明经穴，又是冲脉的起点，两穴相配，可调理冲任；丰隆为足阳明之络，阴陵泉是足太阴之合，二者均为健脾和胃、祛湿化痰之要穴；三阴交为足太阴经穴，可调三阴，理气和血。诸穴共用，可理气化痰，调经种子。

方法 电热针治疗。

操作 选定穴位，皮肤常规消毒。电热针直刺中极 0.8 寸，直刺气冲 0.8 寸，直刺丰隆 0.7 寸，直刺三阴交 0.7 寸，直刺阴陵泉 0.7 寸。接通电热针仪，每个穴位分别给予电流量 50～60mA，以患者舒适为度，留针 40 分钟。

疗程 每日 1 次，30 次为 1 个疗程。疗程间可休息 7～10 天，再进行第 2 个疗程的治疗。一般治疗 2～3 个疗程。

phlegm, regulate menstruation, seeding.

Prescription: Zhongji (RN3), Qichong (ST30), Fenglong (ST40), Sanyinjiao (SP6), Yinlingquan (SP9).

Mechanism of prescription: Zhongji is a meridian acupoint of Ren Channel, Qichong is a meridian acupoint of Yang-Ming Meridian of Foot as well as the start acupoint of Chong Channel, the match of the two acupoints can nurse Chong Channel and Ren Channel; Fenglong is a collateral acupoint of Yang-Ming Meridian of Foot, Yinlingquan is a He acupoint of Tai-Yin Meridian of Foot, the two both are important acupoint to invigorate spleen and stomach, remove Damp and disperse phlegm; Sanyinjiao is an acupoint of Tai-Yin Meridian of Foot, it can regular the three Yin Meridians, tonify Qi-blood. The use of combination of these acupoints can regulate Qi and disperse phlegm, regulate menstruation.

Method: Electrothermal acupuncture treatment.

Operations: Selecting the relevant acupoints, perform routine skin disinfection. Using electrothermal acupuncture needles, vertically puncture into Zhongji and Qichong for 0.8" respectively, Fenglong, Sanyinjiao and Yinlingquan for 0.7" respectively. Turn on the electrothermal acupuncture equipment, apply a current of 50-60mA to each acupoint. The limit is that the patient feels comfortable. Leave the needles in for 40 minutes.

Therapeutic course: Treat once a day, 30 times for a course. Start the treatment for the second course after a break of 7-10 days. Generally treat for 2-3 courses.

下篇　临床论治　Part II: Clinical Treatment

【血瘀证】

治法　行气化瘀，和血通经。

处方　中极（RN3）、归来（ST29）、三阴交（SP6）、子宫（EX-CA1）、气穴（KI13）。

方义　取任脉经穴中极调理冲任，化瘀通经；归来为足阳明胃经穴，能行气化瘀，和血通经，配足太阴经穴三阴交可和血调经；经外奇穴子宫穴、足少阴经穴气穴都是治疗不孕症的效穴。诸穴共用，可行气化瘀，和血通经，治疗不孕症。

方法　电热针治疗。

操作　选定穴位，皮肤常规消毒。电热针直刺中极0.8寸，直刺归来0.8寸，直刺气穴0.7寸，直刺子宫0.8寸，直刺三阴交0.7寸。接通电热针仪，每个穴位分别给予60～70mA的电流量，以患者舒适为度，留针40分钟。

疗程　每日1次，10次为1个疗程。疗程间可休息5～7天，再进行第2个疗程的治疗。一

[Syndrome of Blood Stasis]

Therapeutic method: Activate Qi and remove stasis, regulate blood and dredge meridians.

Prescription: Zhongji (RN3), Guilai (ST29), Sanyinjiao (SP6), Zigong (EX-CA1), Qihai (KI13).

Mechanism of prescription: Use the acupoint Zhongji of Ren Channel to nurse Chong Channel and Ren Channel, remove stasis and dredge meridians; Guilai is a meridian acupoint of Yang-Ming Stomach Meridian of Foot, it can activate Qi and remove stasis, regulate blood and dredge meridians, and can regulate blood and tonify meridians when being matched with the acupoint Sanyinjiao of Tai-Yin Meridian of Foot; the extra nerve point Zigong and the Qi acupoint of Shao-Yin Meridian of Foot are both effective acupoints for treatment of infertilitas feminis. The use of combination of these acupoints can activate Qi and remove stasis, regulate blood and dredge meridians, and treat infertilitas feminis.

Method: Electrothermal acupuncture treatment.

Operations: Selecting the relevant acupoints, perform routine skin disinfection. Using electrothermal acupuncture needles, vertically puncture into Zhongji and Guilai for 0.8" respectively, Qixue for 0.7", Zigong for 0.8", Sanyinjiao for 0.7". Turn on the electrothermal acupuncture equipment, apply a current of 60-70mA to each acupoint. The limit is that the patient feels comfortable. Leave the needles in for 40 minutes.

Therapeutic course: Once a day, 10 times for a course. Start the treatment for the second course after a break of 5-7 days. Generally treat for 2-3 courses.

般治疗 2～3 个疗程。

三、注意事项

1. 在决定治疗之前，要做好全身及妇科检查，首先治疗影响身体健康的疾病，如全身性疾病及炎症，然后再治疗不孕。

2. 注意心理卫生，要养成良好的生活习惯，调理好饮食。

3. 患者应了解必要的性知识，注意安排好性生活。

4. 患者要有良好的心态，不要过度紧张，做到心情舒畅，稳定生活。

四、典型病例

韩某，女，30 岁，已婚，工人，北京人。

主诉：婚后 3 年不孕。病史：患者 13 岁月经初潮，经期多错后，量少色淡，27 岁结婚，不孕，平素纳少，倦怠乏力，月经量少。

刻下症：体弱，面色白，五心烦热，咽干口燥，头晕，心悸，腰膝酸软，舌淡少苔，脉细数。

查体：未见阳性体征。

III. Precautions

1. Take systemic and gynecological examinations before deciding on treatment, first treat diseases affecting physical health such as systemic diseases and inflammations, then treat infertilitas feminis.

2. Pay attention to psychological health, develop good living habits, regulate diets.

3. Patients should know necessary sexual knowledge and well arrange sexual intercourses.

4. Patients should have good attitude, do not overstress, keep peaceful mind and stable life.

IV. Typical Case

Han, female, 30 years old, married, worker, residence: Beijing.

Self-reported symptoms: No pregnancy after 3-year marriage. Medical history: The patient experienced menarche at a year of 13, the menstruation normally delayed, less menstrual blood volume and light color, married at a year of 27, infertility, less daily food intake, tiredness and asthenia, less menstrual blood volume.

Current symptoms: Weak body, pale complexion, dysphoria in chest with palms-soles, dry throat and mouth, dizziness, palpitation, soreness and weakness of waist and knees, light tongue with less fur, thin and rapid pulse.

Physical examination: No positive signs were seen.

辅助检查：妇科检查示"卵巢功能低下"。

【诊断依据】

1. 妇科检查示"卵巢功能低下"。

2. 青年女性，素体虚弱，平素纳少。

3. 月经先期，量少色红。

【证治分析】

病因 肾阴亏虚。

病机 素体肝肾不足，致经血两亏，冲任失滋，胞宫失养，不能受精而不孕。

证候分析 肾阴亏虚，冲任失养，行经后期，量少色红，阴虚内热，虚火上炎，则五心烦热，咽干口燥，头晕心悸。腰为肾之府，肾为作强之官，肾阴亏虚则腰腿失养，故腰酸腿软。舌红少苔，脉细数，为肾阴不足之象。

病位 肾。

病性 肾阴不足。

西医诊断 卵巢功能低下。

中医诊断 不孕。

Auxiliary examination: Gynecological examination showed "poor ovary function".

[Diagnostic Basis]

1. Gynecological examination showed "poor ovary function".

2. Young female, weak body, less food intake.

3. Advanced menstruation, less volume and red.

[Syndrome-treatment Analysis]

Etiology: Depletion and deficiency of kidney Yin.

Pathogenesis: Liver and kidney deficiency, causing depletion of essence and blood, nourishing loss of Chong Channel and Ren Channel, the uterus lacks tonifying therefore leads to infertilitas feminis.

Syndrome analysis: Depletion and deficiency of kidney Yin, nourishing loss of Chong Channel and Ren Channel, delayed menstruation, less volume and red color, Yin deficiency and internal Heat, flaring up of deficiency-Fire, causing dysphoria in chest with palms-soles, dry throat and mouth, dizziness and palpitation. Waist is the place where the kidneys locate, kidney is the organ of strengthening, depletion and deficiency of kidney Yin causes nourishing loss of waist and legs, leading to aching lumbus and limp legs. Red tongue and less tongue fur, thin and rapid pulse are symptoms of kidney Yin deficiency.

Lesion location: Kidney.

Disease nature: Kidney Yin deficiency.

The diagnosis of Western Medicine: Poor ovary function.

The diagnosis of Traditional Chinese Medicine:

Infertilitas feminis.

治法 滋阴益肾，调理冲任。以任脉、足少阴肾经穴为主。

Therapeutic method: Nourish Yin and tonify kidney, nurse Chong Channel and Ren Channel. Mainly focus on Ren Channel and acupoints of the Shao-Yin Kidney Meridian of Foot.

方法 电热针治疗。

Method: Electrothermal acupuncture treatment.

处方 肾俞（BL23）、关元（RN4）、三阴交（SP6）、足三里（ST36）、内关（PC6）、然谷（KI2）、气穴（KI13）、子宫（EX-CA1）、太溪（KI3）。

Prescription: Shenshu (BL23), Guanyuan (RN4), Sanyinjiao (SP6), Zusanli (ST36), Neiguan (PC6), Rangu (KI2), Qixue (KI13), Zigong (EX-CA1), Taixi (KI3).

方义 本方以足太阳经穴肾俞补益肾气，任脉经穴关元调补冲任二脉；取足阳明经穴足三里培补后天，合足太阴脾经穴三阴交助后天以养先天；手厥阴经穴内关为八脉交会穴之一，合足少阴经穴然谷益肾固精；气穴为肾经穴，子宫为经外奇穴，取之可调养胞宫，为治不孕之效穴。诸穴共用，可收滋阴益肾、调理冲任之功。

Mechanism of prescription: In this prescription use the acupoint Shenshu of Tai-Yang Meridian of Foot to replenish and tonify kidney Qi, use the acupoint Guanyuan of Ren Channel to nurse Chong Channel and Ren Channel. Use the acupoint Zusanli of Yangming Meridian of Foot to reinforce acquired construction, and match it with the acupoint Sanyinjiao of Tai-Yin Spleen Meridian of Foot to facilitate acquired construction so as to nourish congenital construction; the acupoint Neiguan of Jue-Yin Meridian of Hand is one of the confluent acupoints of eight Channels, which can tonify kidney and secure essence when being matched with the acupoint Rangu of Shao-Yin Meridian of Foot; Qixue is an acupoint of Kidney Meridian, Zigong is an extra nerve point, they can tonify uterus and are effective acupoints for treatment of infertilitas feminis. The use of combination of these acupoints can nourish Yin and tonify kidney, nurse Chong Channel and Ren Channel.

配穴 腰膝酸软者加肾俞、足三里。

Math acupoints: For patients with soreness and weakness of waist and knees, add Shenshu, Zusanli.

Operations: Selecting the relevant acupoints, perform routine skin disinfection. Using electrothermal acupuncture needles, vertically puncture into Guanyuan, Zusanli, Sanyinjiao, Neiguan, Zigong, Qixue, Taixi, Rangu for 0.8" respectively, obliquely puncture (towards Jizhong) into Shenshu for 0.7". Turn on the electrothermal acupuncture equipment, apply a current of 40mA to each acupoint. The limit is that the patient feels swell and comfortable. Leave the needles in for 40 minutes. (Note: Select 3 pairs of acupoints each time, and use alternately.)

Therapeutic course: Once a day, 90 times for a course. Generally the patient can get pregnant during this period, otherwise continue the acupuncture treatment.

Treatment process: The patient got pregnant after the second month (64 days), so the treatment was stopped.

[Lifestyle Change and Health Maintenance]

1. The acupuncture therapy has good efficacies on infertilitas feminis, however the diagnosis must be confirmed before treatments to exclude infertility caused by men or psychological factors. Take related auxiliary examinations if necessary, to select different therapies against causes.

2. For patients with infertilitas feminis, it is important to know their history of menstruation, delivery, abortion, childbed and sexual intercourses. If any contraception and the method, if any long-term lactation, if any events like obesity and poor development of second sex characters, and if any other chronic diseases, such as tuberculosis, especially abdominal tuberculosis.

3. During acupuncture treatment, psychological

治疗很重要，必须放下包袱，保持平和乐观的心情配合治疗。

更年期综合征

更年期综合征是妇女在绝经前后出现的以自主神经功能失调为主的症候群。绝经年龄一般在45～52岁之间，临床上出现的症状往往因人而异，轻重不一，但多伴有月经紊乱，烦躁易怒，烘热汗出，心悸失眠，头晕耳鸣，健忘，多疑，感觉异常，性欲减退，或面目、下肢浮肿，倦怠无力，或胃痞纳呆，便溏，甚至情志失常，持续时间或长或短，短者半年到1年，长者延续数年之久。

中医认为，本病属于"绝经前后诸症""脏躁""郁证"的范畴。病因是妇女绝经前后肾气渐衰，天癸将竭，精血不足，冲任亏虚，进而出现肾之偏盛偏衰的现象。肾阴不足，阳失潜藏，肝阳上亢，或肾阴不足，营血暗伤，心血亏损；肾阳衰竭，失于温养，脾失健运，痰湿阻滞，痰与气结而致本病。病变脏腑主要在肾，并可累及心、肝、脾三脏。

treatment is very important, patients must lift their concerns and keep a peaceful and optimistic mood to cooperate with treatment.

Menopausal Syndrome

Menopausal syndrome is a syndrome which occurs around menopause, and mainly is the dysfunction of autonomic nerves. The age of menopause generally is between 45-52 years old, the clinical symptoms as well as severities differ among patients, however normally are accompanied with menstrual disorder, irritability, Heat and sweating, palpitation and insomnia, dizziness and tinnitus, amnesia, oversensitiveness, paresthesia, hyposexuality, or swollen face and limbs, fatigue and weakness, or stomach stuffiness and anorexia, sloppy stool, or even emotional disorders, with short term of a half to one year or long term of several years.

Traditional Chinese Medicine believes that this disease belongs to the ranges of "premenopausal and postmenopausal diseases", "hysteria", "stagnation syndrome". Etiology: Around menopause of women, kidney Qi declines gradually, menstruation is about to exhaust, with insufficient essence and blood, depletion and deficiency of Chong Channel and Ren Channel, therefore causes excessive exuberance or excessive deficiency of kidney. Inefficiency of kidney Yin, loss of Yang hide and storage, hyperactivity of liver Yang, or inefficiency of kidney Yin, internal injury of Ying-blood, depletion of heart blood; exhaustion and loss of warm nourishing of kidney Yang, dysfunction of spleen in transportation, Damp-Heat obstruction and stasis, stagnation of phlegm and Qi, causing this disease. The main lesion organ is kidney, and can affect heart, liver and spleen.

一、诊断及辨证要点

1. 肝阳上亢：头晕目眩，心烦易怒，烘热汗出，腰膝酸软，经来量多，或淋漓漏下，舌质红，苔白或少苔，脉弦细或数。

2. 心血亏损：心悸怔忡，失眠多梦，五心烦热，或情志失常，舌红少苔，脉细数。

3. 脾胃虚弱：面色苍白，神倦肢怠，纳少腹胀，大便溏泻，面浮肢肿，舌淡苔薄，脉沉细少力。

4. 痰气郁结：形体肥胖，胸闷吐痰，脘腹胀满，嗳气吞酸，呕恶食少，浮肿便溏，苔腻，脉滑。

5. 肾阴虚：头晕耳鸣，夜寐不安，五心烦热，盗汗自汗，腰膝酸软，足跟痛，便干，尿黄赤，皮肤干燥、瘙痒，舌红苔少，脉细数。

I. Key Points for Diagnosis and Syndrome Differentiation

1. Hperactivity of Liver-Yang: Dizziness, vexation and irritability, Heat and sweating, soreness and weakness of waist and knees, excessive menstrual blood volume, or dripping blood flow, red tongue, whitish or less tongue fur, taut and thin or rapid pulse.

2. Heart-blood depletion: Continuous palpitation, insomnia and dreamful sleep, dysphoria in chest with palms-soles, or emotional disorders, red tongue with less fur, thin and rapid pulse.

3. Weak spleen and stomach: Pale complexion, mental fatigue and limb tiredness, less food intake and abdominal distension, sloppy and thin stool, puffy face and swollen limbs, light tongue with thin fur, deep and thin and weak pulse.

4. Phlegm Qi stagnation: Obesity, chest distress and phlegm, abdominal distention, belching and acid swallowing, vomiting and nausea and less food intake, swelling and sloppy stool, greasy tongue fur, slippery pulse.

5. Yin-deficiency of kidney: Dizziness, disturbed sleep at night, dysphoria in chest with palms-soles, night sweat and spontaneous sweating, soreness and weakness of waist and knees, pain of heel, dry stool, dark and yellowish urine, dry skin, pruritus, red tongue with less fur, thin and rapid pulse.

6. 肾阳虚：面色晦暗，精神萎靡，形寒肢冷，腰膝酸痛，纳呆腹胀，便溏薄，面浮肢肿，尿多或失禁，舌淡或胖嫩、边有齿痕，苔薄白，脉沉细少力。

二、治疗方法

【肝阳上亢证】

治法 平肝潜阳，壮水涵木。

处方 太溪（KI3）、太冲（LR3）、百会（DU20）、风池（GB20）。

方义 肾为先天之本，元气之根，主藏精；肝为藏血之脏，肝肾同源，肾为肝之母。太冲为足厥阴肝经的原穴，太溪为足少阴肾经的原穴，二穴合用，前者平肝潜阳，后者补肾水，共奏滋水涵木之功。百会为督脉之腧穴，又是足太阳经的交会穴，与风池相配，可祛头目眩晕。诸穴共用，平肝潜阳，壮水涵木。

配穴 心烦者加大陵，烘

6. Yang-deficiency of kidney: Gloomy complexion, spirit drooping, cold body and limbs, soreness and weakness of waist and knees, anorexia and abdominal distension, sloppy and thin stool, puffy face and swollen limbs, excessive urination or urinary incontinence, light and fat and tender tongue with teeth prints at edge, thin and whitish tongue fur, deep and thin and weak pulse.

II. Therapeutic Methods

[Syndrome of Hperactivity of Liver-Yang]

Therapeutic method: Calm liver and suppress Yang, enrich Water and nourish Wood.

Prescription: Taixi (KI3), Taichong (LR3), Baihui (DU20), Fengchi (GB20).

Mechanism of prescription: Liver is the organ of blood storage, and liver and kidney originate from the same source, kidney is the parent organ of liver. Taichong is a Yuan acupoint of Jue-Yin Liver Meridian of Foot, Taixi is a Yuan acupoint of Shao-Yin Kidney Meridian of Foot, kidney is the congenital foundation, the root of vitality, and it governs storage of essence. The combination of the two acupoints can enrich Water and nourish Wood: the former calm liver and suppress Yang while the later replenish kidney Water. Baihui is an acupoint of Du Channel as well as the confluent acupoint of Tai-Yang Meridian of Foot, it can eliminate dizziness when being matched with Fengchi. The use of combination of these acupoints can calm liver and suppress Yang, enrich Water and nourish Wood.

Matching acupoints: For vexation add Daling. For

热者加涌泉、照海，腰酸痛者加肾俞、腰眼。

方法 电热针治疗。

操作 选定穴位，皮肤常规消毒。电热针直刺太冲0.7寸，直刺太溪0.7寸，平刺百会0.8寸，直刺照海0.6寸。接通电热针仪，每个穴位分别给予40～50mA的电流量，留针40分钟。

疗程 每天1次，90次为1个疗程。

【心血亏损证】

治法 调和心脾，滋肾宁心。

处方 心俞（BL15）、脾俞（BL20）、肾俞（BL23）、三阴交（SP6）。

方义 心俞为心的背俞穴，是治疗本脏疾病之主穴，能宁心安神，配脾俞、三阴交补中健脾，益生化之源。肾俞与心俞相配，补养精血，引心火下降，交通心肾，使水火相济。诸穴共用，调和心脾，滋肾宁心。

配穴 失眠者加神门、四神聪，心悸者加通里，五心烦

patients with Heat add Yongquan, Zhaohai. For patients with pain and soreness of waist, add Shenshu, Yaoyan.

Method: Electrothermal acupuncture treatment.

Operations: Selecting the relevant acupoints, perform routine skin disinfection. Using electrothermal acupuncture needles, vertically puncture into Taichong and Taixi for 0.7", Baihui for 0.8", Zhaohai for 0.6". Turn on the electrothermal acupuncture equipment, apply a current of 40-50mA to each acupoint. Leave the needles in for 40 minutes.

Therapeutic course: Once a day, 90 times for a course.

[Syndrome of Heart-blood depletion]

Therapeutic method: Reconcile heart and spleen, nourish kidney and calm heart.

Prescription: Xinshu(BL15), Pishu (BL20), Shenshu (BL23), Sanyinjiao (SP6).

Mechanism of prescription: Xinshu is a Back-Shu acupoint of Heart, a main acupoint for treatment of cardiac diseases, it can tranquilize mind and can nourish vital energy and invigorate spleen, tonify the source of generation and transformation when being matched with Pishu and Sanyinjiao. The match of Shenshu and Xinshu can nourish essence and blood, guide the heart Fire down, achieve communication between heart and kidney to enable interaction between Water and Fire. The use of combination of these acupoints can reconcile heart and spleen, nourish kidney and calm heart.

Matching acupoints: For insomnia add Shenmen, Sishencong. For palpitation add Tongli,; for dysphoria

热者加劳宫，神智失常者加人中、大陵。

方法 电热针治疗。

操作 选定穴位，皮肤常规消毒。电热针直刺三阴交0.7寸，向脊柱方向斜刺心俞0.8寸，斜刺脾俞0.8寸，斜刺肾俞0.7寸。接通电热针仪，每个穴位分别给予60～70mA的电流量，以患者舒适为度，留针40分钟。

疗程 每天1次，90次为1个疗程。

【脾胃虚寒证】

治法 温胃健脾。

处方 脾俞（BL20）、胃俞（BL21）、足三里（ST36）、中脘（RN12）、章门（LR13）。

方义 脾俞为足太阴脾经之背俞穴，"脾为后天之本""气血生化之源"，故取脾俞、胃俞配胃募中脘、脾募章门，一司运化，一司受纳，俞募相配，补益脾肾。再合强壮要穴足三里，以助运化，调补后天，强壮身体。

in chest with palms-soles add Laogong. For insanity add Renzhong, Daling.

Method: Electrothermal acupuncture treatment.

Operations: Selecting the relevant acupoints, perform routine skin disinfection. Using electrothermal acupuncture needles, vertically puncture into Sanyinjiao for 0.7", obliquely puncture towards spine into Xinshu and Pishu for 0.8" respectively, Shenshu for 0.7". Turn on the electrothermal acupuncture equipment, apply a current of 60-70mA to each acupoint. The limit is that the patient feels comfortable. Leave the needles in for 40 minutes.

Therapeutic course: Once a day, 90 times for a course.

[Syndrome of Deficiency-Cold of Spleen and Stomach]

Therapeutic method: Warm stomach and invigorate spleen.

Prescription: Pishu(BL20), Weishu(BL21), Zusanli(ST36), Zhongwan(RN12), Zhangmen(LR13).

Mechanism of prescription: Pishu is a Back-Shu acupoint of Tai-Yin Spleen Meridian of Foot, "spleen is the foundation of acquired constitution", "source of generation and transformation of Qi-blood", so use Pishu, Weishu matched with the Mu acupoint Zhongwan of Stomach Meridian, the Mu acupoint Zhangmen of Spleen Meridian, one governs transportation and transformation, one governs reception, the match of Shu-Mu acupoints can nourish spleen and kidney. And match them with the important tonifying acupoint Zusanli to facilitate transportation and transformation, tonify acquired construc-

配穴 腹胀者加下脘、气海；便溏者加天枢、阴陵泉；浮肿者加关元。

方法 电热针治疗。

操作 选定穴位，皮肤常规消毒。电热针向脊柱侧斜刺脾俞0.7寸，斜刺胃俞0.8寸，直刺足三里0.7寸，直刺阴陵泉0.7寸。接通电热针仪，每个穴位分别给予60～70mA的电流量，以患者舒适为度，留针40分钟。

疗程 每天1次，90次为1个疗程。

【痰气郁结证】

治法 健脾益气，除湿化痰。

处方 膻中（RN17）、中脘（RN12）、气海（RN6）、支沟（SJ6）、丰隆（ST40）、三阴交（SP6）。

方义 膻中为手厥阴心包经的募穴，又是气之会穴，功在宽胸理气；"脾为生痰之源"，脾失健运则聚湿生痰，气机受阻，故取膻中、中脘、气海、支沟调气理气，健脾和胃，通三焦，合丰隆、三阴交健脾益气，除湿化痰。

tion, strengthen body.

Matching acupoints: for abdominal distension add Xiawan, Qihai. For sloppy stool add Tianshu, Yinlingquan. For edema add Guanyuan.

Method: Electrothermal acupuncture treatment.

Operations: Selecting the relevant acupoints, perform routine skin disinfection. Using electrothermal acupuncture needles, obliquely puncture towards spine into Pishu for 0.7", Weishu for 0.8", Zusanli for 0.7", vertically puncture into Yinlingquan for 0.7". Turn on the electrothermal acupuncture equipment, apply a current of 60-70mA to each acupoint. The limit is that the patient feels comfortable. Leave the needles in for 40 minutes.

Therapeutic course: Once a day, 90 times for a course.

[Syndrome of Phlegm-Qi Stagnation]

Therapeutic method: Invigorate spleen and tonify Qi, remove Damp and disperse phlegm.

Prescription: Danzhong (RN17), Zhongwan (RN12), Qihai (RN6), Zhigou (SJ6), Fenglong (ST40), Sanyinjiao (SP6).

Mechanism of prescription: Danzhong is a Mu acupoint of Jue-Yin Pericardium Meridian of Hand as well as a confluent acupoint of Qi, its effect is to relive chest distress and regulate Qi; "Spleen is the source of phlegm generation", dysfunction of spleen in transportation leads to Damp accumulation and phlegm generation, obstruction of Qi Dynamic, therefore use Danzhong, Zhongwan, Qihai and Zhigou to regulate and tonify Qi, invigorate spleen and stomach, dredge three Jiaos, and match with Fenglong, Sanyinjiao to invigorate spleen and tonify Qi, remove Damp and disperse phlegm.

Matching acupoints: For loss of appetite add Ganshu, Pishu, Zusanli. For patients with excessive phlegm, add Fengmen, Chize, Hegu. For edema add Guanyuan, Shuifen, Zusanli, Yinlingquan.

Method: Electrothermal acupuncture treatment.

Operations: Selecting the relevant acupoints, perform routine skin disinfection. Using electrothermal acupuncture needles, vertically puncture into Danzhong 0.6", vertically puncture into Zhongwan, Qihai and Zhigou for 0.7" respectively, Fenglong for 0.8", Sanyinjiao, Zusanli and Yinlingquan for 0.7" respectively. Turn on the electrothermal acupuncture equipment, apply a current of 50-60mA to each acupoint. The limit is that the patient feels comfortable. Leave the needles in for 40 minutes. Additionally, use triangular needle to quickly puncture into Chize.

Therapeutic course: Once a day, 90 times for a course.

[Syndrome of Yin Deficiency of Kidney]

Therapeutic method: Nourish kidney Yin and clear deficiency-Heat.

Prescription: Shenshu (BL23), Taixi (KI3), Zhishi (BL52), Yongquan (KI1), Sanyinjiao (SP6).

Mechanism of prescription: Shenshu is an acupoint of Tai-Yang Bladder Meridian of Foot as well as a Back-Shu acupoint of Kidney Meridian, Taixi is a Yuan acupoint of Shao-Yin Kidney Meridian of Foot, the match of two these acupoints has a synergistic effect of

热；取志室、涌泉，有补肾益精血的作用，再配三阴交以扶中土之气，使后天气血生化之源旺盛，先天得到后天的濡养，阴阳、气血协调则脏腑安康。

配穴 失眠多梦者，加心俞、神门、三阴交；心悸、健忘者，加足三里、心俞、百会；皮肤瘙痒者，加风池、大椎、肺俞、血海。

方法 电热针治疗。

操作 选定穴位，皮肤常规消毒。电热针斜刺（向脊柱）肾俞 0.7 寸，斜刺肺俞 0.7 寸，斜刺心俞 0.7 寸，斜刺志室 0.7 寸，直刺三阴交 0.6 寸，直刺足三里 0.7 寸，直刺涌泉 0.7 寸，直刺神门 0.6 寸，平刺百会 0.7 寸。接通电热针仪，每个穴位分别给予 40～50mA 的电流量，以患者舒适为度，留针 40 分钟。

疗程 每天 1 次，90 次为 1 个疗程。

【肾阳虚证】

治法 益肾温阳。

处方 命门（DU4）、关元（RN4）、气海（RN6）、

enhancing efficacies of acupoints for disease treatment, and can nourish kidney Yin, remove deficiency-Heat. The use of Zhishi and Yongquan can nourish kidney and tonify essence and blood, and match Sanyinjiao to strengthen the Middle Qi, flourish the acquired source of generation and transformation of Qi-blood, nourish the congenital with the acquired, and internal organs will be healthy with Yin-Yang harmony and Qi-blood harmony.

Matching acupoints: For patients with insomnia and dreamful sleep, add Xinshu, Shenmen, Sanyinjiao. For palpitation and amnesia add Zusanli, Xinshu, Baihui. For cutaneous pruritus add Fengchi, Dazhui, Feishu, Xuehai.

Method: Electrothermal acupuncture treatment.

Operations: Selecting the relevant acupoints, perform routine skin disinfection. Using electrothermal acupuncture needles, obliquely puncture (towards spine) into Shenshu for 0.7", obliquely puncture into Feishu, Xinshu, Zhishi for 0.7" respectively, vertically puncture into Sanyinjiao for 0.6", and into Zusanli, Yongquan for 0.7" respectively, Shenmen for 0.6", horizonally puncture into Baihui for 0.7". Turn on the electrothermal acupuncture equipment, apply a current of 40-50mA to each acupoint. The limit is that the patient feels comfortable. Leave the needles in for 40 minutes.

Therapeutic course: Once a day, 90 times for a course.

[Syndrome of Yang Deficiency of Kidney]

Therapeutic method: Tonify kidney and warm Yang.

Prescription: Mingmen (DU4), Guanyuan (RN4), Qihai (RN6), Shenshu (BL23), Zusanli (ST36), Rangu

肾俞（BL23）、足三里（ST36）、然谷（KI2）。

方义 命门为督脉之腧穴，善培元补肾；关元、气海为任脉的腧穴，能调气益元，补肾固本和营血；肾俞可益火之源，如阳光一布而阴霾尽消；配然谷益肾温阳，使肾气作强；佐足三里以调整人体机能，先天之肾得以调养，阴阳协和而诸症自愈。

配穴 食欲不振者加中脘、脾俞、足三里；神疲乏力者加曲池、大椎、足三里；浮肿者加三焦俞、肾俞、复溜、水道、膀胱俞。

方法 电热针治疗。

操作 选定穴位，皮肤常规消毒。电热针直刺关元0.8寸，直刺气海0.7寸，直刺复溜0.8寸，直刺然谷0.7寸，直刺水道0.8寸，直刺曲池0.7寸，直刺中脘0.7寸，斜刺命门0.7寸，斜刺脾俞0.7寸，斜刺膀胱俞0.8寸，直刺三焦俞0.7寸。接通电热针仪，每个穴位分别给予电流量40～50mA，以患者舒适为度，

(KI2).

Mechanism of prescription: Mingmen is a Shu acupoint of Du Channel, and it has good efficacy in reinforcing vital essence and nourishing kidney; Guanyuan and Qihai are acupoints of Ren Channel, they can regulate Qi and tonify vital essence, nourish kidney, strengthen foundation and nourish blood; Shenshu can tonify the source of Fire, like the spreading of sunshine to eliminate hazes; it can tonify kidney and warm Yang when being matched with Rangu, strengthen kidney Qi; match with Zusanli to regulate body functions, tonify congenital kidney, achieving Yin-Yang harmony, so symptoms disappear naturally.

Matching acupoints: For patients that lose appetite, add Zhongwan, Pishu, Zusanli. For mental fatigue and asthenia add Quchi, Dazhui, Zusanli. For edema add Sanjiaoshu, Shenshu, Fuliu, Shuidao, Pangguangshu.

Method: Electrothermal acupuncture treatment.

Operations: Selecting the relevant acupoints, perform routine skin disinfection. Using electrothermal acupuncture needles, vertically puncture into Guanyuan for 0.8", Qihai for 0.7", Fuliu for 0.8", Rangu for 0.7", Shuidao for 0.8", Quchi and Zhongwan for 0.7" respectively, obliquely puncture into Mingmen and Pishu for 0.7" respectively, Pangguanshu for 0.8", Sanjiaoshu for 0.7". Turn on the electrothermal acupuncture equipment, apply a current of 40-50mA to each acupoint. The limit is that the patient feels comfortable. Leave the needles in for 40 minutes. (Note: Anterior and posterior acupoints

留针40分钟。（注：前后穴位可分成两组交替使用。）can be divided into two groups for alternate use.)

疗程 每天1次，90次为1个疗程。

Therapeutic course: Once a day, 90 times for a course.

三、注意事项

III. Precautions

1. 更年期是妇女从成熟期进入老年期的一个过渡时期，卵巢功能由活动状态转为衰退状态而出现的一系列症状，对患者要做好耐心细致的思想工作，解除顾虑，增强患者战胜疾病的信心和决心。

1. Menopause is a transitional period for women between maturation period and senescent period, and a series of symptoms occur due to the transition of ovarian functions form active status to degeneration. It is necessary to do patient and meticulous ideological work on patients, lift their concerns, enhance their confidence and determination to defeat diseases.

2. 对更年期综合征较重的患者应配合药物综合治疗，特别要进行心理治疗，开导患者决心配合治疗，一定会收到较好的疗效。

2. For patients with serious menopausal syndrome, matched comprehensive medicine therapy is necessary, especially psychotherapy is required to enlighten patients to cooperate with treatments, then better efficacies will be definitely achieved.

3. 绝经期常有月经紊乱，要特别注意更年期也是女性生殖器肿瘤的好发年龄，必须让患者经常去做妇科检查。

3. There always be menstrual disorder during menopause, and it should be especially noted that menopause is also a frequently occurring period of female genital tumors, so patients must do gynecological examination frequently.

4. 绝经后若有阴道出血，更应引起注意，应及早检查和诊治。

4. Vaginal bleeding after menopause should be paid more attention, and timely examination as well as diagnosis and treatment are required.

5. 在针灸治疗期间，要求患者保持有规律的生活，注意劳逸结合，保证足够的睡眠，避免各种不良刺激，进行适当的体育锻炼。

5. During the acupuncture treatment, patients are required to keep regular lifestyle, pay attention to alternate work with rest, ensure enough sleep, avoid various adverse irritations, have appropriate physical exercise.

四、典型病例

陈某，女，54岁，教师，北京人。

主诉：胸闷心慌，失眠健忘，已有3年。近日加重。

刻下症：善思多虑，多汗，纳食不香，面色萎黄，舌淡，苔白而薄，脉细微弦。

查体：两肺呼吸音粗糙，二尖瓣区及主动脉瓣第二听诊区可闻及二级收缩期杂音。

辅助检查：胸部X片示"肺纹理稍增粗"，其余未见异常。

【诊断依据】

1. 中老年女性，已闭经。

2. 胸闷气短，心悸，多愁善感，失眠健忘，多汗，已有3年，经治不效。

3. 查体及各项检查未发现器质性病变，未见异常体征。

【证治分析】

病因 情志不舒，气机郁滞而致。

病机 劳心过度，思虑伤脾，纳食减少，生化无源，则气血双亏，心脾两虚。

IV. Typical Case

Chen, female, 54 years old, teacher, residence: Beijing.

Self-reported symptoms: Chest tightness and palpitation, insomnia and amnesia, for 3 years. Recently increased.

Current symptoms: Keeping on thinking and worrying, hidrosis, loss of appetite, sallow complexion, light tongue, whitish and thin tongue fur, thin and sightly taut pulse.

Physical examination: Coarse breath sounds in both lungs, Grade 2 systolic noise at mitral valve area and second aortic valve area.

Auxiliary examination: Chest X-ray exam showed "slightly thickening of lung texture", no other abnormalities.

[Diagnostic Basis]

1. Middle-aged and elder women, amenorrhea.

2. Chest distress and shortness of breath, palpitation, sentimentality, insomnia and amnesia, hidrosis, last for 3 years, no improvement by treatments.

3. No organic lesions were found under physical examination and other examinations, no abnormal physical signs.

[Syndrome-treatment Analysis]

Etiology: Emotional upset, Qi Dynamic stagnation.

Pathogenesis: Excessive mind work, thoughtfulness hurting spleen, reduction of food intake, no source of generation and transformation, causing Qi-blood depletion, deficiency of heart and spleen.

证候分析 劳心思虑,心脾两虚,心失所养,故善息多虑,心悸失眠,健忘;脾肾为气血生化之源,脾虚不能健运,故饮食减少;气血生化不足,故面色萎黄,头晕,神疲,易汗。舌淡,脉细为心脾两虚之象,脉弦为肝郁之证。

Syndrome analysis: Excessive mind work and thoughtfulness, deficiency of heart and spleen, loss of heart nourishment, cause keeping on thinking and worrying, palpitation and insomnia, amnesia; spleen and kidney is the source of generation and transformation of Qi-blood, dysfunction of spleen in transportation, causing reducing of food intake; insufficient of generation and transformation of Qi-blood, causing sallow complexion, dizziness, spiritlessness, easy to sweat. Light tongue and thin pulse is the symptoms of heart and spleen deficiency, taut pulse is the symptom of liver stagnation.

病位 心、脾。

病性 虚性。

西医诊断 更年期综合征。

中医诊断 郁证。

治法 健脾益气,养心安神。

方法 电热针治疗。

处方 神门(HT7)、足三里(ST36)、三阴交(SP6)、心俞(BL15)、脾俞(BL20)、章门(LR13)、中脘(RN12)、肾俞(BL23)。

方义 神门、心俞与肾俞相合,益心气而宁心悸。足三里、三阴交分属脾胃两经,合胃募中脘、脾募章门及背俞穴脾俞,共取补益后天之气而益

Lesion location: Heart, spleen.

Disease nature: Deficiency.

The diagnosis of Western Medicine: Menopausal syndrome.

The diagnosis of Traditional Chinese Medicine: Depression syndrome.

Therapeutic method: Invigorate spleen and tonify Qi, nourish heart and tranquilize mind.

Method: Electrothermal acupuncture treatment.

Prescription: Shenmen (HT7), Zusanli (ST36), Sanyinjiao (SP6), Xinshu (BL15), Pishu (BL20), Zhangmen (LR13), Zhongwan (RN12), Shenshu (BL23).

Mechanism of prescription: The combination of Shenmen, Xinshu and Shenshu can tonify heart Qi and claim palpitation down. Zusanli and Sanyinjiao belong to Spleen Meridian and Stomach Meridian respectively, they can replenish and tonify acquired Qi when being

之功效。

配穴 郁闷不舒者,加内关、太冲;失眠者,加神门、四神聪;便溏者,加天枢、阴陵泉。

操作 选定穴位,皮肤常规消毒。电热针直刺足三里、三阴交、中脘各0.7寸,平刺章门0.8寸,直刺内关、天枢、阴陵泉、太冲各0.7寸,斜刺(针尖向脊柱)心俞、脾俞、肾俞各0.8寸。接通电热针仪,每个穴位分别给予50mA的电流量,以患者感到胀而舒适为度,留针40分钟。(注:每次选3组穴给予电热针治疗,余穴用毫针治疗,轮流应用。)

疗程 每日1次,90次为1个疗程。

治疗过程 该患者见效较快,其病程已有3年,但针灸治疗3次后就大有好转,能入睡,头晕已消失。上述穴位轮流选用,共治疗67次,基本恢复正常。为巩固疗效,治疗90次后结束治疗。随访5年,已恢复正常生活及工作。

matched with the Mu acupoint Zhongwan of Stomach Meridian, the Mu acupoint Zhangmen of Spleen Meridian and the Back-Shu acupoint Pishu.

Matching acupoints: For depressed patients add Neiguan, Taichong. For insomnia add Shenmen, Sishencong. For patients with sloppy stool add Tianshu, Yinlingquan.

Operations: Selecting the relevant acupoints, perform routine skin disinfection. Using electrothermal acupuncture needles, vertically puncture into Zusanli, Sanyinjiao, Zhongwan for 0.7" respectively, horizontally puncture into Zhangmen for 0.7", vertically puncture into Neiguan, Tianshu, Yinlingquan, Taichong for 0.7" respectively, obliquely puncture (towards Jizhong) into Xinshu, Pishu, Shenshu for 0.8" respectively. Turn on the electrothermal acupuncture equipment, apply a current of 50mA to each acupoint. The limit is that the patient feels swell and comfortable. Leave the needles in for 40 minutes. (Note: Select 3 pairs of acupoints for electrothermal acupuncture treatment each time, and treat the other acupoints with filiform needles, use alternately.)

Therapeutic course: Treat once a day, 90 times for a course.

Treatment process: Quick returns were obtained on this patient. Her disease course had been 3 years, however her condition achieved a big improvement after only 3 treatments, she could sleep and the dizziness disappeared. The above acupoints were selectively used alternately, and the total number of treatment was 67. The patient basically returned to normal. To consolidate the efficacy, the treatment was ended after 90 treatments.

5-year follow-up, the patient had returned to normal life and work.

【生活调摄】

1. 对患者要做好耐心细致的思想工作，解除顾虑，增强患者战胜疾病的信心和决心。

2. 对更年期综合征较重的患者应配合药物综合治疗，特别要进行心理治疗，开导患者决心配合治疗，一定会收到较好的疗效。

3. 在针灸治疗期间，要求患者保持有规律的生活，注意劳逸结合，保证足够的睡眠，避免各种不良刺激，进行适当的体育锻炼。

子宫肌瘤

子宫肌瘤（子宫平滑肌瘤）是女性生殖器官中最常见的良性肿瘤。

中医认为，本病属于"妇女癥瘕""石瘕""肠覃"等范畴。多因胞宫为寒邪所侵袭、气血受寒、凝结不散或肝郁气滞而血留所致。

一、诊断及辨证要点

1. 子宫肌瘤的发生率：30

[Lifestyle Change and Health Maintenance]

1. It is necessary to do patient and meticulous ideological work on patients, lift their concerns, enhance their confidence and determination to defeat diseases.

2. For patients with serious menopausal syndrome, matched comprehensive medicine therapy is necessary, especially psychotherapy is required to enlighten patients to cooperate with treatments, then better efficacies will be definitely achieved.

3. During the acupuncture treatment, patients are required to keep regular lifestyle, pay attention to alternate work with rest, ensure enough sleep, avoid various adverse irritations, have appropriate physical exercise.

Hysteromyoma

Hysteromyoma (uterine leiomyoma) is the most common benign tumor in female genital organs.

Traditional Chinese Medicine believes that this disease belongs to the range of "women abdominal mass", "stony uterine mass", "female abdominal mass". Most are due to attack of pathogenic cold, Qi-blood affected by Cold, coagulation or liver Qi stagnation leading to blood retention.

I. Key Points for Diagnosis and Syndrome Differentiation

1. The incidence of hysteromyoma: Around 20%

岁以上的妇女约为20%，20岁以下者极少见，以40～50岁发生率最高，占50.2%～60.9%。

2. 症见子宫出血，腹部包块，邻近器官的压迫症状，白带增多不孕，贫血，心脏功能障碍。无症状者约占37.2%。

3. 子宫肌瘤的诱因可能与雌激素刺激过多有关。

二、治疗方法

【气滞血瘀证】

治法 培补元气，行气活血，通经散结。

处方 子宫（EX-CA1）、曲骨（RN2）、横骨（KI11）、三阴交（SP6）。

方义 曲骨是肝经与任脉之交会穴，是治疗妇科疾病的要穴，肾主生殖，配肾经之横骨穴培补元气，行气活血；三阴交是肝、脾、肾经之交会穴，具有通经活络、调理气血之作用；子宫是经外奇穴，主治子宫疾病。诸穴合用，共收培补元气、行气活血、通经散结之功效。

for women over 30 years old, very rare in women under 20 years old, and most frequent in women of 40-50 years old, accounts for 50.2%-60.9%.

2. Symptoms include uterine hemorrhage, abdomen mass, compression symptoms of adjacent organs, leukorrhagia, infertilitas feminis, anemia, cardiac dysfunction. Asymptomatic patients account for around 37.2%.

3. The causes of hysteromyoma may be related to excessive estrogen stimulation.

II. Therapeutic Methods

[Syndrome of Qi Stagnation and Blood Stasis]

Therapeutic method: Replenish vitality, activate Qi and blood circulation, dredge meridians and eliminate stagnation.

Prescription: Zigong (EX-CA1), Qugu (RN2), Henggu (KI11), Sanyinjiao (SP6).

Mechanism of prescription: Qugu is the confluent acupoint of Liver Meridian and Ren Channel, an important acupoint for treatment of gynecological diseases. Kidney governs reproduction, and the acupoint Qugu matched with Henggu of Kidney Meridian can replenish vitality, activate Qi and blood circulation. Sanyinjiao is the confluent acupoint of Liver Meridian, Spleen Meridian and Kidney Meridian, which can dredge meridians and collaterals, nurse Qi-blood. Zigong is an extra nerve point which is mainly used for treatment of untrine diseases. The use of combination of these acupoints can replenish vitality, activate Qi and blood circulation, dredge meridians and eliminate stagnation.

配穴　腰酸痛、白带多者加血海、太溪；情志不舒者加太冲；月经量过多者加血海。

方法　电热针治疗。

操作　选定穴位，皮肤常规消毒。电热针直刺曲骨0.8寸，直刺横骨0.8寸，直刺子宫0.8寸，直刺三阴交0.8寸。接通电热针仪，每个穴位分别给予电流量40～60mA，以患者舒适为度，留针40分钟。

疗程　每日1次，10次为1个疗程。疗程间可休息3～5天，若无不适可连续治疗。

三、注意事项

1. 针刺曲骨、横骨时，先要排空膀胱的尿液，然后再行针刺。

2. 绝经后子宫肌瘤包块增大时，应予以高度重视，要进一步检查。

3. 针刺治疗中，亦可配合中药治疗，以提高疗效。

4. 治疗过程中要注意定期检查。

乳房纤维腺瘤

乳房纤维腺瘤是临床常见

Matching acupoints: For patients with pain and soreness of waist, excessive leukorrhea, add Xuehai, Taixi. For emotional upset add Taichong. For hypermenorrhea add Xuehai.

Method: Electrothermal acupuncture treatment.

Operations: Select acupoints, perform routine skin disinfection. Using electrothermal acupuncture needles, vertically puncture into Qugu, Henggu, Zigong, Sanyinjiao for 0.8" respectively. Turn on the electrothermal acupuncture equipment, apply a current of 40-60mA to each acupoint. The limit is that the patient feels comfortable. Leave the needles in for 40 minutes.

Therapeutic course: Once a day, 10 times for a course. Start the treatment for the second course after a break of 3-5 days, or perform continuous treatment if there is no discomfort.

III. Precautions

1. For acupuncutre of Qugu and Henggu, it is necessary to empty urine in the bladders first.

2. High attention should be paid to postmenopausal uterine fibroids mass enlargement, and further examination is required.

3. During the acupuncture treatment, Chinese Herb Medicine treatment also can be used to improve efficacies.

4. Regular examinations are required during treatment.

Breast Fibroadenoma

Breast fibroadenoma is a clinically common breast

的乳腺疾病，发病率约占乳房良性肿瘤的 3/4。

中医认为，本病属于"乳癖"的范畴。多因情志内伤，肝气郁结，痰凝瘀滞，积聚乳房乳络所致。

一、诊断及辨证要点

1. 好发年龄多在性功能旺盛时期（18～25 岁）。多数学者认为，本病的发生与雌激素作用活跃有密切的关系。

2. 多发部位在乳房的外上象限，内象限次之，内下象限很少。

3. 75% 为单发，少数属多发性。

4. 肿块形状似桃核或鸡卵，肤色不变，扪之质地坚实，表面光滑，边界清楚，不与皮肤及深部胸筋膜粘连，易推动，多不溃破，肿块增长速度较缓慢，一般无痛，个别有轻微胀痛，与月经无关。

5. 全身症状：多伴有心烦易怒，胸闷气短，常善太息，失眠多梦，口苦且质红，脉弱滑等症状。

disease, accounting for around 3/4 of breast benign tumor occurrences.

Traditional Chinese Medicine believes that this disease belongs to the range of "lump in breast". Most are resulted by internal injuries caused by seven emotions, liver Qi stagnation, phlegm stasis, accumulating at breast collaterals at breasts.

I. Key Points for Diagnosis and Syndrome Differentiation

1. It normally occurs in sexual function exuberant period (18-25 years old). Most scholars believe that the incidence of this disease is closely related to the active role of estrogen.

2. Most occur in the outer quadrant of the breast, followed by the inner quadrant, rare in the lower quadrant.

3. 75% are single, few are multiple.

4. The lump shape is like peach pit or egg, skin color unchanged, solid texture when stroking, with smooth surface, clear boundaries, not adhered with skin and deep thoracic fascia, easy to push, normally with no ulceration, slow growing speed, generally with no pain, few with slight pain, and has nothing to do with menstruation.

5. Systemic symptoms: Most are accompanied by vexation and irritability, chest distress and shortness of breath, often with preference for sighing, insomnia and dreamy sleep, bitter taste and red tongue, weak and slippery pulse.

6. 部分患者妊娠期若有迅速增大，则有恶变之虑，要引起重视。

二、治疗方法

【肝郁气滞证】

治法 疏肝解郁，化痰散结。

处方 乳根（ST18）、屋翳（ST15）、膺窗（ST16）、足三里（ST36）、丰隆（ST40）、期门（LR14）、膻中（RN17）。

方义 足阳明胃经"从缺盆下乳内廉"，故方中取本经之合穴足三里、络穴丰隆配乳根、膺窗、屋翳、膻中行气化痰，以解乳络之壅滞。又因肝经分布胁肋，本病是肝郁痰凝所致，故取肝经之募穴、肝脾两经与阴维脉之交会穴期门，以疏肝解郁，化痰散结。诸穴共用，有疏肝郁、行气血、化痰结之功效。

配穴 气滞血瘀，加膈俞、血海；肝郁化火，去足三里，加三阴交、行间；胸闷，

6. For most pregnant women who experience rapid enlargement of lumps, then there will be potential of malignant transformation and attentions should be paid.

II. Therapeutic Methods

[Syndrome of Liver Stasis and Qi Stagnation]

Therapeutic method: Soothe liver Qi stagnation, disperse phlegm and eliminate stagnation.

Prescription: Rugen (ST18), Wuyi (ST15), Yingchuang (ST16), Zusanli (ST36), Fenglong (ST40), Qimen (LR14), Danzhong (RN17).

Mechanism of prescription: The Yang-Ming Stomach Meridian of Foot "from the acupoint Quepen down to the inner side of breast", therefore use the He acupoint Zusanli and the meridian acupoint Fenglong of this meridian matched with Rugen, Yingchuang, Wuyi, Danzhong to activate Qi and disperse phlegm, so as to resolve Qi stasis of Ru Collateral. And since the Liver Meridian distributes among lateral thorax, while this disease is caused by liver stagnation and phlegm stasis, therefore use Qimen, the Mu acupoint as well as the confluent acupoint of Liver Meridian and Spleen Meridian as well as Yinwei Channel, to soothe liver Qi stagnation, disperse phlegm and eliminate stagnation. The use of combination of these acupoints can soothe liver Qi stagnation, promote Qi-blood flow, disperse phlegm and eliminate stagnation.

Matching acupoints: For Qi stagnation and blood stasis add Geshu, Xuehai. For transformation of liver stasis into Fire remove Zusanli and add Sanyinjiao, Xing-

加合谷、内关；月经不调，加三阴交。

方法 电热针治疗。

操作 选定穴位，皮肤常规消毒。电热针斜刺或平刺乳根、膺窗、屋翳、期门各0.7～0.8寸，直刺丰隆0.8寸，平刺膻中0.8寸，直刺足三里、丰隆各0.8寸。接通电热针仪，每个穴位分别给予电热量30～40mA，留针40分钟。

疗程 每日1次，10次为1个疗程。疗程间可休息3～5天，再进行第2个疗程的治疗。

三、注意事项

1. 要保持心情舒畅，避免不良因素的精神刺激。

2. 治疗后肿块缩小不明显者，或更年期妇女患本病而疗效不理想者，均应考虑手术切除。

3. 为了提高疗效，可配合中药治疗。

乳腺癌

乳腺癌是女性常见的恶性肿瘤之一。多发生在40～60岁

jian. For chest distress add Hegu, Neiguan. For menoxenia add Sanyinjiao.

Method: Electrothermal acupuncture treatment.

Operations: Selecting the relevant acupoints, perform routine skin disinfection. Using electrothermal acupuncture needles, obliquely or horizontally puncture into Rugen, Yingchuang, Wuyi, Qimen for 0.7-0.8" respectively, vertically puncture into Fenglong for 0.8", horizontally puncture into Danzhong for 0.8", vertically puncture into Zusanli, Fenglong for 0.8" respectively. Turn on the electrothermal acupuncture equipment, apply a current of 30-40mA to each acupoint. Leave the needles in for 40 minutes.

Therapeutic course: Once a day, 10 times for a course. Start the treatment for the second course after a break of 3-5 days.

III. Precautions

1. Keep good mood, avoid mental stimulation by adverse factors.

2. For patients with unapparent lump reduction after treatment, or patients who develop this disease during menopause with unsatisfactory treatment efficacy, operational excision should be considered.

3. Chinese Herb Medicine treatment can be used to improve efficacies.

Breast Cancer

Breast cancer is one of the common malignant tumors among women. Most occur among women around

绝经期前后的妇女，其发病与女性激素有关。

中医认为，本病属于"乳岩""乳石痈"的范畴。多因忧思郁怒，邪毒蕴结，冲任失调所致。初期为实证、热证，晚期气血耗伤，多为虚实夹杂证。

一、诊断及辨证要点

1. 临床检查

（1）早期为无痛的、单发的小肿块，质硬，表面不甚光滑，与周围组织分界不清，在乳房内不易被推动，多在患者无意中发现，随着肿块的增大，局部皮肤往往凹陷，乳头抬高或回缩内陷。

（2）晚期癌块固定，乳房不能推动，皮肤发生水肿，呈"橘皮样"，继而皮肤破溃，成溃疡（呈菜花样），有恶臭，易出血。

（3）多有淋巴结转移，常转移到同侧腋窝淋巴结，晚期锁骨上淋巴结和对侧腋窝淋巴亦可肿大、变硬。

menopause with an age of 40-60 years old, the incidence of which is associated with female hormones.

Traditional Chinese Medicine believes that this disease belongs to the range of "lump in breast", "hard tumor in breast". Most are caused by deep sorrow and stagnated anger, pathogenic toxin accumulation, disorder of Chong Channel and Ren Channel. Excess syndrome, Heat syndrome at first, later change into syndrome of intermingled deficiency and excess due to consumption of Qi-blood.

I. Key Points for Diagnosis and Syndrome Differentiation

1. Clinical examination

(1) In early phase it is painless, single small lump with hard texture, unsmooth surface, unclear boundaries, and it is hard to be pushed to move within the breast, most are inadvertently found by the patient, normally local skin will be sagging along with enlargement of the lump, the nipple raised or retracted.

(2) During the advanced phase, the lump is immobile, the breast cannot be pushed to move, "orange peel like" edema of skin occurs, followed by skin ruptured into ulcers (cauliflower-like), with foul smell, easy to bleed.

(3) Most are accompanied with lymphatic metastasis, normally transfer to the ipsilateral axillary lymph nodes, in advanced phase the supraclavicular lymph nodes and contralateral axillary lymph nodes also may be

(4) X-ray examination: Sometimes it can facilitate the diagnosis of breast lumps, if the diagnosis of breast cancer is clear, then the X-ray radiography should be done for lungs, skeletons and abdomen (liver). Detailed clinical examinations should be done for skeletons, especially the spine, and take X-ray radiography if necessary.

(5) Pathological examination: Pathological reports are the objective criteria of the diagnosis of this disease. ① For patients with secreta from nipples, cytological examination should be done for the secreta. ② Aspirate tissue cells with needle penetration for smear examination, with which 88% cases can be confirmed. ③ Biopsy should be closely aligned with radical resection of breast cancer, and rapid frozen section also will be done. At the same time, complete all preparation for radical resection of breast cancer, perform the radical resection of breast cancer immediately once cancer is confirmed in the pathological report, and the accuracy of frozen section diagnosis.

2. Syndrome Differentiation

(1) For patients with liver stasis and Qi stagnation, symptoms include rib pain of both sides, pain of breast lump, vexation and irritability, bitter taste and dry throat, dizziness, light red tongue, thin tongue, yellow or thin and whitish tongue fur, taut pulse.

(2) For patients with Yin deficiency of liver and kidney, symptoms include menoxenia, aching lumbus and limp legs, dry eyes, dry mouth, dizziness and tinnitus, red tongue with whitish and less fur, thin pulse.

(3) For patients with toxic Heat and weakened body

块迅速增大，疼痛，或红肿，甚则溃烂翻花，久则气血衰败，正气大亏，消瘦乏力，或发热，口干，心烦，便秘，舌苔白或黄而厚腻，脉弦数或细数。

二、治疗方法

【肝郁气滞兼毒热正虚】

治法 疏肝解郁，扶正祛邪。

处方 神道（DU11）、至阳（DU9）、足三里（ST36）、曲池（LI11）、阿是穴（根据肿块大小，取中心及上、下、左、右共5针）。

方义 乳头属足厥阴肝经，乳房属足阳明胃经，透泻神道、至阳，以疏泄肝经之瘀滞，泻阳明之热毒，二穴皆属督脉，督脉总督诸阳，督脉通调，则诸阳经气亦可和利，而收散结消肿之功。取足阳明胃经的合穴足三里，合治内腑，不仅有和调胃肠，疏理气机，清化湿热之功，还能补益元气，助脾胃以生化气血，从而达到扶正祛邪之目的。

resistance, symptoms include rapid enlargement of breast lump, pain, or red and swollen, even ulcers, and for long time depletion of Qi-blood, serious depletion of healthy Qi, emaciation and asthenia, or fever, dry mouth, vexation, constipation, whitish or yellowish thick and greasy tongue fur, taut and rapid or thin and rapid pulse.

II. Therapeutic Methods

[Liver Stasis and Qi Stagnation, Toxic Heat and Weakened Body Resistance]

Therapeutic method: Soothe liver Qi stagnation, strengthen vital Qi and eliminate pathogenic factors.

Prescription: Shendao (DU11), Zhiyang (DU9), Zusanli (ST36), Quchi (LI11), Ashi acupoints (5 punctures, center, upper, lower, left and right of the lump each, depending on the lump size).

Mechanism of prescription: Nipple belongs to Jue-Yin Liver Meridian of Foot, breast belongs to Yang-Ming Stomach Meridian of Foot, purge Shendao and Zhiyang to sooth stagnation of Liver Meridian, purge Heat toxin of Yang-Ming, the two acupoints are both belong to Du Channel, and Du Channel governs Yang of the whole body, so dredging and soothing of Du Channel can promote harmony of meridian Qi of all Yang so as to disperse stagnation and subside lumps. Use the He acupoint Zusanli of the Yang-Ming Stomach Meridian of Foot to care organs. It not only can regulate intestines and stomach, soothe Qi Dynamic, clear Damp-Heat, and can replenish vitality, help the spleen and stomach to generate Qi-blood, so as to achieve the aim of strength-

配穴　瘀血甚者加血海；正气亏虚者加气海；气滞者加太冲。

Matching acupoints: For patients with serious blood stasis, add Xuehai. For patients with depletion and deficiency of healthy Qi add Qihai. For patients with Qi stagnation add Taichong.

方法　电热针治疗。

Method: Electrothermal acupuncture treatment.

操作　选定穴位，皮肤常规消毒。将电热针直刺肿块中心 0.8 寸，在肿块的上、下、左、右各直刺 1 针达 0.8 寸。接通电热针仪，每个穴位分别给予电流量 80～100mA，温度控制在 42～45℃之间，以患者感到温胀舒适为度，留针 40 分钟。另配以毫针向下斜刺透至阳 0.8～1 寸，留针 3 小时。

Operations: Selecting the relevant acupoints, perform routine skin disinfection. Using electrothermal acupuncture needles, vertically puncture into the lump center for 0.8", one puncture vertically each into upper, lower, left and right of the lump for 0.8" respectively. Turn on the electrothermal acupuncture equipment, apply a current of 80-100mA to each acupoint, maintain the temperature within 42-45℃, and the limit is that the patient feels warmly swell and comfortable. Leave the needles in for 40 minutes. Additionally, using filiform needles, obliquely puncture downward into Zhiyang for 0.8-1", leaving the needles in for 3 hours.

疗程　每隔 1 日治疗 1 次，10 次为 1 个疗程。疗程间休息 3～5 天，再进行第 2 个疗程的治疗。

Therapeutic course: Once every 2 days, 10 times for a course. Start the treatment for the second course after a break of 3-5 days.

三、注意事项

1. 增加营养，忌食酒类等刺激食品。

2. 避免精神刺激，注意生活规律。

3. 遇肿块较大又能适合切除者，应切除病原，再经电热针康复治疗，更能达到早日康

III. Precautions

1. Increase nutrition, avoid stimulating food like alcohol.

2. Avoid mental stimulations, pay attentions to regular lifestyle.

3. For larger lump suitable for resection, the lesion should be resected, then undergo electrothermal acupuncture treatment as rehabilitation treatment so as to achieve

复的目的。

4. 用电热针治疗时，应测量肿瘤体内的温度，使之控制在43～45℃之间。

四、典型病例

王某，女，34岁，职员，北京人。

主诉：发现右乳腺肿块1月余，质硬，如核桃大小。病史：患者做过3次人工流产，月经前乳腺胀痛，可摸到一个肿块，较软，如枣仁大小，月事之后即退。每个月反复出现，以后就未加注意，上个月没有月经，乳房未发生胀痛，可摸到一个大肿块，质硬，触之活动不痛，经西医诊为"乳腺癌"。

刻下症：右侧乳腺肿块，质硬，无压痛，神清，精神可，纳可，二便通畅，舌质红，苔薄白，脉弦。

查体：右侧乳腺外观正常，可触及3cm×4cm大小的硬块，边界清楚，表面不光滑，推之可移动，无压痛。二尖瓣区及主动脉瓣第二听诊区闻及二级收缩期杂音。

辅助检查：活检示"腺癌"。白细胞计数$12×10^9$/L。

the purpose of early rehabilitation.

4. When using electrothermal acupuncture treatment, it is necessary to measure the temperature within the tumor, and control it within 43-45℃.

IV. Typical Case

Wang, female, 34 years old, employee, residence: Beijing.

Self-reported symptoms: Lump in right breast found for more than a month, hard, size similar to walnut. Medical history: The patient underwent 3 times of induced abortion, breast distending pain before menstruation, a touched lump, soft, size of a jujube kernel, disappeared after menstruation. Reappeared each month, the patient paid no attention to it later, and no menstrual bleeding came last month, no breast distending pain occurred, a large lump could be touched, hard, movable when being pushed, no pain, diagnosed as "breast cancer" by Western Medicine.

Current symptoms: Lump in right breast, hard, no tenderness, clear mind, fine mental condition, fine appetite, smooth urination and defecation, red tongue, thin and whitish fur, taut pulse.

Physical examination: Normal appearance of right breast, a hard lump of 3cm×4cm could be palpated, clear boundaries and unsmooth surface, movable when being pushed, no tenderness. Grade 2 systolic noise at mitral valve area and second aortic valve area.

Auxiliary examination: Biopsy indicated "glandular cancer". Leukocyte count $12×10^9$/L. B ultrasound indi-

B 超示肿块大小 3cm×4cm。

【诊断依据】

1. 乳腺肿块活检示"腺癌",白细胞计数 $12×10^9/L$。

2. 乳腺 B 超示肿块大小 3cm×4cm,坚硬。

3. 查体:全身其他部位均未发现阳性体征。

4. 患者做过 3 次人工流产,平素经常情志不舒,抑郁。

5. 既往月经前多有乳房胀痛,月事后消退,现已闭经。

【证治分析】

病因 冲任失调。

病机 《圣济总录》曰:"以任冲二经,上为乳汁,下为月水。"冲任二脉隶属肝肾,堕胎损及肝肾,冲任失调,则经脉失养而成瘤疾。

证候分析 内伤情志,化火而耗损肾阳,肝肾亏损,冲任失调,冲任二脉上为乳汁,下为月水,月经前经血尚未排出,冲任两脉充盈阻滞,乳房内痰浊凝结较甚,故肿块肿大。月经不排出,经络壅滞,

cated the lump size of 3cm×4cm.

[Diagnostic Basis]

1. Breast lump indicated "glandular cancer", leukocyte count $12×10^9/L$.

2. B ultrasound indicated the lump size of 3cm×4cm, hard.

3. Physical examination: No positive signs were found in all other parts.

4. The patients underwent 3 times of induced abortion, often showed emotional upset, depression.

5. Previous history of breast distending pain before menstruation, which disappeared after menstruation, now amenorrhea.

[Syndrome-treatment Analysis]

Etiology: Disorder of Chong Channel and Ren Channel.

Pathogenesis: It is said in *General Medical Collection of Royal Benevolence* that "For the two channels Ren and Chong, the upper is milk, the lower is menstrual blood". Chong Channel and Ren Channel belong to Liver and Kidney, abortions impaired liver and kidney, caused disorders of Chong Channel and Ren Channel, leading to nourishment loss of meridians and channels to develop into chronic illness.

Syndrome analysis: Emotional internal injuries transforming into Fire consuming kidney Yang, depletion and deficiency of liver and kidney, disorders of Chong Channel and Ren Channel, the upper and lower of Chong Channel and Ren Channel are milk and menstrual blood respectively, menstrual blood not yet discharged before menstrual period, Chong Channel and Ren Channel

其势猛增，故肿块增大变硬，闭经。舌淡苔白，脉沉，为气血不足之象。

病位 乳腺。

病性 实性。

西医诊断 乳腺癌。

中医诊断 乳岩（冲任失调）。

治法 补益肝肾，调理冲任，行气化痰，软坚散结。

方法 电热针治疗。

处方 肝俞（BL18）、肾俞（BL23）、关元（RN4）、膻中（RN17）、丰隆（ST40）、三阴交（SP6）、神道（DU11）、至阳（DU9）、屋翳（ST15）、阿是穴。

方义 肝俞、肾俞可补益肝肾；关元、三阴交既可补肾健脾调肝，又能调理冲任；近取屋翳、气会膻中，旨在补气通络；足阳明经之络丰隆，可除湿化痰消肿块；局部取阿是穴有软坚散结、活血化瘀之功。

filled and blocked, serious phlegm stagnation within breast, causing larger lump. Menstrual blood could not be discharged, meridians and collaterals being stagnated, the condition rapidly aggravated, causing enlarging and hardening of the lump, amenorrhea. Light tongue with whitish fur, deep pulse, are all symptoms of deficiency of Qi and blood.

Lesion location: Breast.

Disease nature: Excess.

The diagnosis of Western Medicine: Breast cancer.

The diagnosis of Traditional Chinese Medicine: Mammary cancer (disorder of Chong Channel and Ren Channel).

Therapeutic method: Tonify liver and kidney, nurse Chong Channel and Ren Channel, activate Qi and disperse phlegm, soften hardness and remove stagnation.

Method: Electrothermal acupuncture treatment.

Prescription: Ganshu (BL18), Shenshu (BL23), Guanyuan (RN4), Danzhong (RN4), Fenglong (ST40), Sanyinjiao (SP6), Shendao (DU11), Zhiyang (DU9), Wuyi (ST15), Ashi acupoints.

Mechanism of prescription: Ganshu, Shenshu can tonify liver and kidney; Guanyuan, Sanyinjiao can replenish kidney, invigorate spleen and tonify liver, as well as nurse Chong Channel and Ren Channel. Use Wuyi, Danzhong to replenish Qi and dredge collaterals; the meridian acupoint Fenglong of Yang-Ming Meridian of Foot can remove Damp, disperse phlegm and subside lumps; local Ashi acupoints can remove soften hardness,

操作 选定穴位，皮肤常规消毒。以毫针直刺关元、三阴交、丰隆各 0.6 寸，平刺膻中 0.7 寸。然后用电热针直刺病灶（乳腺肿块）中心 1 针，肿块用 6 支针围刺，距离相等，接通电热针仪，每个穴位分别给予电流量 150mA，半导体针型温度针检测病体温度达 45℃，留针 40 分钟。

疗程 每 5 天 1 次，10 次为 1 个疗程。疗程结束后，视病情决定是否继续进行第 2 个疗程的治疗。

治疗过程 患者 5 天治疗 1 次，治疗 10 次后肿瘤消失。活检复查未见癌细胞。追踪 5 年未见复发。

【生活调摄】

1. 电热针直刺肿块必须慎重，不能将针刺穿健康皮肤以及肿块附近的健康组织，只能刺入肿块中。掌握好方向、深度。

2. 用针较粗，要在局部给予利多卡因 10mL 局部麻醉下

disperse phlegm and remove stagnation, activate blood circulation and remove stasis.

Operations: Selecting the relevant acupoints, perform routine skin disinfection. Using filiform needles, vertically puncture into Guanyuan, Sanyinjiao, Fenlong for 0.6" respectively, horizontally puncture into Danzhong for 0.7". Then using electrothermal acupuncture needles, vertically puncture into the lesion (breast lump) center with 1 needle, and 6 needles for surrounding acupuncture around the lesion with a same distance of every two adjacent needles. Turn on the electrothermal acupuncture equipment, apply a current of 150mA to each acupoint, the lesion temperature reach 45℃ when detecting with semiconductor-type temperature needles. Leave the needles in for 40 minutes.

Therapeutic course: Once every 5 days, 10 times for a course. After the end of the course, decide if continue to perform treatment of the second course according to the patient's conditions.

Treatment process: The patient received treatment once every 5 days, and the tumor disappeared after 10 treatments. No cancer cells were found in reexamination of biopsy. Follow-up for 5 years, no recurrence.

[Lifestyle Change and Health Maintenance]

1. Direct electrothermal acupuncture treatment of lumps should be careful, needles should not be penetrate through healthy skin or healthy tissues around the lump, but only into the lump. Well control directions and depth.

2. The used needles are thick, it is necessary to give local anesthesia with 10ml lidocaine to avoid pain of pa-

进针，避免患者疼痛。

3. 针刺后留针时，以患者感到局部无痛为原则，温度必须达 43～45℃之间，方可有效。

4. 治疗中注意患者的饮食调养。

五、现代临床诊疗

【电热针治疗乳腺癌诊案】

一位晚期乳腺癌患者，瘤体大小为 9.8cm×8cm×3cm，经电热针治疗 2 个疗程，瘤体缩小为 3.5cm×3cm×3.5cm，之后进行局部手术切除，发现瘤体中心坏死，腋窝转移灶液化，转为阴性，瘤体周围出现环形被膜，环绕包围瘤体。(《内蒙古中医药》1987 年第 6 期)

【毫针治疗乳腺癌诊案】

王某，女，32 岁。左侧乳房疼痛，按之有一核桃大的硬块，经上海某医院诊断为乳腺癌，服中药 1 月余未见效果。治取神道透至阳，采用该透针法，留针 3 小时。治疗 10 次后，疼痛已止，硬块缩小，针治 39 次，肿块消失。随访 2 年病已痊愈，未见复发。(《中国

3. For needle retaining after puncturing, the standard is that patient feel no local pain, and the temperature must reach 43-45℃ for effective treatment.

4. Pay attention to the patient's dietetic care during treatment.

V. Modern Clinical Diagnosis and Treatment

[Case of Breast Cancer Treatment Using electrothermal Acupuncture]

A patient with advanced breast cancer, the lump size was 9.8cm×8cm×3cm, and it shrunk down to 3.5cm×3cm×3.5cm after two courses of treatment. Then performed local surgical resection, it was found that the lump center was necrotic, the axillary metastatic lesion was liquefied, transformed into negative, ring-shaped envelope occurred around the lump, surrounding the lump. (*Chinese Medicine of Inner Mongolia*; Issue 6, 1987.)

[Case of Breast Cancer Treatment Using Filiform Needles]

Wang, female, 32 years old. Pain of the left breast, a hard mass with a size of a walnut could be felt when pressing, diagnosed as breast cancer by a hospital in Shanghai, no efficacies after more than 1 month of Chinese Herb Medicine treatment. Use penetrating needling therapy at Shendao and Zhiyang. Leave the needles in for 3 hours. After 10 treatments, the pain was stopped, the hard lump shrunk down, after 39 times of acupuncture, the lump disappeared. Follow-up 2 years, cured, no

针法集锦》)

宫颈癌

宫颈癌是妇女最常见的恶性肿瘤之一,占女性生殖器肿瘤的首位,多发生于45岁以上的妇女。

中医认为,本病属于"阴疮""崩漏""五色带""癥瘕"等范畴。多因七情所伤,肝郁气滞,瘀阻胞脉,痰凝毒结,致冲任受损,并使肝、脾、肾脏功能失常而发。

一、诊断及辨证要点

1. 早期:宫颈癌的临床表现为功能性出血,断经后又出现阴道不规则出血,或排出大量混有血液的恶臭白带,少腹痛,舌红,苔白或黄,脉弦。

2. 晚期:可因肿块压迫而出现腹部酸痛,肛门下坠,尿频、尿急、血尿,或发生尿毒症。

3. 本病多与早婚、早孕、多产、宫颈创伤等因素有关。

recurrence. (*Collection of Chinese Acupuncture*)

Cervical Cancer

Cervical cancer is one of the most common malignant tumors among women, ranked as first in female genital tumors, most of which occur in women over 45 years old.

Traditional Chinese Medicine believes that this disease belongs to the range of "sore of vulva", "metrorrhagia and metrostaxis", "multi-colored leukorrhea", "abdominal mass". Most caused by excess of seven emotions, liver stasis and Qi stagnation, block and stasis of Uterine Channel, phlegm and toxin stagnation, causing injuries of Chong Channel and Ren Channel, as well as dysfunctions of liver, spleen and kidney.

I. Key Points for Diagnosis and Syndrome Differentiation

1. The clinical manifestations of early cervical cancers include functional bleeding, irregular vaginal bleeding after menstrual period ended, or discharge of a large number of stinky leucorrhea containing blood, lateral lower abdominal pain, red tongue with whitish or yellowish fur, taut pulse.

2. In advanced phase there may occur soreness of abdomen, anna dropping, frequent micturition, urgent micturition, hematuria or toxuria due to compression of the lump.

3. This disease is associated with early marriage, early pregnancy, excessive deliveries, cervical trauma and other factors.

4. 外阴白斑（女阴白色病变）是本病的癌前病变，要注意早期发现、早期治疗，针灸可以预防宫颈癌、外阴癌的发生。尤其用电热针治疗本病的癌前病变，效果肯定。

二、治疗方法

【早期】

治法 调理冲任，祛湿解毒。

处方 气海（RN6）、蠡沟（LR5）、行间（LR2）、三阴交（SP6）、阿是穴，根据病变范围取穴。

方义 气海是任脉经穴，通胞宫、理冲任、化湿浊、祛痰毒；蠡沟为肝经之络穴，可宣郁调经，理气和血；行间为肝经之荥穴，可疏肝理气，和血解毒，养阴止崩；三阴交为足三阴经之交会穴，主和气血，调冲任，护胞宫；局部取穴，以活血养血，舒筋活络，改善局部气血。诸穴共用，可收调理冲任，祛湿解毒之功效。

4. Leukoplakia vulva (white lesions of vluva) is the precancerous lesion of this disease, early detection and early treatment are very important. Acupuncture treatment can prevent incidence of cervical cancers and vulvar cancers. Especially the use of electrothermal acupuncture treatment for the precancerous lesion of this disease, can achieve positive effects.

II. Therapeutic Methods

[Early Phase]

Therapeutic method: Nurse Chong Channel and Ren Channel, remove Damp and relieve internal Heat.

Prescription: Qihai (RN6), Ligou (LR5), Xingjian (LR2), Sanyinjiao (SP6); Ashi acupoints, select acupoints depending on the lesion range.

Mechanism of prescription: Qihai is an acupoint of Ren Channel, it can soothe uterus, nurse Chong Channel and Ren Channel, eliminate Damp, remove phelgm toxins. Ligou is a collateral acupoint of Liver Meridian, which can disperse stasis and regulate meridians, regulate Qi and blood. Xinjian is a Xing acupoint of Liver Meridian, which can soothe liver and regulate Qi, harmonize blood and clear toxins, nourish Yin and stop collapse. Sanyinjiao is the confluent acupoint of the three Yin Meridians of Foot, which can harmonize Qi and blood, nurse Chong Channel and Ren Channel, protect uterus. Local selection of acupoints, to activate and nourish blood, relax tendons and activate collaterals, improve local Qi-blood. The use of combination of these acupoints can nurse Chong Channel and Ren Channel,

配穴　宫颈痛者，加太冲、太溪；带下多者，可加丰隆、地机；腹胀者，可加足三里、阳陵泉。

方法　电热针治疗。

操作　选定穴位，皮肤常规消毒。电热针直刺气海、三阴交各 0.7 寸，直刺蠡沟 0.6 寸，直刺足三里、丰隆、地机各 0.8 寸。接通电热针仪，每个穴位分别给予电流量 50～60mA，以患者感到温胀舒适为度，留针 40 分钟。另配以毫针直刺行间、太冲、太溪各 0.5 寸，留针 30 分钟。

疗程　每日 1 次，10 次为 1 个疗程。疗程间休息 3～5 天，再进行第 2 个疗程的治疗。

【晚期】

治法　补气固冲，止血升陷。

处方　气海（RN6）、三阴交（SP6）、大敦（LR1）、脾俞（BL20）、大都（SP2）。

方义　气海为任脉经穴、元气之海，与三阴交合用，有补元气、调养气血、固护冲任的作用；大敦是肝经之井穴，擅长固冲止崩，升举下陷；脾

remove Damp and relieve internal Heat.

Matching acupoints: For cervical pain add Taichong, Taixi. For excessive leukorrhea add Fenglong, Diji. For abdominal distension add Zusanli, Yanglingquan.

Method: Electrothermal acupuncture treatment.

Operations: Selecting the relevant acupoints, perform routine skin disinfection. Using electrothermal acupuncture needles, vertically puncture into Qihai, Sanyinjiao for 0.7" respectively, Ligou for 0.6", Zusanli, Fenglong, Diji for 0.8" respectively. Turn on the electrothermal acupuncture equipment, apply a current of 50-60mA to each acupoint. The limit is that the patient feels warmly swell and comfortable. Leave the needles in for 40 minutes. Additionally, using filiform needles, vertically puncture into Xingjian, Taichong and Taixi for 0.5" respectively. Leave the needles in for 30 minutes.

Therapeutic course: Once a day, 10 times for a course. Start the treatment for the second course after a break of 3-5 days.

[Advanced Phase]

Therapeutic method: Tonify Qi and reinforce Ren, stop bleeding and ascend up collapse.

Prescription: Qihai (RN6), Sanyinjiao (SP6), Dadun (LR1), Pishu (BL20), Dadu (SP2).

Mechanism of prescription: Qihai is an acupoint of Ren Channel, the sea of vitality, which can replenish vitality Qi, tonify Qi-blood, reinforce and nurse Chong Channel and Ren Channel when being matched with Sanyinjiao. Dadun is a Jing acupoint of Liver Meridian, it is good at reinforcing Ren, stop collapse and ascend up collapse. Pishu is a Shu acupoint of Spleen Meridian, Dadu is a Xing acupoint of Spleen Meridian, the match of these two acupoints can replenish spleen and tonify qi, nourish blood and stop leucorrhea. The use of combination of these acupoints can tonify Qi and reinforce Chong, stop bleeding and ascend up collapse.

Matching acupoints: For frequent micturition, hematuria, add Zhongji. For palpitation add Shenmen, Neiguan. For abdominal pain add Guanyuan.

Method: Electrothermal acupuncture treatment.

Operations: Selecting the relevant acupoints, perform routine skin disinfection. Using the electrothermal acupuncture needles, vertically puncture into Qihai for 0.7", Sanyinjiao for 0.8", obliquely puncture toward spine into Pishu for 0.8". Turn on the electrothermal acupuncture equipment, apply a current of 40-60mA to each acupoint. The limit is that the patient feels warmly swell and comfortable. Leave the needles in for 40 minutes. Additionally, using filiform needles, obliquely puncture into Dadun and Dadu for 0.4" respectively. Leave the needles in for 40 minutes. Use surrounding acupuncture for partly central area.

Therapeutic course: Once a day, 10 times for a course. Start the treatment for the second course after a break of 3-5 days.

III. Precautions

1. Diet should be light, and eat more food containing high levels of protein and vitamins, do not eat cold, spicy food.

2. 患者应精神愉快，情志舒畅，忌忿怒、抑郁、惊恐、忧伤。

3. 避风寒水湿，严禁房事，减少剧烈活动。

4. 如出血量大，患者面色苍白，肢冷汗出，应及时救治。

5. 有条件者最好配合中药治疗，效果较好。

2. Patients should keep happy mood and emotional ease, avoid anger, depression, fear, sorrow.

3. Avoid Wind Cold and Water Damp, forbid sexual intercourses, reduce strenuous activities.

4. If excessive bleeding volume, pale complexion, cold limbs and sweating of the patient, timely treatment is required.

5. If possible, it is better to match with Chinese Herb Medicine treatment so as to achieve better efficacies.

男科疾病 Men's diseases

阳痿 Asynodia

阳痿是指成年男子阴茎临房不举，或举而不坚，影响正常性生活的一种疾病。本病有功能性阳痿与器质性阳痿之分。前者约占85%～90%，其原因与多种精神因素有关，为针灸治疗的主要对象。后者是由于解剖原因，或其他疾病及药物的影响所致。

因为本病主要表现为阴茎痿软，故又称"阴痿"，亦称"宗筋弛纵"或"阴器不用"，属于现代医学"男子性功能障碍"的范畴。临床分为虚证、实证两大类，其中以虚证居多。

Asynodia refers to impotence during sexual intercourses or erection with soft penis of adult males, which affects normal sexual intercourses. This disease is divided into functional asynodia and organic asynodia. The former accounts for 85%-90%, the causes of which normally related to various mental issues, and is the main subject of acupuncture treatment. The later is caused by anatomical reasons or influence of other diseases and drugs.

Since this disease mainly presents as soft penis, so is also called "impotence", as well as "slackness of male external genitals" or "inability to produce an erection", it belongs to the range of "male sexual dysfunction" in modern medicine. It is divided into two classes, deficiency syndromes and excess syndromes, most of which are deficiency syndromes.

一、诊断及辨证要点

I. Key Points for Diagnosis and Syndrome Differentiation

1. 肾阳虚衰者，症见阳事不举，精液清冷，夜尿多，小便清长，眩晕耳鸣，神疲乏力，腰酸腿软，畏寒肢冷，舌质淡，脉沉迟。

1. For patients with depletion and deficiency of kidney Yang, symptoms include impotence, thin and cold semen, frequent urination at night, clear abundant urine, dizziness and tinnitus, mental fatigue and asthenia, aching lumbus and limp legs, intolerance of cold and ex-

2. 心脾两虚者，症见性欲淡漠，举而不坚，心悸易惊，失眠健忘，面色萎黄，气短乏力，食少腹胀，大便溏泻，舌质淡，苔薄白或腻，脉细弱。

3. 肝气郁结者，症见阳痿，精神抑郁，胸闷纳差，善太息，胁肋或小腹胀满不舒，或咽中异物感，舌苔薄白，脉弦细。

4. 临床以性交时多不能勃起，但在手淫、夜间憋尿时却能勃起，多勃起无力，或坚而不长为特征。

二、治疗方法

【肾阳虚衰证】

治法 补肾气，壮元阳。

处方 大椎（DU14）、命门（DU4）、肾俞（BL23）、关元俞（BL26）、三阴交（SP6）。

方义 大椎乃诸阳之会，为壮阳益精之要穴。命门、肾俞、关元俞合用，可补肾气，壮元阳。本病多因阴精先伤，

treme chilliness, light tongue, deep and slow pulse.

2. For patients with deficiency of heart and spleen, symptoms include sexual apathy, erection with soft penis, palpitation and easy to be scared, insomnia and amnesia, sallow complexion, short breath and asthenia, less food intake and abdominal distension, thin and sloppy stool, light tongue with thin and whitish or greasy fur, thin and weak pulse.

3. For patients with liver Qi stagnation, symptoms include asynodia, depression, chest distress and poor appetite, reference for sighing, distension of ribs or lower abdomen, or foreign body sensation in throat, thin and whitish tongue fur, thin and taut pulse.

4. Clinical erectile weakness of penis include unable to erect during sexual intercourses but able to erect during masturbating or urine suppressing at night, the features include erectile weakness of penis and hardness for short time.

II. Therapeutic Methods

[Syndrome of Deficiency and Depletion of Kidney Yang]

Therapeutic method: Replenish kidney Qi and strengthen Yuan Yang.

Prescription: Dazhui (DU14), Mingmen (DU4), Shenshu (BL23), Guanyuanshu (BL26), Sanyinjiao (SP6).

Mechanism of prescription: Dazhui is the confluent acupoint for Yang of the whole body, is an important acupoint for strengthening Yang and tonifying essence. The combination of Mingmen, Shenshu and Guanyuan-

后损及阳，故取三阴交补肝肾之阴以治本。诸穴相伍，温阳而不损阴，肾阳复振，则病易愈。

配穴 头晕耳鸣者，加风池、印堂；胸闷纳差者，加中脘；精液清冷者加腰阳关。

方法 电热针治疗（温补法）。

操作 选定穴位，常规皮肤消毒。电热针向下斜刺大椎0.7寸，直刺命门0.6寸，直刺肾俞0.7寸，直刺关元俞0.8寸。接通电热针仪，每个穴位分别给予电流量70mA。另配以毫针直刺三阴交0.8寸，向下斜刺印堂0.5寸，直刺中脘0.7寸，留针40分钟。快针风池，不留针。

疗程 每日1次，10次为1个疗程，疗程间休息3～5天，再继续进行第2个疗程的治疗。

【心脾两虚证】

治法 宁心安神，健脾养心。

shu can replenish kidney Qi and strengthen Yuan Yang. This disease is mostly caused by that Yin essence got hurt and subsequently damage Yang, so use Sanyinjiao to replenish Yin of liver and kidney so as to effect a permanent cure. The match of these acupoints can warm Yang without damage of Ying, and the disease will be easily cured if kidney Yang revitalized.

Matching acupoints: For dizziness and tinnitus add Fengchi, Yintang. For chest distress and poor appetite, add Zhongwan. For patients with cold and thin semen, add Yaoyangguan.

Method: Electrothermal acupuncture treatment (warm tonifying).

Operations: Selecting the relevant acupoints, perform routine skin disinfection. Using the electrothermal acupuncture needles, obliquely puncture downward into Dazhui for 0.7", vertically puncture into Minmen for 0.6", Shenshu for 0.7", Guanyuanshu for 0.8". Turn on the electrothermal acupuncture equipment, apply a current of 70mA to each acupoint. Additionally, using the filiform needles, vertically puncture into Sanyinjiao for 0.8", obliquely puncture into Yintang for 0.5", vertically puncture into Zhongwan for 0.7", leaving the needles in for 40 minutes. Quickly puncture into Fengchi, do not leave the needle in.

Therapeutic course: Treat once a day, 10 times for a course, and start the treatment for the second course after a break of 3-5 days.

[Syndrome of Deficiency of Heart and Spleen]

Therapeutic method: Calm heart and tranquilize mind, invigorate spleen and nourish heart.

处方 心俞（BL15）、内关（PC6）、三阴交（SP6）、足三里（ST36）、关元（RN4）。

方义 足三里是胃经的合穴，乃全身壮阳要穴，可健脾益胃，以助气血生化之源；心俞与内关、三阴交同用，补益心脾，养血安神；关元温阳益气，强壮宗筋。诸穴合用，收健脾胃、养心神之功效。

配穴 心悸健忘者，加神门；腹胀便溏者，加脾俞、中脘；神疲肢冷者，加中极、命门。

方法 电热针治疗（温补法）。

操作 选定穴位，常规皮肤消毒。电热针向下斜刺关元0.8寸，直刺足三里0.8寸，直刺三阴交0.8寸，直刺中脘0.7寸。接通电热针仪，每个穴位分别给予电流量60mA。另配以毫针直刺内关、神门各0.5寸，留针40分钟。快针心俞，不留针，后加艾条灸，每穴10分钟。

Prescription: Xinshu (BL15), Neiguan (PC6), Sanyinjiao (SP6), Zusanli (ST36), Guanyuan (RN4).

Mechanism of prescription: Zusanli is a He acupoint of Stomach Meridian, an important acupoint for systemic Yang strengthening, it can invigorate spleen and tonify stomach, so as to facilitate the source of generation and transformation of Qi-blood. Use Xinshu together with Neiguan and Sanyinjiao can tonify heart and spleen, nourish blood and tranquilize mind; Guanyuan can warm Yang and tonify Qi, strengthen male external genital. The use of combination of these acupoints can astringe and invigorate spleen and stomach, nourish mind.

Matching acupoints: For palpitation and amnesia add Shenmen. For abdominal distension and sloppy stool add Pishu and Zhongwan. For patients with mental fatigue and cold limbs add Zhongji, Mingmen.

Method: Electrothermal acupuncture treatment (warm tonifying).

Operations: Selecting the relevant acupoints, perform routine skin disinfection. Using electrothermal acupuncture needles, obliquely puncture downward into Guanyuan for 0.8", vertically puncture into Zusanli and Sanyinjiao for 0.8" respectively, Zhongwan for 0.7". Turn on the electrothermal acupuncture equipment, apply a current of 60mA to each acupoint. Additionally, using filiform needles, vertically puncture into Neiguan and Shenmen for 0.5" respectively. Leave the needles in for 40 minutes. Quickly puncture into Xinshu, do not leave the needle in. Then add moxa-roll moxibustion, 10 minutes for each acupoint.

疗程　每日1次，10次为1个疗程，疗程间休息3～5天，再继续进行第2个疗程的治疗。

【肝气郁结证】

治法　疏肝理气，调养宗筋。

处方　肝俞（BL18）、期门（LR14）、太冲（LR3）、曲骨（RN2）、曲泉（LR8）。

方义　肝俞为肝脉之气转输之处，太冲是肝经的原穴，曲骨是肝经与任脉之交会穴，三穴共用，可疏肝理气，调养宗筋。配肝之募穴期门，可增强疏肝理气之功，亦可活血通脉。用肝之合穴曲泉，可养血柔肝，疏肝而不伐肝。

配穴　肝脾失调者，加脾俞；肝胃不和者，加胃俞；肝郁化热者，加阳陵泉、丘墟。

方法　电热针治疗（平补平泻法）。

操作　选定穴位，常规皮肤消毒。电热针向脊柱侧斜刺肝俞、脾俞各0.8寸，斜刺期门0.7寸。接通电热针仪，每

Therapeutic course: Treat once a day, 10 times for a course, and start the treatment for the second course after a break of 3-5 days.

[Syndrome of Liver-Qi Stagnation]

Therapeutic method: Soothe liver and regulate Qi, tonify male external genital.

Prescription: Ganshu (BL18), Qimen (LR14), Taichong (LR3), Qugu (RN2), Ququan (LR8).

Mechanism of prescription: Ganshu is the place for transformation and transportation of Qi of Liver Channel, Taichong is a Yuan acupoint of Liver Meridian, Qugu is the confluent acupoint of Liver Meridian and Ren Channel, the use of combination of these three acupoints can soothe liver and regulate Qi, tonify male external genital. The match of Qimen, a Mu acupoint of Liver, can soothe liver and regulate Qi, as well as activate blood and dredge channels. Use the He acupoint Ququan of Liver to nourish blood and tonify liver, soothe liver without damage.

Matching acupoints: For liver and spleen disorders add Pishu. For liver-stomach disharmony add Weishu. For liver stasis transforming into Heat add Yanglingquan, Qiuxu.

Method: Electrothermal acupuncture treatment (mild tonifying and attenuating).

Operations: Selecting the relevant acupoints, perform routine skin disinfection. Using electrothermal acupuncture needles, obliquely puncture toward spine into Ganshu, Pishu for 0.8" respectively, obliquely

· 631 ·

个穴位分别给予电流量 60mA。另配以毫针直刺曲骨 0.7 寸，直刺曲泉 0.8 寸，留针 40 分钟。

疗程 每日 1 次，10 次为 1 个疗程，疗程间休息 3～5 天，再继续进行第 2 个疗程的治疗。

三、注意事项

1. 针灸是治疗功能性阳痿的有效方法，施术时取穴要准确，手法要温和适中。针刺关元或中极时，要使针感到达阴茎或会阴部，以提高疗效。对器质性阳痿则非单独运用针灸方法所能奏效的，必须配合相应的措施，还要消除病因。

2. 本病疗程长，针灸治疗要坚持，按疗程进行，病情好转亦需巩固治疗，以达彻底治愈。

3. 配合心理治疗和体疗，有助于提高疗效。要使患者心情开朗，消除对房事的顾虑和焦虑心理。

4. 治疗期间应清心寡欲，避免房事，治疗后房事亦应有

puncture into Qimen for 0.7". Turn on the electrothermal acupuncture equipment, apply a current of 60mA to each acupoint. Additionally, using the filiform needles, vertically puncture into Qugu for 0.7", Ququan for 0.8", leaving the needles in for 40 minutes.

Therapeutic course: Treat once a day, 10 times for a course, and start the treatment for the second course after a break of 3-5 days.

III. Precautions

1. Acupuncture therapy is an effective approach for functional asynodia treatment. For acupuncture, the acupoint locating should be accurate and the skill should be mild and appropriate. When puncturing Guanyuan or Zhongji, the feeling of needle puncturing must be spread to penis or perineum, so as to improve efficacies. For organic asynodia, the use of acupuncture therapy alone is not enough, it must be matched with corresponding measures as well as elimination of causes.

2. This disease has a long treatment course, so the key point of acupuncture therapy is persistence and performing as per courses, and to achieve complete cure, it still needs consolidation treatment after condition improvement.

3. Match with psychological therapy and physical therapy to improve efficacies. Make patients feel cheerful, eliminate concerns on sexual intercourses and anxious mood.

4. During treatment, it is necessary to purify mind and limit desires, avoid sexual intercourses, and after

所节制，切勿恣情纵欲。

5. 女方对男方的病情要体谅理解，切勿指责和鄙视，以有利于患者的精神调养。

四、典型病例

张某，男，44岁，工程师，北京人。

主诉：婚后阴茎不能勃起已3年。病史：患者3年前刚结婚不久，在行房时突遇惊慌之事，当时早泄，以后每逢行房就阳痿不举，经多方诊治，疗效不显。

刻下症：阳痿不举，胆怯多疑，心悸易惊，夜寐不宁，面色白，舌红，苔薄白，脉弦。

查体：未见阳性体征。

辅助检查：未见异常。

【诊断依据】

1. 中年男子，急性起病，3年不愈。

2. 原因清楚，房事中突遇意外，惊恐伤肾。

3. 查体未发现生殖、泌尿系统器质性病变，刻下症纯属功能性障碍。

4. 各项检查未见异常。

treatment sexual intercourses also should be limited, do not indulge in carnal pleasure without restraint.

5. The wife should be considerate for the husband's condition, do not blame and despise the husband so as to facilitate the patient's mental rehabilitation.

IV. Typical Case

Zhang, male, 44 years old, engineer, residence: Beijing.

Self-reported symptoms: Unable to erect for 3 years after marriage. Medical history: 3 years ago, when the patient just married, he suddenly met scary matters during sexual intercourse and suffered a premature ejaculation at the time, later he suffered from asynodia at each time of sexual intercourse, and got non-significant efficacies after various therapies.

Current symptoms: Asynodia, timid and suspicious, palpitation and easy to be scared, disturbed sleep at night, pale complexion, red tongue with whitish and thin fur, taut pulse.

Physical examination: No positive signs were seen.

Auxiliary examination: No abnormalities.

[Diagnostic Basis]

1. Middle-aged male, acute onset, unhealed for 3 years.

2. Clear cause: The patient met accident during sexual intercourse, scare and fear impairing kidney.

3. No organic lesions of reproductive system and urinary system were found in the physical examination, the current syndrome belonged to functional disorder.

4. No abnormalities found in various examinations.

【证治分析】

病因 惊恐伤肾。

病机 房事之中突遇意外，惊恐伤肾。

证候分析 惊则气乱，恐则气下，气机逆乱，肾气失司，而致宗筋弛纵，发为阳痿。

病位 肾。

病性 虚性。

西医诊断 阳痿、神经衰弱。

中医诊断 阳痿。

治法 补肾安神。

方法 电热针治疗。

处方 百会（DU20）、四神聪（EX-HN1）、神门（HT7）、肾俞（BL23）、命门（DU4）、关元（RN4）、三阴交（SP6）。

方义 百会、四神聪可镇静安神，益聪定志；神门是心经的原穴，心主神明，取神门以补心气，安神定志；肾俞可补肾壮阳；关元、三阴交可补益下元，助阳以起痿。

配穴 胆怯者加间使；失眠易惊者加风池、足三里。

[Syndrome-treatment Analysis]

Etiology: Scare impairing kidney.

Pathogenesis: The patient met an accident during sexual intercourse, scare and fear impairing kidney.

Syndrome analysis: Scare causes disorder of Qi, fear causes downward flow of Qi, Qi Dynamic disturbance, loss of kidney Qi control, leading to male external genital dysfunction which present as asynodia.

Lesion location: Kidney.

Disease nature: Deficiency.

The diagnosis of Western Medicine: Asynodia and neurasthenia.

The diagnosis of Traditional Chinese Medicine: Asynodia.

Therapeutic method: Replenish kidney and tranquilize mind.

Method: Electrothermal acupuncture treatment.

Prescription: Baihui (DU20), Sishencong (EX-HN1), Shenmen (HT7), Shenshu (BL23), Mingmen (DU4), Guanyuan (RN4), Sanyinjiao (SP6).

Mechanism of prescription: Baihui, Sishencong can calm and tranquilize mind, tonify Cong and consolidate Zhi; Shenmen is a Yuan acupoint of Heart Meridian, heart governs mental activities, so use Shenmen to tonify heart Qi, tranquilize mind and consolidate Zhi; Shenshu can replenish kidney and strengthen Yang; Guanyuan, Sanyinjiao can tonify lower origin, facilitate Yang to resolve impotence.

Matching acupoints: For timidity add Jianshi. For insomnia and easy to be frightened, add Fengchi, Zusanli.

操作 选定穴位，皮肤常规消毒。电热针平刺百会、四神聪各0.6寸，直刺神门、三阴交、足三里、间使、关元各0.7寸，斜刺（针尖向脊柱）肾俞、关元俞各0.7寸。接通电热针仪，每穴分别给予电流量30～40mA，留针40分钟。（注：每次选3组穴给予电热针治疗，余者用毫针治疗。）

Operations: Selecting the relevant acupoints, perform routine skin disinfection. Using electrothermal acupuncture needles, horizontally puncture into Baihui, Sishencong for 0.6" respectively, vertically puncture into Shenmen, Sanyinjiao, Zusanli, Jianshi, Guanyuan for 0.7" respectively, obliquely puncture (with the needle tip towards spine) into Shenshu, Guanyuanshu for 0.7" respectively. Turn on the electrothermal acupuncture equipment, apply a current of 30-40mA to each acupoint. Leave the needles in for 40 minutes. (Note: Selecting 3 pairs of acupoints for electrothermal acupuncture treatment each time, and treat the other acupoints with filiform needles.)

疗程 每日1次，10次为1个疗程，疗程间休息3～5天，再继续进行第2个疗程的治疗。

Therapeutic course: Treat once a day, 10 times for a course, and start the treatment for the second course after a break of 3-5 days.

治疗过程 该患者在治疗过程中，效果较明显，经23次治疗后，症状全部消失，性生活正常，又继续巩固治疗20天后结束治疗。随访2年，已有一男孩（14个月）。

Therapeutic process: The patient achieved obvious effects during treatment, all symptoms disappeared after 23 treatments, and he completed the treatment after 20 days of consolidation therapy. Follow-up for 2 years, had fathered a boy (14 months old).

【生活调摄】

1. 调畅情志，使患者心情开朗，消除对房事的顾虑和焦虑心理。

2. 治疗期间应清心寡欲，避免房事，治疗后房事亦应有所节制，切勿恣情纵欲。

[Lifestyle Change and Health Maintenance]

1. Make patients regulate mood, let them feel cheerful, eliminate concerns on sexual intercourses and anxious mood.

2. During treatment, it is necessary to purify mind and limit desires, avoid sexual intercourses, and after treatment sexual intercourses also should be limited, do not indulge in carnal pleasure without restraint.

早泄

早泄是指性交时间极短即行排精，甚至性交前即泄精的病症。

中医认为，早泄的发生与心、肝、肾功能失调有关。多因心有所欲，相火妄动；或纵欲伤肾，精气不固；或肝经湿热，扰动精室所致。病有虚实之分。

一、诊断及辨证要点

1. 君相火旺者，症见欲念时起，阳事易举，临房早泄，或心烦失眠，梦中遗精，腰酸头晕，口燥咽干，舌质红，苔少，脉细数。

2. 肾气不固者，症见性欲减退，临房早泄，精神萎靡，腰酸腿软，畏寒肢冷，或兼阳痿，自汗，气短，舌质淡，脉沉细。

3. 肝经湿热者，症见早泄，阴茎易举，阴囊热痒，尿黄不爽，胸闷胁痛，口苦纳呆，苔黄腻，脉弦滑而数。

Premature Ejaculation

Premature ejaculation refers to ejaculation after a very short time of sexual intercourse, or even ejaculate before sexual intercourses.

Traditional Chinese Medicine believes that the development of premature ejaculation is related to dysfunctions of heart, liver and kidney. Most are caused by desires and hyperactivity of ministerial Fire; or indulge in carnal pleasure without restraint injuring kidney, non-consolidation of essence Qi; or Damp-Heat of Liver Channel interfering seminal chamber. This disease includes deficiency and excess syndromes.

I. Key Points for Diagnosis and Syndrome Differentiation

1. For patients with blazing monarchic and ministerial Fire, symptoms include rise of desire from time to time, easy erection during sexual intercourses, premature ejaculation, or vexation and insomnia, spermatorrhea during dream, soreness of waist and dizziness, dry mouth and throat, red tongue with less fur, thin and rapid pulse.

2. For patients with non-consolidation of kidney Qi, symptoms include hyposexuality, spiritlessness, aching lumbus and limp legs, intolerance of cold and extreme chilliness, or accompanied with asynodia, spontaneous sweating, short breath, light tongue, deep and thin pulse.

3. For patients with Damp-Heat of Liver Channel, symptoms include premature ejaculation, easy erection of penis, hot and itching scrotum, yellow urine and unsmooth urination, chest distress and rib pain, bitter taste

and poor appetite, yellow and greasy tongue fur, taut, slippery and rapid pulse.

4. 发病与大脑皮层和脊髓性神经中枢功能紊乱,以及外生殖器及泌尿系统炎症刺激等因素有密切的关系。

4. The incidence is closely related to factors such as cerebral cortex and spinal nerve center dysfunctions as well as stimulations of external genitalia and urinary tract inflammations.

5. 仅对在每次性交或大多数性交过程中经常发生早泄者方可诊断为本病。

5. This disease can only be confirmed if the premature ejaculation occurs in each time or most of the sexual intercourses.

二、治疗方法

【君相火旺证】

治法 清心降火。

处方 心俞(BL15)、劳宫(PC8)、然谷(KI2)、地机(SP8)、肾俞(BL23)、太溪(KI3)、三阴交(SP6)。

方义 劳宫是心包经的荥穴,主治本经热证,与心俞相配,可清降君火,宁心安神;然谷是足少阴经之荥穴,配地机可清虚火,坚肾阴;取肾俞、太溪、三阴交以滋阴潜阳。诸穴共用,有清心降火、滋阴固精的作用。

配穴 失眠者,加神门;头晕者,加百会;性功能亢进

II. Therapeutic Methods

[Syndrome of Blazing Monarchic and Ministerial Fire]

Therapeutic method: Clear heart and decline Fire.

Prescription: Xinshu (BL15), Laogong (PC8), Rangu (KI2), Diji (SP8), Shenshu (BL23), Taixi (KI3), Sanyinjiao (SP6).

Mechanism of prescription: Laogong is a Xing acupoint of Pericardium Meridian, which mainly can treat Heat syndrome of this meridian, clear and decline monarchic Fire as well as tranquilize mind and nourish vital energy when being matched with Xinshu; Rangu is a Xing acupoint of Shao-Yin Meridian of Foot, which can clear Defficiency-Fire and reinforce kidney Fire when being matched with Diji. Use Shenshu, Taixi, Sanyinjiao to nourish Yin and suppress Yang. The use of combination of these acupoints can clear and decline monarchic Fire, nourish Yin and reinforce essence.

Matching acupoints: For insomnia add Shenmen. For dizziness add Baihui. For sexual function hyperfunc-

者，加太冲。

方法 电热针治疗。

操作 选定穴位，常规皮肤消毒。电热针向脊柱侧斜刺肾俞 0.8 寸，直刺三阴交 0.8 寸。接通电热针仪，每个穴位分别给予电流量 70mA。另配以毫针向脊柱侧斜刺心俞 0.8 寸，直刺劳宫 0.3 寸，直刺然谷 0.5 寸，直刺地机 0.8 寸，留针 40 分钟。

疗程 每天 1 次，10 天为 1 个疗程，疗程间休息 3 天。

【肾气不固证】

治法 补肾气，固精关，止早泄。

处方 肾俞（BL23）、京门（GB25）、太溪（KI3）、阴谷（KI10）、关元（RN4）。

方义 肾俞、京门分别是足少阴肾经的俞、募穴，俞募相配以固肾气；太溪是肾经的原穴，可滋补元阳和元阴；阴谷是肾经的合穴，长于补益肾气；加补足三阴与任脉之会关元以助下元之气，加强固摄之功。诸穴合用，可补肾气，固精关，止早泄。

tion add Taichong.

Method: Electrothermal acupuncture treatment.

Operations: Selecting the relevant acupoints, perform routine skin disinfection. Using electrothermal acupuncture needles, obliquely puncture toward spine into Shenshu for 0.8", vertically puncture into Sanyinjiao for 0.8". Turn on the electrothermal acupuncture equipment, apply a current of 70mA to each acupoint. Additionally, using the filiform needles, obliquely puncture toward spine into Xinshu for 0.8", vertically puncture into Laogong for 0.3", Rangu for 0.5", Diji for 0.8", leaving the needles in for 40 minutes.

Therapeutic course: Once a day, 10 days as a course. Rest for 3 days between courses.

[Syndrome of Non-consolidation of Kidney Qi]

Therapeutic method: Replenish kidney Qi, consolidate seminal gate, stop premature ejaculation.

Prescription: Shenshu (BL23), Jingmen (GB25), Taixi (KI3), Yingu (KI10), Guanyuan (RN4).

Mechanism of prescription: Shenshu and Jingmen are respectively the Shu acupoint and Mu acupoint of Shao-Yin Kidney Meridian of Foot, the match of Shu and Mu acupoint can reinforce kidney Qi; Taixi is a Yuan acupoint of Kidney Meridian, it can nourish Yuan Yang and Yuan Yin; Yingu is a He acupoint of Kidney Meridian, it is good at tonify kidney Qi; add the confluent acupoint of three Yin Meridians of Foot and Ren Channel, Guanyuan, to promote Qi of lower origin, reinforce effects of nourishment. The use of combination of these acupoints can replenish kidney Qi, consolidate seminal gate, stop premature ejaculation.

Matching acupoints: For spontaneous sweating add Yinxi, Zusanli; For shortness of breath add Feishu. For urorrhagia add Pangguangshu. For hyposexuality add Shenque.

Method: Electrothermal acupuncture treatment (warm tonifying).

Operations: Selecting the relevant acupoints, perform routine skin disinfection. Using electrothermal acupuncture needles, obliquely puncture toward spine into Shenshu for 0.8", obliquely puncture into Yingu for 0.7", vertically puncture into Jingmen for 0.7". Turn on the electrothermal acupuncture equipment, apply a current of 70mA to each acupoint. Additionally, using the filiform needles, obliquely puncture downward into Guanyuan, make the feeling of needle puncturing spread to perineum, vertically puncture into Taixi for 0.5", leaving the needles in for 40 minutes.

Therapeutic course: Once a day, 10 days as a course. Rest for 3 days between courses.

[Damp-Heat Syndrome of Liver Meridian]

Therapeutic method: Purge Damp-Heat, consolidate seminal gate.

Prescription: Ganshu (BL18), Xinjian (LR2), Fenglong (ST40), Pangguangshu (BL28), Ciliao (BL32).

Mechanism of prescription: Xingjian is a Xing acupoint of Liver Meridian, it can purge Heat of this meridian, and can enhance the effect of clearing liver and purging Heat when being matched with Ganshu; downward flow of Damp-Heat, interference of seminal cham-

热。诸穴合用，共收清泻湿热、安定精关之功效。

配穴 小便热痛者，加三阴交；烦躁不寐者，加神门。

方法 毫针治疗（泻法）。

操作 选定穴位，常规皮肤消毒。用毫针向脊柱侧斜刺肝俞、膀胱俞、次髎各 0.8 寸，直刺丰隆 0.7 寸，直刺行间 0.5 寸，留针 30 分钟。

疗程 每天 1 次，10 次为 1 个疗程，疗程间休息 3 天。

三、注意事项

1. 针灸是治疗早泄的有效方法，施术时取穴要准确，手法要温和适中。针刺关元或中极时，要使针感到达阴茎或会阴部，以提高疗效。本病疗程长，针灸治疗要坚持，按疗程进行，病情好转亦需巩固治疗，以达彻底治愈。

2. 配合心理治疗和体疗，有助于提高疗效。要使患者心

ber, therefore purge Pangguangshu and Ciliao to clear Damp-Heat of Lower Jiao; Fenlong can remove Damp and clear Heat. The use of combination of these acupoints can purge Damp-Heat, consolidate seminal gate.

Matching acupoints: For patients feeling hot and painful when urinating, add Sanyinjiao. For vexation and sleeplessness add Shenmen.

Method: Filiform needle acupuncture treatment (attenuating).

Operations: Selecting the relevant acupoints, perform routine skin disinfection. Using the filiform needles, obliquely puncture toward spine side into Ganshu, Pangguangshu, Ciliao for 0.8" respectively, vertically puncture into Fenlong for 0.7", Xingjian for 0.5", leaving the needles in for 30 minutes.

Therapeutic course: Once a day, 10 times for a course. Rest for 3 days between courses.

III. Precautions

1. Acupuncture therapy is an effective approach for premature ejaculation treatment. For acupuncture, the acupoint locating should be accurate and the skill should be mild and appropriate. When puncturing Guanyuan or Zhongji, the feeling of needle puncturing must be spread to penis or perineum, so as to improve efficacies. This disease has a long treatment course, so the key point of acupuncture therapy is persistence and performing as per courses, and to achieve complete cure, it still needs consolidation treatment after condition improvement.

2. Match with psychological therapy and physical therapy to improve efficacies. Make patients feel cheer-

情开朗，消除对房事的顾虑和焦虑心理。

3. 治疗期间应清心寡欲，避免房事，治疗后房事亦应有所节制，切勿恣情纵欲。

4. 女方对男方的病情要体贴，切勿指责和鄙视，以有利于患者的精神调养。

四、典型病例

冯某，男，38岁，工人，北京人。

主诉：婚后早泄1年多，经治不愈。

刻下症：精神抑郁，腰酸腿软，一交即泄，平素多头晕目眩，时常口苦咽干，舌红苔薄，脉弦。

查体：未见阳性体征。

辅助检查：未见异常。

【诊断依据】

1. 中年男性，少年无知，犯手淫日久，婚后1年多，阳举而不坚，一交即泄。

2. 查体和各项检查未见异常。

3. 平素多精神抑郁，腰酸腿软，倦怠乏力之虚象。

ful, eliminate concerns on sexual intercourses and anxious mood.

3. During treatment, it is necessary to purify mind and limit desires, avoid sexual intercourses, and after treatment sexual intercourses also should be limited, do not indulge in carnal pleasure without restraint.

4. The wife should be considerate for the husband's condition, do not blame and despise the husband so as to facilitate the patient's mental rehabilitation.

IV. Typical Case

Feng, male, 38 years old, worker, residence: Beijing.

Self-reported symptoms: Premature ejaculation for more than a year after getting married, unhealed by treatment.

Current symptoms: Depression, aching lumbus and limp legs, ejaculation at the beginning of sexual intercourses, in normal times often had dizziness, bitter taste and dry throat, red tongue with thin fur, taut pulse.

Physical examination: No positive signs were seen.

Auxiliary examination: No abnormalities.

[Diagnostic Basis]

1. Middle-aged male, had a long history of masturbation due to being young and innocent, married for more than 1 year, erection with soft penis, ejaculation at the beginning of sexual intercourses.

2. No abnormalities found in physical examination and other examinations.

3. Often suffered from symptoms of deficiency syndrome including depression, aching lumbus and limp

4. 生殖器官无异常。

【证治分析】

病因　肾虚肝郁。

病机　肾脏本虚，固摄无力，加之精神抑郁，郁久化火，扰动精宫，发生早泄。

证候分析　肝藏血，肾藏精，肝血依赖肾精滋养，肾得肝血而精充，肾精不足，肝失滋养，气机失于条达，则精神抑郁；肾虚精失不固，故一交即泄；腰为肾之府，肾虚腰失所养，故腰酸腿软；肾精不足，水不涵木，肝阳上亢则头晕目眩；阴虚生内热，故口苦咽干。舌红、脉弦皆为阴虚内热之象。

病位　肝、肾。

病性　虚性。

西医诊断　早泄、性神经衰弱。

中医诊断　早泄。

治法　疏肝解郁，填精固本。

legs, fatigue and asthenia.

4. No reproductive organ abnormalities.

[Syndrome-treatment Analysis]

Etiology: Kidney deficiency and liver stasis.

Pathogenesis: Deficiency of kidney base, insufficient nourishment, together with depression, long-time stasis transforming into Fire which interfere with seminal chamber, leading to premature ejaculation.

Syndrome analysis: Liver stores blood, kidney stores essence, liver blood replies on kidney essence for nourishment, kidney essence becomes sufficient when get liver blood, while liver loses nourishment with insufficient kidney essence, Qi Dynamic loses free circulation, leading to depression; kidney deficiency and non-consolidation of essence, leading to ejaculation at the beginning of sexual intercourses; waist is where kidney located in, kidney deficiency causes nourishment loss of waist, leading to aching lumbus and limp legs; insufficient kidney essence, Water not nourishing Wood, hyperactivity of liver Yang, leading to dizziness; Yin deficiency generates inner Heat, leading to bitter mouth and dry throat. Red tongue and taut pulse are both symptoms of Yin deficiency and inner Heat.

Lesion location: Liver, kidney.

Disease nature: Deficiency.

The diagnosis of Western Medicine: Premature ejaculation and sexual neurasthenia.

The diagnosis of Traditional Chinese Medicine: Premature ejaculation.

Therapeutic method: Soothe liver Qi stagnation, refill essence and reinforce foundation.

方法 电热针治疗。

处方 内关（PC6）、关元（RN4）、三阴交（SP6）、膻中（RN17）、太溪（KI3）、太冲（LR3）。

方义 内关、膻中可宽胸理气，调理气机以解肝郁；太冲可清泻肝火；关元可培补肾气以固摄精液；太溪、三阴交可滋补肾阴以填精固本。

配穴 潮热盗汗者，加合谷、复溜；腰膝酸软者，加腰阳关、肾俞。

操作选定 穴位，皮肤常规消毒。电热针直刺内关、三阴交、关元、太溪、太冲、合谷、复溜、腰阳关各 0.7 寸，斜刺（针尖向脊柱）肾俞 0.7 寸。接通电热针仪，每个穴位分别给予 40 mA 的电流量，以患者感到胀而舒适为度，留针 40 分钟。（注：每次选 3 组穴给予电热针治疗，交替使用，余穴用毫针治疗。）

疗程 每天 1 次，10 次为 1 个疗程，疗程间休息 3 天。

治疗过程 该患者经 17 天的治疗后，症状基本消失，但因患病已久，故继续巩固治

Method: Electrothermal acupuncture treatment.

Prescription: Neiguan (PC6), Guanyuan (RN4), Sanyinjiao (SP6), Danzhong (RN17), Taixi (KI3), Taichong (LR3).

Mechanism of prescription: Neiguan and Danzhong can relive chest distress and regulate Qi, regulate Qi Dynamic to soothe liver stasis; Taichong can slightly disperse liver Fire; Guanyuan can reinforce kidney Qi so as to nourish semen; Taichong, Sanyinjiao can tonify kidney so as to refill essence and reinforce foundation.

Matching acupoints: For tidal fever and night sweating add Hegu, Fuliu. For aching lumbus and limp knees add Yaoyangguan, Shenshu.

Operations: Selecting the relevant acupoints, perform routine skin disinfection. Using electrothermal acupuncture needles, vertically puncture into Neiguan, Sanyinjiao, Guanyuan, Taixi, Taichong, Hegu, Fuliu, Yaoyangguan for 0.7" respectively, obliquely (with the needle tip towards spine) into Shenshu for 0.7". Turn on the electrothermal acupuncture equipment, apply a current of 40mA to each acupoint. The limit is that the patient feels swell and comfortable. Leave the needles in for 40 minutes. (Note: Select 3 pairs of acupoints for electrothermal acupuncture treatment each time, use alternately, and treat the other acupoints with filiform needles.)

Therapeutic course: Once a day, 10 times for a course. Rest for 3 days between courses.

Treatment process: After 17 days of treatment, the patient's symptoms almost all disappeared, however, he continued to take consolidation therapy due to long-term

疗，3个月后结束治疗，病情稳定。随访2年，夫妻生活正常。

【生活调摄】

1. 治疗期间应停止房事。

2. 本病为功能性，因此在治疗的同时须做好患者的思想工作，使之消除顾虑。

遗精

男子非性生活而致精液外泄者称为遗精。

中医认为，遗精的形成乃精关不固所致。有梦而遗者称"梦遗"，多为实证；无梦而遗或清醒时精液自流者称"滑精"，多为虚证。多由于思虑过度，恣情纵欲，劳伤心肾，阴精亏耗，心阳独亢，水火不济，心肾不交，相火内炽，扰动精室所致。

一、诊断及辨证要点

1. 心肾不交者，症见梦境纷纭，阳事易举，梦中遗泄，

course of disease, and he ended the treatment 3 months later, with stable conditions. Follow-up for 2 years, normal sexual intercourses.

[Lifestyle Change and Health Maintenance]

1. Sexual intercourses should be stopped during treatment.

2. This is a functional disease, therefore it is necessary to do ideological work on patients, lift their concerns.

Spermatorrhea

Spermatorrhea refers to seminal fluid leakage of men due to causes other than sexual intercourses.

Traditional Chinese Medicine believes that the development of spermatorrhea is caused by insecurity of seminal gate. Spermatorrhea with dreams is called "nocturnal emission", most of which belong to excess syndrome; spermatorrhea without dreams or spontaneous seminal fluid leakage is called "premature ejaculation", most of which belong to deficiency syndrome. Most are caused by worry beyond measure, indulgence in carnal pleasure without restraint, overstrain injuring heart and kidney, depletion and consumption of Yin essence, individual excess of heart Yang, imbalance of Water and Fire, disharmony of heart and kidney, inner burning of ministerial Fire interfering seminal chamber.

I. Key Points for Diagnosis and Syndrome Differentiation

1. For patients with disharmony between heart and kidney, symptoms include dreamy sleep, easy erection

夜寐不安，心悸神倦，腰酸，耳鸣，尿赤，舌红，脉细数。

2. 湿热下注者，症见遗精频作，身倦纳呆，口苦且渴，小便黄赤，热涩不爽，舌苔黄腻，脉濡数。

3. 肾气不固者，症见无梦而遗，甚则见色则精流，滑泄不禁，精液清稀，头晕目眩，面色白，腰酸膝软，畏寒肢冷，舌淡苔白，脉细弱。

二、治疗方法

【心肾不交证】

治法　交通心肾，摄精止遗。

处方　内关（PC6）、关元（RN4）、三阴交（SP6）、志室（BL52）、大赫（KI12）。

方义　关元是足三阴与任脉之会，可补益肾气；配志室、大赫以宁志安宫，固摄精关；内关可清心宁神；三阴交是足三阴经之会穴，有调阴精、资生化之功。诸穴合用，旨在交

during sexual intercourses, nocturnal emission, disturbed sleep at night, palpitation and fatigue on face, soreness of waist, tinnitus, dark urine, red tongue, thin and rapid pulse.

2. For patient with downward flow of Damp-Heat, symptoms include frequent spermatorrhea, physical fatigue and poor appetite, bitter mouth and thirsty, yellowish red urine, Heat and unsmooth, yellowish and greasy tongue fur, soft and rapid pulse.

3. For patients with non-consolidation of kidney Qi, symptoms include spermatorrhea without dreams, even ejaculation seeing beauties, slippery and thin semen, dizziness, pale complexion, aching lumbus and limp knees, intolerance of cold and extreme chilliness, light tongue with whitish fur, thin and weak pulse.

II. Therapeutic Methods

[Syndrome of Disharmony Between Heart and Kidney]

Therapeutic method: Unobstruct transportation between heart and kidney, obtain essence and stop spermatorrhea.

Prescription: Neiguan (PC6), Guanyuan (RN4), Sanyinjiao (SP6), Zhishi (BL52), Dahe (KI12).

Mechanism of prescription: Guanyuan is the confluent acupoint of three Yin Meridians of Foot with Ren Channel, which can replenish kidney and tonify Qi; it can calm mind and Gong, reinforce seminal gate when being matched with Zhishi, Dahe; Neiguan can purify mind and relieve restlessness. The use of combination of

通心肾，摄精止遗。

配穴 梦境纷纭者，加心俞、神门；腰酸腿软者，加肾俞、太溪。

方法 电热针治疗（补法）。

操作 选定穴位，常规皮肤消毒。电热针向脊柱侧斜刺志室 0.8 寸，直刺三阴交 0.7 寸，向脊柱侧斜刺心俞 0.8 寸。接通电热针仪，每个穴位分别给予电流量 80mA。另配以毫针直刺内关 0.5 寸，向下斜刺关元 3 寸，要求针感到达会阴部，直刺大赫 0.8 寸，留针 40 分钟。

疗程 每天 1 次，10 次为 1 个疗程，疗程间如无不适可进行第 2 个疗程的治疗。

【湿热下注证】

治法 清利湿热，安宁精室。

处方 中极（RN3）、阴陵泉（SP9）、三阴交（SP6）、足三里（ST36）。

方义 中极是膀胱经的募穴，可清湿热之邪；阴陵泉是脾经之合穴，泻之能利湿

these acupoints can unobstruct transportation between heart and kidney, obtain essence and stop spermatorrhea.

Matching acupoints: For dreamy sleep add Xinshu, Shenmen. For aching lumbus and limp legs add Shenshu, Taixi.

Method: Electrothermal acupuncture treatment (tonifying).

Operations: Selecting the relevant acupoints, perform routine skin disinfection. Using electrothermal acupuncture needles, obliquely puncture toward spine into Zhishi for 0.8", vertically puncture into Sanyinjiao for 0.7", obliquely puncture toward spine into Xinshu for 0.8". Turn on the electrothermal acupuncture equipment, apply a current of 80mA to each acupoint. Additionally, using the filiform needles, vertically puncture into Neiguan for 0.5", obliquely puncture downward into Guanyuan for 3", make the feeling of needle puncturing spread to perineum, vertically puncture into Dahe for 0.8", leaving the needles in for 40 minutes.

Therapeutic course: Treat once a day, 10 times for a course, and start the treatment for the second course if there is no discomfort.

[Syndrome of Downward Flow of Damp-Heat]

Therapeutic method: Dredge and disperse Damp-Heat, calm essence chamber.

Prescription: Zhongji (RN3), Yinlingquan (SP9), Sanyinjiao (SP6), Zusanli (ST36).

Mechanism of prescription: Zhongji is a Mu acupoint of Bladder Meridian, and it can clear toxins of Damp-Heat; Yinlingquan is a He acupoint of Spleen

热；三阴交和中极都是足三阴之交会穴，可调三阴；足三里是胃经之合穴，可强脾胃，助运化。诸穴合用，共收清利湿热、安宁精神之功。

配穴 小便热赤者加阳陵泉；脘闷纳呆者加中脘、脾俞。

方法 毫针治疗（泻法）。

操作 选定穴位，常规皮肤消毒。用毫针直刺三阴交0.6寸，向下斜刺中极3寸，使针感到达会阴部，直刺阴陵泉0.6寸，提插泻法，留针30分钟。

疗程 每天1次，10次为1个疗程，疗程间如无不适可进行第2个疗程的治疗。

【肾气不固证】

治法 补肾壮阳，固涩精关。

处方 关元（RN4）、太溪（KI3）、肾俞（BL23）、志室（BL52）、命门（DU4）。

方义 关元是任脉与足三阴之交会穴，是人身元气的根本，可补益元阳，与肾经原穴

Meridian, and it can regular the three Yins; Sanyinjiao and Zhaoji are both confluent acupoints of the three Yin Meridians of Foot, and they can regulate the three Yins; Zusanli is a He acupoint of Stomach Meridian, and it can strengthen stomach and facilitate transportation and transformation. The use of combination of these acupoints can dredge and disperse Damp-Heat, calm mind.

Matching acupoints: For hot and dark urine add Yanglingquan. For abdominal tightness and anorexia add Zhongwan, Pishu.

Method: Filiform needle acupuncture treatment (attenuating).

Operations: Selecting the relevant acupoints, perform routine skin disinfection. Using the filiform needles, vertically puncture into Sanyinjiao for 0.6", obliquely puncture downward into Zhongji for 3", make the feeling of needle puncturing spread to perineum, vertically puncture into Yinlingquan for 0.6", lifting-thrusting and attenuating method. Leave the needles in for 30 minutes.

Therapeutic course: Treat once a day, 10 times for a course, and start the treatment for the second course if there is no discomfort.

[Syndrome of Non-consolidation of Kidney Qi]

Therapeutic method: Replenish kidney and strengthen Yang, reinforce seminal gate.

Prescription: Guanyuan (RN4), Taixi (KI3), Shenshu (BL23), Zhishi (BL52), Mingmen (DU4).

Mechanism of prescription: Guanyuan, the confluent acupoint of Ren Meridian and three Yin Meridians of Foot, is the basis of body vitality, can nourish Yuan Yang,

太溪和背俞穴肾俞相配，可补肾固精；志室可宁志安宫；督脉总督一身之阳，取命门旨在振奋阳气。诸穴合用，共取补肾壮阳、固涩精关之功效。

配穴 少气自汗者，加肺俞、足三里；腰膝酸软者，加三阴交。

方法 电热针治疗（温补法）。

操作 选定穴位，常规皮肤消毒。电热针向脊柱侧斜刺肺俞、肾俞、志室各0.8寸。接通电热针仪，每个穴位分别给予电流量80mA。另配以毫针向下斜刺关元3寸，使针感到达会阴部，直刺足三里0.7寸，直刺三阴交0.6寸，直刺太溪0.4寸，留针40分钟。

疗程 每天1次，10次为1个疗程，疗程间休息3天。

三、注意事项

1. 针灸是治疗遗精的有效方法，施术时取穴要准确，手法要温和适中。针刺关元或中

and it can replenish kidney and inforce essence when being matched with the Yuan acupoint Taixi and the Back-Shu acupoint Shenshu of Kidney Meridian; Zhishi can calm mind and Gong; Du Channel governs Yang of the whole body, so use of Mingmen is aimed to promote Yang Qi. The use of combination of these acupoints can replenish kidney and strengthen Yang, reinforce seminal gate.

Matching acupoints: For weak breath and spontaneous sweating add Feishu, Zusanli. For aching lumbus and limp knees add Sanyinjiao.

Method: Electrothermal acupuncture treatment (warm tonifying).

Operations: Selecting the relevant acupoints, perform routine skin disinfection. Using electrothermal acupuncture needles, obliquely puncture toward spine into Feishu, Shenshu, Zhishi for 0.8" respectively. Turn on the electrothermal acupuncture equipment, apply a current of 80mA to each acupoint. Additionally, using the filiform needles, obliquely puncture downward into Guanyuan for 3", make the feeling of needle puncturing spread to perineum, vertically puncture into Zusanli for 0.7", Sanyinjiao for 0.6", Taixi for 0.4", leaving the needles in for 40 minutes.

Therapeutic course: Once a day, 10 times for a course. Rest for 3 days between courses.

III. Precautions

1. Acupuncture therapy is an effective approach for spermatorrhea treatment. For acupuncture, the acupoint locating should be accurate and the skill should be mild

极时，要使针感到达阴茎或会阴部，以提高疗效。本病疗程长，针灸治疗要坚持，按疗程进行，病情好转亦需巩固治疗，以达彻底治愈。

2. 配合心理治疗和体疗，有助于提高疗效。要使患者心情开朗，消除对遗精的顾虑和焦虑心理。

四、典型病例

齐某，男，31岁，未婚，职员，北京人。

主诉：每夜梦遗3～4次，已2个月。

刻下症：多因工作压力大，思虑或劳思过度而发病。症见头晕不寐，心悸健忘，饮食减少，大便溏泻，面黄神疲，舌淡，苔薄白，脉细。

查体：未见阳性体征。

辅助检查：未见异常。

【诊断依据】

1. 中年男性，查体未发现器质性病变，生殖、泌尿系统正常。

2. 素体健康，但由于工作压力大，多因思虑过度而致心

and appropriate. When puncturing Guanyuan or Zhongji, the feeling of needle puncturing must be spread to penis or perineum, so as to improve efficacies. This disease has a long treatment course, so the key point of acupuncture therapy is persistence and performing as per courses, and to achieve complete cure, it still needs consolidation treatment after condition improvement.

2. Match with psychological therapy and physical therapy to improve efficacies. Make patients feel cheerful, eliminate concerns on spermatorrhea and anxious mood.

IV. Typical Case

Qi, male, 31 years old, unmarried, employee, residence: Beijing.

Self-reported symptoms: 3-4 times of spermatorrhea each night, lasting for 2 months.

Current symptoms: Mostly caused by heavy work stress, thoughtfulness or worry beyond measure. Symptoms included dizziness and sleepless, palpitation and amnesia, less food intake, thin and sloppy stool, yellowish complexion and spiritlessness, light tongue with thin and whitish fur, thin pulse.

Physical examination: No positive signs were seen.

Auxiliary examination: No abnormalities.

[Diagnostic Basis]

1. Middle-aged male, no organic lesions were found in the physical examination, with normal reproductive system and urinary system.

2. Healthy body, deficiency of heart and spleen caused by worry beyond measure and heavy work stress.

脾虚损。

3. 既往无特殊病史可记载。

4. 查体和各项检查未发现阳性体征。

【证治分析】

病因 气不摄精。

病机 思虑过度，劳伤心脾，明消中气，暗耗心血，脾虚气陷不摄，心气虚则神浮不舍，心脾两虚，气不摄精，故见遗精。

证候分析 思虑劳倦伤及心脾，气虚下陷，不能摄精，故见遗精；心血亏虚，心神失养，神不守舍，故头晕失眠，心悸健忘，精神倦怠；血虚不能上荣于头面，故面黄少华；脾虚失其健运，则食少便溏。舌淡、脉细均为气血衰少之象。

病位 心、脾。

病性 虚性。

西医诊断 遗精、神经衰弱。

中医诊断 遗精。

治法 补益心脾，固摄下元。

3. No recordable previous special medical history.

4. No positive signs found in physical examination and other examinations.

[Syndrome-treatment Analysis]

Etiology: Qi cannot nourish essence.

Pathogenesis: Worry beyond measure, overstrain injuring heart and spleen, outward consumption of Middle-Jiao Qi with inward consumption of heart blood, spleen deficiency and Qi collapse without nourishment, thoughtfulness, cause mind loosing, deficiency of heart and spleen, Qi unable to nourish essence, subsequently lead to spermatorrhea.

Syndrome analysis: thoughtfulness and spiritlessness injury heart and spleen, Qi deficiency and collapse unable to nourish essence, therefore lead to spermatorrhea; depletion and deficiency of heart blood, nourishment loss of mind, mind loosing, lead to dizziness and insomnia, palpitation and amnesia, spiritual burnout; blood deficiency causing blood could not go up to the face, leading to lusterless complexion; losing transport because of spleen deficiency, lead to less food intake and sloppy stool. Light tongue and thin pulse are both symptoms of depletion and reduction of Qi-blood.

Lesion location: Heart, spleen.

Disease nature: Deficiency.

The diagnosis of Western Medicine: Spermatorrhea and neurasthenia.

The diagnosis of Traditional Chinese Medicine: Spermatorrhea.

Therapeutic method: Tonify heart and spleen, reinforce and nourish lower origin.

Method: Electrothermal acupuncture treatment.

Prescription: Xinshu (BL15), Pishu (BL20), Shenshu (BL23), Guanyuan (RN4), Zusanli (ST36), Sanyinjiao (SP6).

Mechanism of prescription: Xinshu and Pishu can tonify Qi of heart and spleen; Zusanli and Sanyinjiao can strengthen spleen and stomach to nourish the source of generation and transformation for Qi-blood; Guanyuan is the confluent acupoint of three Yin Meridians and Ren Meridian, it can tonify kidney and strengthen Yang, reinforce vital essence and foundation when being matched with Shenshu.

Matching acupoints: For disturbed sleep and sleepless at night, add Shenmen. For dizziness and serious palpitation, add Fengchi, Neiguan.

Operations: Selecting the relevant acupoints, perform routine skin disinfection. Using electrothermal acupuncture needles, vertically puncture into Zusanli, Sanyinjiao for 0.7" respectively, obliquely (with the needle tip towards spine) into Xinshu, Pishu for 0.7" respectively, vertically puncture into Shenmen, Neiguan for 0.6" respectively. Turn on the electrothermal acupuncture equipment, apply a current of 40mA to each acupoint. The limit is that the patient feels swell and comfortable. Leave the needles in for 40 minutes. (Note: select 3 pairs of acupoints for electrothermal acupuncture treatment each time, use alternately, and treat the other acupoints with filiform needles.)

Therapeutic course: Each course consists of 10

每日或隔日1次。

治疗 过程该患者治疗5次后，一切症状消失，夜能安眠，没有梦遗，继续治疗以巩固疗效，20次后结束治疗。随访，治疗半年后结婚。

【生活调摄】

1. 本病为功能性，因此在治疗的同时须做好患者的思想工作，使之消除顾虑。

2. 清淡饮食，规律作息，做适量的运动。

不射精症

不射精症，是指阴茎能勃起性交，但不能达到性欲高潮，也不出现射精的一种病症。

本病中医称为"精闭""精瘀症"。多因肾精不足，不能上济于心，致阴虚火旺，心肾失交，精关不开；或因肝郁化火，精关疏泄失调；或因肾阳虚衰，气化失利，无力推动排出；或因瘀血阻滞精道，碍精排出所致。本症有虚有实，也有虚实夹杂，多与心、肝、肾有关。

treatments, once a day or every two days.

Treatment process: After 5 days' treatment, all symptoms of this patient disappeared, he could sleep well without nocturnal emission, he continued the treatment so as to consolidate the efficacy, and completed after 20 treatments. Follow-up, he got married a half year after the treatment.

[Lifestyle Change and Health Maintenance]

1. This is a functional disease, therefore it is necessary to do ideological work on patients, lift their concerns.

2. Light diet and regular life schedules, and do appropriate exercises.

Anejaculation

Anejaculation refers to a disease that the penis can erect for sexual intercourses but cannot reach orgasm as well as ejaculate.

In Traditional Chinese Medicine this is called "sperm closure", "syndrome of sperm stasis". Most are caused by deficiency of kidney essence, unable to nourish heart, therefore lead to hyperactivity of Fire and Yin deficiency, loss of communication between heart and kidney, closure of seminal gate; or caused by transformation of liver stasis into Fire, disorder of seminal gate soothing; or caused by depletion and deficiency of kidney Yang, loss of Qi transportation, unable to promote ejaculation; or caused by that the stagnated blood obstructs seminal channel, and impede discharge of semen. This syndrome includes deficiency and excess syndrome, syndrome of intermingled deficiency and excess, and most are related to heart, liver, kidney.

一、诊断及辨证要点

I. Key Points for Diagnosis and Syndrome Differentiation

1. 阴虚火旺者，症见性欲亢进，阳强不射精，五心烦热，头晕耳鸣，盗汗，口干，便秘，尿黄，舌质嫩红，少苔或无苔，脉细数。

1. For patients with hyperactivity of Fire and Yin deficiency, symptoms include sexual hyperesthesia, persistent erection of penis without ejaculation, dysphoria in chest with palms-soles, dizziness and tinnitus, sweating at night, dry mouth, constipation, yellow urine, tender and red tongue with less or no fur, thin and rapid pulse.

2. 肝郁化火者，症见性欲亢进，性交持久而不射精，性情急躁，两胁胀满，善太息，抑郁不乐，或小腹胀满，舌质暗红，苔黄，脉弦数。

2. For patients suffered from transformation of liver stasis into Fire, symptoms include sexual hyperesthesia, persistent erection of penis without ejaculation, quick temper, swell of bilateral ribs, Preference for sighing, depression, or abdominal distension, dark and red tongue with yellow fur, taut and rapid pulse.

3. 肾虚者，症见性交时间短而不射精，阳事举而不坚，性欲减退，腰膝酸软，或形寒肢冷，或夜尿多，大便溏，甚者五更泻，面色晦暗，头昏乏力，精神萎靡不振，舌质淡，苔白，脉沉细或沉迟。

3. For patients with kidney deficiency, symptoms include short time of intercourses without ejaculation, erection with soft penis, hyposexuality, soreness and weakness of waist and knees, or cold body and limbs, or frequent urination at night, sloppy stool, or even predawn diarrhea, gloomy complexion, dizziness and asthenia, spiritlessness, light tongue with whitish fur, deep and thin pulse or deep and slow pulse.

4. 瘀血阻滞者，症见阴茎勃起正常，但性交不能射精，伴有小腹坠痛胀满，阴部胀痛，舌质紫黯且有瘀斑，脉涩。

4. For patients with blood stasis, symptoms include normal ejection without ejaculation, accompanied with bearing-down pain and swell of lower abdomen, swelling pain of private parts, dark purple tongue with ecchymosis, uneven pulse.

二、治疗方法

【阴虚火旺证】

治法 滋阴补肾降火。

处方 大赫（KI12）、气海（RN6）、横骨（KI11）、三阴交（SP6）、太冲（LR3）、复溜（KI7）。

方义 取足厥阴经穴之大赫以滋阴补肾，取任脉之气海以补益阴精，两穴相配可治本，所谓"壮水之主，以制阳光"；三阴交、复溜可滋阴降火；横骨补肾而通精道；太冲可泻上元之肝火，以治其标。诸穴共用，以取滋阴、补肾、降火之功，阴平阳秘，则精道自通。

配穴 阳强不倒者，加涌泉；盗汗者，加阴郄。

方法 毫针治疗（平补平泻法）。

操作 选定穴位，常规皮肤消毒。用毫针直刺大赫 0.6 寸，直刺气海 0.6 寸，直刺三阴交 0.7 寸，直刺复溜 0.5 寸，直刺太冲 0.5 寸，直刺横骨 0.6

II. Therapeutic Methods

[Syndrome of Hyperactivity of Fire and Yin Deficiency]

Therapeutic method: Nourish Yin, replenish kidney and decline Fire.

Prescription: Dahe (KI12), Qihai (RN6), Henggu (KI11), Sanyinjiao (SP6), Taichong (LR3), Fuliu (KI7).

Mechanism of prescription: Use the acupoint Dahe of Jue-Yin Meridian of Foot to nourish Yin and replenish kidney, use the acupoint Qihai of Ren Channel to tonify Yin essence, the match of these two acupoints can effect a permanent cure, namely "strengthen Water governor to suppress Yang"; Sanyinjiao and Fuliu can nourish Yin and decline Fire; Henggu can replenish kidney and soothe seminal channel; Taichong can dredge liver Fire of upper origin as a temporary solution. The use of combination of these acupoints can nourish Yin, replenish kidney, decline Fire, Yin and Yang reach balance then the seminal channel will be unobstructed naturally.

Matching acupoints: For persistent erection of penis add Yongquan. For sweating at night add Yinxi.

Method: Filiform needle acupuncture treatment (mild tonifying and attenuating).

Operations: Selecting the relevant acupoints, perform routine skin disinfection. Using the filiform needles, vertically puncture into Dahe and Qihai for 0.6" respectively, Sanyinjiao for 0.7", Fuliu and Taichong for 0.5", Henggu for 0.6", Yongquan and Yinxi for 0.5",

寸，直刺涌泉 0.5 寸，直刺阴郄 0.5 寸，留针 30 分钟。

疗程 每天 1 次，10 天为 1 个疗程，疗程间如无不适可进行第 2 个疗程的治疗。

【肝郁化火证】

治法 泻肝火，滋肾水。

处方 中极（RN3）、肾俞（BL23）、行间（LR2）、三阴交（SP6）、太冲（LR3）、水道（ST28）。

方义 取行间、太冲以泻肝火；中极、三阴交可条达精窍；肾俞配三阴交可滋阴补肾，以制上元之阳。诸穴合用，取泻肝火、滋肾水、通络利窍之功效。

配穴 胁肋胀痛者，加期门；失眠多梦者，加厥阴俞。

方法 毫针治疗（泻法）。

操作 选定穴位，常规皮肤消毒。用毫针直刺中极 3 寸，使针感到达会阴部，直刺行间 0.4 寸，直刺三阴交 0.8 寸，直刺太冲 0.5 寸，自肋间隙向外斜刺期门 0.5 寸，向脊柱侧斜刺肾俞、厥阴俞各 0.7 寸，留针 30 分钟。

leaving the needles in for 40 minutes.

Therapeutic course: Treat once a day, 10 days as a course, and start the treatment for the second course if there is no discomfort.

[Syndrome of Liver Stasis Transforming into Fire]

Therapeutic method: Dredge liver Fire, nourish kidney Water.

Prescription: Zhongji (RN3), Shenshu (BL23), Xingjian (LR2), Sanyinjiao (SP6), Taichong (LR3), Shuidao (ST28).

Mechanism of prescription: Use Xinjian and Taichong to dredge liver Fire; Zhongji and Sanyinjiao can soothe seminal orifice; Shenshu together with Sanyinjiao can nourish Yin and replenish kidney to suppress Yang of upper origin. The use of combination of these acupoints can dredge liver Fire, nourish kidney Water, and soothe collaterals and orifices.

Matching acupoints: For distending pain in ribs add Qimen. For insomnia and dreamy sleep add Jueyinshu.

Method: Filiform needle acupuncture treatment (attenuating).

Operations: Selecting the relevant acupoints, perform routine skin disinfection. Using the filiform needles, vertically puncture into Zhongji for 3", make the feeling of needle puncturing spread to perineum, vertically puncture into Xingjian for 0.4", Sanyinjiao for 0.8", Taichong for 0.5", obliquely puncture from the intercostal space outward into Qimen for 0.5", obliquely puncture toward spine into Shenshu, Jueyinshu for 0.7"

疗程 每天1次，10天为1个疗程，疗程间如无不适可进行第2个疗程的治疗。

【肾虚证】

治法 温肾阳，滋肾阴。

处方 关元（RN4）、肾俞（BL23）、三阴交（SP6）、腰阳关（DU3）、太溪（KI3）。

方义 肾为水火之宅，内寄真阴、真阳，两者相互制约，相互依存。肾阳是动力，阳气虚则不能射精，故以温肾阳为主，滋肾阴为辅。取足少阴肾经之太溪与肾的背俞穴肾俞以壮肾；三阴交为脾经穴，取其后天养先天之意；关元为任脉穴，任主一身之阴，腰阳关为督脉穴，督主一身之阳，两穴相配，使阴生阳长。诸穴合用，肾气得补，阳气得振，则精道自通。

配穴 五更泻者，加大肠俞、足三里；阴茎不举或举而不坚者，加次髎；小便频数者，加膀胱俞。

respectively. Leave the needles in for 30 minutes.

Therapeutic course: Treat once a day, 10 days as a course, and start the treatment for the second course if there is no discomfort.

[Kidney Deficiency Syndrome]

Therapeutic method: Warm kidney Yang and nourish kidney Yin.

Prescription: Guanyuan (RN4), Shenshu (BL23), Sanyinjiao (SP6), Yaoyangguan (DU3), Taixi (KI3).

Mechanism of prescription: Kidney is the place of Water and Fire, there stores true Yin and true Yang, these two restrict each other and depend on each other. Kidney Yang is the power, deficiency of Yang Qi will disenable ejaculation, so warm kidney Yang supplemented by nourishment of kidney Yin. Use Taixi of Shao-Yin Kidney Meridian and the Back-Shu acupoint Shenshu of Kidney to reinforce kidney; Sanyinjiao is an acupoint of Spleen Meridian, it can nourish congenital foundation with acquired construction; Guanyuan is an acupoint of Ren Channel, the later governs Yin of the whole body, Yaoyangguan is an acupoint of Du Channel, while Du governs Yang of the whole body, so the match of these two acupoints can facilitate generation of Yin and Yang. The use of combination of these acupoints can replenish kidney Qi and promote Yang Qi, then the seminal channel will be unobstructed naturally.

Matching acupoints: For predawn diarrhea add Dachangshu, Zusanli; For erectile problems or erection with soft penis, add Ciliao. For frequent and rapid micturition add Pangguangshu.

Method: Electrothermal acupuncture treatment (warm tonifying).

Operations: Selecting the relevant acupoints, perform routine skin disinfection. Using electrothermal acupuncture needles, obliquely puncture downward into Guanyuan, make the feeling of needle puncturing spread to perineum, obliquely puncture toward spine into Shenshu, Yaoyangguan for 0.8" respectively, vertically puncture into Zusanli for 0.8", Sanyinjiao for 0.7", obliquely puncture toward spine into Dachangshu for 0.8", vertically puncture into Ciliao for 0.8". Turn on the electrothermal acupuncture equipment, apply a current of 70-80mA to each acupoint. Leave the needles in for 40 minutes. (Note: Above acupoints can be divided into two groups to use alternately.)

Therapeutic course: Once a day, 10 times for a course. Start the treatment for the second course after a break of 3 days, or perform continuous treatment if there is no discomfort.

[Syndrome of Blood Stasis]

Therapeutic method: Soothe liver and regulate Qi, activate blood circulation and remove stasis.

Prescription: Qugu (RN2), Jimai (LR12), Ququan (LR8), Sanyinjiao (SP6), Geshu (BL17), Taichong (LR3).

Mechanism of prescription: This syndrome is caused by Qi stagnation and blood stasis which obstruct essence. Therefore use the acupoints Ququan, Jimai, Taichong to soothe and dredge liver Qi; Geshu is a Hui acupoint of blood, it can activate blood circulation and

穴，取之以补脾气，脾气足则血运有力；曲骨是任脉穴，任为任养之本，主生殖，与上穴相配，可使针效直达病所，肝气条达，瘀血得化，脉道通畅，射精自趋正常。

配穴 精神紧张者，加神门、内关；睡眠欠佳者，加神门。

方法 毫针治疗（泻法）。

操作 选定穴位，常规皮肤消毒。用毫针直刺曲骨 0.6 寸，直刺急脉 0.8 寸，直刺曲泉 0.5 寸，直刺三阴交 0.7 寸，向脊柱侧斜刺膈俞 0.8 寸，直刺神门 0.4 寸，直刺内关 0.5 寸，留针 30 分钟，提插泻法。

疗程 每天 1 次，10 次为 1 个疗程。疗程间如无不适可连续治疗；若有倦怠，可休息 3 天再进行第 2 个疗程的治疗。

三、注意事项

1. 针刺中极、关元时，针感必须到达会阴部或龟头。

2. 治疗中亦要配合心理治

remove stasis; Sanyinjiao is an acupoint of Spleen Meridian, it can replenish spleen Qi, and sufficient spleen Qi can lead to strong blood circulation; Qugu is an acupoint of Ren Channel, Ren is the basis of nourishment which governs reproduction, so the match of this acupoint with Shangxue can let the acupuncture effects reach lesions, liver Qi spread out freely, and disperse stagnated blood, soothe Channels, therefore the ejaculation tends to be normal.

Matching acupoints: For psychentonia add Shenmen, Neiguan. For poor sleep add Shenmen.

Method: Filiform needle acupuncture treatment (attenuating).

Operations: Selecting the relevant acupoints, perform routine skin disinfection. Using the filiform needles, vertically puncture into Qugu for 0.6", Jimai for 0.8", Ququan for 0.5', Sanyinjiao for 0.7", obliquely puncture toward spine into Geshu for 0.8", Shenmen for 0.4", Neiguan for 0.5", leaving the needles in for 30 minutes, Use lifting-thrusting and attenuating method.

Therapeutic course: Once a day, 10 times for a course. Perform continuous treatment if there is no discomfort; if burnout, take a break of 3 days and start the treatment for the second course.

III. Precautions

1. When puncturing Zhongji and Guanyuan, the feeling of needle puncturing must be spread to perineum or balanus.

2. The treatment should be matched with psycho-

疗，让患者消除思想顾虑，保持乐观的情绪，对治疗要有信心，决心配合治疗。

3. 治疗过程中节房事、禁手淫，要清心寡欲。

4. 生活规律，加强体力活动和适当的体育锻炼。

5. 饮食宜清淡，少食或不食辛辣助阳之食物。

无精子症

多次精液检查均未发现精子者，称为无精子症，属精子缺乏症的范畴。多种原因引起的睾丸组织萎缩及生殖细胞病变可导致本病的发生。本病是造成男性不育症的常见原因之一。目前尚缺少有效的治疗方法。

中医认为，本病属于"无子"的范畴。多因先天禀赋不足，或后天虚损太过，以致肾精不足、命门火衰所致。

一、诊断及辨证要点

肾精不足，命门火衰者，症见精液稀薄，无精子，腰酸腿软，阴茎勃起无力，畏寒肢

logical therapy, free patients' misgivings and enlighten patients to keep optimistic attitude, have confidence in treatments as well as cooperate with treatments.

3. During treatment, it is necessary to restrain sexual interourses, forbid masturbation, purify mind and limit desires.

4. Regular lifestyle, enhance physical activity and appropriate physical exercise.

5. Light diet, eat less or no spicy food which strengthen Yang.

Azoospermia

For no sperm found in several sperm examinations, it is called azoospermia, which belongs to the range of sperm deficiency. This disease can be caused by testicular tissue atrophy and germ cell diseases due to various causes. This disease is one of the common causes for male infertility. Currently there are no efficient therapies.

Traditional Chinese Medicine believes that this disease belongs to the range of "childless". Most are caused by inadequate inherent endowment or excessive consumption leading to deficiency of kidney essence and Fire decline of Mingmen.

I. Key Points for Diagnosis and Syndrome Differentiation

For patients with deficiency of kidney essence and Fire decline of Mingmen, the symptoms include thin semens, absence of sperms, aching lumbus and limp

冷，头晕耳鸣，精神不振，面色白，舌质淡，脉沉细。

二、治疗方法

【肾精不足，命门火衰】

治法 补先天之肾气，补后天之本。

处方 关元（RN4）、肾俞（BL23）、命门（DU4）、三阴交（SP6）、太溪（KI3）。

方义 关元是任脉穴，任为任养之本，主生殖，人体精、津、血、液皆由任脉所司，故取关元以大补阴精；命门为督脉之穴，督脉主一身之阳，与关元相配，可使阴生阳长；太溪是肾之原穴，肾俞是肾之背俞穴，取之可补先天之肾气；三阴交是脾经穴，取之可补后天之本。诸穴合用，可使阴生阳长，气血充足则精自生。

配穴 纳差便溏者，可加足三里、中脘；夜不寐者，加神门。

legs, erectile weakness of penis, intolerance of cold and extremities' chilliness, dizziness and tinnitus, lassitude, pale complexion, light tongue, deep and thin pulse.

II. Therapeutic Methods

[Deficiency of Kidney Essence, Fire Decline of Mingmen]

Therapeutic method: Replenish congenital kidney Qi and foundation of acquired constitution.

Prescription: Guanyuan (RN4), Shenshu (BL23), Mingmen (DU4), Sanyinjiao (SP6), Taixi (KI3).

Mechanism of prescription: Guanyuan is an acupoint of Ren Channel, while the later is the basis of nourishment and governs reproduction, the essence, saliva, blood and fluid of human body are all governed by Ren Channel, so use the acupoint Guanyuan to greatly nourish Yin essence; Mingmen is an acupoint of Du Channel, while the later governs Yang of the whole body, so the match of Mingmen and Guanyuan can facilitate the generation of Yin and Yang; Taixi is a Yuan acupoint of Kidney, Shenshu a Back-Shu acupoint of Kidney, the use of these two can replenish congenital kidney Qi; Sanyinjiao is an acupoint of Spleen Meridian, it can replenish the foundation of acquired constitution. The use of combination of these acupoints can facilitate the generation of Yin and Yang, achieve sufficient Qi and blood, subsequently nourish generation of essence.

Matching acupoints: For poor appetite and sloppy stool add Zusanli, Zhongwan. For insomnia add Shenmen.

方法　电热针治疗（温补法）。

操作　选定穴位，常规皮肤消毒。电热针直刺关元、命门各0.8寸，向脊柱侧斜刺肾俞0.8寸，直刺三阴交0.7寸，直刺足三里0.8寸，直刺中脘0.8寸，直刺神门0.5寸。接通电热针仪，每穴分别给予电流量70～80mA，留针40分钟。（注：上述穴位前后分成两组，交替使用。）

疗程　每天1次，10天为1个疗程，疗程间如无不适可进行第2个疗程的治疗。

三、注意事项

1. 治疗期间禁止性生活，心态要平和，精神要乐观，要树立治愈的信心。

2. 洗澡时不宜在高温或蒸汽池中浸泡过久，避免经常在高温环境中作业。

3. 衣裤宜宽松舒适，避免下身穿紧身裤，防止造成睾丸上提，温度升高，影响精子的生长。

4. 宜多食韭菜和韭花、猪羊肉等，不宜饮酒。

Method: Electrothermal acupuncture treatment (warm tonification).

Operations: Selecting the relevant acupoints, perform routine skin disinfection. Using electrothermal acupuncture needles, vertically puncture into Guanyuan and Mingmen for 0.8" respectively, obliquely puncture toward spine into Shenshu for 0.8", vertically puncture into Sanyinjiao for 0.7", Zusanli and Zhongwan for 0.8" respectively, Shenmen for 0.5". Turn on the electrothermal acupuncture equipment, apply a current of 70-80mA to each acupoint. Leave the needles in for 40 minutes. (Note: Divide anterior and posterior acupoints into two groups for alternate use.)

Therapeutic course: Treat once a day, 10 days as a course, and start the treatment for the second course if there is no discomfort.

III. Precautions

1. Sexual intercourses are forbidden during treatment, and it is necessary to keep peace mind, optimistic attitude and establish confidence in cure.

2. It is inappropriate to soak in high-temperature or steamy bath for too long, as well as to avoid frequent work under high-temperature environments.

3. Clothing should be loose and comfortable, avoid wear tight trousers, otherwise will cause testis lifting and temperature rising subsequently affecting growth of sperms.

4. Eat more leek and leek flowers, pig and sheep meat, better not drink.

Semen Abnormalities

Normal semen is white or gray opaque fluid. An average of 3-5ml each time, self-liquefied after being excreted out of body for about 30 minutes, more than 60 million of sperm per milliliter with active sperm accounting for over 60%, abnormal ones less than 20%. Ones not comply with above standards are called semen abnormalities. Semen abnormalities include azoospermia, less sperm, non-liquefaction of semen, less semen, excessive sperm death, etc. Most are caused by congenital testicular hypoplasia, testes damage due to parotitis, prostatitis, epididymitis, vesiculitis, tuberculosis of epididymis, varicocele and other diseases.

Traditional Chinese Medicine believes that this disease belongs to the range of "cold semen", "thin semen", "childless", etc. Most are caused by depletion and deficiency of kidney essence, hyperactivity of Fire and Yin deficiency or downward flow of Damp-Heat of liver and gallbladder.

I. Key Points for Diagnosis and Syndrome Differentiation

1. For patients with kidney deficiency, infertility after many years of marriage, less or thin semen, or less or no sperm or dead sperm, soreness and weakness of waist and knees, dizziness and tinnitus, poor memory, intolerance of cold and extremities' chilliness, clear abundant urine, thin and sloppy stool, light tongue with thin and

沉细。

2. 阴虚火旺者，性欲亢进，精液量少，精液稠而不化，五心烦热，腰膝酸软，头晕耳鸣，口干，苔黄腻，脉滑数；或大便秘结，舌质红，少苔或无苔，脉细数。

3. 肝胆湿热者，性生活尚可，精液不液化，精子少或全无，口苦，头晕而沉重，阴囊潮湿或阴囊红肿，小腹胀痛，尿痛，小便黄赤而热，舌质红，苔黄腻，脉滑数或弦数。

二、治疗方法

【阴虚证】

治法　补肾健脾，益精养血。

处方　关元（RN4）、肾俞（BL23）、三阴交（SP6）、太溪（KI3）。

方义　肾藏精，主生殖，故取肾之原穴太溪以补肾；关元属任脉，任主一身之阴，又为足三阴经的交会穴，故取关元以大补阴精；肾俞是肾的背俞穴，取之以壮肾；三阴交是脾经穴，取之以调脾胃。诸穴合用，共奏补肾健脾、益精养血

whitish fur, deep and thin pulse.

2. For patients with hyperactivity of Fire and Yin deficiency, sexual hyperesthesia, less semen, thick and non-liquefied semen, dysphoria in chest with palms-soles, soreness and weakness of waist and knees, dizziness and tinnitus, dry mouth, yellowish and greasy tongue fur, slippery and rapid pulse; or constipation, red tongue with less or no fur, thin and rapid pulse.

3. For patients with Damp-Heat of liver and gallbladder, acceptable sexual life, non-liquefaction of semen, less or no sperm, bitter taste, dizziness and heavy head, damp scrota or red and swollen scrota, distending pain of abdomen, painful micturition, yellowish red and hot urine, red tongue with yellowish and greasy fur, slippery rapid or taut rapid pulse.

II. Therapeutic Methods

[Syndrome of Yin Deficiency]

Therapeutic method: Reinforce kidney and invigorate spleen, tonify essence and nourish blood.

Prescription: Guanyuan (RN4), Shenshu (BL23), Sanyinjiao (SP6), Taixi (KI3).

Mechanism of prescription: Kidney stores essence and governs reproduction, therefore use the Yuan acupoint Taixi of Kidney to tonify kidney; Guanyuan belongs to Ren Channel, Ren governs Yin of the whole body, and also is the confluent acupoint of three Yin Meridians of Foot, therefore use Guanyuan to greatly nourish Yin essence; Shenshu is a Back-Shu acupoint of Kidney, it can reinforce kidney; Sanyinjiao is an acupoint

之功效。

方法 电热针治疗（温补法）。

配穴 形寒肢冷者加命门、腰阳关；纳差、便溏者，加足三里。

操作 选定穴位，常规皮肤消毒。电热针直刺关元 0.8 寸，直刺足三里 0.8 寸，直刺三阴交 0.6 寸，向脊椎侧斜刺肾俞 0.8 寸，向脊椎侧斜刺腰阳关 0.7 寸，向脊椎侧斜刺命门 0.8 寸。接通电热针仪，每个穴位分别给予电流量 70～80mA。上述穴位分成两组，轮流交替使用。另配以毫针直刺太溪 0.5 寸，留针 40 分钟。

疗程 每天 1 次，10 天为 1 个疗程，疗程间如无不适可进行第 2 个疗程的治疗。

【阴虚火旺证】

治法 滋阴降火。

处方 关元（RN4）、气海（RN6）、太溪（KI3）、涌泉（KI1）。

方义 关元、气海都是任脉穴，取之以大补阴精；太溪

of Spleen Meridian, it can tonify spleen and stomach. The use of combination of these acupoints can reinforce kidney and invigorate spleen, tonify essence and nourish blood.

Method: Electrothermal acupuncture treatment (warm tonifying).

Matching acupoint: For cold body and limbs add Mingmen, Yaoyangguan; for poor appetite and sloppy stool add Zusanli.

Operations: Preparing the selected acupoints, perform routine skin disinfection. Using electrothermal acupuncture needles, vertically puncture into Guanyuan and Zusanli for 0.8" respectively, Sanyinjiao for 0.6", obliquely puncture toward spine into Shenshu for 0.8" and Yaoyangguan for 0.7", Mingmen for 0.8". Turn on the electrothermal acupuncture equipment, apply a current of 70-80mA to each acupoint. Divide the above acupoints into two groups for alternate use. Additionally, using filiform needles, vertically puncture into Taixi for 0.5", leaving the needles in for 40 minutes.

Therapeutic course: Treat once a day, 10 days as a course, and start the treatment for the second course if there is no discomfort.

[Syndrome of Hyperactivity of Fire and Yin Deficiency]

Therapeutic method: Nourish Yin and decline Fire.

Prescription: Guanyuan(RN4), Qihai (RN6), Taixi (KI3), Yongquan (KI1).

Mechanism of prescription: Guanyuan and Qihai are both acupoints of Ren Channel, they can greatly replenish Yin essence. Taixi is a Yuan acupoint of Shao-Yin Meridian of Foot, Yongquan is a Jing acupoint of Shao-Yin Meridian of Foot, the match of these two can nourish Yin and decline Fire. Taichong is a Yuan acupoint of Jue-Yin Liver Meridian of Foot, it can calm the hyperactivity of liver Fire. The use of combination of these acupoints can nourish Yin and decline Fire.

Matching acupoints: For insomnia and dreamy sleep add Shenmen, Sanyinjiao; for sweating at night added Yinxi, Fuliu.

Method: Electrothermal acupuncture treatment (mild tonifying and attenuating).

Operations: Preparing the selected acupoints, perform routine skin disinfection. Using electrothermal acupuncture needles, vertically puncture into Guanyuan, Qihai and Sanyinjiao for 0.8" respectively. Turn on the electrothermal acupuncture equipment, apply a current of 50mA to each acupoint. Additionally, using filiform needles, vertically puncture into Shenmen and Taixi for 0.5" respectively, Fuliu and Yinxi for 0.6" respectively, Yongquan for 0.5", leaving the needles in for 40 minutes.

Therapeutic course: Treat once a day, 10 times for a course, and if there is no discomfort, perform 3 continuous courses.

[Syndrome of Damp-Heat of Liver and Gallbladder]

Therapeutic method: Clear Damp-Heat of Middle Jiao.

Prescription: Zhongji (RN3), Taichong (LR3), Ligou (LR5), Shuidao (ST28), Pangguangshu (BL28),

道（ST28）、膀胱俞（BL28）、足三里（ST36）。

方义 本证是湿热下注所致，故取足厥阴肝经的原穴太冲，以清肝经之热；取足阳明经之足三里、蠡沟、水道，以清利中焦湿热；取膀胱俞，使湿热从小便排出。其湿热去，则精液自复原。

配穴 精液清冷者，加命门；阴茎痛者，加中极、横骨、三阴交。

方法 毫针治疗（泻法）。

操作 选定穴位，常规皮肤消毒。用毫针向下斜刺中极0.8寸，使针感到达龟头部，直刺水道0.8寸，直刺太冲0.5寸，直刺三阴交0.7寸，直刺横骨0.6寸，直刺行间0.4寸，向脊柱侧斜刺膀胱俞0.8寸。行提插泻法，留针30分钟。

疗程 每天1次，10次为1个疗程，疗程间可休息3～5天。

三、注意事项

1. 首先要鼓励患者消除顾

Zusanli (ST36).

Mechanism of prescription: This syndrome is caused by downward flow of Damp-Heat, so use the Yuan acupoint Taichong of Jue-Yin Liver Meridian of Foot to clear Heat of Liver Meridian. Use the acupoints Zusanli, Ligou and Shuidao of Yang-Ming Meridian of Foot to clear Damp-Heat of Middle Jiao. Use Pangguangshu to discharge Damp-Heat through urine. The semen will recover to normal once damp-heat being removed.

Matching acupoints: For thin and cold semen add Mingmen; for penis pain add Zhongji, Henggu, Sanyinjiao.

Method: Filiform needle acupuncture treatment (reduction in acupuncture).

Operations: Preparing the selected acupoints, perform routine skin disinfection. Using the filiform needles, obliquely puncture downward into Zhongji for 0.8", make the feeling of needle puncturing spread to balanus, vertically puncture into Shuidao for 0.8", Taichong for 0.5", Sanyinjiao for 0.7", Henggu for 0.6", Xingjian for 0.4", obliquely puncture toward spine into Pangguangshu for 0.8". Use the method of lifting-thrusting and attenuating, leaving the needles in for 30 minutes.

Therapeutic course: Once a day, 10 times for a course. Rest for 3-5 days between courses.

III. Precautions

1. First encourage patients to lift their concerns,

虑，树立治愈的信心，努力配合治疗。

2. 在治疗期间，嘱咐患者节制房事，切忌恣情纵欲，重伤肾精。

3. 对偏于热证的患者，在治疗期间应忌烟酒及辛辣助阳之品，如辣椒、大蒜、胡椒、葱、八角、小茴香等。

四、典型病例

汪某，男，36岁，农民，河南人，已婚。

主诉：结婚5年未育。

刻下症：婚久不育，性欲减弱，经检查提示精子数少，活动力不强。常有腰酸腿软，手足清冷，面色白，大便稀薄，小便清长，舌淡，苔薄白，脉沉细。

查体：未见阳性体征。

辅助检查：精液检查示"精液量3mL，精子存活率15%，存活精子不能呈直线运动"。

【诊断依据】

1. 中年男性，发育正常，生殖器官未发现异常。

2. 精液检查示"精液量3mL，精子存活率15%，存活精子不能呈直线运动"。

establish confidence in cure, and make every effort to cooperate with the treatment.

2. During treatment, ask patients to control sexual intercourses, do not indulge in carnal pleasure without restraint leading to greatly damage of kidney essence.

3. For patients tending to Heat syndrome, smoking and drinking as well as intake of spicy food that can reinforce Yang, such as chili, garlic, pepper, shallot, star anise, cumin, should be forbidden.

IV. Typical Case

Wang, male, 36 years old, farmer, residence: Henan, married.

Self-reported symptoms: No child after 5 years of marriage.

Current symptoms: Long-time marriage without child, hyposexuality, less sperm with weak activity indicated by examinations. Often accompanied with aching lumbus and limp legs, cold hands and feet, pale complexion, thin sloppy stool, clear abundant urine, light tongue with thin and whitish fur, deep and thin pulse.

Physical examination: No positive signs were seen.

Auxiliary examination: Semen examination showed "3ml of semen, sperm survival rate of 15%, survived sperm could not move linearly".

[Diagnostic Basis]

1. Middle-aged male, normal development, no abnormalities of reproductive organs found.

2. Semen examination showed "3ml of semen, sperm survival rate of 15%, survive sperm could not move linearly".

3. 其他常规检查未见异常。

4. 查体未发现各部器官异常或病变。

【证治分析】

病因 肾气虚弱。

病机 禀赋不足,肾气衰弱,肾阴不足,无精可藏,又因房劳伤精,阴精暗耗,而精少精薄。

证候分析 肾主藏精,又主生殖,肾气枯竭,无源化生精子,则见精子数少,活动力弱;腰为肾之府,肾虚则腰酸腿软;阳气不能温煦形体,故畏寒肢冷,面色白,大便稀薄,小便清长。舌淡,苔薄白,脉沉细,皆为阳虚之象。

病位 肾。

病性 虚性。

西医诊断 不育症。

中医诊断 不育。

治法 补肾壮阳,益精填髓。

方法 电热针治疗。

处方 肾俞(BL23)、命

3. No abnormalities found in other routine examinations.

4. No abnormalities or lesions of various organs found in physical examination.

[Syndrome-treatment Analysis]

Etiology: Weakness of kidney Qi.

Pathogenesis: Inadequate endowment, weakness of kidney Qi, kidney Yin deficiency, no essence to be stored, while essence impairment caused by excessive sexual intercourses and inward consumption of Yin essence led to less and thin semen.

Syndrome analysis: Kidney governs storage of essence as well as reproduction, exhaustion of kidney Qi leads to no source for generation and transformation into sperm, therefore causes less sperm and weak activity of sperm. The waist is where kidney located in, kidney deficiency causes aching lumbus and limp legs. Yang Qi cannot warm the cold hands and feet, therefore causes intolerance of cold and extremities' chilliness, pale complexion, thin sloppy stool, clear abundant urine. Light tongue, whitish and thin fur, deep and thin pulse are all symptoms of Yang deficiency.

Lesion location: Kidney.

Disease nature: Deficiency.

The diagnosis of Western Medicine: Infertility.

The diagnosis of Traditional Chinese Medicine: Infertility.

Therapeutic method: Replenish kidney and strengthen Yang, tonify essence and fill marrow.

Method: Electrothermal acupuncture treatment.

Prescription: Shenshu (BL23), Mingmen (DU4),

门（DU4）、关元（RN4）、三阴交（SP6）、太溪（KI3）。

方义 肾藏精，主生殖，故取太溪以补肾；关元属任脉，任主一身之阴，又是三阴之会穴，故取关元以大补阴精；肾俞是肾的背俞穴，取之以壮肾；三阴交为脾经穴，取之以调脾胃，益肾养阴，健脾以资生化之源。

配穴 形寒肢冷者，加命门、腰阳关；纳差便溏者，加足三里；腰酸腿软者，加关元俞。

操作 选定穴位，皮肤常规消毒。电热针直刺关元、足三里、三阴交各0.7寸，斜刺（针尖向脊柱）肾俞、关元俞各0.8寸。接通电热针仪，每个穴位分别给予电流量40mA，以患者感到胀而舒适为度，留针40分钟。（注：每次选3组穴给予电热针治疗，余穴用毫针治疗。）

疗程 每天1次，10天为1个疗程，疗程间如无不适可进行第2个疗程的治疗。

治疗过程 该患者治疗经

Guanyuan (RN4), Sanyinjiao (SP6), Taixi (KI3).

Mechanism of prescription: Kidney stores essence and governs reproduction, therefore use Taixi to tonify kidney. Guanyuan belongs to Ren Channel, Ren governs Yin of the whole body, and also is the confluent acupoint of three Yins, therefore use Guanyuan to greatly nourish Yin essence. Shenshu is a Back-Shu acupoint of Kidney, it can reinforce kidney. Sanyinjiao is an acupoint of Spleen Meridian, it can tonify spleen and stomach, nourish kidney and Yin, invigorate spleen to facilitate source of generation and transformation.

Matching acupoint: For cold body and limbs add Mingmen, Yaoyangguan; for poor appetite and sloppy stool add Zusanli; and for aching lumbus and limp legs add Guanyuanshu.

Operations: Preparing the selected acupoints, perform routine skin disinfection. Using electrothermal acupuncture needles, vertically puncture into Guanyuan, Zusanli, Sanyinjiao for 0.7" respectively, obliquely (with the needle tip towards spine) into Shenshu, Guanyuanshu for 0.8" respectively. Turn on the electrothermal acupuncture equipment, apply a current of 40mA to each acupoint, and the limit is that the patient feels swell and comfortable, leaving the needles in for 40 minutes. (Note: Select 3 pairs of acupoints for electrothermal acupuncture treatment each time, and treat the other acupoints with filiform needles.)

Therapeutic course: Treat once a day, 10 days as a course, and start the treatment for the second course if there is no discomfort.

Treatment process: The treatment process of that

过较顺利，疗效较好，治疗 20 次后症状基本消失，较前精力充沛，面色红润，情绪及心志较平和。为巩固效果，连续治疗 90 次，在此期间停止房事。治疗结束后，追踪观察 1 年，未见复发。精液复查示"精子数达 $23.7×10^9$/L，精子存活率为 65%，有 60%的精子形态正常"，故停止治疗，嘱患者每天自灸关元、气海各 15 分钟。4 个月后，其妻子怀孕，足月顺产一名男婴。

【生活调摄】

1. 治疗过程中，停止房事，配合治疗。

2. 做好患者的思想工作，要心志平和，不要紧张，要有信心和决心配合治疗。

3. 必须坚持治疗 90 次以上方可取效。

前列腺炎

前列腺炎是男性泌尿系统的常见病之一，有急性和慢性之分。前者以膀胱刺激症状、终末血尿、会阴部疼痛为主要症状；后者以排尿延迟，尿后

patient was smooth with good efficacies, and the symptoms basically disappeared after 20 times of treatment, the patient was more energetic than before, with red complexion, relatively peaceful mind and mood. In order to consolidate effects, the patient received 90 times of continuous treatment, and he stopped sexual intercourses during this period. After the end of treatment, follow-up for 1 year, no recurrence was found. Semen re-examination indicated "$23.7×10^9$/L of sperm with a survival rate of 65%, and 60% sperm were morphologically normal", therefore stopped treatment and asked the patient to do acupuncture of Guanyuan and Qihai for 15 minutes respectively by himself. Four months later, his wife got pregnant and gave birth to a baby boy with a full-term normal delivery.

[Lifestyle Change and Health Maintenance]

1. During the treatment, stop sexual intercourses and cooperate with treatments.

2. Do ideological work on patients, make them keep peaceful mind and mood and don't be nervous, establish confidence and determination to cooperate with treatments.

3. The treatment must be adhered to at least 90 times to take effect.

Prostatitis

Prostatitis is one of the common male urinary system diseases, which is divided into acute and chronic ones. For the former, its main symptoms are bladder irritation symptoms, terminal hematuria and perineum pain. The main symptoms of the later are urination delay, urine

滴尿，或滴出白色前列腺液，或引起遗精、早泄、阳痿等为主要症状。

中医认为，本病属于"白淫""尿精""精浊"等范畴。多因嗜食肥甘，酿成中焦湿热，流注下焦；或因房劳不节，肾气虚衰，湿热之邪乘虚而入所致。与肝、脾、肾三脏功能失调有关。

一、诊断及辨证要点

1. 急性前列腺炎

湿热蕴结者，症见寒战高热，全身酸痛，饮食欠佳，头痛，神疲乏力；大便秘结，尿频、尿急，终末血尿；会阴部坠痛，并向腰骶部、前阴及大腿部放射；舌苔黄腻，脉滑数。

2. 慢性前列腺炎

（1）寒滞肝脉者，症见少腹与睾丸隐隐作痛，遇寒则甚，得热则舒，腹寒阴冷，小便色清，尿时不畅，尿后有白色黏液滴出，舌苔白，脉沉或迟。

dropping after urination, or dropping of white prostatic fluid, or spermatorrhea, premature ejaculation, asynodia.

Traditional Chinese Medicine believes that this disease belongs to the range of "white ooze""spermaturia", "turbid semen". Most are caused by preference to fat and sweet food leading to Damp-Heat of Lower Jiao flowing downward; or caused by indignation in sexual intercourses leading to deficiency and failure of kidney, subsequently causing swooping in of Damp-Heat toxins. Related to dysfunctions of liver, spleen and kidney.

I. Key Points for Diagnosis and Syndrome Differentiation

1. Acute Prostatitis

For patients with Damp-Heat stagnation, symptoms include shiver and high fever, soreness of the whole body, poor appetite, headache, mental fatigue and asthenia; constipation, frequent micturition, urgent micturition, terminal hematuria; bearing-down pain of perineum radiating towards lumbosacral portion, front genital organs and thigh; yellowish and greasy tongue fur, slippery and rapid pulse.

2. Chronic Prostatitis

(1) For patients with accumulation of Cold in Liver Channel, symptoms include dull pain of lateral lower abdomen and testis, worsen in case of cold and ease in case of warmness, cold abdomen and coldness of external genitals, urine with clear color, unsmooth urination, dropping of white mucus after urination, whitish tongue fur, deep or slow pulse.

（2）肝肾阴虚者，症见腰膝酸软，倦怠乏力，五心烦热，盗汗，遗精，头晕目眩，会阴部隐痛，有时尿道有灼热感，舌质红，苔薄黄，脉细数。

（3）肾阳不足者，症见小便淋漓不爽，排尿无力，面色白，神气怯弱，腰以下冷，腰膝酸软，倦怠少力，舌质淡，苔白，脉沉细。

（4）湿热下注者，症见小便短小急迫且有疼感，尿色黄，甚者血尿，口苦咽干，外阴湿热，会阴部疼痛，舌质红，舌苔黄，脉数滑。

二、治疗方法

【急性前列腺炎】

治法 清肝泻热，化湿利尿。

处方 中髎（BL33）、阴陵泉（SP9）、曲骨（RN2）、蠡沟（LR5）、大敦（LR1）。

方义 中髎可清泻下焦之实热；取阴陵泉有利尿祛湿之效；小腹与前阴胀坠痛是因湿热阻滞肝络，造成肝气之疏泄

(2) For patients with deficiency of liver Yin and kidney Yin, symptoms include soreness and weakness of waist and knees, fatigue and asthenia, dysphoria in chest with palms-soles, sweating at night, spermatorrhea, dizziness, dull pain of perineum, sometimes with urination with feeling of burning, red tongue, yellow and greasy thin tongue fur, thin and rapid pulse.

(3) For patients with deficiency of kidney Yang, symptoms include dripping and unsmooth urination, weak micturition, pale complexion, timid and weak-willed expression, cold below waist, soreness and weakness of waist and knees, fatigue and asthenia, light tongue with whitish fur, deep and thin pulse.

(4) For patients with downward flow of dampness-heat, symptoms include short and urgent urination with feeling of pain, yellow urine or even blood urine, bitter taste and dry throat, Damp-Heat of external genital organs, perineum pain, red tongue with yellow fur, rapid and slippery pulse.

II. Therapeutic Methods

[Acute Prostatitis]

Therapeutic method: Clear liver and purge Heat, remove Damp and facilitate urination.

Prescription: Zhongliao (BL33), Yinlingquan (SP9), Qugu (RN2), Ligou (LR5), Dadun (LR1).

Mechanism of prescription: Zhongliao can clear and purge the excess Damp of Lower Jiao. Use Yinlingquan to facilitate urination and remove damp; distending bearing-down pains of lower abdomen and front genital

不利，故取井穴大敦、络穴蠡沟，以清泻肝经邪热，疏调经气，用以解除少腹与前阴之疼痛。诸穴共用，取清肝泻热、化湿利尿之功。

organs are caused by obstruction of Liver Collateral by damp-heat, leading to unsuccessful soothing and dredging of liver Qi, therefore use the Jing acupoint Dadun and the collateral acupoint Ligou to clear and dredge Heat toxins of Liver Meridian, soothe and regulate meridian Qi, so as to resolve pains of lateral lower abdomen and front genital organs. The use of combination of these acupoints can clear liver and purge Heat, remove Damp and facilitate urination.

配穴 血尿者加血海；小便不利者加水道。

Matching acupoints: For hematuria add Xuehai; for unsmooth urination add Shuidao.

方法 毫针治疗（泻法）。

Method: Filiform needle acupuncture treatment (reduction in acupuncture).

操作 选定穴位，常规皮肤消毒。用毫针直刺中髎1.5寸，使针感到达少腹部，向下斜刺曲骨0.8寸，使针感到达会阴部，平刺蠡沟0.5寸，向上斜刺大敦0.2寸，直刺血海0.5寸，直刺水道0.8寸，留针30分钟。

Operations: Preparing the selected acupoints, perform routine skin disinfection. Using the filiform needles, vertically puncture into Zhongliao for 1.5", obliquely puncture downward into Qugu for 0.8", make the feeling of needle puncturing spread to lower abdomen, horizontally puncture into Ligou for 0.5", obliquely puncture upward into Dadun for 0.2", vertically puncture into Xuehai for 0.5", Shuidao for 0.8", leaving the needles in for 30 minutes.

疗程 每天1次，10天为1个疗程，疗程间如无不适可进行第2个疗程的治疗。

Therapeutic course: Treat once a day, 10 days as a course, and start the treatment for the second course if there is no discomfort.

【慢性前列腺炎】

（1）寒滞肝脉证

[Chronic Prostatitis]

(1) Syndrome of Accumulation of Cold in Liver Channel

治法 温经散寒，培补下元。

Therapeutic method: Warm meridians and dissipate cold, reinforce lower origin.

处方 大敦（LR1）、曲骨

Prescription: Dadun (LR1), Qugu (RN2),

（RN2）、关元（RN4）。

方义 寒滞肝经，故在肝经所过之少腹、前阴等处作痛，治以温散足厥阴肝经之邪。故以灸其井穴大敦以祛本经之寒滞；取合穴曲泉以疏调肝气；本病多因下元不足所致，故温补关元，以益下元，而治其本。

配穴 小便不利者，加阴陵泉，使气化复常，小便通利。

方法 电热针治疗（温补法）。

操作 选定穴位，常规皮肤消毒。电热针直刺曲泉0.8寸，直刺关元0.8寸，直刺阴陵泉0.8寸。接通电热针仪，每个穴位分别给予电流量80mA，留针40分钟。温灸大敦20～30分钟。

疗程 每日1次，5次为1个疗程，疗程间可休息3天。

（2）湿热下注证

治法 清热化湿，益阴利窍。

处方 中极（RN3）、阴陵泉（SP9）、三阴交（SP6）、会阴（RN1）。

Guanyuan (RN4).

Mechanism of prescription: Stagnation of Cold in Liver Meridian, leading to pain of lower abdomen and front genital organs where the Liver Meridian passing by, the therapy is to warm up so as to dissipate toxins of Jue-Yin Liver Meridian of Foot. So use the Jing acupoint Dadun to remove the Cold stagnation of this meridian. Use the He acupoint Ququan to soothe and regulate liver Qi. This disease normally is caused by deficiency of lower origin, so warm and nourish Guanyuan to tonify lower origin so as to affect a permanent cure.

Matching acupoints: For unsmooth urination add Yinlingquan to recover Qi transportation and soothe urination.

Method: Electrothermal acupuncture treatment (warm tonifying).

Operations: Prepare selecting the relevant acupoints, perform routine skin disinfection. Using electrothermal acupuncture needles, vertically puncture into Ququan for 0.8", Guanyuan for 0.8", Yinlingquan for 0.8". Turn on the electrothermal acupuncture equipment, apply a current of 80mA to each acupoint, leaving the needles in for 40 minutes. Warm moxibustion of Dadun for 20-30 minutes.

Treatment course: Once a day, 5 times for a course. Rest for 3 days between courses.

(2) Syndrome of downward flow of Damp-Heat

Therapeutic method: Clear Heat and remove Damp, tonify Yin and soothe orifices.

Prescription: Zhongji (RN3), Yinlingquan (SP9), Sanyinjiao (SP6), Huiyin (RN1).

方义 取中极、阴陵泉以清利湿热,取三阴交先用泻法清利湿邪,后以温补法治阴亏。

配穴 痰多者加丰隆;神疲乏力者加足三里。

方法 电热针治疗(泻法)。

操作 选定穴位,常规皮肤消毒。电热针斜刺中极 3 寸,使针感到达会阴部,直刺阴陵泉 0.8 寸,直刺三阴交 0.8 寸。接通电热针仪,每个穴位分别给予电流量 50～80mA,留针 40 分钟。

疗程 每日 1 次,5 次为 1 个疗程。疗程间休息 3 天,再进行第 2 个疗程的治疗。

(3)脾肾亏虚证

治法 补益脾肾,以利下元。

处方 肾俞(BL23)、膀胱俞(BL28)、脾俞(BL20)、足三里(ST36)、三阴交(SP6)、太溪(KI3)、关元俞(BL26)。

方义 脾肾亏虚,故取肾俞、膀胱俞、脾肾、足三里以培补脾肾;取三阴交、太溪以养阴;取关元俞能益肾,又能

Mechanism of prescription: Use Zhongji, Yinlingquan to clear Damp-Heat, use Sanyinjiao to clear Damp toxins with attenuating then to treat Yin depletion with warm tonifying.

Matching acupoints: For excessive phlegm add Fenglong, for mental fatigue and asthenia add Zusanli.

Method: Electrothermal acupuncture treatment (attenuating).

Operations: Preparing the selected acupoints, perform routine skin disinfection. Using electrothermal acupuncture needles, obliquely puncture into Zhongji for 3", make the feeling of needle puncturing spread to perineum, vertically puncture into Yinlingquan for 0.8", Sanyinjiao for 0.8". Turn on the electrothermal acupuncture equipment, apply a current of 50-80mA to each acupoint, leaving the needles in for 40 minutes.

Therapeutic course: Treat once a day, 5 times for a course. Start the treatment for the second course after a break of 3 days.

(3) Syndrome of Depletion and Deficiency of Spleen and Kidney

Therapeutic method: Tonify spleen and kidney to nourish lower origin.

Prescription: Shenshu (BL23), Pangguangshu (BL28), Pishu (BL20), Zusanli (ST36), Sanyinjiao (SP6), Taixi (KI3), Guanyuanshu (BL26).

Mechanism of prescription: Depletion and deficiency of spleen and kidney, so use Shenshu, Pangguangshu, Pishu, Zusanli to tonify spleen and kidney. Use Sanyinjiao, Taixi to nourish Yin. Use Guanyuanshu

治下腹之痛。诸穴合用，可奏补益脾肾而利下元之功。

配穴 盗汗者加阴郄；五心烦热者加间使。

方法 电热针治疗（温补法）。

操作 选定穴位，常规皮肤消毒。电热针向脊柱侧斜刺肾俞、膀胱俞、脾俞、关元俞各 0.8 寸，直刺足三里 0.8 寸，直刺三阴交 0.8 寸。接通电热针仪，每个穴位分别给予电流量 70～80mA。另配以毫针直刺太溪 0.4 寸，留针 40 分钟。

疗程 每天 1 次，10 次为 1 个疗程。疗程间休息 3 天，再进行第 2 个疗程的治疗。

（4）肾阳不足证

治法 温补肾阳，通利小便。

处方 肾俞（BL23）、三焦俞（BL22）、气海（RN6）、中极（RN3）、三阴交（SP6）。

方义 多因年老体弱，久病伤肾，肾阳不足，造成膀胱气化无权而病。故取肾俞、太溪以温补肾阳；配三焦俞可通调三焦，化气行水；取气海以温通下元，行气利水；中极为

to tonify kidney and treat pain of lower abdomen. The use of combination of these acupoints can tonify spleen and kidney to nourish lower origin.

Matching acupoints: For sweating at night add Yinxi, For dysphoria in chest with palms-soles add Jianshi.

Method: Electrothermal acupuncture treatment (warm tonifying).

Operations: Preparing the selected acupoints, perform routine skin disinfection. Using electrothermal acupuncture needles, obliquely puncture toward spine into Shenshu, Pangguangshu, Pishu, Guanyuanshu for 0.8" respectively; vertically puncture into Zhusanli, Sanyinjiao for 0.8". Turn on the electrothermal acupuncture equipment, apply a current of 70-80mA to each acupoint. Additionally, using filiform needles, vertically puncture into Taixi for 0.4", leaving the needles in for 40 minutes.

Therapeutic course: Once a day, 10 times for a course. Start the treatment for the second course after a break of 3 days.

(4) Syndrome of Kidney Yang Deficiency

Therapeutic method: Warm and tonify kidney Yang, dredge urination.

Prescription: Shenshu (BL23), Sanjiaoshu (BL22), Qihai (RN6), Zhongji (RN3), Sanyinjiao (SP6).

Mechanism of prescription: Old and poor in health, long-term diseases impairing kidney, deficiency of kidney Yang, leading to failure of Qi transformation in bladder, subsequently leading to diseases. Therefore use Shenshu, Taixi to warm and tonify kidney Yang; the match with Sanjiaoshu can dredge and regulate three

膀胱之募，补之可助膀胱之气化，泻之能利关门之开启；三阴交是肝、脾、肾三经之会，补之可补益三脏，泻之可疏肝健脾、利水通淋，故取二穴先补后泻，有标本兼顾之意。诸穴合用，有补肾气、调三焦、利膀胱、通小便之效。

Jiaos, transform Qi and transport Water. Use Qihai to warm and dredge lower origin, transform Qi and smooth Water; Zhongji is a Mu acupoint of Bladder, tonifying of Zhongji can facilitate the Qi transformation of bladder, and attenuating can facilitate the opening of Guanmen; Sanyinjiao is the confluent acupoint of Liver, Spleen and Kidney Meridians, tonifying of Sanyinjiao can tonify these three organs, attenuating can soothe liver and invigorate spleen, increase Water and treat stranguria, so use these two acupoints in an order of tonifying followed by attenuating in order to treat symptoms as well as to effect a permanent cure. The use of combination of these acupoints can replenish kidney Qi, regulate three Jiaos, soothe bladder and dredge urination.

配穴 阳痿滑精者，加归来、曲骨；浮肿者，加水分、足三里。

方法 电热针治疗（先补后泻）。

操作 选定穴位，常规皮肤消毒。电热针向脊柱侧斜刺肾俞、三焦俞各0.8寸，直刺气海0.8寸，向下斜刺中极3寸，使针感到达会阴部，直刺三阴交0.7寸，直刺归来0.8寸，直刺曲骨0.7寸。接通电热针仪，每个穴位分别给予电流量50～80mA。另配以毫针直刺太溪0.4寸，留针40分钟。

Matching acupoints: For asynodia and premature ejaculation add Guilai, Qugu; for edema add Shuifen, Zusanli.

Method: Electrothermal acupuncture treatment (tonifying followed by attenuating).

Operations: Preparing the selected acupoints, perform routine skin disinfection. Using electrothermal acupuncture needles, obliquely puncture toward spine into Shenshu, Sanjiaoshu for 0.8" respectively, vertically puncture into Qihai for 0.8", obliquely puncture downward into Zhongji for 3", make the feeling of needle puncturing spread to perineum, vertically puncture into Sanyinjiao for 0.7", Guilai for 0.8", Qugu for 0.7". Turn on the electrothermal acupuncture equipment, apply a current of 50-80mA to each acupoint. Additionally, using filiform needles, vertically puncture into Taixi for 0.4", leaving the needles in for 40 minutes.

疗程　每天 1 次，10 天为 1 个疗程。疗程间休息 3 天，再进行第 2 个疗程的治疗。

三、注意事项

1. 急性期针灸疗效较好，能迅速缓解疼痛。对肾虚者要适当配合中药以补气养血。

2. 针刺后或晚间做局部热敷。

3. 治疗期间禁忌房欲，以免过劳。

四、典型病例

孙某，男，56 岁，职员，北京人。

主诉：小便涩滞，淋漓不畅已 2 年。

刻下症：小便频数，尿不尽，短涩淋漓，偶尔刺痛，小腹坠胀，面色白，舌淡，脉细。

查体：未见阳性体征。

辅助检查：尿常规检查示"红细胞（++），白细胞（++），脓细胞（++），上皮细胞少许"。

【诊断依据】

1. 中老年男性，小便淋

Therapeutic course: Once a day, 10 days for a course. Start the treatment for the second course after a break of 3 days.

III. Precautions

1. The acupuncture therapy has better efficacies during acute period, can alleviate pains rapidly. For patients with kidney deficiency, it is necessary to match with Chinese Herb Medicine so as to replenish Qi and nourish blood.

2. Local hot compress after acupuncture or in the evening.

3. Sexual intercourses are forbidden during treatment so as to avoid defatigation.

IV. Typical Case

Sun, male, 56 years old, employee, residence: Beijing.

Self-reported symptoms: Stranguria and dripping urine for 2 years.

Current symptoms: Frequent and rapid urination, endless urine, short astringent and dripping, occasional prickling, bearing-down distension of lower abdomen, pale complexion, light tongue, and thin pulse.

Physical examination: No positive signs were seen.

Auxiliary examination: Routine urine examination indicated "erythrocyte (++), leukocyte (++), pyocyte (++), a few epithelial cells".

[Diagnostic Basis]

1. Aged man, dripping and endless urine for 2 years,

漓不尽，有2年病史，时好时发，多于劳累后加重。

2. 查体未发现器质性病变。

3. 面色白，少腹多坠胀。

4. 尿常规检查发现红细胞、白细胞及脓细胞，伴发尿道炎症。

【证治分析】

病因 脾肾虚亏。

病机 脾虚则中气下陷，肾虚则下元不固，因此小便淋漓不尽。

证候分析 脾虚则中气耗伤，气虚下陷，则少腹坠胀；气虚不能摄纳，故尿有余沥，面色白。舌淡，脉虚细，为气血亏虚之象，此为气淋。

病位 脾、肾。

病性 虚性。

西医诊断 慢性前列腺炎、尿道炎。

中医诊断 气淋。

治法 补益脾肾，以利下元。

onset time to time, normally aggregated after overwork.

2. No organic lesions were found in the physical examination.

3. Pale complexion, usually with bearing-down distension of lateral lower abdomen.

4. Erythrocytes, leukocytes and pyocytes were found in the routine urine examination, accompanied with urethral inflammation.

[Syndrome-treatment Analysis]

Etiology: Deficiency and depletion of spleen and kidney.

Pathogenesis: Spleen deficiency causes Middle-Jiao Qi collapse, leading to dripping and endless urine.

Syndrome analysis: Spleen deficiency causes Middle-Jiao Qi consumption and impairment, deficiency and collapse of Qi, leading to bearing-down distension of lateral lower abdomen. Qi deficiency causes unable to intake food, leading to dripping urine and pale complexion. Light tongue, feeble and thin pulse, are symptoms of depletion and deficiency of Qi-blood, and this is called "Stranguria due to disturbance of Qi".

Lesion location: Spleen, kidney.

Disease nature: Deficiency.

The diagnosis of Western Medicine: Chronic prostatitis, urethritis.

The diagnosis of Traditional Chinese Medicine: "Stranguria due to disturbance of Qi".

Therapeutic method: Tonify spleen and kidney to nourish lower origin.

方法 电热针治疗。

处方 肾俞（BL23）、膀胱俞（BL28）、脾俞（BL20）、足三里（ST36）、三阴交（SP6）、太溪（KI3）、关元俞（BL26）。

方义 脾肾亏虚之证，可取肾俞、膀胱俞、脾俞、足三里以培补脾肾，三阴交、太溪以养阴，关元俞既能益肾，又能治下腹痛，诸穴共用，取补益脾肾而利下元之功。

配穴 小便不利者，加阴陵泉；汗多者，加阴郄。

操作 选定穴位，皮肤常规消毒。电热针直刺足三里、三阴交、太溪各0.7寸，斜刺肾俞、膀胱俞、脾俞、关元俞各0.7寸，接通电热针仪，每个穴位分别给予电流量40mA，以患者感到胀而舒适为度，留针40分钟。（注：上述穴位分成两组，每次取3组穴，轮流交替应用，留针40分钟，每日1次。）

疗程 每天1次，10天为1个疗程，疗程间如无不适可进行第2个疗程的治疗。

治疗 过程连续针治5次，小腹坠胀、小便淋漓不尽

Method: Electrothermal acupuncture treatment.

Prescription: Shenshu (BL23), Pangguangshu (BL28), Pishu(BL20), Zusanli (ST36), Sanyinjiao (SP6), Taixi (KI3), Guanyuanshu (BL26).

Mechanism of prescription: Syndrome of depletion and deficiency of spleen and kidney, can use Shenshu, Pangguangshu, Pishu, Zusanli to tonify spleen and kidney. Use Sanyinjiao, Taixi to nourish Yin. Guanyuanshu can tonify kidney as well as treat pain of lower abdomen, the use of combination of these acupoints can tonify spleen and kidney to nourish lower origin.

Matching acupoints: For unsmooth urination add Yinlingquan; for hydrosols add Yinxi.

Operations: Preparing the selected acupoints, perform routine skin disinfection. Using electrothermal acupuncture needles, vertically puncture into Zusanli, Sanyinjiao, Taixi for 0.7" respectively, obliquely puncture into Shenshu, Pangguangshu, Pishu, Guanyuanshu for 0.7" respectively. Turn on the electrothermal acupuncture equipment, apply a current of 40mA to each acupoint, and the limit is that the patient feels swell and comfortable, leaving the needles in for 40 minutes. (Note: Divide above acupoints into two groups for alternate use, each time use 3 pairs of acupoints, leave the needles in for 40 minutes, once a day.)

Therapeutic course: Treat once a day, 10 days as a course, and start the treatment for the second course if there is no discomfort.

Therapeutic course: Acupuncture treatment for continuous 5 times, bearing-down distension of lower

之症大有改观。继续治疗 20 次，症状基本消失，尿常规检查正常。为巩固效果，又治疗 10 次，痊愈出院。随访 2 年，未见复发。

【生活调摄】

1. 治疗期间，令患者注意卫生。

2. 忌食一切辛辣之品，可多食绿豆粥、莲子、梨、苹果等。

3. 针灸治疗急性发作或急性期患者，能迅速缓解疼痛，疗效满意。对肾虚者要适当配合中药以补气养血，提高疗效。

abdomen, dripping and endless urine were greatly improved. Continued to treat for 20 times, symptoms basically disappeared, results of routine urine examination indicated as normal. In order to consolidate effects, treated for another 10 times and the patient was cured and discharged. 2-year follow-up, no recurrence.

[Lifestyle Change and Health Maintenance]

1. During treatment, let the patient pay attention to hygiene.

2. Do not eat any spicy food, eat more mung bean porridge, lotus nuts, pears, apples, etc.

3. For patients within acute onset period or acute period, acupuncture therapy can rapidly alleviate pains with satisfying efficacies. For patients with kidney deficiency, it is necessary to match with Chinese Herb Medicine to replenish Qi and nourish blood, so as to improve efficacies.

皮外骨伤科疾病 / Diseases of dermasurgery and orthopedics

皮肤鳞状细胞癌 / Squamous Cell Carcinoma of Skin

皮肤鳞状细胞癌,简称"鳞癌",又名"棘细胞癌"或"表皮样癌"。本病起于上皮细胞,是皮肤癌中最常见的一种类型,约占皮肤的30%。其发展较快、破坏性大、恶性程度高,可以深入结缔组织、软骨、骨膜,也可以转移到附近的淋巴结或发生内脏转移。

鳞癌类似中医文献中的"翻花疮",其病恶肉增殖,推之不动,破烂紫斑,渗流血水,秽气熏熏,愈久愈大,越溃越坚,终属败证,是一种预后较差、比较难愈的恶性疾患。

一、诊断及辨证要点

1. 本病高发年龄为50~60岁之间,男女比例为2∶1。

Squamous cell carcinoma of skin, "squamous carcinoma" for short, is also called "prickle cell carcinoma" or "epidermoid carcinoma". This disease originates from epithelial cells, which is one of the most common tissue types, accounting for around 30% of the skin. This disease develops fast with great destructiveness and high degree of malignancy, can develop into connective tissues, cartilages, periosteum, as well as transfer to nearby lymph nodes or develop visceral metastases.

Squamous carcinoma is similar to "everted flower ulcer" in literatures of Traditional Chinese Medicine, it presents as proliferation of malign flesh which immobile when being pushed, broken and ulcerated purple spots oozing bloody water, strong mephitis, which increase over time and harden along with ulcerating and finally become incurable. This is a malignant non-healing disease with poor prognosis.

I. Key Points for Diagnosis and Syndrome Differentiation

1. The age with high incidence of this disease is between 50-60 years old, and the ratio of male to female is 2:1.

2. 本病多由角化病、黏膜白斑或癌前疾病转变而成。它可以发生于皮肤及黏膜的任何部位，尤其容易发生于皮肤黏膜连接处、面部、下唇、手背、乳房及外阴部等处。

3. 病灶局部表现

（1）初期：初起皮肤损害是一个干燥的疣状小结节，基底较硬，表面呈暗红色或有毛细血管扩张，损害逐渐扩大，表面常有角化物而不易剥脱，用力剥离则易出血，剥离后会复出长角质物质。

（2）中期：癌瘤中央可以发生溃疡，溃疡的边缘可显著隆起及充血，表面有许多鳞屑，损害逐渐扩大。

（3）后期：经过几周或几个月之后，可以发生带痂的溃疡面，剥离痂后所出现的溃疡面是坚硬的，并有颗粒状突起，损害逐渐发展，可和深部组织粘连，成为坚硬的肿瘤，边缘翻起，损害表面溃疡而成菜花样瘤块，有众多的颗粒状突起，其间含有脓液，有接触性出血，味恶臭。

4. 全身状态：病情发展较快，后期有难以忍受的剧烈疼痛或瘙痒，伴有食少纳差、全

2. This disease mostly is transformed from keratosis, leukoplakia or precancerous diseases. It can occur on any part of skin and mucosa, especially at junctions of skin and mucosa, face, lower lip, back of hands, breast and vulva, etc.

3. Local manifestation of lesions

(1) Early phase: The early skin lesion is a dry verrucous tubercule with a hard base, its surface is dark red or has telangiectasis, and the lesion enlarges gradually which normally has keratosis substances uneasy to peel off on the surface, it is easy to bleed if being peeled off with excessive force, and other keratosis substances will grow again later.

(2) Middle phase: There can be ulceration in the center of the tumor with significant uplift and congestion of the ulcer edge, and there are many scales on the surface. The lesion gradually enlarges.

(3) Advanced phase: After several weeks or several months, there can be ulcer with scab on it, the ulcer surface appears after the scab being peeled off, which is hard with granular protrusions. The lesion enlarges gradually and can adhere to deep tissues to form a hard tumor with edge turned up, and the ulcer edge ulcerates into cauliflower-like tumor mass with many granular protrusions on it, which contains pus, accompanied with contact bleeding, stinky smell.

4. Systemic conditions: The condition progresses rapidly, there are intolerable sharp pain or itching during the advanced phase, accompanied with less food intake

身乏力、消瘦、舌质淡、苔白腻、脉沉缓。或因出血不止，症见形瘦面、心神不宁、头昏眼花、舌质淡、苔薄白、脉沉细等。

5. 辨证类型

（1）脾虚湿滞型：肿块如堆粟，表面破溃，疮面有渗液，边缘高起坚硬，翻如花状，伴食少纳差、乏力倦怠、消瘦、舌质淡、苔白腻、脉沉缓。

（2）气血两虚型：皮肤瘤块破溃后不易收口，边缘隆起，中央溃疡，隆起部呈菜花状，伴形瘦、心神不宁、头昏眼花、舌质淡、苔薄白、脉沉细。

6. 病理诊断：取活检，病理切片检验示"鳞状细胞癌"。

二、治疗方法

【脾虚湿滞证】

治法　温经散结，健脾化湿。

处方　阿是穴（瘤体局部1点或数点为穴）。

配穴　公孙（SP4）、三阴

and poor appetite, systemic asthenia, emaciation, light tongue with whitish and greasy fur, deep and slow pulse. Or symptoms like skinny and soft body, unease, dizziness, light tongue with whitish and thin fur, deep and thin pulse, etc., are caused by endless bleeding.

5. Types of symptom differentiation

(1) Spleen deficiency and Damp stagnation: The lump is like accumulated millets with broken and ulcerated surface, there is seepage on the ulcer surface, the edge is uplifted and hard, turns up like flower, accompanied with less food intake and poor appetite, asthenia and fatigue, emaciation, light tongue with whitish and greasy fur, deep and slow pulse.

(2) Qi-blood deficiency: The skin tumor mass is uneasy to close after ulcerated, with edge uplift and center ulceration, the uplift part is cauliflower-like, accompanied with skinny and soft body, unease, dizziness, light tongue with whitish and thin fur, deep and thin pulse.

6. Pathological diagnosis: Perform biopsy, and the pathological smear test indicates "squamous cell carcinoma".

II. Therapeutic Methods

[Syndrome of Spleen Deficiency and Damp Stagnation]

Therapeutic method: Warm meridians and eliminate stagnation, invigorate spleen and remove Damp.

Prescription: Ashi acupoints (1 or several points on local parts of the tumor are the acupoints).

Matching acupoints: Gongsun（SP4）, Sanyin-

交（SP6）。

方义 主穴根据瘤体大小，局部取1点或数点，与阿是穴相似。应用电热针治疗，既能起到温经通脉、理气活血的作用，又能通过皮部经络的传导，调整整体机能。选配公孙和三阴交，前者为足太阴脾经的络穴，与足阳明胃经联系紧密，又为八脉交会穴之一，后者是足三阴经的交会穴，二者合用，可加强健脾化湿、舒筋通络、理气活血、软坚散结的作用。

方法 电热针治疗。

操作 选定穴位，皮肤常规消毒。在瘤体处采用电热针治疗，按每平方厘米2针进行选穴治疗。接通电热针仪，每穴分别给予电流量100～140mA（相当于43～45℃），留针40分钟。用艾条温和灸公孙、三阴交，每穴15分钟，以皮肤潮红稍润为度。

疗程 根据瘤体大小，每日或隔日1次，10次为1个疗程，疗程间休息3～5天。

【气血两虚证】

治法 温经散结，补益气血。

jiao (SP6).

Mechanism of prescription: For the main acupoint, one or several points, similar to Ashi acupoints. The use of electrothermal acupuncture treatment can warm meridians and soothe channels, as well as regulate overall functions through conduction of skin meridians and collaterals. Selectively match Gongsun and Sanyinjiao, the former is a meridian acupoint of Tai-Yin Spleen Meridian of Foot that has close connection with Yang-Ming Stomach Meridian of Foot, and also one of the confluent acupoints of eight channels, while the later is the confluent acupoint of three Yin meridians of foot. The match of these two can strengthen the effects of invigorating spleen and removing Damp, relaxing tendons and activating collaterals, regulating Qi and activating blood as well as softening hardness and eliminating stagnation.

Method: Electrothermal acupuncture treatment.

Operations: Prepare selected acupoints, perform routine skin disinfection. Apply electrothermal acupuncture treatment at the tumor, select acupoints for treatment as per 2 needle punctures per squire centimeter. Turn on the electrothermal acupuncture equipment, apply a current of 100-140mA (equivalent to 43-45℃) each acupoint, leaving the needles in for 40 minutes. Moxa-roll moxibustion of Gongsun and Sanyinjiao for 15 minutes each, the limit is flushing and slightly glowing skin.

Therapeutic course: Depending on tumor size, once a day or once every two days, 10 times for a course. Rest for 3-5 days between courses.

[Syndrome of Qi-blood Deficiency]

Therapeutic method: Warm meridians and elimi-

处方 阿是穴（瘤体局部取 1 点或数点）。

配穴 膈俞（BL17）、膻中（CV17）。

方义 阿是穴的临床意义如前所述。配穴膈俞，为血之会穴，此穴施灸，主治一切痈疽、恶疮、发背、妇人乳痛等证；膻中为气之会穴，有益气、理气之功。两穴合用，重在补血益气、行气活血，从而达到治病之目的。

方法 电热针治疗。

操作 阿是穴的施术方法同上。膈俞、膻中用艾条温灸，每穴 15 分钟，以皮肤潮红稍润为度。

疗程 同脾虚湿热证。

三、注意事项

1. 在治疗期间注意患者的营养摄入，忌食辛辣刺激性食物。

2. 电热针施术时，必须避免穿透健康组织，要求距健康组织 2mm，针刺过程注意针尖的方向，忌穿过健康皮肤。

nate stagnation, tonify Qi-blood.

Prescription: Ashi acupoints (take 1 or several points on local parts of the tumor).

Matching acupoints: Geshu（BL17）, Danzhong（CV17）.

Mechanism of prescription: The clinical significance of Ashi acupoints is as described above. Matching acupoints: Geshu is the confluent acupoint of blood, acupuncture and moxibustion of this acupoint can treat all ulcers, malignant sores, carbuncle on the back, breast pain of women; Danzhong is the confluent acupoint of Qi, it can tonify Qi and regulate Qi. The match of these two is focused on replenish blood and tonify Qi, activate Qi and blood circulation, so as to achieve the purpose of treatment.

Method: Electrothermal acupuncture treatment.

Therapeutic course: The operation on Ashi acupoints is the same as above. Moxa-roll moxibustion of Geshu and Danzhong for 15 minutes each, the limit is flushing and slightly glowing skin.

Therapeutic course: The same as above.

III. Precautions

1. During treatment, pay attention to nutrition intake of patients, spicy and irritating food is forbidden.

2. When performing electrothermal acupuncture, must avoid penetrating healthy tissues, a distance of 2mm from health tissues is required; pay attention to direction of needle tips during puncturing, it is forbidden to penetrate healthy skin.

3. 根据瘤体大小选穴，要注意在瘤体中电热针之间不能相遇，避免短路或烧伤。

4. 每次治疗前必须严格检查电热针、电热针仪，查看线路是否完好，确认针没损坏再施术。

5. 在治疗前，患者要选好合适的体位，避免留针时间长而引起患者不适或疲劳感。

四、评述

电热针治皮肤癌是根据中医理论和历史文献对有关肿瘤的论述而应用之，是中医针灸治癌的一个组成部分，配合艾灸即可达到温阳健脾、益气补血、疏通经络、祛瘀散结的目的。更重要的是，电热针保持并发展了火针的特点，克服了现代医学加温手段之不足，把热效应直接引入瘤体中心，热辐射途径由组织深部到体表，从根本上改变了加温肿瘤的途径。并能根据肿瘤部位和大小之异，从不同方向进行多点针刺，使瘤体内散热均匀、瘤体中心组织炭化，瘤体温度可达 43～50℃（癌细胞不能生存的温度），且不损伤正常组织。

3. Select acupoints depending on tumor size, note that the electrothermal needles mustn't contact with each other within the tumor so as to avoid short circuit or burn.

4. Before each treatment, must strictly check the electrothermal needles, the device of electrothermal needles to see if the lines are intact, perform acupuncture after confirmed that there are no needle damages.

5. Before treatment, the patient should choose proper body position to avoid patient comfort or fatigue caused by long time of needle leaving in.

IV. Comments

The application of electrothermal acupuncture for skin cancers is as per description related to tumors in Traditional Chinese Medicine theories and historical literatures, and is a part of acupuncture and moxibustion treatment for cancers in Traditional Chinese Medicine. When matching with moxa-moxibustion, it can warm Yang and invigorate spleen, tonify Qi and replenish blood, soothe meridians and collaterals, remove stasis and disperse stagnation. What's more important is that electrothermal acupuncture keeps and develops the features of fire needle acupuncture, conquers the disadvantages of heating approaches in Modern Medicine. It can introduce the heat effect directly into the tumor center with the heat radiation pathway from deep in the tissue to body surface, therefore fundamentally change the way of heating cancer, and perform multi-point needle puncturing from different directions depending on parts of tumor and tumor size, to facilitate even heat dissipation within the tumor and carbonization of center tissues with a tumor temperature up to 43-50℃ (a temperature that cancer cells cannot survive with), and do not damage normal tissues.

中医治疗皮肤癌，多用中药内服或外敷，《圣济总录》"瘿有可针割，而瘤慎不破耳"，《东医宝鉴》"翻出一肉，突如菌，如蛇形，长数寸……若误用针刀蚀灸必危，慎之"均有相关论述。但是，电热针的问世突破了"慎之"这一禁区。实践证明，电热针治疗皮肤癌疗效较好，且在肿瘤消退之后，局部愈合良好，不留瘢痕，甚至可转为正常皮肤组织。根据这些特点，电热针适合治疗颈面及外阴等部位皮肤的恶性肿瘤，既能使癌瘤完全缓解，又能保证器官功能、容貌和外形美观。

The approaches for treatment of skin cancers in Traditional Chinese Medicine, mostly are oral administration or external application of Chinese Herb Medicine. It is generally believed that, "Goiters can be cut by needles, but tumors should be carefully treated and cannot be broken"(*General Medical Collection of Royal Benevolence*), "A mass of flesh turns up, protrudes out like a fungi, snake-shaped, with a lengths of several inches...if treat it with burning moxibustion mistakenly then it will be dangerous, so it must be done with care" (*Valuable Compendium of Eastern Medicine,*). However, the advent of electrothermal needle broke through this restricted area. Practice has proved that the electrothermal acupuncture treatment has good efficacies on skin cancers, and after tumor regression the local healing is good, no scar left, or even can return to normal skin tissues. According to these characteristics, the electrothermal acupuncture treatment is suitable for treatment of malignant tumors at sites like neck and face as well as external genital organs. The outcome is that it can completely relieve cancer tumors as well as ensure organ functions, appearance and good shapes.

电热针治癌，同现代医学的加温治癌的机理基本一致。目前，关于加温治癌的机理公认的有以下几种：①肿瘤组织有效血流量明显低于正常组

The mechanism of electrothermal acupuncture treatment for cancers is basically the same as that of heating treatment for cancer in Modern Medicine. Currently, generally accepted mechanisms of heating treatment for cancer are as followed: ① The effective blood flow of

织，因此，其较正常组织散热慢而蓄热高；肿瘤组织血流灌注量少，可致营养乏于正常组织。这两点是其致死的原因所在。②癌瘤组织的含氧量及酸碱度均较正常组织低，故对高温的敏感性高。③加热后癌瘤组织内线粒体髓鞘样变和空泡化，导致呼吸抑制而死亡。溶酶体活性增强，促使癌细胞自溶崩解。

现代医学加温治癌机制研究表明，加热对癌细胞有明显的选择破坏作用。因此，在加热治癌的同时，对正常组织几乎没有什么损害。电热针对皮肤鳞癌的疗效机制也在于此。

指间关节扭伤

指间关节扭伤，是指指间关节在外力作用下引起的指间关节肿胀，活动功能障碍的一种伤筋病症。多由撞击、压轧等外伤，或间接暴力致手指过度背伸、掌屈和扭转而引起。

中医认为，本病属于"指骱伤筋"的范畴。

cancer tissues is significantly lower than that of normal tissues, therefore their heat dissipation is slower than that of normal tissues, with higher heat accumulation. The volume of blood perfusion is less, causing that their nutrition is less than that of normal tissues. These two are causes of death. ② The oxygen content and pH of cancer tissues are both lower than those of normal tissues, so they have high sensitivity to high temperatures. ③ After heating, change and vacuolation of myelin sheath like structures in the mitochondria within cancer tissues lead to respiratory depression and subsequent death. The activity of lysosomes increase, promoting autolysis and disintegration of cancer cells.

Study on the mechanism of heating treatment for cancer in Modern Medicine demonstrated that, heating has obvious selective disruptive effects on cancer cells. Therefore, it almost has no impairment on normal tissues when heating for cancer treatment. This is also the efficacy mechanism of electrothermal acupuncture treatment for skin squamous carcinoma.

Sprain of Interphalangeal Joint

Sprain of interphalangeal joint refers to a tendon injury with interphalangeal joint swelling and activity dysfunctions caused by external forces. Most are caused by traumas such as impact and press-rolling, or indirect violence leading to excessive dorsiflexion, pendulum and twist of fingers.

Traditional Chinese Medicine believes that this disease belongs to the range of "finger diastasis injuring tendon".

一、治疗方法

【血瘀证】

治法 舒筋活络，活血止痛。

处方 阿是穴、八邪（EX-UE9）。

方义 八邪为经外奇穴，阿是穴以痛为输，具有调气血、舒筋活络、止痛的功效。

方法 电热针治疗。

操作 选定穴位，皮肤常规消毒。电热针斜刺或平刺阿是穴和八邪各 0.5～0.7 寸，接通电热针仪，每个穴位分别给予 35～40mA 的电流量，以患者舒适为度（局部温热或胀感），留针 40 分钟。

疗程 每日 1 次，5 次为 1 个疗程。若无不适可进行第 2 个疗程的治疗。一般治疗 4～5 个疗程即可恢复。

二、注意事项

1. 治疗过程中注意休息，保护患肢，不再做剧烈运动，但可以保持功能活动，甚至训练。

2. 患肢经过治疗，疼痛、

I. Therapeutic Methods

[Syndrome of Blood Stasis]

Therapeutic method: Relax tendons and activate collaterals, activate blood and alleviate pain.

Prescription: Ashi, Baxie (EX-UE9).

Mechanism of prescription: Baxie is an external nerve acupoint, for Ashi, takes pain point as acupoint, they can tonify Qi-blood, relax tendons and activate collaterals, alleviate pain.

Method: Electrothermal acupuncture treatment.

Operations: Prepare selected acupoints, perform routine skin disinfection. Using electrothermal acupuncture needles, obliquely or horizontally puncture into Ashi and Baxie for 0.5-0.7" respectively, turn on the electrothermal acupuncture equipment, apply a current of 35-40mA to each acupoint, and the limit is that the patient feels comfortable (local feeling of swell or warm) leaving the needles in for 40 minutes.

Therapeutic course: Treat once a day, 5 times for a course. Start the treatment for the second course if there is no discomfort. Generally cured after 4-5 courses.

II. Precautions

1. During treatment, pay attention to rest, protect affected limbs, no longer do strenuous exercises, but can maintain functional activities, and even trainings.

2. After treatment, pain and swelling of the affected

肿胀得以改善，此时亦不要剧烈运动，还要注意保温，适当进行功能训练。

3. 接治患者前必须排除骨质损伤。

腕关节扭伤

腕关节扭伤是指腕关节周围软组织损伤而引起局部疼痛、肿胀、活动受限的一种伤筋病症。多因腕关节用力过度致扭伤或跌扑而发病。

中医认为，本病属于"腕缝伤筋"的范畴

一、治疗方法

【血瘀证】

治法 舒筋通络，活血化瘀，消肿止痛。

处方 阳池（SJ4）、阳谷（SI5）、阳溪（LI5）。

方义 阳池为手少阳三焦经的原穴，能舒筋止痛，是治疗腕部伤筋疼痛的常用穴；阳谷是手太阳小肠经经穴，能疏通筋络，消肿止痛；阳溪手阳明大肠经经穴，是治疗腕部肿胀的要穴。诸穴合用，可收疏通筋络、活血化瘀、消肿止痛

limb is improved, at this time strenuous exercises are also forbidden, and it is also necessary to keep warm, have proper functional trainings.

3. Before treatment of the patient, bone damage must be excluded first.

Sprain of Waist Joint

Sprain of wrist joint refers to a tendon injury with local pain, swelling and limited activities caused by injuries of soft tissues surrounding the wrist joint. Most are caused by overexertion of wrist joint leading to sprain or tumble.

Traditional Chinese Medicine believes that this disease belongs to the range of "tendon injuries caused by wrist joint".

I. Therapeutic Methods

[Syndrome of Blood Stasis]

Therapeutic method: Relax tendons and activate collaterals, activate blood circulation and remove stasis, relieve swelling and pain.

Prescription: Yangchi (SJ4), Yanggu (SI5), Yangxi (LI5).

Mechanism of prescription: Yangchi is a Yuan acupoint of Shao-Yang Three-Jiao Meridian of Hand, it can relax tendons and alleviate pain, is a commonly used acupoint in treatment of tendon injuries and pain of wrist. Yanggu is a meridian acupoint of Tai-Yang Small Intestine Meridian of Hand, it can relax tendons and activate collaterals, relieve swelling and pain. Yangxi is a meridian acupoint of Yang-Ming Large Intestine Merid-

的功效。

配穴 扶正加足三里、三阴交、曲池。根据扭伤部位，可加外关、手三里、养老。

方法 电热针治疗。

操作 选定穴位，皮肤常规消毒。电热针斜刺阳池、阳谷、阳溪各 0.6～0.7 寸，直刺曲池、足三里、三阴交各 0.7 寸，直刺外关、养老各 0.6 寸。接通电热针仪，每个穴位分别给予 30～40mA 的电流量，以患者感到局部舒适为度，留针 40 分钟。（注：每次选 4 个穴位轮番使用。）

疗程 每日 1 次，10 次为 1 个疗程。疗程间可休息 3～5 天，再进行第 2 个疗程的治疗。一般治疗 1～2 个疗程。

二、注意事项

1. 接治时一定要先排除腕骨骨折或脱位，细心诊查。

2. 扭伤当天针刺时要选远端穴，不宜用电热针或毫针针刺局部，注意扶正祛邪。

ian of Hand, it is an important acupoint in treatment of wrist swelling. The use of the combination of these three acupoints can relax tendons and activate collaterals, relieve swelling and pain.

Matching acupoints: To strengthen vital Qi add Zusanli, Sanyinjiao, Quchi. Add Waiguan, Shousanli, Yanglao depending on site of sprain.

Method: Electrothermal acupuncture treatment.

Operations: Selecting the relevant acupoints, perform routine skin disinfection. Using electrothermal acupuncture needles, obliquely puncture into Yangchi, Yanggu, Yangxi for 0.6-0.7" respectively, vertically puncture into Quchi, Zusanli, Sanyinjiao for 0.7" respectively, Waiguan and Yanglao for 0.6" respectively. Turn on the electrothermal acupuncture equipment, apply a current of 30-40mA to each acupoint, and the limit is that the patient feels locally comfortable, leaving the needles in for 40 minutes. (Note: Select 4 acupoints each time, use alternatively.）

Therapeutic course: Once a day, 10 times for a course. Start the treatment for the second course after a break of 3-5 days. Generally treat for 1-2 courses.

II. Precautions

1. Before treatment, fracture or dislocation of carpus must be excluded first, diagnose and exam carefully.

2. If perform acupuncture treatment at the day of sprain, chose distal acupoints, do not use electrothermal needles or filiform needles to puncture locally, pay attention to strengthening vital Qi and eliminating pathogenic

3. 肿胀缓解后，要逐渐增加活动量，进行功能训练，保证腕关节功能的恢复。

菱形肌劳损

菱形肌劳损，多因颈部突然后伸，上肢突然上举等动作（如端盆泼水、打球投篮、迎风扬谷等以及长期低头伏案工作）致伤。伤后多为单侧颈部酸痛，有负重感，其痛由背向颈部放散，每遇颈部旋转或后伸时疼痛加重。在患侧的肩胛骨内缘和下角处有明显压痛。重者每于深呼吸、咳嗽、打喷嚏时疼痛加剧。患者颈部呈强直状，以躯干代替颈部扭转。

中医认为，本病属于"伤筋"的范畴。常因颈部、上肢活动不当，使筋脉劳损，气滞血瘀，经脉阻闭所致。

一、治疗方法

【气滞血瘀证】

治法 调气活血，舒筋散寒。

处方 风池（GB20）、大椎（DU14）、后溪（SI3）、昆

factors.

3. After relief of swelling, add amount of exercises gradually, have functional trainings to ensure the recovery of wrist joint functions.

Strain of Rhomboid Muscle

Strain of rhomboid muscle is mostly caused by activities like sudden extension of the neck, sudden upthrow of two upper limbs (such as holding basin for splashing water, shooting when playing basketball, winnowing facing the wind, and long-time bending over desk for work). After injury, most are unilateral neck pain with a load-bearing feel, the pain radiates from back to the neck, and gets agitated at each time of neck rotation or stretching backwards. Obvious tenderness at the inner and lower edges of the scapula at the affected side. In severe cases, the pain will get agitated when taking a deep breath, coughing, and sneezing. The patient's neck is stiff and the trunk replaces the neck to rotate.

Traditional Chinese Medicine believes that this disease belongs to the range of "tendon injuries". Often caused by improper activities of neck and upper limbs leading to tendon and vessel strains, Qi stagnation and blood stasis, obstruction of meridian and channel.

I. Therapeutic Methods

[Syndrome of Qi Stagnation and Blood Stasis]

Therapeutic method: Regulate Qi and activate blood, relax tendons and disperse cold.

Prescription: Fengchi (GB20), Dazhui (DU14), Houxi (SI3), Kunlun (BL60).

仑（BL60）。

方义 本方取手太阳小肠经穴后溪与足太阳膀胱经穴昆仑相配，上下互应，以通太阳之经气而除颈背部强痛；取风池、大椎以舒筋活络，通阳除痹。诸穴合用，共收调气活血、舒筋散寒之功效。

配穴 肩胛疼痛者，加肩外俞；肩痛者，加肩髃；若要扶正，加曲池、足三里、三阴交。

方法 电热针治疗。

操作 选定穴位，皮肤常规消毒。电热针直刺后溪0.6寸，斜刺昆仑0.7寸，直刺肩髃、曲池、足三里、三阴交各0.7寸，斜刺肩外俞0.7寸。接通电热针仪，每个穴位分别给予40～50mA的电流量，以患者感到局部温热或胀感为度，留针40分钟。（注：每次选4个穴位，轮番应用。）

疗程 每日1次，10次为1个疗程。若有不适可休息3～5天；如无不适可进行第2个疗程的治疗，至痊愈为止。一

Mechanism of prescription: In this prescription use the match of the meridian acupoint Houxi of Tai-Yang Small Intestine Meridian of Hand and the meridian acupoint Kunlun of Tai-Yang Bladder Meridian of Foot to echo up and down, so as to dredge the meridian Qi of Tai-Yang, subsequently relive the pain of neck and back. Use Fengchi and Dazhui to relax tendons and activate collaterals, activate Yang and remove pain or numbness. The use of combination of these acupoints can regulate Qi and activate blood, relax tendons and disperse cold.

Matching acupoints: For scapula pain add Jianwaishu; for shoulder pain add Jianyu; for strengthen vital Qi add Quchi, Zusanli, Sanyinjiao.

Method: Electrothermal acupuncture treatment.

Operations: Selecting the relevant acupoints, perform routine skin disinfection. Using electrothermal acupuncture needles, vertically puncture into Houxi for 0.6", obliquely puncture into Kunlun for 0.7", vertically puncture into Jianyu, Quchi, Zusanli, Sanyinjiao for 0.7" respectively, obliquely puncture into Jianwaishu for 0.7". Turn on the electrothermal acupuncture equipment, apply a current of 40-50mA to each acupoint, and the limit is that the patient feels locally warm or swelling, leaving the needles in for 40 minutes. (Note: Select 4 acupoints each time, use alternatively.)

Therapeutic course: Once a day, 10 times for a course. If there is any discomfort, take a break for 3-5 days; start the treatment for the second course if there is no discomfort. Generally treat for 2 courses.

般治疗 2 个疗程。

二、注意事项

1. 治疗期间注意休息，避免过劳。

2. 避免上肢及颈部强劲负重活动，但可以保持功能训练。

3. 局部注意保暖，注意体位，减少伏案工作，适当增加活动。

胸壁挫伤

胸壁挫伤，多由于外来的暴力直接撞击胸壁，或人体在运动中碰在硬物上，而致胸壁软组织、骨膜等受伤。伤后疼痛明显，部位较局限，肋骨及肋间隙处可有明显的压痛点，局部可见肿胀、青紫瘀斑等异常改变。若伤后治疗不当或伤后未治，均可使瘀血散而未尽，或结而不化，成为陈伤，致病情缠绵不愈。

中医认为，本病属于"胸胁内伤"的范畴。多由暴力伤及气血，使胸壁部气血瘀滞、经络不通所致。

II. Precautions

1. During treatment, pay attention to rest and avoid overwork.

2. Avoid heavy load-bearing activities of neck and upper limbs, but can keep having functional trainings.

3. Pay attention to keeping local warm, body positions, reduce work bearing over desk and appropriately add activities.

Contusion of Thoracic Wall

Contusion of thoracic wall, most are caused by that external force impact the thoracic wall directly, or the human body collides with hard objects when moving, causing injuries of soft tissues, periosteum of thoracic wall. After injury, the pain is obvious, the painful site is relatively limited, there are obvious tenderness points, and abnormal changes like swelling and green and purple ecchymosis can be seen locally. Improper treatment or no treatment after injuries both can cause incomplete dispersing of blood stasis, or stagnation without dispersion transferred into old injury, causing lingering unhealing of the disease.

Traditional Chinese Medicine believes that this disease belongs to the range of "internal injuries of sternal ribs". Most are caused by that external force impairs Qi-blood, cause stagnation and stasis of Qi-blood and obtrusion of meridians and collaterals at the portion of thoracic wall.

I. Therapeutic Methods

[Syndrome of Qi Stagnation and Blood Stasis]

Therapeutic method: Relive chest distress and regulate Qi, activate blood and alleviate pain.

Prescription: Ashi, Neiguan (PC6), Lieque (LU7).

Mechanism of prescription: Ashi is the place where the Qi-blood of the injured part stagnates, acupuncture of Ashi can remove stagnated Qi, disperse blood stasis and alleviate pain. Neiguan is a collateral acupoint of Jue-Yin Pericardium Meridian of Hand as well as the confluent acupoint of Yin-Wei Channel. Lieque is a collateral acupoint of Tai-Yin Lung Meridian of Hand as well as the confluent acupoint of Ren Channel, and they are important acupoints for treatment of chest diseases, so the use of these acupoints combined can relive chest distress and regulate Qi, activate blood and alleviate pain.

Matching acupoints: For chest distress add Danzhong; for shortness of breath add Qihai; for severe blood stasis add Xuehai.

Method: Electrothermal acupuncture treatment.

Operations: Selecting the relevant acupoints, perform routine skin disinfection. Using electrothermal acupuncture needles, horizontally puncture into Ashi for 0.6-0.7", obliquely puncture upward into Neiguan and Lieque for 0.7" respectively. Turn on the electrothermal acupuncture equipment, apply a current of 35-40mA to each acupoint, and the limit is that the patient feels locally comfortable (feeling of swelling or warm), leaving the

疗程 每日1次，7次为1个疗程。一般治疗1个疗程即可痊愈。若还需继续治疗，可不休息连续治疗5～7天。

二、注意事项

1. 如遇严重者可配合活血化瘀、行气止痛药物治疗，以提高疗效。

2. 多做深呼吸，在不引起剧烈疼痛的情况下，多做上肢活动和扩胸运动。

肩关节周围炎

肩关节周围炎，是由于肩关节周围肌肉、肌腱、滑囊、关节囊等软组织病变引起的肩部疼痛和运动受限的病症。

中医认为，本病属于"肩凝症""冻结肩"等范畴。因为多发生在50岁以上的患者，也称"五十肩"。

一、诊断及辨证要点

1. 多发生在中年人或老年人，多继发于肱二头肌腱鞘炎或上肢外伤。

2. 肩部疼痛，开始时较轻，以后逐渐加重，昼轻夜

needles in for 40 minutes.

Treat once a day, 7 times for a course. Generally cured after 1 course. If it is needed to continue the treatment, it can treat for 5-7 days continuously without break.

II. Precautions

1. In severe cases, it can match with drugs intended to activate blood circulation and remove stasis as well as activate Qi and alleviate pain, so as to improve efficacies.

2. Do more deep breath, and do more upper limb activities and chest expansion exercises in the premise that do not cause strong pains.

Scapulohumeral Periarthritis

Scapulohumeral periarthritis refers to the disease of shoulder pain and limited activities caused by lesions of soft tissues surrounding the shoulder joints such as muscle, muscle tendons, bursa synovialis, joint capsules.

Traditional Chinese Medicine believes that this disease belongs to the range of "shoulder periarthritis", "frozen shoulder". It is also called "fifty shoulder" since it generally occurs among patients over 50 years old.

I. Key Points for Diagnosis and Syndrome Differentiation

1. Most are occur among middle-aged or elder person, normally secondary to biceps tenosynovitis or upper limb trauma.

2. Shoulder pain, it is slight at first, then aggravates gradually, less pain during the day and aggravates at

重，不能睡于患侧，疼痛可向颈、耳、肩胛、前肢和手放射。

3. 肩部活动受限，以上臂外展、内旋、外旋较为明显，严重者不能做穿衣服、梳头、洗脸等动作。

4. 体征：肩部肿胀不明显，肩前、肩后、肩峰下三角肌止点处有压痛，以结节间沟处较为明显，可见三角肌萎缩。

5. X线检查：常规X线检查无特殊发现，后期可见肩部骨质疏松，无髓破坏，可在肩峰下见到钙化阴影。

二、治疗方法

【风寒痹证】

治法　疏散风寒，温经通脉。

处方　肩髃（LI15）、肩髎（SJ14）、肩外俞（SI14）、曲池（LI11）、合谷（LI4）、外关（SJ5）。

方义　肩周炎的范围大小不等，有很多经脉通过肩部，但以手三阳经、足少阳经及手太阴经所过处为主，故取上述各经过肩部的腧穴，以温经

night, unable to sleep towards the affected side, the pain can radiates towards neck, ears, scapula, upper limbs and hands.

3. The activities of shoulder are limited, which are obvious in outstretching, rotating inward and rotating outward, in severe cases the patient cannot do activities such as put on clothes, comb hair and wash face.

4. Physical signs: The swelling of shoulder is not obvious, and there is tenderness at anterior shoulder, posterior shoulder, the end point of deltoid under the acromion, and it is more apparent at the inter-tubercular sulcus, with visible deltoid atrophy.

5. X-ray examination: No special findings in routine X-ray examination, during the advanced phase, osteoporosis of the shoulder can be seen, with no marrow damage, and shadows of calcification can be found under the acromion.

II. Therapeutic Methods

[Wind-Damp Arthralgia Syndrome]

Therapeutic method: Dredge and disperse Wind-Damp, warm meridians and soothe channels.

Prescription: Jianyu (LI15), Jianliao (SJ14), Jianwaishu (SI14), Quchi (LI11), Hegu (LI4), Waiguan (SJ5).

Mechanism of prescription: The range of scapulohumeral periarthritis varies, and many meridians and channels pass through the shoulder, among which the main parts are where three Yang Meridians of Hand, Shao-Yang Meridian of Foot and Tai-Yin Meridian of

通脉，疏散风寒；再选取曲池、外关，以疏通阳明、少阳之气。

配穴 上臂痛者加臂臑；肩胛痛者加曲垣、天宗。

方法 电热针治疗。

操作 选定穴位，皮肤常规消毒。电热针直刺肩髃、肩髎、肩井、肩外俞各 0.7 寸，直刺曲池、外关、合谷各 0.6 寸，直刺臂臑 0.8 寸。接通电热针仪，每个穴位分别给予 50mA 的电流量，以患者舒适为度，留针 40 分钟。（注：根据肩周疼痛部位的大小，选 3～4 个穴轮流应用。）

疗程 每日 1 次，10 次为 1 个疗程。疗程间可休息 3～5 天，根据病情需要再决定是否进行第 2 个疗程的治疗。一般治疗 1～2 个疗程即可恢复健康。

三、注意事项

1. 近胸腔的穴位（如肩井、肩外俞、曲垣等），注意不可向内深刺，以免造成气胸或伤及肺脏。

2. 在治疗过程中，要求患

Hand, so use the acupoints of above meridians that pass through the shoulder, to warm meridians and soothe channels, dredge and disperse Wind-Damp. And use Quchi, Waiguan to soothe Qi of Yang-Ming and Shao-Yang Meridians.

Matching acupoints: For pain of upper arms add Binao; for pain of scapula add Quyuan, Tianzong.

Method: Electrothermal acupuncture treatment.

Operations: Selecting the relevant acupoints, perform routine skin disinfection. Using electrothermal acupuncture needles, vertically puncture into Jianyu, Jianliao, Jianjing, Jianwaishu for 0.7" respectively, Quchi, Waiguan, Hegu for 0.6" respectively, Binao for 0.8". Turn on the electrothermal acupuncture equipment, apply a current of 50mA to each acupoint, and the limit is that the patient feels comfortable, leaving the needles in for 40 minutes. (Note: Depending on the size of pain site around the shoulder, select 3-4 acupoints for alternatively use.)

Therapeutic course: Once a day, 10 times for a course. Rest for 3-5 days between courses, decide if perform the second course depending on the disease conditions. Generally cured after 1-2 courses.

III. Precautions

1. For acupoints close to the thorax (such as Jianjing, Jianwaishu, Quyuan), note that deep puncture inward is forbidden to avoid pneumothorax or lung damage.

2. During treatment, patients are required to keep

者坚持功能锻炼，以利于肩关节的功能早日恢复。虽然锻炼中会疼痛但也要坚持，之后疼痛会逐渐减轻。

3. 在肩周疼痛部位每日给予局部热敷2次，以助行气活血，通络止痛。

肱二头肌短头肌腱损伤

肱二头肌是支配屈肘和前臂旋后的主要肌肉，其短头肌起于肩胛喙突，下端止于桡骨粗隆。短头肌腱短而宽，无沟槽及滑膜鞘的保护，若肩关节脱位，肱骨外踝颈骨折，或肩部外展，屈肘时活动不当，均导致肱二头肌短头肌腱拉伤。其临床表现是肩关节前方及肩胛喙突部有明显压痛点，局部肿胀，可见瘀斑，屈肘和前臂旋后活动受限。

中医认为，本病属于"肩部伤筋"的范畴。因外力损伤筋脉，使气血瘀滞，经络不通所致。

doing exercises to promote the early recovery of functions of shoulder joint. Although there will be pain during exercises, patients should persist in it and the pain will reduce gradually later.

3. Perform local hot compress at the pain sites of shoulder twice a day, to facilitate to activate collaterals and alleviate pain.

Tendon Injuries of Short Head of Biceps Brachii

Biceps brachii is the main muscle that governs elbow flexion and inward rotation of forearm, and its short head originates from the scapula coracoids with the lower end ends at the radial tuberosity. The tendon of the short head is short and wide, without protection from groove and synovial sheath. Dislocation of shoulder joint, humeral lateral malleolus fracture, or shoulder outstretching, improper activities during elbow flexion, all can cause tendon injury of short head of biceps brachii. Its clinical manifestation include obvious tenderness points in front of the shoulder joint and at the scapula coracoids, local swelling, ecchymosis, limited elbow flexion and inward rotation of forearm.

Traditional Chinese Medicine believes that this disease belongs to the range of "tendon injuries of shoulder". Caused by tendon and vessel strains by external forces, leading to stagnation and stasis of Qi-blood, obstruction of meridians and collaterals.

一、治疗方法

【血瘀证】

治法 活血通络,舒筋止痛。

处方 肩髎(SJ14)、肩前、合谷(LI4)、阿是穴。

方义 取阿是穴以散局部瘀血、通经止痛;取肩前、肩髎以调肩部气血;合谷为手阳明大肠经的原穴,功擅活血化瘀,行气止痛,为治疗上肢疼痛的要穴。诸穴共用,可收活血通络、舒筋止痛之功。

方法 电热针治疗。

操作 选定穴位,皮肤常规消毒。电热针直刺阿是穴、肩前、合谷各0.7寸,向下(极泉方向)透刺肩髎0.8寸。接通电热针仪,每个穴位分别给予电流量40mA,以局部温热或胀而舒适为度,留针40分钟。

疗程 每日1次,20次为1个疗程。疗程间若无不适可连续治疗,不必休息。一般治疗1个疗程。

I. Therapeutic Methods

[Syndrome of Blood Stasis]

Therapeutic method: Activate blood and collaterals, relax tendons and alleviate pain.

Prescription: Jianliao (SJ14), Jianqian, Hegu (LI4), Ashi.

Mechanism of prescription: Use Ashi to disperse local blood stasis, dredge meridians and alleviate pain. Use Jianqian, Jianliao to regulate Qi-blood of the shoulder; Hegu, a Yuan acupoint of Yang-Ming Large Intestine of Hand, is good at activating blood circulation and removing stasis, activating Qi and alleviating pain and an important acupoint for treatment of upper limb pains. The use of combination of these acupoints can activate blood and collaterals, relax tendons and alleviate pain.

Method: Electrothermal acupuncture treatment.

Operations: Selecting the relevant acupoints, perform routine skin disinfection. Using electrothermal acupuncture needles, vertically puncture into Ashi, Jianqian, Hegu for 0.7" respectively, penetrate Jianliao downward (towards Jiquan) for 0.8". Turn on the electrothermal acupuncture equipment, apply a current of 40mA to each acupoint, and the limit is that the patient feels partial warm or swelling and comfortable, leaving the needles in for 40 minutes.

Therapeutic course: Treat once a day, 20 times for a course. Perform continuous treatment without break if there is no discomfort. Generally treat for a course.

二、注意事项

1. 在治疗过程中，避免上肢负重及外展、旋后等活动，逐渐开始轻轻活动，保持功能。

2. 在伤后急性期，应屈肘90°，用三角巾将前臂悬挂于胸前，4 周后解除，开始进行功能训练。

3. 要注意局部保温。

三角纤维软骨盘损伤

三角纤维软骨盘损伤，是在外力作用下致腕关节软骨盘受损的一种病症。

中医认为，本病属于"腕缝伤筋"的范畴。

一、诊断及辨证要点

1. 初期：局部肿胀，疼痛局限在腕关节尺侧，活动功能障碍。

2. 后期：肿胀减退，腕部疼痛，乏力，握力减退。

3. 在旋前、尺侧或背伸支撑时疼痛加重。

4. 查体：软骨盘挤压试验阳性，做腕关节旋转或挤压捻转时常可听见清脆的响声。

II. Precautions

1. During treatment, avoid activities like load-bearing as well as outstretching and rotating backwards of upper limbs, start from slight activities gradually to protect functions.

2. During the acute period after injury, flex the elbow for 90°, hung the forearm with triangular bandage on the chest, remove 4 weeks later, and start functional exercises.

3. Pay attention to local warming.

Injuries of Triangular Fibrous Cartilage Plate

Injuries of triangular fibrous cartilage plate refers to the disease that external forces cause injuries of wrist joint cartilage plate.

Traditional Chinese Medicine believes that this disease belongs to the range of "tendon injuries caused by wrist joint".

I. Key Points for Diagnosis and Syndrome Differentiation

1. Early phase: Local swelling, the pain is limited to the wrist joint side towards ulna, activity dysfunction.

2. Advanced phase: Swelling relieves, pain of wrist, weak, reduced grip strength.

3. The pain aggravates when rotating forward, ulnar or dorsal stretch supporting.

4. Physical examination: Positive in cartilage plate compression test, crisp sound often audible during rotating or squeezing and twirling of wrist joint.

5. 可由于长期反复的桡腕关节背伸、前臂旋前，使三角软骨盘受到磨损和牵拉，进而发展为慢性炎症。

二、治疗方法

【痹证】

治法 舒筋活络，消肿止痛。

处方 腕骨（SI4）、阳谷（SI5）、阳池（SJ4）。

方义 腕骨、阳谷分别为手太阳小肠经的原穴、经穴，可舒筋活血止痛，善治腕外侧痛脱如拔，难以握举。阳池为手太阳三焦经的原穴，是治疗腕部伤筋疼痛的常用穴。三穴共用，可收舒筋活络、消肿止痛之功效。

方法 电热针治疗。

操作 选定穴位，皮肤常规消毒。电热针直刺腕骨、阳谷、阳池各0.6寸，接通电热针仪，每个穴位分别给予电流量35～40mA，以患者局部温热或胀而舒适为度，留针40分钟。

5. It can be caused by long-term repeated dorsal stretching of radial wrist joint and rotating forward of forearm leading to wear and traction of the triangular cartilage plate, subsequently developing into chronic inflammation.

II. Therapeutic Methods

[Arthralgia Syndrome]

Therapeutic method: Relax tendons and activate collaterals, remove swelling and alleviate pain.

Prescription: Wangu (SI4), Yanggu (SI5), Yangchi (SJ4).

Mechanism of prescription: Wangu, Yanggu respectively are Yuan acupoint and meridian acupoint of Tai-Yang Small Intestine Meridian of Hand, and they can relax tendons, activate blood and alleviate pain, and good at treatment of pain like being pulled at lateral wrist and incapability of griping of wrist. Yangchi is a Yuan acupoint of Tai-Yang Three-Jiao Meridian of Hand, is a commonly used acupoint in treatment of tendon injuries and pain of wrist. The use of combination of these three acupoints can relax tendons and activate collaterals, remove swelling and alleviate pain.

Method: Electrothermal acupuncture treatment.

Operations: Selecting the relevant acupoints, perform routine skin disinfection. Using electrothermal acupuncture needles, vertically puncture into Wangu, Yanggu, Yangchi for 0.6" respectively, turn on the electrothermal acupuncture equipment, apply a current of 35-40mA to each acupoint, and the limit is that the patient feels local swell or warm and comfortable, leaving the

疗程　每日1次，20次为1个疗程。疗程间若无不适可连续治疗，不必休息。一般治疗1个疗程。

三、注意事项

1. 伤后应减少关节活动，疼痛减轻后可开始进行功能训练，慢慢增加活动量。

2. 挫伤严重者可采取针药结合法，给予活血止痛、舒筋活络的药物，以提高疗效。

腰肌扭伤

腰肌损伤是以腰部软组织突然损伤引起的腰部疼痛，活动受限为主症的伤筋病症。多在负重情况下因姿势不正、用力不当或跌打闪仆所致，有时在日常生活中突然弯腰或转身也可引起。受伤时，可有闪电或撕脱感，甚者可听到组织撕裂声，随即腰部剧痛，不能继续用力，呈典型的"板腰"，僵硬畸形，行走不便，腰部前屈、后伸运动受限严重，扭伤处的横突部位有明显压痛。

中医认为，本病属于"腰痛""闪挫"的范畴。多由于

needles in for 40 minutes.

Therapeutic course: Treat once a day, 20 times for a course. Perform continuous treatment without break if there is no discomfort. Generally treat for 1 course.

III. Precautions

1. After injury, joint activities should be reduced, and functional exercises can start after pain relief, increase activity amount gradually.

2. For severe contusions, use the combination of acupuncture and medicine therapy, give patients drugs that can activate blood and alleviate pain as well as relax tendons and activate efficacies.

Sprain of Psoas

Sprain of psoas refers to a kind of tendon injuries, its primary symptoms include waist pain and limited activities caused by sudden injuries of waist soft tissues. Most are caused by improper position, inappropriate forcing during load bearing or falling, sometimes also can caused by sudden bending down or turn-back during daily life. Upon injury, there can be feeling of electricity or avulsion, or even audible sound of tissue tearing, closely followed by intense waist pain, weakness, like the typical "plate-like waist", stiff and deformity, walking difficulties, serious limitation of flexing forward and stretching backward of waist, as well as obvious tenderness at the transverse process of the injured area.

Traditional Chinese Medicine believes that this disease belongs to the range of "waist pain", "sudden strain

剧烈运动或持重不当，跌仆及过度扭转等原因，引起筋脉损伤，经气运行受阻，气血壅滞局部而成。

一、治疗方法

【气滞血瘀证】

治法 调理气血，舒筋通络，活血止痛。

处方 肾俞（BL23）、委中（BL40）、大肠俞（BL25）、气海俞（BL24）、关元俞（BL26）。

方义 采用局部取穴与循经取穴相结合的方法，取肾俞、大肠俞、委中以达到调理气血、疏通经络、活血止痛的目的。

方法 电热针治疗。

操作 选定穴位，皮肤常规消毒。先用毫针刺后溪0.5寸，令患者做弯腰活动，至腰活动自如为止（一般20～30分钟）。之后取俯卧位，电热针直刺肾俞、大肠俞、气海俞、关元俞各0.7寸，直刺委中0.7寸，接通电热针仪，每个穴位分别给予30～40mA的电流量，以患者感到温热或胀感为度，留针40分钟。

or contusion". Most are caused by intense activities or improper load bearing, falling and excessive twisting, leading to tendon and vessel strains, obstruction of meridian Qi circulation, stagnation and stasis of Qi-blood.

I. Therapeutic Methods

[Syndrome of Qi Stagnation and Blood Stasis]

Therapeutic method: Nurse Qi-blood, relax tendons and activate collaterals, activate blood and alleviate pain.

Prescription: Shenshu(BL23), Weizhong(BL40), Dachangshu (BL25), Qihaishu(BL24), Guanyuanshu (BL26).

Mechanism of prescription: Utilize the approach that combine local acupoint selecting with acupoint selecting along meridians, use Shenshu, Dachangshu, Weizhong to nurse Qi-blood, soothe and dredge mechanism of prescription, activate blood and alleviate pain.

Method: Electrothermal acupuncture treatment.

Operations: Selecting the relevant acupoints, perform routine skin disinfection. Using filiform needles, puncture into Houxi for 0.5" at first, then let the patient perform waist bending until the waist can do activities without limitations (normally 20-30 minutes). Then let the patient lie at a prone position, using electrothermal acupuncture needles, vertically puncture into Shenshu, Dachangshu, Qihaishu, Guanyuanshu for 0.7" respectively, vertically puncture into Weizhong for 0.7". Turn on the electrothermal acupuncture equipment, apply a current of 30-40mA to each acupoint, and the limit is that the patient feels warm or swelling, leaving the needles in for 40 minutes.

疗程 每日1次，一般治疗3～5次即可痊愈。

二、注意事项

1. 针刺治疗前必须明确诊断，排除骨折和关节的器质性病变。

2. 若有皮肤外伤者，伤处不宜针刺。

3. 要求患者治疗过程中注意功能训练，保证腰的生理功能的恢复。

梨状肌损伤综合征

由于梨状肌刺激或压迫坐骨神经而引起的臀腿痛，称为梨状肌综合征。梨状肌起始于第2～4骶椎前的骶前孔外侧和骶结节韧带，其肌纤维穿出坐骨大孔后，抵止于股骨大转子。髋关节急剧外旋，梨状肌猛烈收缩，或髋关节突然内收、内旋，使梨状肌受到牵拉，均可使梨状肌遭受损伤。损伤后，由于充血、水肿、痉挛，肥厚的梨状肌刺激或压迫坐骨神经而引起臀腿痛。

一、诊断及辨证要点

1. 臀部及下肢沿坐骨神

Therapeutic course: Once a day, generally cured after 3-5 times of treatment.

II. Precautions

1. Before acupuncture treatment, the practitioner must perform clear diagnosis to exclude fractures and organic ankle lesions.

2. For patients with skin trauma, the injured site is not suitable for acupuncture.

3. During treatment, patients are required to pay attention to functional exercises, to ensure the recovery of waist physiological functions.

Syndrome of Piriformis Injuries

Pains of buttock and legs caused by stimulations of piriformis or compression of sciatic nerves are called syndrome of piriformis injuries. Piriformis originates from the lateral anterior sacral foramina in front of the sacral vertebrae 2-4 and sacrotuberous ligament, its muscle fibers arrive at the greater trochanter of femur after going through the greater sciatic foramen. Sharp outward rotation of hip joint, violent contraction of piriformis, or sudden adduction, inward rotation of hip joint leading to traction of piriformis, all can cause injury of piriformis. After injuries, due to congestion, edema and spasm, the thick piriformis stimulates or compress sciatic nerves, therefore causes pains of buttock and legs.

I. Key Points for Diagnosis and Syndrome Differentiation

1. Radiative pains along distrusting area of sciatic

经分布区放射性疼痛，可因劳累或受风寒湿邪侵袭而致疼痛加重。

2. 严重患者可自觉臀部呈"刀割样"或"烧灼样"疼痛，不能入睡，影响日常生活，甚至走路呈跛行。

3. 查体：①患者腰部无明显压痛和畸形，活动不受限，梨状肌部位有压痛和放射性疼痛，局部能触及条索状隆起，有钝厚感，或者肌腹呈弥漫性肿胀，肌束变硬、坚韧、弹性减低。②沿坐骨神经可有压痛，直腿抬高试验多为阳性。

4. 有梨状肌牵拉伤病史。

二、治疗方法

【血瘀证】

治法　活血化瘀，消肿止痛。

处方　阿是穴、环跳（GB30）、阳陵泉（GB34）。

方义　环跳为足少阳胆经与足太阳膀胱经之交会穴，且位于梨状肌部位，与阿是穴相配，能活血化瘀，消肿止痛，解除梨状肌的痉挛与水肿。

方法　电热针治疗。

操作　选定穴位，皮肤常

nerves of buttock and lower limbs, the pain can aggravate due to fatigue or invasion of Wind, Cold, Damp toxins.

2. In severe cases, patents may feel "knife cutting like" or "burning" pains of buttock, cannot sleep, which effects daily life or even causes limp.

3. Physical examination: ① No obvious tenderness or malformation at patient's waist, no activity limitations, tenderness and radiation pains at part of piriformis, string-like uplift can be touched locally with feeling of blunt and thick, or diffuse swelling at muscle belly, muscle bundles become firm and tenacious with reduced flexibility. ② There can be tenderness along sciatic nerves, normally positive in the straight-leg raising test.

4. Medical history of piriformis strain injuries.

II. Therapeutic Methods

[Syndrome of Blood Stasis]

Therapeutic method: Activate blood circulation and remove stasis, relieve swelling and pain.

Prescription: Ashi, Huantiao (GB30), Yanglingquan (GB34).

Mechanism of prescription: Huantiao is the confluent acupoint of Shao-Yang Gall Meridian of Foot and Tai-Yang Bladder Meridian of Foot, and is located at piriformis, when being matched with Ashi, it can activate blood circulation and remove stasis, relieve swelling and pain, as well as solve spasm and edema of piriformis.

Method: Electrothermal acupuncture treatment.

Operations: Selecting the relevant acupoints, per-

规消毒。电热针直刺环跳 1.2 寸，直刺阿是穴 0.8 寸。接通电热针仪，每个穴位分别给予 60～70mA 的电流量，以患者感到局部有温热或胀感而向下肢传导，并感到舒适为度，留针 40 分钟。

疗程 每日 1 次，20 次为 1 个疗程。因该病恢复得较慢，故需治疗 1～2 个疗程方能痊愈。

三、注意事项

1. 在治疗过程中注意休息，避免下肢外展及用力旋转活动。

2. 电热针治疗的同时亦可配合活血化瘀、消肿止痛之中药，以提高疗效。

3. 疼痛减轻后，要注意功能训练和局部保温。

踝关节扭伤

踝关节扭伤，是全身关节扭伤中最为常见的一种伤筋病症。临床表现为踝关节周围肿胀、疼痛、行走困难、皮下瘀血等。多由高处坠落，或在不平的路面上行走、跳跃，或下

form routine skin disinfection. Using electrothermal acupuncture needles, vertically puncture into Huantiao for 1.2", Ashi for 0.8". Turn on the electrothermal acupuncture equipment, apply a current of 60-70mA to each acupoint, and the limit is that the patient feels locally warm or swelling which conducts to the lower limbs, leaving the needles in for 40 minutes.

Therapeutic course: Treat once a day, 20 times for a course. Since healing of this disease is slow, it normally needs 1-2 courses to be cured.

III. Precautions

1. During treatment, pay attention to rest, avoid outstretching and hard rotating of lower limbs.

2. While performing electrothermal acupuncture treatment, it can match with Chinese Herb Medicine intended to activate blood circulation and remove stasis as well as disperse swelling and alleviate pain, so as to improve efficacies.

3. After pain relieving, pay attention to functional exercises and local warm.

Sprain of Ankle Joint

Sprain of ankle joint is the most common tendon injury among sprains of systemic joints. The clinical manifestations include swelling around ankle joint, pain, walking difficulties, subcutaneous bleeding and so on. Most are caused by falling from high place, or walking or jumping on uneven road surfaces, or step miss while

楼梯时踩空等，使足踝突然翻转而致。

中医认为，本病属于"踝缝伤筋"的范畴。

一、治疗方法

【气滞血瘀证】

治法 调理气血，舒筋通络，消肿止痛。

处方 解溪（ST41）、昆仑（BL60）、丘墟（GB40）。

方义 解溪为足阳明胃经穴，能舒筋止痛，是治疗踝关节疼痛之要穴。昆仑为足太阳膀胱经穴，有通络止痛的作用，主治踝部如裂疼痛。丘墟为足少阳胆经的原穴，亦为治疗踝部肿痛的常用穴。三穴共用，具有调理气血、疏通经络、消肿止痛的功效。

配穴 根据扭伤部位的大小，可配申脉、金门、悬钟、照海、商丘、阿是穴等。

方法 电热针治疗。

操作 选定穴位，皮肤常规消毒。电热针直刺解溪0.6寸，直刺昆仑0.7寸，直刺丘

going downstairs, leading to sudden ankle rotation.

Traditional Chinese Medicine believes that this disease belongs to the range of "tendon injuries caused by ankle joint".

I. Therapeutic Methods

[Syndrome of Qi Stagnation and Blood Stasis]

Therapeutic method: Nurse Qi-blood, relax tendons and activate collaterals, disperse swelling and alleviate pain.

Prescription: Jiexi (ST41), Kunlun (BL60), Qiuxu (GB40).

Mechanism of prescription: Jiexi is an acupoint of Yang-Ming Stomach Meridian of Foot, an important acupoint for treatment of ankle joint pains, which can relax tendons and alleviate pain. Kunlun, an acupoint of Tai-Yang Bladder Meridian of Foot, is good at treatment of ankle pain which feel like cracking, which can activate collaterals and alleviate pain. Qiuxu, a Yuan acupoint of Shao-Yang Gall Meridian of Foot, is also a commonly used acupoint for treatment of ankle swelling. The use of combination of these three acupoints can nourish Qi-blood, relax tendons and activate collaterals, disperse swelling and alleviate pain.

Matching acupoints: match with Shenmai, Jinmen, Xuanzhong, Zhaohai, Shangqiu, Ashi depending on the size of sprained site.

Method: Electrothermal acupuncture treatment.

Operations: Selecting the relevant acupoints, perform routine skin disinfection. Using electrothermal acupuncture needles, vertically puncture into Jiexi for

墟 0.7 寸，直刺申脉 0.7 寸，直刺金门 0.6 寸，直刺悬钟、照海、商丘各 0.7 寸。接通电热针仪，每个穴位分别给予电流量 30mA，以患者感到局部舒适为度，留针 40 分钟。（注：每次选 3～4 个穴位，轮流使用。）

疗程 每日 1 次，一般治疗 3～5 次即可痊愈。

二、注意事项

1. 减少扭伤关节的活动。

2. 疼痛缓解后注意局部保温，加强功能训练。

3. 首次针刺给予低温（30mA），第 3 天可给予 40mA。

足跟腱扭伤

足跟腱扭伤，是指在间接暴力作用下致使跟部肌腱过度牵拉撕裂所产生的一种伤筋病症。临床表现为局部疼痛，不能行走或行走不便，轻度肿胀，可见局部瘀斑，压痛明显，触摸跟腱处变细，足主动跖屈无力。常因跟腱受到骤然猛力牵拉，如从高处跳下前足着地，或肩负过重勉强行走，或剧烈奔跑等致伤。

0.6", Kunlun for 0.7", Qiuxu for 0.7", Shenmai for 0.7", Jinmen for 0.6", Xuanzhong, Zhaohai, Shangqiu for 0.7" respectively. Turn on the electrothermal acupuncture equipment, apply a current of 30mA to each acupoint, and the limit is that the patient feels locally comfortable, leaving the needles in for 40 minutes. (Note: Select 3-4 acupoints each time, use alternatively.)

Therapeutic course: Once a day, generally cured after 3-5 times of treatment.

II. Precautions

1. Reduce activities of the injured joint.

2. After pain relief, pay attention to keeping local warm, strengthen functional exercises.

3. Apply low temperature (30mA) for the first time of acupuncture, and at the third day 40 mA can be applied.

Achilles Tendon Sprain

Achilles tendon sprain refers to a tendon injury caused by indirect violence leading to excessive tractive tearing of heel tendon. The clinical manifestations include non-walking or difficulties in walking, slight swelling, visible local ecchymosis, obvious tenderness, touched Achilles tendon thinning, active plantar flexion weakness of foot. Normally are caused by sudden violent traction, such as jumping from a high place with feet touching the ground first, or barely walking with excessive load over shoulder, or violent running.

Traditional Chinese Medicine believes that this disease belongs to the range of "tendon injuries of heel".

I. Therapeutic Methods

[Syndrome of Blood Stasis]

Therapeutic method: Activate blood and remove stasis, activate collaterals and alleviate pain.

Prescription: Ashi, Taixi (KI3), Kunlun (BL60), Xuanzhong (GB39).

Mechanism of prescription: Ashi is the reaction point of diseases, takes pain point as acupoint, which is an important acupoint for treatment of meridian and channel pain as well as injuries. Taixi is a meridian acupoint of Shao-Yang Kidney Meridian of Foot, which can relax tendons and activate collaterals, treat local swelling. Kunlun, a meridian acupoint of Tai-Yang Bladder Meridian of Foot, is an important acupoint for treatment of pains of ankles and heels. Xuanzhong is an acupoint of Shao-Yang Gall Meridian of Foot, which can dredge meridians and alleviate pain. Use these acupoints together, combine selection of near and far acupoints, to achieve the effects of activating blood and removing stasis, activating collaterals and alleviating pain.

Matching acupoints: Match Jiaoxin, Fuliu according to injured parts.

Method: Electrothermal acupuncture treatment.

Operations: Selecting the relevant acupoints, perform routine skin disinfection. Using electrothermal acupuncture needles, vertically puncture into Ashi, Taixi, Kunlun for 0.7" respectively, Jiaoxin, Fuliu for 0.8" respectively. Turn on the electrothermal acupuncture

给予 25～30mA 的电流量，以患者感到局部舒适为度，留针 40 分钟。（注：2 天后可给予 40～50mA 的电流量，仍留针 40 分钟。）

疗程 每日 1 次，一般治疗 7～10 次即可痊愈。

二、注意事项

1. 在治疗过程中要减少局部活动，必要时可配合舒筋活络、活血止痛的药物，以提高疗效。

2. 局部疼痛缓解后，要增加功能训练，从少量活动逐渐加量，以利于功能的恢复。

3. 要注意局部保温，避免风、寒、湿邪的侵袭。

足跟外侧皮神经损伤

足跟外侧皮神经损伤，是由于足跟外伤，关节超出正常活动范围，使外侧皮神经移位而致的一种伤筋病症。临床表现为跛行，足跟不能着地，踝关节背伸受限，足跟外侧皮神经投影部位可触及滚动的纤细条索，压痛明显，可向踝上放射。多由足部外伤后，踝关节内翻过度而致。

中医认为，本病属于"筋

equipment, apply a current of 25-30mA to each acupoint, and the limit is that the patient feels locally comfortable, leaving the needles in for 40 minutes. (Note: Apply a current of 40-50mA after 2 days, still leave the needles in for 40 minutes.)

Therapeutic course: Once a day, generally cured after 7-10 times of treatment.

II. Precautions

1. Reduce local activities during treatment, use drugs intended to relax tendons and activate collaterals as well as to activate blood and alleviate pain if necessary, so as to improve efficacies.

2. After relief of local pain, it is necessary to increase functional exercises gradually from a small amount to facilitate the recovery of functions.

3. Pay attention to local warming, avoid invasion of Wind, Cold, Damp toxins.

Heel Lateral Cutaneous Nerve Injuries

Heel lateral cutaneous nerve injuries refers to a tendon injury caused by that the joints excess the normal activity range due to heel trauma, leading to displacement of lateral cutaneous nerves. The clinical manifestations include claudication, heel unable to be on the ground, limited ankle dorsiflexion limited, rolling string can be touched at the projection site of heel lateral cutaneous nerve, obvious tenderness which can radiate upwards. Most are caused by ankle overpronation after foot trauma.

Traditional Chinese Medicine believes that this dis-

出槽"的范畴。

一、治疗方法

【痹证】

治法 舒筋活络，消肿止痛。

处方 阿是穴、金门（BL63）、昆仑（BL60）。

方义 昆仑为足太阳膀胱经穴，能舒筋止痛，是治疗足踝疼痛的要穴；金门为足太阳经之郄穴，可疏通经络，治疗踝部肿胀、疼痛。阿是穴是以痛为输，为治疗经脉伤痛的常用穴。诸穴共用，可收舒筋活络、消肿止痛之功效。

方法 电热针治疗。

操作 选定穴位，皮肤常规消毒。电热针直刺阿是穴、昆仑、金门各0.7寸，接通电热针仪，每个穴位分别给予25～30mA的电流量，以患者感到局部舒适为度，留针40分钟。（注：前2天给予25～30mA的电流量，肿胀消失后改为40mA的电流量，留针40分钟。）

疗程 每日1次，一般治疗5～6次即可痊愈。

ease belongs to the range of "tendon off-position".

I. Therapeutic Methods

[Arthralgia Syndrome]

Therapeutic method: Relax tendons and activate collaterals, remove swelling and alleviate pain.

Prescription: Ashi, Jinmen (BL63), Kunlun (BL60).

Mechanism of prescription: Kunlun, an acupoint of Tai-Yang Bladder Meridian of Foot and an important acupoint for treatment of ankle swelling and pains, which can relax tendons and alleviate pain. Ashi takes pain point as acupoint, is a commonly used acupoint for treatment of meridian and channel pain as well as injuries. The use of combination of these acupoints can relax tendons and activate collaterals, remove swelling and alleviate pain.

Method: Electrothermal acupuncture treatment.

Operations: Selecting the relevant acupoints, perform routine skin disinfection. Using electrothermal acupuncture needles, vertically puncture into Ashi, Kunlun, Jinmen for 0.7" respectively. Turn on the electrothermal acupuncture equipment, apply a current of 25-30mA to each acupoint, and the limit is that the patient feels locally comfortable, leaving the needles in for 40 minutes. (Note: Apply a current of 25-30mA for the first 2 days, after the swelling disappear, apply a current of 40mA and leave the needles in for 40 minutes.)

Therapeutic course: Once a day, generally cured after 5-6 treatments.

二、注意事项

1. 伤后注意休息，在治疗过程中减少活动，注意保温。

2. 可配合营养神经的药物治疗，以提高疗效。

3. 注意适量的功能训练，逐渐增加活动量，以促进功能恢复。

腓肠肌损伤

腓肠肌是小腿后面的主要肌肉，起于股骨两髁，止于跟骨结节。肌肉强力收缩，踝关节过度背伸或长期慢性损伤，均可导致腓肠肌损伤。

急性损伤多见于跟腱部和联合部断裂伤，受损局部有肿胀、疼痛、压痛以及广泛皮下出血等症；慢性损伤多见于股骨髁的附着部或跟腱部位，局部疼痛，肌肉萎缩，筋脉僵硬，而肿胀不明显。

中医认为，本病属于"伤筋"的范畴。多因外伤劳损、伤筋、伤脉，以致气血瘀滞，筋脉不通所致。

II. Precautions

1. Pay attention to rest after injury, during treatment reduce activities and keep warm.

2. Medicine therapies intended to nourish nerves can be matched to improve efficacies.

3. Pay attention to appropriate amount of functional exercises, and increase amount gradually so as to facilitate function recovery.

Gastrocnemius Injuries

Gastrocnemius is the main muscle behind the calf, starting from two femoral condyles till the calcaneal tubercles. Strong muscle contraction, excessive ankle dorsiflexion and long-term chronic injuries, all can cause injuries of gastrocnemius.

Acute injuries most are seen in Achilles tendon and joint site ruptures, with symptoms like local swelling, pain, tenderness and extensive subcutaneous hemorrhage at injured part; chronic injuries most are seen in femoral condyle attachment sites and heel tendons, with local pain, amyotrophia, tendon and muscle stiffness, while swelling not obvious.

Traditional Chinese Medicine believes that this disease belongs to the range of "tendon injuries". Most are caused by traumatic strain, tendon and vessel injuries, leading to Qi-blood stagnation and stasis, obstruction of tendon and vessels.

一、治疗方法

【痹证】

治法 伸筋活血,解痉止痛。

处方 委中(BL40)、承山(BL57)、阳陵泉(GB34)、阿是穴。

方义 腓肠肌为足太阳经筋所结之处,故取阿是穴与足太阳膀胱经穴承山、委中相伍,可舒筋止痛,通经活络;阳陵泉为足少阳胆经的合穴,又为筋之会穴,是治疗筋脉损伤之要穴,有伸筋活血、解痉止痛之功效。

方法 电热针治疗。

操作 选定穴位,皮肤常规消毒。电热针直刺阿是穴、委中、承山各0.8寸,接通电热针仪,每个穴位分别给予电流量40mA,以患者感到局部舒适为度,留针40分钟。(注:伤后局部有肿胀时,给予电流量40mA,肿胀消退后给予60mA。)

疗程 每日1次,10次为1个疗程。一般治疗1~2个

I. Therapeutic Methods

[Arthralgia Syndrome]

Therapeutic method: Stretch tendons and activate blood circulation, relieve spasm and alleviate pain.

Prescription: Weizhong (BL40), Chengshan (BL57), Yanglingquan (GB34), Ashi.

Mechanism of prescription: Gastrocnemius is the junction of meridians and collaterals from Tai-Yang Meridian of Foot, so use Ashi matched with the acupoints Chengshan and Weizhong from Tai-Yang Bladder Meridian of Foot to relax tendons and alleviate pain, dredge meridians and collaterals. Yanglingquan is a He acupoint from Shao-Yang Gallbladder Meridian of Foot and a confluent acupoint of tendons, as well as an important acupoint for treatment of tendon and vessel strains, it can stretch tendons and activate blood circulation, relieve spasm and alleviate pain.

Method: Electrothermal acupuncture treatment.

Operations: Selecting the relevant acupoints, perform routine skin disinfection. Using electrothermal acupuncture needles, vertically puncture into Ashi, Weizhong, Chengshan for 0.8" respectively. Turn on the electrothermal acupuncture equipment, apply a current of 40mA to each acupoint, and the limit is that the patient feels locally comfortable, leaving the needles in for 40 minutes. (Note: If it is after injury, give a current of 40mA, then give a current of 60mA after swelling subsides.)

Therapeutic course: Once a day, 10 times for a course. Generally cured after 1-2 courses.

疗程即可痊愈。

二、注意事项

1. 在治疗过程中，避免负重、行走以及踝关节背伸等活动。

2. 患肢注意保温。

3. 患肢局部肿胀消退后，可逐渐增加功能训练，促进功能恢复。

颈椎病

颈椎病，又称颈椎骨关节炎、增生性颈椎炎、颈神经根综合征、颈椎间盘突出症等。本病是因长期颈椎劳损、骨质增生、椎间盘突出、韧带增厚压迫颈脊髓、神经根和血液循环功能障碍所致的综合征。

中医认为，本病属于"痹证""痿证""头痛""眩晕""项强""项筋急"等范畴

一、诊断及辨证要点

1. 颈型（痹阻型）

（1）头、颈、肩疼痛等异常感觉，伴有相应的压痛点。

（2）X线示颈椎曲度改变，

II. Precautions

1. During treatment, avoid activities such as load bearing, walking and ankle dorsiflexion.

2. Keep warm for affected limbs.

3. After local swelling of the affected limb being subsided, it is possible to increase functional exercises gradually to facilitate function recovery.

Cervical Spondylosis

Cervical spondylosis, also called cervical osteoarthritis, proliferative cervical spondylosis, cervical nerve root syndrome, protrusion of cervical intervertebral disc, etc. This disease is a syndrome caused by long-time cervical strain, hyperostosis, protrusion of intervertebral disc, suppression of cervical spinal cord and nerve root by ligament thickening as well as blood circulation dysfunction.

Traditional Chinese Medicine believes that this disease belongs to the range of "arthralgia syndrome", "flaccidity syndrome", "headache", "vertigo", " stiff neck", "neck muscular contracture", etc.

I. Key Points for Diagnosis and Syndrome Differentiation

1. Neck mode (stagnation)

(1) Abnormal feelings like headache, neck pain and shoulder pain, accompanying corresponding tenderness points.

(2) X-ray exam shows change of cervical flexion

或椎间关节不稳,具有"双边""双突""切凹""增生"的特征。

(3)除外颈扭伤(落枕)、肩周炎、风湿性肌纤组织炎,以及非椎间盘退行性所致的颈部疼痛。

2. 神经根型

(1)具有典型的根型症状(麻木、疼痛),并且其范围与颈脊神经所支配的区域相一致。

(2)压痛试验或上肢牵拉试验阳性。

(3)X线示颈椎曲度改变、不稳或骨翼形成。

(4)临床症状与X线显示的异常所见在节段上相一致。

(5)除外颈椎结核、肿瘤等病变,以及胸部出口综合征、肩周炎、网球肘、肱二头肌腱鞘炎等以上肢疼痛为主的疾患。

3. 脊髓型

(1)临床可见脊髓受压迫表现,分为中央及周围两型。中央型症状先从上肢开始,周围型症状先从下肢开始,又分轻、中、重度。

(2)X线显示椎体后缘多有骨质增生、椎管矢状径出现狭窄。

degree, or unstable intervertebral joint, with symptoms of "double edges", "double protrusions", "concaves", "hyperostosis".

(3) Except for neck sprain (stiff neck), scapulohumeral periarthritis, rheumatic muscle fibrositis, and neck pains not caused by intervertebral disc degeneration.

2. Nerve root type

(1) With nerve root-type symptoms (numbness, pain), and the range of which is consistent to that governed by cervical spinal nerves.

(2) Positive in tenderness test or traction test of upper limbs

(3) X-ray exam shows change of cervical flexion degree, unstableness or formation of bone wings.

(4) In the respect of segments, the clinical symptoms are consistent with the abnormalities shown in the X-ray exam.

(5) Except for lesions like external cervical tuberculosis and tumors, as well as upper limb pain based diseases such as thoracic outlet syndrome, scapulohumeral periarthritis, tennis elbow, biceps tenovaginitis.

3. Spinal marrow type

(1) Clinically seen spine marrow compression, divided into two types of central and surrounding. For the central type, the symptoms start from upper limbs, while for the surrounding type from lower limbs, which are divided into mild, moderate and severe types.

(2) X-ray exam normally shows vertebral posterior osteoproliferation, stenosis in the sagittal diameter of spinal canal.

（3）除外肌萎缩型脊髓侧索硬化症、脊髓肿瘤、脊髓损伤、继发性粘连性蛛网膜炎、多发性末梢神经炎。

（4）个别鉴别诊断困难者可做脊髓造影检查。

（5）有条件者可做 CT 扫描检查。

4. 椎动脉型

（1）曾有猝倒发作，并伴有颈源性眩晕。

（2）旋颈性试验阳性。

（3）X 线显示椎间盘节失稳或钩椎关节骨质增生。

（4）除外耳源性和眼源性眩晕。

（5）除外椎动脉 I 段（进入颈 6 横突孔以前的椎动脉段）和椎动脉Ⅲ段（出颈椎进入颅内以前的椎动脉段）受压所引起的基底动脉供血不全。

（6）除外神经官能症、颅内肿瘤等。

（7）确诊本病应根据椎动脉造影检查。

（8）椎动脉血流图及彩超仅有参考价值。

5. 交感神经型

（1）临床表现有头晕、眼花、耳鸣、手麻、心动过速、

(3) Except amyotrophic lateral sclerosis, spine cord tumors, secondary adhesive arachnoiditis, multiple peripheral neuritis.

(4) For some cases with difficulties in diagnosis, myelography is available.

(5) If possible, CT scans can also be done.

4. Vertebral artery type

(1) Previous cataplexy onset, accompanying cervical vertigo.

(2) Positive in neck rotation test.

(3) X-ray exam shows intervertebral disc instability or osteoproliferation of uncovertebral joint.

(4) Except otogenic and ophthalmic vertigo.

(5) Except veretebrobasilar insufficiency caused by compression of Segment Ⅰ (the part of vertebral artery before it enters into the transverse foramen 6) and Segment III (the part of vertebral artery from where it gets out of the cervical vertebra till where it enters into the cranium) of the vertebral artery.

(6) Except neurosis, intracranial tumors, etc.

(7) The diagnosis confirmation of this disease should depend on arteriography.

(8) Rheography and color Doppler ultrasonography are only for reference.

5. Sympathetic type

(1) Clinical manifestations include a series of sympathetic symptoms such as dizziness, blurred sight, tinni-

心前区疼痛等一系列交感神经症状。

（2）X线显示失稳或退变，椎动脉造影阴性。

二、治疗方法

【颈型】

治法 祛风散寒，调和营卫。

处方 大椎（DU14）、天柱（BL10）、肩外俞（SI14）、悬钟（GB39）、后溪（SI3）。

方义 大椎是督脉穴，又是诸阳之会；督脉为阳脉之海；天柱为足太阳膀胱经穴，肩外俞是手太阳小肠经穴，三穴相配，能祛风散寒，宣通后项部及肩部之经气，可缓解颈肌发僵或痉挛、肩背疼痛。悬钟为足少阳胆经穴，髓会悬钟与通督脉的八会穴后溪共用，可疏通后项部经气，使督脉与少阳经在颈部及四肢的气血得以畅通。诸穴共用，可取祛风散寒、调和营卫之功效。

配穴 表邪严重者，加合谷、风池；表虚者，加足三里、

tus, hand numbness, bradycardia, precordial pain.

(2) X-ray exam shows instability or degeneration, negative in vertebral angiography.

II. Therapeutic Methods

[Cervical type]

Therapeutic method: Expel Wind and disperse Cold, tonify Ying and Wei for balance.

Prescription: Dazhui (DU14), Tianzhu (BL10), Jianwaishu (SI14), Xuanzhong (GB39), Houxi (SI3).

Mechanism of prescription: Dazhui is an acupoint of Du Channel, as well as the confluent point of all Yangs. Du Channel is the sea of Yang Channels. Tianzhu is an acupoint of Tai-Yang Bladder Meridian of Foot, Jianwaishu is an acupoint of Tai-Yang Small Intestine Meridian of Hand, the match of these three acupoints can expel Wind and disperse Cold, dredge the meridian Qi of back neck and shoulder, relieve stiffness or spasm of neck muscles, shoulder and back pains. Xuanzhong is an acupoint of Shao-Yang Gallbladder Meridian of Foot, when being used together with one of the eight influential acupoints, Houxi, which can dredge Du Channel, can dredge the meridian Qi of back neck, enable smooth circulation of the Qi-blood of Du Channel and Shao-Yang Meridian at neck and limbs. The use of combination of these acupoints can expel Wind and disperse Cold, tonify Ying and Wei for balance.

Matching acupoints: For severe exterior pathogenic factors, add Hegu, Fengchi; for exterior deficiency,

列缺；颈部前后不能俯仰者，加昆仑、列缺；颈不能回顾者，加支正、后溪；头痛者，加太阳、百会、风府。

方法 电热针治疗。

操作 选定穴位，皮肤常规消毒。电热针向下斜刺大椎0.7寸，直刺（针尖向脊柱）天柱0.7寸，向脊柱方向斜刺肩外俞0.7寸，直刺悬钟0.7寸，直刺后溪0.6寸，直刺合谷0.6寸，直刺（针尖向脊柱）风池0.7寸，直刺足三里0.8寸，平刺列缺0.7寸，直刺昆仑0.6寸，直刺支正0.7寸，直刺太阳0.6寸，向后平刺百会0.6寸，直刺（针尖向脊柱）风府0.6寸。接通电热针仪，每个穴位分别给予30～50mA的电流量，以患者舒适为度，留针40分钟。（注：根据病情，每次选取3～5个穴位，轮番使用。）

疗程 每天1～2次（上、下午各1次），30次为1个疗程。疗程间可休息3～5天，再进行第2个疗程的治疗。一般治疗2～3个疗程。

【神经根型】

治法 祛风散寒，舒筋活络。

add Zusanli, Lieque; for incapability of neck moving upwards and downwards, add Kunlun, Lieque; for incapability of neck turning back, add Zhizheng, Houxi; for headache, add Taiyang, Baihui, Fengfu.

Method: Electrothermal acupuncture treatment.

Operations: Selecting the relevant acupoints, perform routine skin disinfection. Using electrothermal acupuncture needles, obliquely puncture downward into Dazhui for 0.7", vertically puncture (with the needle tip towards spine) into Tianzhu for 0.7", obliquely puncture toward spine into Jianwaishu for 0.7", vertically puncture into Xuanzhong for 0.7", Houxi for 0.6", Hegu for 0.6", vertically puncture (with the needle tip towards spine) into Fengchi for 0.7", vertically puncture into Zusanli for 0.8", horizontally puncture into Lieque for 0.7", vertically puncture into Kunlun for 0.6", Zhizheng for 0.7", Taiyang for 0.6", horizontally puncture backward into Baihui for 0.6", vertically puncture (with the needle tip towards spine) into Fengfu for 0.6". Turn on the electrothermal acupuncture equipment, apply a current of 30-50mA to each acupoint, and the limit is that the patient feels comfortable, leaving the needles in for 40 minutes. (Note: Based on disease conditions, select 3-5 acupoints each time, use alternatively.)

Therapeutic course: 1-2 times a day (one in the morning, and one in the afternoon), 30 times for a course. Start the treatment for the second course after a break of 3-5 days. Generally treatment lasts for 2-3 courses.

[Nerve root type]

Therapeutic method: Expel Wind and disperse Cold, relax tendons and activate collaterals.

处方 大椎（DU14）、风池（GB20）、哑门（DU15）、天柱（BL10）、肩井（GB21）、外关（SJ5）、相应颈椎病变部位的夹脊穴。

方义 取诸阳之会的大椎穴及相应之夹脊穴，能祛风散寒通络，配足少阳胆经穴肩井、阳维之会天柱，能宣痹通络。外关是手少阳经之络穴，配上述诸穴以求活血通络之效。诸穴共用，有祛风散寒、舒筋活络除痹之功效。

配穴 双手麻木者，加肩髃、曲池、手三里、阳池、八邪；颈活动受限者，加昆仑、列缺；胸闷纳呆者，加中脘。

方法 电热针治疗。

操作 选定穴位，皮肤常规消毒。电热针直刺大椎0.7寸，向脊中斜刺相应夹脊穴各0.6寸，平刺肩井0.7寸，向脊中直刺风池、天柱各0.6寸，直刺肩髃0.7寸，直刺手三里0.7寸，斜刺阳池0.6寸，直刺昆仑0.6寸，斜刺列缺0.7寸，直刺中脘0.7寸。接通

Prescription: Dazhui（DU14）, Fengchi (GB20), Yamen (DU15), Tianzhu (BL10), Jianjing (GB21), Waiguan (SJ5), and acupoint Jiaji of the corresponding cervical vertebral lesion.

Mechanism of prescription: Use the confluent acupoint of all Yangs, Dazhui and its corresponding Jiaji acupoint, can expel Wind and disperse Cold, soothe collaterals, and when being matched with the acupoint Jianjing of Shao-Yang Gallbladder Meridian of Foot and the confluent acupoint of Yangwei Channel, Tianzhu, can relieve stagnation and soothe collaterals. Waiguan is a collateral acupoint of Shao-Yang Meridian of Hand, it can activate blood and soothe collaterals when being matched with the above acupoints. The use of combination of these acupoints can expel wind and disperse cold, relax tendons and activate collaterals.

Matching acupoints: For hand numbness, add Jianliao, Quchi, Shousanli, Yangchi, Baxie; for limited neck movement, add Kunlun, Lieque; for chest distress and anorexia, add Zhongwan.

Method: Electrothermal acupuncture treatment.

Operations: Selecting the relevant acupoints, perform routine skin disinfection. Using electrothermal acupuncture needles, vertically puncture into Dazhui for 0.7", obliquely puncture toward Jizhong into the corresponding Jiaji acupoints for 0.6" respectively, horizontally puncture into Jianjing for 0.7", vertically puncture toward Jizhong into Fengchi, Tianzhu for 0.6" respectively, vertically puncture into Jianliao for 0.7", Shousanli for 0.7", obliquely puncture into Yangchi for 0.6", vertically

电热针仪，每个穴位分别给予 40～50mA 的电流量，以患者舒适为度，留针 40 分钟。（注：上述穴位，每次根据病情选用 3 对，轮流交替使用，余者给予毫针治疗。）

疗程 每天 1～2 次（上、下午各 1 次），30 次为 1 个疗程。疗程间可休息 3～5 天，再进行第 2 个疗程的治疗。一般治疗 2～3 个疗程。

【脊髓型】

治法 活血化瘀，舒筋活络。

处方 大椎（DU14）、颈百劳（EX-HN15）、肩髃（LI15）、养老（SI6）、条口（ST38）、膈俞（BL17）及相应夹脊穴。

方义 痹证日久，督脉受累，致气血瘀阻，故取阳经交会穴大椎及相应夹脊穴（颈病变部位）或百劳穴，以通利诸阳之经脉，调和督脉气血，使颈椎局部气滞血瘀得以消散。复取肩井与经筋结聚之肩髃，使少阳、阳明经气得通。养老乃手太阳经的郄穴，能舒筋通络，是历代治疗颈椎病之经验穴；条口是阳足明经穴，阳明

puncture into Kunlun for 0.6", obliquely puncture into Lieque for 0.7", vertically puncture into Zhongwan for 0.7". Turn on the electrothermal acupuncture equipment, apply a current of 40-50mA to each acupoint, and the limit is that the patient feels comfortable, leaving the needles in for 40 minutes. (Note: For acupoints above, select 3 pairs of acupoints each time, and use alternatively, treat others with filiform needles.)

Therapeutic course: 1-2 times a day (one in the morning, and one in the afternoon), 30 times for a course. Start the treatment for the second course after a break of 3-5 days. Generally treatment lasts for 2-3 courses.

[Spinal cord type]

Therapeutic method: Activate blood circulation and remove stasis, relax tendons and activate collaterals.

Prescription: Dazhui (DU14), Jingbailao (EX-HN15), Jianyu (LI15), Yanglao (Si6), Tiaokou (ST38), Geshu (BL17), the corresponding acupoint Jiaji.

Mechanism of prescription: Long-term arthralgia syndrome affects Du Channel therefore leads to Qi-blood stagnation and stasis, so use the confluent acupoint Dazhui of Yang meridians and the corresponding Jiaji acupoint (lesion site of neck) or Bailao to soothe meridians and collaterals of all Yangs, regulate Qi-blood of Du Channel, so as to disperse the Qi stagnation and blood stasis of local cervical vertebra. And then use Jianjing and the confluent site of meridians and tendons, Jianyu, to dredge meridian Qi of Shao-Yang and Yang-Ming meridians. Yanglao is a Xi acupoint of Tai-Yang Meridian

经多气多血,二者合用能理气活血。膈俞是血会,取之以除血分之瘀滞。诸穴合用,能活血化瘀,疏通脉络之瘀阻。

of Hand, it can relax tendons and activate collaterals, is a historically used experienced acupoint for cervical spondylosis treatment. Tiaokou is a meridian acupoint of Yang-Ming Meridian of Foot, Yang-Ming Meridian is full of Qi and blood, so the combination of these two can regulate Qi, activate blood. Geshu is the confluent acupoint of blood, it can remove the stagnation of blood system. The use of combination of these acupoints can activate blood circulation and remove stasis, sooth retention of stasis in channels and collaterals.

配穴 皮肤枯燥、瘙痒、指甲凹陷无光泽、指尖麻木者,加足三里、三阴交、阳陵泉,以养血荣筋;头晕眼花、视物不清、失眠健忘、惊悸、面色无华者,加心俞、肝俞、足三里,以养血安神明目。

Matching acupoints: For dry skin, itching, for depressed fingernails without luster, fingertip numbness, add Zusanli, Sanyinjiao and Yanglingquan to nourish blood and tendons; for dizziness and blurred sight, insomnia and amnesia, palpitation due to fear, gloomy complexion, add Xinshu, Ganshu, Zusanli to nourish the blood, calm the mind and improve eyesight.

方法 电热针治疗。

Method: Electrothermal acupuncture treatment.

操作 选定穴位,皮肤常规消毒。电热针直刺大椎、颈百劳、肩髃各 0.7 寸,向上斜刺养老 0.7 寸,斜刺(针尖向脊柱)膈俞 0.7 寸。接通电热针仪,每个穴位分别给予电流量 40~50mA,以患者舒适为度,留针 40 分钟。(注:每次选 3 组穴轮流交替使用,除电热针之外还可用毫针治疗。)

Operations: Selecting the relevant acupoints, perform routine skin disinfection. Using electrothermal acupuncture needles, vertically puncture into Dazhui, Jingbailao, Jianyu for 0.7" respectively, obliquely puncture upward into Yanglao for 0.7", obliquely puncture (with the needle tip towards spine) into Geshu for 0.7". Turn on the electrothermal acupuncture equipment, apply a current of 40-50mA to each acupoint, and the limit is that the patient feels comfortable, leaving the needles in for 40 minutes. (Note: Select 3 pairs of acupoints each time, and use alternatively, and filiform needles can also be used in addition to electrothermal needles.)

疗程 每日 1 次,30 次为

Therapeutic course: Treat once a day, 30 times for

1个疗程。疗程间可休息5～7天，如无不适可继续针治。

三、注意事项

1. 避免过强的手法治疗。睡觉时应选用舒适的枕头。

2. 避免长期伏案工作，应经常活动颈部。

3. 做一些有利于颈椎的运动，如游泳。

腰椎间盘突出症

腰椎间盘退行性变化或受伤之后，腰椎间盘纤维环破裂引起椎间盘向椎管内后方突出，压迫神经根导致腰痛及一系列神经症状者，称为腰椎间盘突出症。

中医认为，本病属于"腰腿痛""腰痛连膝"等范畴。

一、诊断及辨证要点

1. 常有外伤或慢性腰痛病史，多发于青壮年。

2. 腰痛严重者站立、睡眠、翻身均困难，影响生活和工作。咳嗽、喷嚏、用力排便时疼痛症状加重，卧床休息后疼痛

a course. There can be 5-7 days for rest between courses. Perform continuous treatment without break if there is no discomfort.

III. Precautions

1. Avoid too strong treating approach. Comfortable pillows should be chosen for sleep.

2. Avoid long-time work bearing over desk, and move the neck frequently.

3. Do some activities good to cervical vertebra, like swimming.

Protrusion of Lumbar Intervertebral Disc

After degenerative changes or injuries, rupture of intervertebral disc annulus fibrosus causes rearward protrusion of intervertebral discs within the spinal canal therefore compress nerve roots, leading to waist pain and a serious of neurologic symptoms, which is called protrusion of lumbar intervertebral disc.

Traditional Chinese Medicine believes that this disease belongs to the ranges of "pain in waist and lower extremities", "waist pain radiated towards knees".

I. Key Points for Diagnosis and Syndrome Differentiation

1. History of frequent trauma or chronic waist pain, normally seen in young and middle-aged adults.

2. For patients with severe waist pain, they have difficulties in standing, sleeping and turning over, affecting daily life and work. The pain symptom aggravates when coughing, sneezing and forcible defecating, and the pain

减轻。

3. 下肢放射性疼痛，多为单侧下肢痛，由臀部开始沿大腿后侧、腘窝向下放射至小腿外侧至足跟部或足背外侧，活动或腹压增加时加重，卧床休息后减轻。

4. 体征：可有脊柱侧弯，多数突向患侧，腰生理前突减小或消失；脊柱运动受限，多为腰部活动不对称受限，以后伸活动受限明显；腰部压痛、叩击痛，多在腰4～5或腰5～骶1之间突出，疼痛放散到患肢，腰后伸时按压痛点则疼痛更加严重；直腿抬高试验、足过度背屈试验、屈颈试验阳性；下肢跟腱反射异常，若腰4神经根受压，跟腱反射减弱；腰5神经根受压，跟腱反射正常或减弱；骶1神经根受压，跟腱反射减弱或消失；皮肤感觉异常，多有小腿前外或后外、足背或足外侧感觉障碍，重者可超过此范围；伸踇指肌力减弱；可见大腿、小腿肌肉萎缩。

relieve after rest on bed.

3. Radioactive pain of lower extremities, most are unilateral pain, radiate from the buttock along the back of thigh as well as the popliteal fossa downwards to the lateral calf until the foot heel or the lateral dorsum of foot, which aggravate with increase of abdominal pressure and relieve after rest on bed.

4. Physical signs: There may be scoliosis, most of which protrude towards the affected side, the psychological protrusion of waist reduces or disappears; limited spine movements, most of which are asymmetric limited movements of waist, and future obvious limited stretching movements; tenderness and percussion pain, mostly occurs at the protrusion between the Lumbar Vertebral 4-5 or between the Lumbar Vertebral 5 - Sacral Vertebra 1, the pain radiates towards affected extremities, and the pain aggravates if press the tenderness point with waist stretching backwards; positive in the straight-leg raising test, the excessive foot dorsiflexion test and the neck flexion test; abnormal Achilles tendon reflex of lower extremities, and the Achilles tendon reflex reduces if the nerve root of the Lumbar Vertebral 4 is compressed; the Achilles tendon reflex is normal or reduced when the nerve root of the Lumbar Vertebral 1 is compressed; the Achilles tendon reflex is reduced or disappears when the nerve root of the Sacral Vertebral 5 is compressed; abnormal skin sense, mostly accompanying with sensory disorders of anterior lateral or posterior lateral calf, dorsum of foot or lateral foot, in severe cases the range may excesses the above, weakened muscle strength for stretching of the big toe; visible thigh and calf amyotro-

5. X线检查：一般无改变，正位片可见脊柱侧弯，侧位片可见生理前突消失，病变椎间隙变窄，相邻椎体边缘有骨赘增生。

6. 临床上根据症状特点，可分为如下3型：

（1）单侧型：髓核突出和神经根受压只限于一侧，绝大多数患者属此型。

（2）双侧型：髓核自后纵韧带两侧突出，两侧神经根受压，双下肢交替出刻下症状，继而发展为双下肢都有症状，但无马尾神经受压症状。

（3）中央型：突出物在中央，直接压迫马尾神经，出现马鞍区麻木和大小便功能障碍。

7. 根据病因及症状可辨证为3个证型：

（1）气滞血瘀型：有明显外伤史，伤后即出现腰部疼痛，活动受限，脊柱侧弯，腰之一侧有明显压痛，并向下肢放射，咳嗽则疼痛加重。后期可见下肢麻木，肌肉萎缩，舌质

5. X-ray examination: No general changes, scoliosis can be seen in the posteroanterior radiograph, and disappearance of the psychological protrusion can be seen in the lateral radiograph, the intervertebral space of affected vertebral bodies is narrowed, with proliferation of osteophytes at edges of adjacent vertebral bodies.

6. Based on characteristics of symptoms, it can be clinically divided into three types as followed:

(1) Unilateral type: Herniation of nucleus pulposus and nerve root compression are limited to one side, and most patients are belonging to this group.

(2) Bilateral type: The nucleus pulposus protrude from the two sides of the longitudinal ligaments, the two-side nerve roots are compressed, symptoms occur at the two lower extremities alternatively and subsequently develops into that there are symptoms at both lower extremities, without symptoms of caudal equina compression.

(3) Central type: The protrusion is at the center and directly compresses the caudal equina, causing saddle area numbness as well as urination and defecation dysfunction.

7. It can be identified as three types as per etiology and symptoms:

(1) Qi stagnation and blood stasis type: History of obvious trauma, waist pain which occurs immediately after injury, limited movement, scoliosis, obvious tenderness at one side of the waist which radiates towards lower extremities and aggravates when coughing. Later numbness of lower extremities, amyotrophia, dark red

黯红，脉沉。

（2）风寒湿阻型：无明显外伤史，腰腿部逐渐出现重着疼痛，转侧不利，渐渐加重，亦有椎旁压痛和放射痛，天气变化则疼痛加重，得热则缓解，舌质淡，苔白腻，脉沉缓。

（3）肾虚型：素体先天不足，肾精亏损，以致腰腿疼痛，酸重无力，缠绵不愈，肾阳虚者伴有恶寒肢冷，面色浮白，气喘；肾阴虚者伴有头晕目眩，耳鸣，面部潮红，口干咽燥，五心烦热。

二、治疗方法

【血瘀证】

治法　舒筋活络，活血止痛。

处方　大肠俞（BL25）、关元俞（BL26）、阳陵泉（GB34）、委中（BL40）、阿是穴。

方义　大肠俞、关元俞均位于腰骶部，是足太阳膀胱经治腰骶疼痛之要穴，与阿是穴相配，有舒筋活络、活血止痛之功。

tongue and deep pulse can be seen.

(2) Wind-Cold-Damp stagnation type: No history of obvious trauma, pain occurs gradually at waist and thigh, rigid turning around, which aggravates gradually, accompanying paravertebral tenderness and radioactive pain which aggravates with weather changes and relieves with heat, light tongue with whitish and greasy fur, deep and slow pulse.

(3) Kidney deficiency type: Congenitally deficient body, depletion of kidney essence, leading to waist and thigh pains, soreness and heaviness as well as weakness, lingering without heal, for patients with kidney Yang deficiency accompanying with intolerance of cold and extreme chilliness, pale complexion, short of breath; for patients with kidney Yin deficiency accompanying with dizziness, tinnitus, flash complexion, dry mouth and throat, dysphoria in chest with palms-soles.

II. Therapeutic Methods

[Syndrome of Blood Stasis]

Therapeutic method: Relax tendons and activate collaterals, activate blood and alleviate pain.

Prescription: Dachangshu(BL25), Guanyuanshu(BL26), Yanglingquan (GB34), Weizhong (BL40), Ashi acupoints.

Mechanism of prescription: Dachangshu, Guanyuanshu are both at lumbosacral portion and are important acupoints for treatment of pains at lumbosacral portion, which are from Tai-Yang Bladder Meridian of Foot, and they can relax tendons and activate collaterals, activate blood and alleviate pain when being matched

配穴 臀部疼痛者，加环跳；大腿后侧疼痛者，加殷门；大腿外侧疼痛者，加风市；小腿后侧疼痛者，加承山；腰痛明显者，加压痛点、气海、上髎、次髎；股前痛明显者，加伏兔、梁丘；气滞血瘀者，加血海、膻中、足三里；风寒湿者，加风门、风市、阴陵泉；肾阳虚者，加关元、命门；肾阴虚者，加太溪、三阴交。

方法 电热针治疗。

操作 选定穴位，皮肤常规消毒。电热针直刺大肠俞、关元俞各0.8寸，直刺阿是穴、委中、阳陵泉各0.7寸，直刺环跳、殷门、风市、承山各0.7寸。接通电热针仪，每个穴位分别给予电流量40～50mA，以患者感到舒适或温热为度，留针40分钟。（注：每次选3组穴给予电热针治疗，根据病情及症状将穴位划分成小组，轮流交替使用。）

疗程 每日1～2次（上、下午各1次），根据病情的轻重不同而定。60次为1个疗程，疗程间可休息7～10天，之后

Matching acupoints: For buttock pain add Huantiao; for pain of back thigh add Yinmen; for pain of lateral thigh add Fengshi; for pain of posterior calf add Chengshan; for obvious waist pain add the point of tenderness, Qihai, Shangliao, Ciliao; for obvious pain in the anterior region of thigh, add Futu, Liangqiu; For Qi stagnation and blood stasis, add Xuehai, Danzhong, Zusanli; For Wind-Cold-Damp add Fengmen, Fengshi, Yinlingquan; for kidney Yang deficiency add Guanyuan, Mingmen; for kidney Yin deficiency, add Taixi, Sanyinjiao.

Method: Electrothermal acupuncture treatment.

Operations: Selecting the relevant acupoints, perform routine skin disinfection. Using electrothermal acupuncture needles, vertically puncture into Dachangshu, Guanyuanshu for 0.8" respectively, vertically puncture into Ashi, Weizhong, Yanglingquan for 0.7" respectively, vertically puncture into Huantiao, Yinmen, Fengshi, Chengshan for 0.7" respectively. Turn on the electrothermal acupuncture equipment, apply a current of 40-50mA to each acupoint, and the limit is that the patient feels comfortable or warm, leaving the needles in for 40 minutes. (Note：Select 3 pairs of acupoints for electrothermal acupuncture treatment each time, group the acupoints as per conditions and symptoms, and use alternatively.)

Therapeutic course: 1-2 times a day (one in the morning, and one in the afternoon), depending on severity of conditions. 60 times for a course, and start the treatment for the second course after a break of 7-10 days.

再进入第 2 个疗程的治疗。一般治疗 1～2 个疗程。

三、注意事项

1. 急性期避免手法治疗。针灸治疗期间可卧床休息，睡硬板床较好。

2. 做腰部的轻微运动，有助于膨出的椎间盘的恢复，必须在医生的指导下进行。

3. 注意下肢及腰部的保暖，不宜受寒。

增生性骨性关节病

增生性骨性关节病又称骨性关节炎，是一种退行性疾病。本病多见于中年之后，老年女性比男性多见。起病慢，临床特征是关节疼痛、肿胀和功能受限，早期呈间断性发作，以后逐渐变成持续性。目前其发病机制尚不十分清楚，一般认为是多种因素引起的软骨破坏所致。

中医认为，本病属于"痹证"的范畴。

一、诊断及辨证要点

1. 慢性病程，原发性的年龄多在 50 岁以上，继发性的年

Generally treatment lasts for 1-2 courses.

III. Precautions

1. Avoid manipulation therapy during the acute period. During the acupuncture treatment, patients can rest on bed, better a hard bed.

2. Do slight waist movements that are helpful to recovery of protruded intervertebral discs, which must be carried out under the guidance of a doctor.

3. Pay attention that keep lower extremities as well as waist warm, which better not exposed to cold.

Proliferative Osteoarthritis

Proliferative osteoarthritis, also called osteoarthritis, is a degenerative disease. It is mostly seen in adults after their middle age, more elder females than males. Slow disease development, its clinical symptoms include pain, swelling and limited functions of joints, which is intermittent attack during the early phase, and later gradually become persistent. The pathogenesis is unknown currently, and generally it is believed that it's caused by cartilage destruction due to multiple causes.

Traditional Chinese Medicine believes that this disease belongs to the range of "arthralgia syndrome".

I. Key Points for Diagnosis and Syndrome Differentiation

1. Chronic disease course, normally the onset age for primary ones is over 50 years old while an age around

龄多为 40 岁左右。

2. 发病部位：多见于脊柱、颈椎、腰椎。下肢多发生在膝、髋、踝和第 1 趾关节；上肢多见于肘、远侧指间关节和第 1 腕掌关节。受累关节常为少数，下肢负重关节症状明显。

3. 主要症状：关节疼痛、肿胀，功能障碍，渐进性加重，并由发作性变为持续性，脊柱可有神经压迫症状。

4. 查体可见关节骨性粗大或肿胀，明显的压痛，可触及骨赘，功能活动受限。可有关节畸形或固定。

5. X 线表现为关节有不对称狭窄，关节面下囊性变，关节面硬化或变形，边缘骨质增生和骨桥、关节腔游离体等。CT、MRI 等可作更精确的诊断。

6. 本病尚需注意与创伤性关节炎、大骨节病相鉴别。前者有严重的外伤史与劳损病史，后者为地方性疾病。

7. 中医辨证

（1）气虚风湿痹阻：关节疼痛，活动不利，受累关节可由 1～2 个发展成更多个，少

40 years old for secondary ones.

2. Disease site: Normally are at spine, cervical vertebra, lumbar vertebra. For lower extremities the lesions normally are at knees, hip, ankles and 1st toe joint; for upper extremities most are at elbows, distal interphalangeal joint and the 1st palm joint. Affected joints normally are less, and symptoms are obvious at the load-bearing joints of lower extremities.

3. Main symptoms: Pain, swelling and function failures of joints, which aggravate gradually and develop from paroxysmal one into persistent one, while there may be compressive symptoms at the spine.

4. In the physical examination, osseous thickening or swelling can be seen with obvious tenderness and touchable osteophyte, limited functional activities. Joint malformation or fixation can be seen.

5. X-ray examination shows asymmetric joint stenosis, cystic lesions under articular surface, hardness or malformation of articular surface, edge osteoproliferation and loose bodies of bone bridge as well as within articular cavity. More exact diagnosis can be done with CT, MRI, etc.

6. For this disease, attention should be paid to the differentiation it from traumatic arthritis and Kashin-Beck disease. The former has a medical history of severe trauma and strain, while the later is a local disease.

7. Syndrome differentiation of Traditional Chinese Medicine

(1) Qi deficiency and Wind-Damp stagnation: Joint pain, rigid movements, affected joints can be developed from 1-2 into several ones, short of breath and laziness to

气懒言，乏力，心悸，失眠，舌淡，苔白，脉缓。

（2）劳损感寒湿邪：关节疼痛剧烈，但持续性发展，常与职业有关，或多见于膝、踝等负重关节，可有气血虚亏症状，舌淡，脉弱。

（3）阳虚血凝：关节呈针刺、刀割样疼痛，痛处微肿，皮色较暗，或形寒肢冷，腰膝酸软，行走时足软欲跌，舌淡胖，可有瘀斑，脉细弱。

二、治疗方法

【颈椎】

治法 祛风散寒，舒筋通络。

处方 大椎（DU14）、风池（GB20）、天柱（BL10）、肩井（GB21）、外关（SJ5）、相应病变颈椎之夹脊穴。

方义 取诸阳之会大椎穴及相应夹脊穴，能祛风散寒通络；配足少阳胆经之肩井、阳维之会风池及天柱，能宣痹通络；外关为手少阳经之络穴，配合上述诸穴以收活血通络之功。诸穴合用，有祛风散寒、舒筋通络除痹之功。

speak, asthenia, palpitation, insomnia, light tongue with whitish fur, slow pulse.

(2) Strain with Cold-Damp toxins: Intensive joint pain with continuous progress, normally associated with occupation, or generally are seen at load-bearing joints like knees and ankles, there may be symptoms of Qi-blood deficiency, light tongue, weak pulse.

(3) Yang deficiency and blood coagulation: Needle prickling or knife cutting like pains at joints, slight swelling of painful parts, relatively darker skin color, or cold body and limbs, soreness and weakness of waist and knees, soft feet tending to falling while walking, light and fat tongue, possible ecchymosis, thin and weak pulse.

II. Therapeutic Methods

[Cervical Vertebra]

Therapeutic method: Expel wind and disperse cold, relax tendons and activate collaterals.

Prescription: Dazhui(DU14), Fengchi (GB20), Tianzhu (BL10), Jianjing (GB21), Waiguan (SJ5), and acupoint Jiaji of the corresponding cervical vertebral lesion.

Mechanism of prescription: Use the confluent acupoint of all Yangs, Dazhui and its corresponding Jiaji acupoint, can expel Wind and disperse Cold, soothe collaterals, and when matched with the acupoint Jianjing of Shao-Yang Gallbladder Meridian of Foot and the confluent acupoints of Yangwei Channel, Fengchi and Tianzhu, can relieve stagnation and soothe collaterals; Waiguan is a collateral acupoint of Shao-Yang Meridian of Hand,

方法　电热针治疗。

操作　选定穴位，皮肤常规消毒。选6个穴位给予电热针治疗，每穴根据部位给予40～60mA的电流量，留针40分钟。配穴可用毫针治疗，留针40分钟。

疗程　每日1次，20次为1个疗程。疗程间可休息3～5天，再进行第2个疗程的治疗。一般治疗3～4个疗程即可控制病情。

【腰椎】

治法　温补肾阳，理气止痛。

处方　命门（DU4）、腰阳关（DU3）、肾俞（BL23）、大肠俞（BL25）、十七椎（EX-BE8）。

方义　命门、腰阳关是督脉穴，可温经助阳、祛风除湿、舒筋活络，是治疗腰痛之要穴；十七椎是经外奇穴，肾俞、大肠俞是足太阳膀胱经穴，三穴合用，既能温补肾阳以助命门、腰阳关，又能理气

which can activate blood and soothe collaterals when matched with the above acupoints. The use of combination of these acupoints can expel Wind and disperse Cold, relax tendons and activate collaterals.

Method: Electrothermal acupuncture treatment.

Operations: Selecting the relevant acupoints, perform routine skin disinfection. Select 6 acupoints for electrothermal acupuncture treatment, apply a current of 40-60mA to each acupoint as per its location, leaving the needles in for 40 minutes. The matching acupoints can be treated with filiform needles, leaving the needles in for 40 minutes.

Therapeutic course: Treat once a day, 20 times for a course. Start the treatment for the second course after a break of 3-5 days. Generally the condition can be controlled after 3-4 courses of treatment.

[Lumbar Vertebra]

Therapeutic method: Warm and tonify kidney Yang, regulate Qi and alleviate pains.

Prescription: Mingmen(DU4), Yaoyangguan(DU3), Shenshu(BL23), Dachangshu(BL25), Shiqizhui(EX-BE8).

Mechanism of prescription: Yaoyangguan, an acupoint of Du Channel, is an important acupoint for treatment of waist pains, which can warm meridians and facilitate Yang, remove Wind and Damp, relax tendons and activate collaterals; Shiqizhui is an external nerve acupoint, Shenshu and Dachangshu are meridian acupoints of Tai-Yang Bladder Meridian of Foot, the combi-

止痛。诸穴合用，可使肾阳得助，寒湿得除，筋脉得舒，气机得调，从而达到痛缓痛消之目的。

nation of these three can warm and tonify kidney Yang to facilitate Mingmen and Yaoyangguan, as well as regulate Qi and alleviate pains. The use of combination of these acupoints can benefit kidney Yang, remove Cold-Damp, relax tendons and channels, regulate Qi Dynamic, therefore relieve and alleviate pains.

配穴 关节酸胀疼痛者，加大椎、外关、气海、关元；关节畸形疼痛者，加大杼、血海、丰隆、阳陵泉；膝关节病变者，加膝眼、梁丘、血海、鹤顶、阴陵泉、阳陵泉；踝关节病变者，加解溪、丘墟、太溪、昆仑、交信；肩关节病变者，加肩髎、肩髃、肩贞、中渚；腕关节病变者，加外关、阳溪、阳池、腕骨；肘关节病变者，加曲池、天井、小海、手三里、合谷。

Matching acupoints: For soreness and swelling as well as pains of joints, add Dazhui, Waiguan, Qihai, Guanyuan; for malformation and pain of joints, add Dazhu, Xuehai, Fenglong, Yanglingquan; For lesions of knee joints, add Xiyan, Liangqiu, Xuehai, Heding, Yinlingquan, Yanglingquan; For lesions of ankle joints, add Jiexi, Qiuxu, Taixi, Kunlun, Jiaoxin; For lesions of shoulder joints, add Jianliao, Jianyu, Jianzhen, Zhongzhu; for lesions of wrist joints, add Waiguan, Yangxi, Yangchi, Wangu; for lesions of elbow joints, add Quchi, Tianjing, Xiaohai, Shousanli, Hegu.

方法 电热针治疗。

操作 选定穴位，皮肤常规消毒。选3组穴给予电热针治疗，每穴根据部位给予40～60mA的电流量，留针40分钟。配穴可用毫针治疗，留针40分钟。

Method: Electrothermal acupuncture treatment.

Operations: Selecting the relevant acupoints, perform routine skin disinfection. Select 3 pairs of acupoints for electrothermal acupuncture treatment, apply a current of 40-60mA to each acupoint as per its location, leaving the needles in for 40 minutes. The matching acupoints can be treated with filiform needles, leaving the needles in for 40 minutes.

疗程 每日1次，20次为1个疗程。疗程间可休息3～5天，再进行第2个疗程的治疗。一般治疗3～4个疗程即

Therapeutic course: Treat once a day, 20 times for a course. Start the treatment for the second course after a break of 3-5 days. Generally the condition can be controlled after 3-4 courses of treatment.

可控制病情。

三、注意事项

1. 在针刺治疗中，要根据患者的病变部位，将穴位按主次分组，交替轮流运用，每次要有6针是电热针。

2. 针刺方向要根据穴位的部位来决定。如颈椎、胸椎、腰椎部的穴位，针刺方向要向脊中（督脉），避免直刺而造成气胸。

3. 不管是平刺、斜刺还是直刺，都要把能发热的针体刺入穴中，一般达0.7～0.8寸深，避免烧伤皮肤。

4. 患者要注意节制饮食，适当运动，避免体重超标，造成关节过度负荷，应进行有关的肌肉锻炼以增强关节的稳定性，对关节疾病应早期治疗，提早预防关节变形。

III. Precautions

1. During needle acupuncture treatment, the acupoints should be grouped into primary and secondary ones depending on the lesion site of the patients for alternative use, while there should be 6 times of puncture that are done with electrothermal needles.

2. The direction of puncture depends on acupoint sites. For example, for acupoints at cervical vertebra, thoracic vertebra and lumbar vertebra, the direction needs to be toward Jizhong (Du Channel), to avoid pneumothorax caused by vertical puncture.

3. Whether for vertical puncture, oblique puncture or horizontal puncture, the heating needle must be punctured into the acupoints, normally a depth of 0.7-0.8", so as to avoid skin burns.

4. Patients should pay attention to diet control, and do appropriate exercises, avoid excessive weight leading to overload of joints, and they should do some relative muscle exercises so as to enhance joint stability, and for joint diseases early treatment should be done to avoid joint malformation.

五官科疾病

眼睑跳动症

眼睑跳动症，是因眼轮肌抽搐痉挛而引起的胞睑皮肤不自主地抽搐瞤动的眼病。根据发病的程度不同，分为间歇性和持续性两种。间歇性眼睑跳动是因为精神疲劳或神经紧张，如屈光不正、贫血或月经不调等因素导致某一肌束发生跳动性痉挛，一般多可自愈；若疲劳或精神紧张不能缓解而继续加重，则可转为持续性眼睑痉挛，亦可见于老年人的自发性眼睑痉挛，原因多不明确。另外，部分角膜炎患者或面神经痉挛的患者亦可兼见此症。

中医认为，本病属于"胞轮振跳""目瞤""眼眉跳"等范畴。多因劳瞻过度，损伤心脾；或素体阴虚，日久生风；或风热外束，邪留胞睑，至筋脉失养而发。本病多发于上胞，有内风、外风之别。血虚生风者属虚，外邪而至者为外风，属实。

ENT diseases

Eyelid Subsultus

Eyelid subsultus is an eye disease caused by involuntarily twitching of eyelid skin due to orbicularis oculi muscle spasm and twitching. It can be divided as intermittent and persistent types depending on attack degree. Intermittent eyelid subsultus is caused by mental fatigue or psychentonia, factors like ametropia, anemia or menoxenia lead to beating spasm of a muscle bundle, which can be self-healed generally; if the fatigue or psychentonia cannot be relieved and aggravates gradually, it can then develop into persistent eyelid spasm, which can also be seen in spontaneous eyelid spasm of elders, with causes normally unknown. Additionally, some patients with keratitis or facial nerve spasm can also have this disease.

Traditional Chinese Medicine believes that this disease belongs to the range of "twitching of eyelid","eyelid spasm","eyebrow twitching", etc. Most are caused by overuse of eyes impairing heart and spleen; or by Yin deficiency of body, causing generation of Wind after a long period; or by exterior restriction of Wind-Heat, retention of pathogenic toxins at eyelids, leading to nourishment loss of tendons and channels. This disease normally is seen at upper eyelids, and is divided into endogenous

Wind and exogenous Wind. Wind generation by blood deficiency belongs to deficiency syndromes, Wind led by exogenous pathogenic toxins is called exogenous Wind, which belongs to excess syndromes.

I. Key Points for Diagnosis and Syndrome Differentiation

1. Deficiency syndrome: Attack after overuse of eyes, with relatively violent twitching, accompanying symptoms of blood deficiency like palpitation, insomnia, and it is Wind generation from blood deficiency.

2. Excess syndrome: With obvious external causes, for example, attack from Wind toxins causes sudden onset of eyelid twitching, accompanying headache, eyelid redness and swelling or itching, and it is caused by exogenous Wind.

II. Therapeutic Methods

[Deficiency Syndrome]

Therapeutic method: Tonify Qi of heart and spleen, nourish blood circulation and dredge collaterals, dredge Wind and remove pathogenic toxins.

Prescription: Cuanzhu (BL2), Yuyao (EX-HN4), Taiyang (EX-HN5, Jiaosun (SJ20), Chengqi (ST1), Yintang (EX-HN3), Neiting (ST44).

Mechanism of prescription: Cuanzhu is a meridian acupoint of Tai-Yang Meridian of Foot, dredge collaterals and improve eyesight; Taiyang, Yuyao, Yintang are external nerve acupoints as well as highly-effective acupoints for dredging collaterals, dispersing Wind and

为足阳明经穴，可调补气血，强壮后天。诸穴共用，可补益心脾，养血通络，疏风散邪。

配穴 劳倦太过者加心俞、脾俞；肝肾阴虚者加肝俞、肾俞、行间、照海。

方法 电热针治疗。

操作 选定穴位，皮肤常规消毒。电热针斜刺攒竹、鱼腰、太阳、角孙各 0.6 寸，斜刺印堂 0.7 寸，斜刺内庭 0.7 寸，斜刺承泣 0.7 寸，向脊柱方向斜刺心俞、脾俞、肝俞、肾俞各 0.7 寸。接通电热针仪，每个穴位分别给予 40～60mA 的电流量，留针 40 分钟。（注：每次在眼区选 3 个穴位，轮番使用。）

疗程 隔日 1 次，10 天为 1 个疗程。一般治疗 2～3 个疗程即可痊愈。疗程间可不休息。

【实证】

治法 清热散风，通调气血。

处方 合谷（LI4）、太阳（EX-HN5）、睛明（BL1）、瞳子髎（GB1）、四白（ST2）、

soothe stasis; Jiaosun is a confluent acupoint of Shao-Yang Meridian of Hand and of Foot; Neiting is a meridian acupoint of Yang-Ming Meridian of Foot, which can tonify Qi-blood and strengthen acquired construction. The use of combination of these acupoints can tonify Qi of heart and spleen, nourish blood circulation and dredge collaterals, dredge Wind and remove pathogenic toxins.

Matching acupoints: For excessive fatigue add Xinshu, Pishu; for Yin deficiency of liver and kidney, add Ganshu, Shenshu, Xingjian, Zhaohai.

Method: Electrothermal acupuncture treatment.

Operations: Selecting the relevant acupoints, perform routine skin disinfection. Using electrothermal acupuncture needles, obliquely puncture into Cuanzhu, Yuyao, Taiyang, Jiaosun for 0.6" respectively, obliquely puncture into Yintang for 0.7", obliquely puncture into Neiting 0.7", Chengqi for 0.7", obliquely puncture toward spine into Xinshu, Pishu, Ganshu, Shenshu for 0.7" respectively. Turn on the electrothermal acupuncture equipment, apply a current of 40-60mA to each acupoint, leaving the needles in for 40 minutes. (Note: Select 3 acupoints each time, use alternatively at eye parts.）

Therapeutic course: Once every two days, 10 days for a course. Generally cured after 2-3 courses. No breaks between courses.

[Excess Syndrome]

Therapeutic method: Clear Heat and disperse Wind, dredge and tonify Qi-blood.

Prescription: Hegu（LI4）, Taiyang (EX-HN5), Jingming (BL1), Tongziliao (GB1), Sibai (ST2), Jiache (ST6).

颊车（ST6）。

方义 合谷为手阳明经的原穴，可通调气血；太阳是经外奇穴，睛明是膀胱经之穴，配瞳子髎以散胞睑之风邪；四白、颊车为胃经穴，有升清降浊、清热疏风之功效。诸穴合用，可奏清热散风、通调气血之功能。

配穴 上眼睑跳动者，加攒竹、阳白；下眼睑跳动者，加承泣、曲池；心烦易怒者，加内关、神门。

方法 电热针治疗。

操作 选定穴位，皮肤常规消毒。电热针直刺合谷0.7寸，斜刺太阳0.7寸，直刺睛明、四白各0.6寸，斜刺颊车、瞳子髎各0.7寸。接通电热针仪，每个穴位分别给予电流量20～30mA，留针30分钟。（注：每次选3～4个穴，轮番使用。）

疗程 隔日1次，20次为1个疗程。一般治疗1～2个疗程。疗程间可不休息。

Mechanism of prescription: Hegu is a Yuan acupoint of Yang-Ming Meridian of Hand, it can dredge and tonify Qi-blood; Taiyang is an external nerve acupoint, Jingming is an acupoint of Bladder Meridian, they can disperse the Wind pathogenic toxin of eyelid when being matched with Tongziliao; Sibai and Jiache are acupoints of Stomach Meridian, they can ascend lucidity and descend turbidity, clear Heat and disperse Wind. The use of combination of these acupoints can clear Heat and disperse Wind, dredge and tonify Qi-blood.

Matching acupoints: For twitching of upper eyelids add Cuanzhu, Yangbai; for twitching of lower eyelids add Chengqi, Quchi; for vexation and irritability add Neiguan, Shenmen.

Method: Electrothermal acupuncture treatment.

Operations: Selecting the relevant acupoints, perform routine skin disinfection. Using electrothermal acupuncture needles, vertically puncture into Hegu for 0.7", obliquely puncture into Taiyang for 0.7", vertically puncture into Jingming, Sibai for 0.6" respectively, obliquely puncture into Jiache, Tongziliao for 0.7" respectively. Turn on the electrothermal acupuncture equipment, apply a current of 20-30mA to each acupoint, leaving the needles in for 30 minutes. (Note: Select 3-4 acupoints each time, use alternatively.)

Therapeutic course: Once every two days, 20 times for a course. Generally treatment lasts for 1-2 courses. No breaks between courses.

III. Precautions

1. For oblique puncture of acupoints at eye area, attention should be paid to needling direction and depth, mild manipulation is required, and it is necessary to press and hold the needle hole for 2-3 minutes when removing the needle so as to avoid subcutaneous ecchymosis.

2. When puncturing, avoid needle twisting as well as thrusting and attenuating, pay attention to Qi gain, and the actions should be gentle.

3. During spring and winter, instructions should be given to patients so as to avoid attacks from exogenous Wind toxins leading to disease aggravation.

4. Reduce stress, pay attention to keep peaceful mind and mood while avoiding being nervous, sleep regularly, so as to facilitate the stability of conditions.

Iridocyclitis

Uveitis which occurs at anterior ocular segment is called iridocyclitis. The main symptoms of this disease include eye pain, photophobia, lacrimation, hypopsia, may accompanying ciliary body congestion, Yang-based aqueous humor shining, deposits at posterior wall of cornea and miosis, etc. Posterior iris adhesions after a long disease course without treatment, or even pupil closure leading to blindness in severe cases. The main causes of this disease are infections of bacteria, virus, rickettsia or protozoa, or it also can cause by allergic reactions due to exogenous factors as well as immune reactions due to autoantigens.

Traditional Chinese Medicine believes that this dis-

孔紧小"的范畴，后期陈旧性虹膜睫状体炎属"瞳神干缺"之症。常因肝胆实火，或脾胃湿热，或肝肾阴虚，虚火上炎，邪热上犯于目，重灼黄仁而致病。

一、诊断及辨证要点

1. 肝胆火炽者，眼痛拒按，热泪频流，羞明难睁，胞轮红赤，黄仁污秽，瞳仁紧小，口苦咽干，脉弦数。

2. 脾胃湿热者，瞳神紧小，热泪胶黏，胞睑肿胀，黄仁晦浊，舌红苔腻，脉濡数。

3. 肝肾阴虚者，虚火上炎，瞳神紧小，胞轮淡红，时轻时重，久治难消，腰膝酸软，口干咽燥，舌红少苔，脉弦数。

二、治疗方法

【肝胆火炽证】

治法　清肝泻火，散热明目。

处方　大敦（LR1）、太冲

ease belongs to the range of "pupil tightening", and the later old iridocyclitis belongs to "chronic iridocyclitis". The disease often is caused by excess Fire of liver and spleen, or Damp-Heat of spleen and stomach, or Yin deficiency of liver and spleen, flaring up of deficiency-Fire, leading to severe burn of pupils.

I. Key Points for Diagnosis and Syndrome Differentiation

1. For patients with exuberant Fire of liver and gallbladder, pain eyes with refusal to pressing, frequent hot tears, photophobia and hard to open eyes, red eyelids, dirty yellow area of eye, tightening and small pupil, bitter taste and dry throat, taut and rapid pulse.

2. For patients with Damp-Heat of spleen and stomach, tightening and small pupil, sticky hot tears, swelling eyelids, dark and cloudy yellow area of eye, red tongue with greasy fur, soft and rapid pulse.

3. For patients with Yin deficiency of liver and spleen, flaring up of deficiency-Fire, tightening and small pupil, light red eyelids, severity varying, unable to be relieved after long-term treatment, soreness and weakness of waist and knees, dry mouth and throat, red tongue with less fur, taut and rapid pulse.

II. Therapeutic Methods

[Syndrome of Exuberant Fire of Liver and Gallbladder]

Therapeutic method: Clear liver and disperse Fire, remove Heat and improve eyesight.

Prescription: Dadun (LR1), Taichong (LR3), Tong-

(LR3)、瞳子髎（GB1）、风池（GB20）、睛明（BL1）。

方义 大敦为足厥阴肝经的井穴，太冲为足厥阴肝经的原穴，两穴均有清肝明目之功；瞳子髎、风池均属足少阳胆经穴，具有清热消肿、散郁明目之功效；睛明属足太阳膀胱经穴，可泻火解热。诸穴配合，可收清肝泻火、散热明目之功。

配穴 头痛者加合谷；目痛较重者加内庭、承泣。

方法 电热针治疗。

操作 选定穴位，常规皮肤消毒。电热针直刺太冲、睛明各 0.6 寸，向丝竹空方向斜刺瞳子髎 0.6 寸，直刺内庭、承泣各 0.6 寸，直刺合谷 0.6 寸。接通电热针仪，每个穴位分别给予 20～30mA 的电流量，以患者舒适为度，留针 40 分钟。另配以三棱针点刺大敦出血。

疗程 隔日 1 次，20 次为 1 个疗程。疗程间可休息 5～7 天，根据病情决定是否进行第 2 个疗程的治疗。一般治疗 2～3

ziliao (GB1), Fengchi (GB20), Jingming (BL1).

Mechanism of prescription: Dadun is a Jing acupoint of Jue-Yin Liver Meridian of Foot, Taichong is a yuan acupoint of Jue-Yin Liver Meridian of Foot, these two acupoints both can clear liver and improve eyesight; Tongziliao and Fengchi are both belong to Shao-Yang Gall Meridian of Foot, and both can clear Heat and disperse swelling, remove stagnation and improve eyesight; Jingming belongs to Tai-Yang Bladder Meridian of Foot, which can disperse Fire and clear Heat. The use of the combination of these acupoints can clear liver and disperse Fire, remove Heat and improve eyesight.

Matching acupoints: For headache add Hegu; for severe eye pain add Neiting, Chengqi.

Method: Electrothermal acupuncture treatment.

Operations: Selecting the relevant acupoints, perform routine skin disinfection. Using electrothermal acupuncture needles, vertically puncture into Taichong, Jingming for 0.6" respectively, obliquely puncture toward Sizhukong into Tongziliao for 0.6", vertically puncture into Neiting, Chengqi for 0.6", and Hegu for 0.6" respectively. Turn on the electrothermal acupuncture equipment, apply a current of 20-30mA to each acupoint, and the limit is that the patient feels comfortable, leaving the needles in for 40 minutes. Additionally, use triangular needle to quickly puncture into Dadun till bleeding.

Therapeutic course: Once every two days, 20 times for a course. Rest for 5-7 days between courses, decide if perform the second course depending on the disease conditions. Generally the condition can be basi-

个疗程即可基本控制病情。

【脾胃湿热证】

治法 健脾泻胃，清热利湿，明目止痛。

处方 承泣（ST1）、丰隆（ST40）、内庭（ST44）、合谷（LI4）、丝竹空（SJ23）。

方义 内庭是足阳明胃经穴，有清脾胃湿热，通阳明腑气之功效；丰隆、承泣共属胃经，共用有清热祛湿明目之效；合谷可清头目，又能止痛；丝竹空可调畅气机，疏利水道，使湿邪下趋膀胱，从小便而解。诸穴共用，可健脾泻胃，解热利湿，明目止痛。

配穴 睛痛不止者，加瞳子髎、太阳；目睛混赤者，加内迎香、足三里、三阴交。

方法 电热针治疗。

操作 选定穴位，皮肤常规消毒。电热针直刺承泣、内庭各 0.5～0.6 寸，直刺丰隆 0.7 寸，直刺合谷、太阳各 0.6～0.7 寸，向目背方向斜刺丝竹空 0.7 寸，向鱼腰方

cally controlled after 2-3 courses of treatment.

[Syndrome of Spleen and Stomach Damp-Heat]

Therapeutic method: Invigorate spleen and attenuate stomach, clear Heat and remove Damp, improve eyesight and alleviate pain.

Prescription: Chengqi (ST1), Fenglong (ST40), Neiting (ST44), Hegu (LI4), Sizhukong (SJ23).

Mechanism of prescription: Neiting is a meridian acupoint of Yang-Ming Stomach Meridian of Foot, it can clear Damp-Heat of spleen and stomach, activate organ Qi of Yang-Ming Meridian; Fenglong and Chengqi are both belong to Stomach Meridian, their combination can clear Heat, remove Damp and improve eyesight; Hegu can clear brain and eyes, as well as alleviate pains; Sizhukong can regulate and soothe Qi Dynamic, dredge Shuidao, make the Damp toxins flow downwards bladder, and expel them out of body through urine. The use of combination of these acupoints can invigorate spleen and attenuate stomach, clear Heat and remove Damp, improve eyesight and alleviate pain.

Matching acupoints: For endless eye pain add Tongziliao, Taiyang; for turbidity and redness of eyes, add Neiyingxiang, Zusanli, Sanyinjiao.

Method: Electrothermal acupuncture treatment.

Operations: Selecting the relevant acupoints, perform routine skin disinfection. Using electrothermal acupuncture needles, vertically puncture into Chengqi, Neiting for 0.5-0.6" respectively, vertically puncture into Fenglong for 0.7", vertically puncture into Hegu, Taiyang for 0.6-0.7" respectively, obliquely puncture to-

向斜刺瞳子髎 0.7 寸。接通电热针仪，每个穴位分别给予 15～20mA 的电流量，以患者舒适为度，留针 40 分钟。另配以三棱针点刺内迎香出血。

疗程 隔日 1 次，20 次为 1 个疗程。疗程间可休息 7～10 天，一般治疗 1～2 个疗程即能控制病情。

【肝肾阴虚证】

治法 滋阴清热，退赤明目。

处方 太溪（KI3）、太冲（LR3）、睛明（BL1）、攒竹（BL2）、瞳子髎（GB1）。

方义 太溪为肾之原穴，太冲是肝之原穴，温补两穴可滋补肝肾以扶正；睛明可清目窍浮游之火；攒竹、瞳子髎功在清肝泻火，退赤明目。诸穴共用，补泻兼用，扶正祛邪，可收滋阴清热、退赤明目之功效。

配穴 目赤色淡、瞳神干缺、病程较长者，加三阴交；

ward Mubei into Sizhukong for 0.7", obliquely puncture toward Yuyao into Tongziliao for 0.7". Turn on the electrothermal acupuncture equipment, apply a current of 15-20mA to each acupoint, and the limit is that the patient feels comfortable, leaving the needles in for 40 minutes. Additionally, use triangular needle to quickly puncture into Yingxiang till bleeding.

Therapeutic course: Once every two days, 20 times for a course. Start the treatment for the second course after a break of 7-10 days. Generally the condition can be controlled after 1-2 courses of treatment.

[Syndrome of Yin Deficiency of Liver and Kidney]

Therapeutic method: Nourish Yin and clear Heat, relieve Redness and improve eyesight.

Prescription: Taixi (KI3), Taichong (LR3), Jingming (BL1), Cuanzhu (BL2), Tongziliao (GB1).

Mechanism of prescription: Taixi is a Yuan acupoint of Kidney, Taichong is a Yuan acupoint of Liver, warm replenishment of these two acupoints can nourish liver and kidney to strengthen vital Qi; Gingming can clear floating Fire of eyes, Cuanzhu, Tongziliao can clear liver and disperse Fire, relive Redness and improve eyesight. Use all acupoints together, utilize both tonifying and attenuating methods to strengthen vital Qi and eliminate pathogenic factors, so as to achieve the efficacies of nourish Yin and clear Heat, relieve Redness and improve eyesight.

Matching acupoints: For red eyes with light color, chronic iridocyclitis, long disease course, add Sanyinjiao;

目赤较重、发病急骤者，加合谷、内庭。

方法 电热针治疗。

操作 选定穴位，皮肤常规消毒。电热针直刺太溪、太冲、三阴交各 0.6 寸，接通电热针仪，每个穴位分别给予 40～50mA 的电流量，以患者舒适为度，留针 40 分钟。其中，睛明、攒竹、瞳子髎、合谷、内庭用泻法。

疗程 隔日 1 次，20 次为 1 个疗程。疗程间可休息 7～10 天，一般治疗 1～2 个疗程即能控制病情。

三、注意事项

1. 有血友病及出血倾向者，不宜施行点刺放血术。

2. 治疗期间以清淡饮食为宜，少吃腥荤油炸食品；勿劳瞻视，慎房事，休息利于恢复。

3. 本病属眼科急症，散瞳是第一要务，故在针治的同时要及早使用 1% 的阿托品滴眼扩瞳。

for severe red eyes, sudden and urgent disease attack, add Hegu, Neiting.

Method: Electrothermal acupuncture treatment.

Operations: Selecting the relevant acupoints, perform routine skin disinfection. Using electrothermal acupuncture needles, vertically puncture into Taixi, Taichong, Sanyinjiao for 0.6" respectively. Turn on the electrothermal acupuncture equipment, apply a current of 40-50mA to each acupoint, and the limit is that the patient feels locally comfortable, leaving the needles in for 40 minutes. Use attenuating method for Jingming, Cuanzhu, Tongziliao, Hegu, Neiting.

Therapeutic course: Once every two days, 20 times for a course. Start the treatment for the second course after a break of 7-10 days. Generally the condition can be controlled after 1-2 courses of treatment.

III. Precautions

1. For patients with hemophilia and bleeding trend, it is not proper to perform swift pricking blood therapy.

2. During treatment, patients better have bland diet, eat less meat and fish as well as fried food; do not overuse eyes, control sexual intercourses, have enough rest, so as to facilitate recovery.

3. This disease belongs to the range of ophthalmologic emergency, and pupil dilation is the top priority, so it is necessary to dilate the pupil with 1% atropine eye drops as soon as possible while performing needle acupuncture treatment.

Retinal Pigment Degeneration

Retinal pigment degeneration is a hereditary degenerative disease of retina pigment epithelium. Its onset normally begins since childhood, the earliest symptom is nyctalopia, and the vision becomes incomplete along with disease progressing, and the patient generally become blind gradually after middle age. At the early phase, the eye ground may totally normal, and then changes occur gradually, such as bone cell-like pigmentation at peripheral area around the retina, wax-yellow atrophy of optic nerve heads, stenosis of vessels into a line-like shape. Very few patients may have all symptoms of this disease, however with no pigmentary changes of the eye ground.

Traditional Chinese Medicine believes that this disease belongs to the range of "sparrow's eye due to high Wind". Most are caused by kidney Yang deficiency, deficiency and overuse of kidney, weak Yang unable to compete with Yin; or caused by that spleen deficiency and Qi weakness, Qing-Yang unable to be ascended and transported to eyes, Eye Collateral stagnation and loss of nourishment.

I. Key Points for Diagnosis and Syndrome Differentiation

1. For patients with kidney Yang deficiency, unable to see things after sunset, developed in the childhood, cold body and limbs, urorrhagia at night, light tongue, thin pulse and weakness.

2. For patients with spleen deficiency and Qi weak-

能睹物,视野变窄,不能久视,兼身疲劳倦,体乏无力,舌淡,脉细。

3. 目络瘀滞者,夜不睹物,视野变窄,如以管窥物,白天行动亦很艰难,眼底血管变细呈线状。

二、治疗方法

【元阳不足证】

治法 益气升阳,温通目络。

处方 百会(DU20)、太溪(KI3)、球后(EX-HN7)。

方义 百会是督脉穴,督脉为诸阳之海,维系一身之阳气,故针刺百会可益气升阳。太溪为足少阴肾经的原穴,热针补太溪可补肾气,壮肾阳,故以二穴为主补益元阳。球后通目络,可开窍明目。三穴相伍,可收益气升阳、温通目络之功。

配穴 夜尿频而多者,加中极;畏寒肢冷者,加肾俞、足三里、三阴交。

方法 电热针治疗。

ness, unable to see things at dark places, narrowing of vision, unable to looking for a long time, as well as body fatigue, asthenia and weakness, light tongue, thin pulse.

3. For patients with Eye Collateral stagnation and stasis, unable to see things at night, narrowing of vision leading to narrow field like seeing things from a tube, difficulties in actions even in the daytime, thinning of vessels at eye ground into a line-like shape.

II. Therapeutic Methods

[Syndrome of Kidney Yang Deficiency]

Therapeutic method: Tonify Qi and ascend Yang, warm and dredge Eye Collateral.

Prescription: Baihui (DU20), Taixi (KI3), Qiuhou (EX-HN7).

Mechanism of prescription: Baihui is an acupoint of Du Channel, Du Channel is the sea of Yangs that governs all Yang-Qi of the whole body, so needle puncture of Baihui can tonify Qi and ascend Yang. Taixi is a Yuan acupoint of Shao-Yang Kidney Meridian of Foot, replenishment of Taixi with heat needle can nourish kidney Qi, reinforce kidney Yang, so mainly use these two acupoints to tonify kidney Yang. Qiuhou is connected with Eye Collateral, it can induce resuscitation and improve eyesight. The use of the combination of these three acupoints can tonify Qi and ascend Yang, warm and dredge Eye Collateral.

Matching acupoints: For frequent and excessive micturition at night add Zhongji; for intolerance of cold and extreme chilliness add Shenshu, Zusanli, Sanyinjiao.

Method: Electrothermal acupuncture treatment.

Operations: Selecting the relevant acupoints, perform routine skin disinfection. Using electrothermal acupuncture needles, horizontally puncture along the skin into Baihui for 0.6″, horizontally puncture into Taixi, Qiuhou for 0.7″ respectively, vertically puncture into Zhongji for 0.7″. Turn on the electrothermal acupuncture equipment, apply a current of 40-50mA to each acupoint, and the limit is that the patient feels warmly swell and comfortable, leaving the needles in for 40 minutes. Quickly puncture into Shenshu, do not leave the needle in.

Therapeutic course: Once every two days, 30 times for a course. Start the treatment for the second course after a break of 7-10 days. Generally cured basically after 1-2 courses.

[Syndrome of Spleen Deficiency and Qi Weakness]

Therapeutic method: Invigorate spleen and tonify Qi, soothe meridians and induce resuscitation.

Prescription: Taibai (SP3), Chengqi (ST1), Zusanli (ST36), Jingming (BL1), Qiuhou (EX-HN7).

Mechanism of prescription: Replenish the Yuan acupoint Taibai of Spleen Meridian and the He acupoint Zusanli of Stomach Meridian with warm needles, with a focus on invigorating spleen and tonifying Qi, and can soothe meridians and collaterals, regulate Qi-blood, transport Qing-Yang directly to eyes when being matched with the meridian acupoint Chengqi, the meridian acupoint Jingming of Bladder Meridian, and the extra acupoint Qiuhou of the Eyes. The use of combination of these five acupoints can invigorate spleen and tonify Qi,

配穴　胞睑开合无力者，加脾俞、胃俞；不能久视者，加血海、三阴交。

方法　电热针治疗。

操作　选定穴位，皮肤常规消毒。电热针直刺太白、足三里、三阴交、血海各0.6～0.7寸，斜刺承泣0.6寸，向视神经方向斜刺球后0.7寸，向椎体方向斜刺脾俞、胃俞各0.7寸。接通电热针仪，每个穴位分别给予电流量40～60mA，以患者舒适为度，留针40分钟。（注：每次选5组穴，交替应用。）

疗程　隔日1次，30次为1个疗程。疗程间可休息7～10天。一般治疗1～2个疗程即可基本恢复健康。

【目络郁滞证】

治法　舒筋通络，调和气血。

处方　睛明（BL1）、合谷（LI4）、球后（EX-HN7）。

方义　睛明是膀胱经穴，取效于开郁导滞，通利眼络；取眼部奇穴球后，功在通畅目络，调气和血；取合谷清利头

soothe meridians and induce resuscitation.

Matching acupoints: For weakness of eyelid opening and closing add Pishu, Shenshu; for incapability of long-time looking add Xuehai, Sanyinjiao.

Method: Electrothermal acupuncture treatment.

Operations: Selecting the relevant acupoints, perform routine skin disinfection. Using electrothermal acupuncture needles, vertically puncture into Taibai, Zusanli, Sanyinjiao, Xuehai for 0.6-0.7" respectively, obliquely puncture into Chengqi for 0.6", obliquely puncture toward optic nerve into Qiuhou for 0.7", obliquely puncture toward view frustum into Pishu, Weishu for 0.7" respectively. Turn on the electrothermal acupuncture equipment, apply a current of 40-60mA to each acupoint, and the limit is that the patient feels comfortable, leaving the needles in for 40 minutes. (Note: Select 5 pairs of acupoints each time, and use alternatively.)

Therapeutic course: Once every two days, 30 times for a course. Start the treatment for the second course after a break of 7-10 days. Generally cured basically after 1-2 courses.

[Syndrome of Eye Collateral Stagnation and Stasis]

Therapeutic method: Relax tendons and activate collaterals, regulate Qi-blood.

Prescription: Jingming (BL1), Hegu (LI4), Qiuhou (EX-HN7).

Mechanism of prescription: Jingming is a meridian acupoint of Bladder Meridian, which can remove stagnation and disperse stasis, soothe Eye Collateral, regulate Qi-blood; use Hegu to clear eyes; Sanyinjiao

目；三阴交能疏通肝、脾、肾经之滞塞。诸穴共用，经脉调畅，气血冲和，目无郁滞而复明。

配穴 久视目胀者，加丝竹空；羞明干涩者，加涌泉。

方法 电热针治疗。

操作 选定穴位，皮肤常规消毒。直刺睛明、球后、合谷、涌泉各0.6寸，直刺三阴交0.7寸。接通电热针仪，每个穴位分别给予30～50mA的电流量，以患者感到胀或温热舒适为度，留针40分钟。（注：每次选3～4组穴，交替应用。）

疗程 隔日1次，20次为1个疗程。疗程间可休息7～10天。一般治疗2～3个疗程。

三、注意事项

1. 针刺眼区穴位时不要提插、捻转，手法要轻，以免损伤目络而致出血。

2. 本病是慢性眼病，必须坚持长期治疗，因此，要做好患者配合医师治疗的思想工

can dredge the stasis of Liver, Spleen, Kidney Meridians. The use of combination of these acupoints can regulate meridians and channels, tonify Qi-blood, remove stagnation and stasis to recover eyesight.

Matching acupoints: For eyeball distention after long-time looking, add Sizhukong; for photophobia and dry eyes add Yongquan.

Method: Electrothermal acupuncture treatment.

Operations: Selecting the relevant acupoints, perform routine skin disinfection. Using electrothermal acupuncture needles, vertically puncture into Jingming, Qiuhou, Hegu, Yongquan for 0.6" respectively, into Sanyinjiao for 0.7". Turn on the electrothermal acupuncture equipment, apply a current of 30-50mA to each acupoint, and the limit is that the patient feels swelling or warm and comfortable, leaving the needles in for 40 minutes. (Note: Select 3-4 pairs of acupoints each time, and use alternatively.)

Therapeutic course: Once every two days, 20 times for a course. Start the treatment for the second course after a break of 7-10 days. Generally treatment lasts for 2-3 courses.

III. Precautions

1. For puncture of acupoints at eye area, manipulations like lifting and thrusting, twisting are forbidden, and mild manipulation is required, so as to avoid bleeding caused by Eye Collateral injuries.

2. This disease is a chronic eye disease, patients must adhere to long-term treatment, therefore ideological work on patients must be done to cooperate with

作，医患配合坚持治疗，方能取效。

3. 该病后期可并发视神经萎缩，或管状视野（视野变窄），为了提高疗效，可以配合中西药物同时治疗。

视神经萎缩

视神经萎缩是视神经纤维受各种病因损害，而发生变性和传导功能障碍所导致的退行性病变，为眼科难治疾病之一。以视功能严重损害乃至丧失，视盘颜色变白，视野明显缩小，甚至呈管状为其主要特征。

中医认为，本病属于"青盲"的范畴。多因暴盲之"视瞻昏渺""视瞻有色"等症失治、误治而成。

一、诊断及辨证要点

1. 临床分原发性和继发性两种，原发性萎缩的眼底表现为视盘颜色灰白或蜡黄，边界模糊，筛板不暴露，其发病原因较为复杂。一般来说，儿童患者，以脑部肿痛或颅内炎症

physicians. Efficacies only can be achieved at premise of cooperation between physicians and patients as well as adherence to treatment.

3. The concurrent disease optic atrophy, or tubular vision (narrowed vision) may occur at later phase, and to improve efficacies, Traditional Chinese Herb Medicine and Western Medicine treatment can also be used.

Optic Atrophy

Optic atrophy is a degenerative disease caused by that damage of optic nerve fibers due to various causes leads to degeneration and conduction dysfunction, and it is one of the ophthalmic refractory diseases. Its main features include severe impairment or even loss of visual functions, whitening of optic nerve heads, obvious narrowing of vision or even tubular vision.

Traditional Chinese Medicine believes that this disease belongs to the range of "glaucoma". Most are caused by loss of treatment or wrong treatment for syndromes of sudden blind such as "blurred vision", "tinted vision", etc.

I. Key Points for Diagnosis and Syndrome Differentiation

1. It is clinically divided into two types, primary ones and secondary ones. For primary atrophy, features of eye ground are grey-white or wax-yellow optic nerve heads, blur borders, lamina cribrosa not exposed, and its cause is complex. Generally, for child patients most are caused by brain swelling and pain or intracranial inflam-

mation; for young patients most are caused by hereditary causes; for middle-aged patients most are caused by optic neuritis or trauma of optic nerves, swelling and pain of intracranial optic chiasma area; for elder patients the disease is often associated with glaucoma or vascular diseases.

2. For patients with liver and kidney deficiency, no external symptoms of eyes, blur vision or blindness, dizziness and tinnitus, dreamy sleep, aching lumbus and limp knees, thin and rapid pulse; or body and extreme chilliness, urorrhagia at night, down diarrhea, deep and weak pulse.

3. For patients with Qi stagnation and blood stasis, emotional upset, eye swelling and dull pain, dizziness and hypochondriac pain, bitter taste and dry throat, dark tongue with ecchymosis, weak and thin pulse.

II. Therapeutic Methods

[Liver and Kidney Deficiency, Qi Stagnation and Blood Stasis]

Therapeutic method: Soothe liver and regulate Qi, activate blood circulation and soothe collaterals.

Prescription: Fengchi (GB20), Yangbai (GB14), Hegu (LI4), Taiyang (EX-HN5), Yiming (EX-HN14).

Mechanism of prescription: Eyes are openings of liver, liver governs soothing and dredging, emotional upset or obstruction of meridian Qi can both cause Qi-blood retention. Bladder and liver are exterior and interior organs corresponding to each other, the acupoint Fengchi and Yangbai of Shao-Yin Meridian of Foot can

阳明大肠经的原穴，有解郁清热之作用；太阳、翳明为经外奇穴，长于疏风通络，活血明目，擅治目疾。诸穴共用，可收疏肝理气、活血通络之功效。

配穴 胸闷气短者，加章门、膻中、胆俞；胁痛者，加阳陵泉、膈俞；善太息者，加内关、膻中。

方法 电热针治疗。

操作 选定穴位，皮肤常规消毒。电热针向对侧眼眶内下缘斜刺风池 0.7 寸，向眼部斜刺阳白 0.7 寸，直刺合谷 0.7 寸，直刺太阳、翳风各 0.7 寸。接通电热针仪，每个穴位分别给予 20～30mA 的电流量，留针 40 分钟。

疗程 隔日 1 次，30 次为 1 个疗程。疗程间可休息 7～10 天。一般需要治疗 2～3 个疗程以上。

三、注意事项

1. 针刺眼部穴位时，手法要轻，不能捻针和提插，应熟

regulate Qi of Bladder Meridian and can relax tendons and activate collaterals, clear brain and eyes; Hegu is a Yuan acupoint of Yang-Ming Large Intestine Meridian of Hand, it can remove stasis and clear Heat; Taiyang and Yiming are external nerve acupoints, can soothe Wind and dredge collaterals, activate blood and improve eyesight, they are good at treatment of eye diseases. The use of combination of these acupoints can soothe liver and regulate Qi, activate blood circulation and dredge collaterals.

Matching acupoints: For chest distress and shortness of breath add Zhangmen, Danzhong, Danshu; for hypochondriac pain add Yanglingquan, Geahu; for reference for sighing add Neiguan, Danzhong.

Method: Electrothermal acupuncture treatment.

Operations: Preparing the selected acupoints, perform routine skin disinfection. Using electrothermal acupuncture needles, obliquely puncture into Fengchi for 0.7" at the lower edge of the contralateral eyes, obliquely puncture toward the eye into Yangbai for 0.7", vertically puncture into Hegu for 0.7", Taiyang, Yifeng for 0.7" respectively. Turn on the electrothermal acupuncture equipment, apply a current of 20-30mA to each acupoint, leaving the needles in for 40 minutes.

Therapeutic course: Once every two days, 30 times for a course. Start the treatment for the second course after a break of 7-10 days. Generally treatment lasts for 2-3 courses or more.

III. Precautions

1. For puncture of acupoints at eye area, mild manipulation is required, and manipulations like lifting and

练地一次到位（得气）后留针。

2. 进针方向和深度要适度，不能伤害眼球，手法要轻。

3. 因为本病多使视力急骤下降或失明，易使患者产生较大的精神压力，故应做好患者的思想工作，要有信心配合治疗。

夜盲

在明亮的环境下视力较好，或可保持正常的视觉，但在昏暗处表现为视障加重、行动困难者称为夜盲。夜盲的种类很多，大体上可分为先天性与后天性、静止性和进行性以及完全性和不完全性等类型。先天性夜盲属常染色体显性遗传或隐性遗传眼病，除色盲外，视力、视野、眼底都无异常；后天性夜盲常因全身疾病（如维生素A缺乏、肝硬化、甲状腺功能亢进、药物中毒）或某些眼底病（如弥漫性视网膜脉络膜萎缩、视神经萎缩等）所致。

中医认为，本病属于"肝虚雀目"的范畴。发生于小

thrusting, twisting are forbidden, the puncturing should be successful at one try skillfully (Qi acquired) then leave the needle in the body.

2. The direction and depth of needling should be appropriate without injuring eyeball, and mild manipulation is required.

3. Since this disease normally cause sudden decrease of eyesight or blindness, which can bring great mental stress to patients, so it is necessary to do ideological work on patients and establish confidence to cooperate with treatments.

Nyctalopia

Better or normal vision in bright environments, while visual impairment aggravating and difficulties in action at dark place, this is called nyctalopia. The types of nyctalopia are various, which can be basically divided as congenital and acquired, quiescent and progressive as well as complete and incomplete. Congenital nyctalopia is a eye disease caused by autosomal dominant inheritance or recessive inheritance, and in addition to achromatopsia, eyesight, vision, eye ground are all normal; acquired nyctalopia is normally caused by systemic diseases (such as vitamin A deficiency, cirrhosis, hyperthyroidism, drug poisoning) or some eye-ground diseases (such as diffuse areolar retinochoroidal atrophy, optic atrophy, etc.).

Traditional Chinese Medicine believes that this disease belongs to the range of "sparrow's eye due to liver

儿者，称"小儿雀目"，亦称"雀目内障"。多因先天禀赋不足，或后天营养失调，致精气亏乏，肝血不足，肝气不能升运于目而病。故本病多属虚证，与肝、肾、脾三脏虚损、经脉滞塞、经气不能运精于目有关。

一、诊断及辨证要点

1. 肝血不足者，双眼干涩，目眨羞明，入暮视昏，舌淡，脉细。

2. 脾气虚弱者，黄昏视物不见，羞明不适，频频眨目，目睛干燥，并见精神萎靡，便溏，舌淡，脉虚。

二、治疗方法

【肝血不足证】

治法 补肝健脾，开窍明目。

处方 太冲（LR3）、三阴交（SP6）、睛明（BL1）、瞳子髎（GB1）。

方义 本方以温补太冲而养肝益血、清头明目为主，辅以三阴交健脾生血、调和肝

deficiency". It is called "sparrow's eye for pediatrics" or "cataract of sparrow's eye" for those occurs among pediatrics. Most are caused by inadequate inherent endowment or acquired malnutrition leading to depletion and deficiency of essence Qi, liver blood deficiency, liver Qi unable to be ascended and transported to eyes. Therefore most are belong to the range of deficiency syndrome, and are related with deficiency and damage of liver, kidney, spleen, stasis and obstruction of meridians and channels, meridian Qi unable to transport essence to eyes.

I. Key Points for Diagnosis and Syndrome Differentiation

1. For patients with liver blood deficiency, dry eyes, eye blinking and photophobia, blurred vision since sunset, light tongue, thin pulse.

2. For patients with spleen Qi deficiency and weakness, unable to see things at dusk, photophobia and discomfort, frequent blinking, eye dryness, as well as spiritlessness, sloppy stool, light tongue, feeble pulse.

II. Therapeutic Methods

[Syndrome of Liver Blood Deficiency]

Therapeutic method: Replenish liver and invigorate spleen, induce resuscitation and improve eyesight.

Prescription: Taichong (LR3), Sanyinjiao (SP6), Jingming (BL1), Tongziliao (GB1).

Mechanism of prescription: This prescription focuses on warming of Taichong so as to nourish liver and tonify blood, clear brain and improve eyesight, supple-

脾，并刺睛明、瞳子髎以开窍明目、通经络。诸穴共用，可补肝健脾、开窍明目，使夜盲自愈。

配穴 羞明重者加足三里、肝俞；白睛、黑睛干燥者加尺泽、太渊。

方法 电热针治疗。

操作 选定穴位，皮肤常规消毒。电热针直刺三阴交、足三里、睛明各0.7寸，直刺太冲、尺泽各0.7寸，直刺太渊0.6寸，向脊柱方向斜刺肝俞0.7寸。接通电热针仪，每个穴位分别给予40～50mA的电流量，以患者舒适为度，留针40分钟。（注：每次选4～5组穴，交替使用。）

疗程 隔日1次，20次为1个疗程。疗程间可休息7～10天。一般需要治疗2～3个疗程，严重者需要治疗5个疗程。

【脾气虚弱证】

治法 健脾益肾，醒神明目。

mented by Sanyinjiao to invigorate spleen and generate blood, tonify liver and spleen, while puncture Jingming and Tongziliao to induce resuscitation and improve eyesight, dredge channels and collaterals. The use of combination of these acupoints can replenish liver and invigorate spleen, induce resuscitation and improve eyesight, so as to achieve self-healing of nyctalopia.

Matching acupoints: For severe photophobia add Zusanli, Ganshu; for dryness of white as well as black area of the eye add Chize, Taiyuan.

Method: Electrothermal acupuncture treatment.

Operations: Selecting the relevant acupoints, perform routine skin disinfection. Using electrothermal acupuncture needles, vertically puncture into Sanyinjiao, Zusanli, Jingming for 0.7" respectively, vertically puncture into Taichong, Chize for 0.7" respectively, vertically puncture into Taiyuan for 0.6", obliquely puncture toward spine into Ganshu for 0.7". Turn on the electrothermal acupuncture equipment, apply a current of 40-50mA to each acupoint, and the limit is that the patient feels comfortable, leaving the needles in for 40 minutes. (Note: Select 4-5 pairs of acupoints each time, and use alternatively.)

Therapeutic course: Once every two days, 20 times for a course. Start the treatment for the second course after a break of 7-10 days. Generally 2-3 treatment courses are needed, for severe cases 5 treatment courses are needed.

[Syndrome of Spleen Qi Deficiency and Weakness]

Therapeutic method: Invigorate spleen and tonify kidney, induce resuscitation and improve eyesight.

处方 脾俞（BL20）、三阴交（SP6）、睛明（BL1）、攒竹（BL2）、丰隆（ST40）、承泣（ST1）。

方义 本方以膀胱经穴脾俞、脾经穴三阴交健脾益气，和胃消积为主，辅以胃经穴承泣、络穴丰隆调和脾胃，助其化源，同时用睛明、攒竹升运清阳达于目窍以收效。

配穴 便溏者加足三里；食欲不振者加胃俞；夜盲较重者加球后。

方法 电热针治疗。

操作 选定穴位，皮肤常规消毒。电热针向脊柱方向斜刺脾俞、胃俞各0.7寸，直刺丰隆0.7寸，直刺足三里0.7寸，直刺承泣、球后各0.7寸，平刺鱼腰0.7寸，平刺攒竹0.6寸。接通电热针仪，每个穴位分别给予40～50mA的电流量，以患者感到胀或温热舒适为度，留针40分钟。

疗程 隔日1次，20次为1个疗程。疗程间可休息7～

Prescription: Pishu (BL20), Sanyinjiao (SP6), Jingming (BL1), Cuanzhu (BL2), Fenglong (ST40), Chengqi (ST1).

Mechanism of prescription: This prescription focuses on use of the acupoint Pishu from Bladder Meridian and the meridian acupoint Sanyinjiao from Spleen Meridian to invigorate spleen and tonify Qi, regulate stomach to remove stasis, supplemented by the meridian acupoint Chengqi and the collateral acupoint Fenglong of Stomach Meridian to regulate spleen and stomach so as to facilitate their resource transformations, while use Jingming and Cuanzhu to ascend and transport Qing-Yang into eyes in order to achieve efficacies.

Matching acupoints: For sloppy stool add Zusanli; for poor appetite add Weishu; for severe nyctalopia add Qiuhou.

Method: Electrothermal acupuncture treatment.

Operations: Selecting the relevant acupoints, perform routine skin disinfection. Using electrothermal acupuncture needles, obliquely puncture toward spine into Pishu, Weishu for 0.7" respectively, vertically puncture into Fenglong for 0.7", Zusanli for 0.7", Chengqi and Qiuhou for 0.7" respectively, horizontally puncture into Yuyao for 0.7", Cuanzhu for 0.6". Turn on the electrothermal acupuncture equipment, apply a current of 40-50mA to each acupoint, and the limit is that the patient feels swelling or warm and comfortable, leaving the needles in for 40 minutes.

Therapeutic course: Once every two days, 20 times for a course. Start the treatment for the second

10天。一般需要治疗2～3个疗程，严重者需要治疗5个疗程。

三、注意事项

1. 针刺睛明、承泣、球后时，注意不要伤害眼球，忌行提插、捻转等手法，起针后要按压针孔2～3分钟，以防出血。

2. 针刺太渊时要避开桡动脉及静脉，防止出血。

3. 针刺球后时，嘱患者目向上视，用拇、食指轻轻固定眼球，针尖略向上方刺入，绝不能做提插、捻转等手法。起针后要按压针孔5分钟，可防止出血。

4. 嘱患者多食鸡肝、羊肝、猪肝之品，对本病的治疗有益处。

course after a break of 7-10 days. Generally 2-3 treatment courses are needed, for severe cases 5 treatment courses are needed.

III. Precautions

1. When puncturing Jingming, Chengqi, Qiuhou, note do not injury eyeballs, manipulations like lifting and thrusting, twisting are forbidden, and it is necessary to press and hold the needle hole for 2-3 minutes after the needle being removed so as to avoid bleeding.

2. When puncturing Taiyuan the radial artery and veins must be avoided to prevent hemorrhage.

3. When puncturing Qiuhou, instruct patient to look upward, gently fix the eyeball with the thumb and the index finger, puncture into skin with the needle tip slightly upward, manipulations like lifting and thrusting, twisting are strictly forbidden. It is necessary to press and hold the needle hole for 5 minutes after the needle being removed, so as to avoid bleeding.

4. Instruct patients eat more food like chicken livers, sheep livers, pig livers, which are helpful to this disease.

保健与美容

Health and beauty

预防慢性支气管炎和支气管哮喘

Prevention of Chronic Bronchitis

慢性支气管炎和支气管哮喘都是呼吸系统的常见病。慢性支气管炎多见于中老年人，50岁以上的人群中发病率为10%～15%，以咳嗽、咯痰或喘促为主要表现；支气管哮喘发病年龄不限，以胸憋气急突然发作、喉中哮鸣、脸色青紫、咳嗽、吐大量泡沫黏液为主要表现。二者均有半夜发作的特点，随着病情逐渐发展而加重，可导致肺气肿和肺心病。因此对此类疾病的预防和保健在防止其发生和传变方面有着重要意义。

中医认为，以上两种疾病属于"咳嗽""痰饮""喘证""哮证"等病症范畴。其发病都与"外感""内伤"关系密切。"外感"是指感受六淫之气，"内伤"指脏腑功能失调，主要是肺、脾、肾三脏功能失调。二者互为因果，导致疾病

Chronic bronchitis and bronchial asthma are common ailment of respiratory system. Chronic bronchitis is often observed at middle age or elder people; at the age of more than 50 years old, the incidence of disease is about 10%-15%. Cough, cough up phlegm, dyspnea and tachypnea are obvious symptoms. There is no age limitation for occurrence of asthma. Clinical observation indicates that there is sudden occurrence of symptom, leading to difficulty in breathing, pale face, abrupt coughing with formulation of foam and mucus and wheezes. There is a tendency that a system will occur at midnight and facilitate gradual symptom development, leading to possible pulmonary emphysema and pulmonary heart disease. Therefore, it is important to prevent the occurrence of the symptom.

Traditional Chinese Medicine regards the two types of disease mentioned above are in the categories of "coughing", "phlegm and retained fluid", "athematic" and "heavy breathing". The occurrence of the disease has close linkage with "exogenous pathogenic syndrome" and "internal disorder". "Exogenous pathogenic syndrome" are affected by the six climate pathogenic factors. "Internal disorder" means disfunction or lack of

的发生与发展,电热针对本病的预防和保健注重调理脏腑功能,提高机体抗病能力,即扶正抗邪,以达未病先防或既病防变之目的。

一、预防方法

(一)电热针疗法

处方 大椎(GV14)、风门(BL12)、肺俞(BL13)、脾俞(BL20)、肾俞(BL23)、关元(BL23)、足三里(ST36)。

方义 大椎为诸阳之会,可振奋阳气,通阳解表;风门为膀胱经穴,能卫外固表;肺俞宣行肺卫之气,清肺肃肺;脾俞健运脾胃,温化痰饮;肾俞益肾壮阳,培本固元,关元为培补先天之本的要穴,足三里为培补后天之本的要穴。诸穴合用,既可增强机体卫外功能,又能调节脏腑功能,从而达到扶正祛邪的目的。

coordination of organs, mainly lung, spleen and kidney. Both exogenous pathogenic syndrome and internal disorder cause the disease and its progression. electrothermal acupuncture is to prevent the exacerbation of the disease, enhance the function of organs and the immune system for strengthening the body resistance in order to expel the pathogenic factor. Therefore, electrothermal acupuncture can achieve the purpose of prevention of symptom and further exacerbation of the symptom development.

Ⅰ. Prevention Method

(Ⅰ) Electrothermal acupuncture

Prescription: Dazhui (GV14), Fengmen (BL12), Feishu (BL13), Pishu (BL20), Shenshu (BL23), Guanyuan (BL23), Zusanli (ST36).

Mechanism of prescription: Dazhui is the nexus of all Yang pulses, which can boost the Yang Qi and get the Yang Qi through and relieve exterior syndrome. Fengmen is the acupoint of Bladder Meridian to strengthen the exterior defense. Feishu can coordinate the Qi of lung, clean and smooth out the lung; Pishu can strengthen spleen and stomach, gradually melt phlegm and retained fluid. Shenshu can boost up the function of kidney, strengthen Yang, and to firm the Yuan Qi. Both Guanyuan and Zusanli can enhance postnatal physical functions and are the important acupoints. Zusanli can be used in combination with other acupoints and adjust the disfunction of internal organs, so that it can achieve the purpose of expelling the pathogenic factor.

方法 电热针（补法）。每次选用4～6组穴，常规消毒，大椎向下斜刺0.5寸，风门、肺俞、脾俞向脊柱方向斜刺0.5寸，肾俞直刺0.8～1.0寸，关元直刺0.6～0.8寸，足三里直刺0.6～0.8寸，得气后接通电热针仪分别给予电流60mA，待患者感到舒适或温热时留针。

疗程 每日或隔日1次，10次为1个疗程，每次留针30～40分钟。

（二）耳针疗法

处方 肺、支气管、脾、肾、肾上腺、神门。

方法 每次选3～4个穴，皮肤常规消毒，选埋针或压王不留行籽，先选一侧耳，每日按压数次，保留3～4天（夏天耳针不能超过3天）更换1次，左右耳交替。

（三）艾灸疗法

（1）艾炷瘢痕灸

处方 肺俞（BL13）、膏肓俞（BL43）、脾俞（BL20）、肾俞（BL23）。

方法 选用艾炷（状如桃

Methods: Electrothermal acupuncture (tonifying method). Each time select 4-6 pairs of acupoints, conduct conventional alcohol disinfection. Apply an oblique needling towards Dazhui for 0.5"; identify Fengmen, Feishu, Pishu and apply an oblique needling towards spine for 0.5", apply perpendicular insertion of needle towards Shenshu for 0.8-1.0", Guanyuan for 0.6-0.8", and Zusanli for 0.6-0.8". After obtainment of Qi, turn on the electrothermal equipment, apply electrical current of 60mA and retain the needle upon feeling of warmth and comfortableness by the patient.

Therapeutic course: Everyday or every other day, 10 times as one course, each time the needle retention is 30-40 minutes.

(Ⅱ) Auriculotherapy

Prescription: Lung, bronchus, spleen, kidney, adrenal gland and Shenmen.

Methods: Select 3-4 acupoints each time, conduct conventional alcohol disinfection and choose ear needle embedding or ear bean. Select one side of ear (right or left ear), push a few times a day and retain for 3-4 days (should not exceed for 3 days during summer), and then change once, interchange between left and right ear.

(Ⅲ) Moxibustion

(1) Cicatricial moxibustion with artemisia

Prescription: Feishu(BL13)、Gaohuangshu (BL43)、Pishu (BL20)、Shenshu (BL23).

Methods: Select a large moxa cone, use garlic juice

仁大小），先用蒜汁涂于皮肤穴位上，立即将艾炷黏附于上，用火点燃，待艾火燃尽，除去艾灰，另换1粒，每穴灸4～5粒（壮），灸后贴淡水膏或胶布，5～7天化脓，形成灸疮，50天左右灸疮愈合，结痂脱落，此法适用于慢性支气管炎和支气管哮喘的缓解期。每灸2次，或三伏天施灸。

（2）艾炷隔姜灸

处方 神阙（CV8）。

方法 取白芥子3克、半夏3克、麻黄5克、公丁香0.5克、细辛2克、麝香少许，将诸药共研末，贮瓶备用。神阙穴常规消毒后，取药粉适量，填满脐窝（神阙穴），将鲜姜片1片，厚约0.3cm，中心都用针穿刺数孔，盖在药末上，姜片上再放上艾炷（柱高1cm，柱底直径1cm），用火点燃施灸，每次3～5壮，隔日治疗1次。10次为1疗程。疗程间休息7天，此法可治疗慢性气管炎迁延期及缓解期的治疗。

to paint acupoints and skin. Immediate paste moxa cone and ignite. After the burning, remove the moxa ashes, and switch to a new one. Each acupoint can have 4-5 peach kernel moxa cone. After the moxibustion, use adhesive bandage. The wound will have maturated for 5-7 days formulating post-moxibustion sore. It will be healed for about 50 days and form a scab and then falling. This method is applicable for chronic bronchitis and mitigation of bronchial asthma. Each time moxa cone can be applied twice or it can be applied during the dog days (the hottest weeks of the summer based on Chinese lunar calendar).

(2) Aizhuge ginger moxibustion

Prescription: Shenque (CV8).

Methods: Take Sinapis semen 3g, pinelliae rhizoma 3g, ephedrae herba 5g, caryophylli flos 0.5g, asari radix et rhizoma 2g, moschus (a little), mill them into powder and store them in a bin. Conduct conventional alcohol disinfection at the acupoint of Shenque, take the above milled power and fill them in umbilicus (Shenque acupoint). Take a fresh piece of ginger with 0.3cm of thickness and open several holes on it, and then put it on the milled powder. Then put the moxa cone on top of this piece of ginger (the height is of the moxa cone is about 1cm and the diameter at the bottom of the cone is about 1cm), ignite and apply moxa stick moxibustion. 3-5 cones each time 10 times for a course, and treat every other day. Rest for 7days between coures. This method is applicable for the prevention and health maintainance of chronic bronchitis during delaying or releasing period.

（3）艾条温和灸

处方 大椎（GU14）、风门（BL12）、肺俞（BL13）、膏肓俞（BL43）。

方法 将艾条点燃的一端对准穴位施灸，约10～15分钟，以达局部皮肤红润温热舒适为度。每次选用1～2个穴位，每日或隔日1次，10次为1个疗程。此法可作为中老年人体虚易患感冒并引起呼吸系统疾病患者的预防保健。

（4）穴位贴敷疗法

处方 肺俞（BL13）、心俞（BL15）、膈俞（BL17）。

方法 取炙白芥子21g，延胡索21g，甘遂12g，细辛12g共研细末，制成散剂，装瓶内备用，以上为1人3次用药量。加生姜汁调成糊状，加麝香少许，分别摊在6块5cm²的油纸上，贴敷于上述穴位，以胶布固定，一般贴敷6～8小时后取下。若贴敷后局部有烧灼疼痛感，可提前取下，多在三伏天贴敷，每隔10天贴敷1次，即初伏、中伏、末伏各1次，共贴敷3次，此法最适于慢性支气管炎及支气管哮喘冬季发作者，连贴3年者效果好。

(3) Mild moxibustion with moxa rolls

Prescription: Dazhui(GU14), Fengmen(BL12), Feishu (BL13), Gaohuangshu (BL43).

Methods: Apply moxa rolls and use the ignited end to burn the located acupoints for 10-15min until the skin turns to reddish and feels warm. Select 1-2 acupoint each time and conduct the treatment every day or every other day. One course of treatment is 10 days, and this is a prevention method for middle aged or elderly people who have tendency to catch cold and suffer respiratory problems.

(4) Acupoints sticking

Prescription: Feishu(BL13), Xinshu(BL15), Geshu (BL17).

Methods: Take sinapis semen 21g, corydalis rhizoma 21g, kansui radix 12g, asari radix et rhizoma 12g and mill them into power and then store them into a bin. The above should amounting to one person with 3 times of applications. Add ginger juice and a little bit of moschus and make them into paste. Then put them on 6 pieces of oil paper (about 5cm²) and apply this paper on the above prescribed acupoints. Use rubberized fabric to stick them and leave them for 6-8 hours and then peel them off. If there is a feeling of burning, it can be peeled off before the prescribed hours. This method has often been applied during the dog days, and it may apply every other 10 days, namely apply each time at the beginning of the dog day, in the middle of the dog days and the end of the dog days for a total of three times. This is most applicable for patients with chronic bronchitis and bronchial asthma

二、注意事项

在以电热针及灸法预防保健同时，还要注意御寒锻炼，尽量避免过敏物刺激，提倡戒烟。

三、现代临床研究

冬病夏治消喘膏防治喘息性气管炎和支气管哮喘的临床研究，据中国中医科学院广安门医院报道，采用复方灸白芥子灸治疗未病289例，年龄最大80岁，最小5岁，以20～50岁者居多，未组病例。一般病程较长，曾用过多种方法治疗，接上法敷灸后，随访1～3年，289例中，治愈40例，显效98例，好转104例，无效47例；显效以上率仅47.8%，总有效率为83.7%。敷灸1、2、3年的疗效比较，显效以上率分别为34.4%、46.7%、69.9%。且疗效随敷灸年限而逐渐提高，以连续灸治3年的疗效较好，经统计学处理后$P < 0.005$，有显著性差异；寒证型较好，热证型次之，而寒热

and with a tendency to experience symptoms during winter. If apply this method continuously for three years, the patient usually experiences obvious improvement.

II. Cautions

While using the electrothermal acupuncture and moxa cone for health improvement, it is also recommended to exercise regularly and avoid contact with allergic materials and stop smoking.

III. Modern clinic research

Treat winter disease during summer through the Chinese medication paste can usefully prevent asthmatic bronchitis and bronchial asthma and is proven by clinical research. According to Guang'anmen Hospital, China Academy of Chinese Medical Sciences, the adoption of compound sinapis semen moxibustion methods cured about 289 cases. Among which the oldest is 80 years old and the youngest is 5 years old. The age group of 20-50 years old forms the largest group of samples. Among the 289 cases, the patients have been using multiples treatment methods, and then combined with moxibustion and acupoints sticking. It is discovered that within the 1-3 years of follow-up, 40 cases have been cured, 98 cases with obvious improvement, 104 cases of improvement, and 47 cases with non-improvement. The percentage of above obvious improvement was about 47.8% and the overall improvement reached 83.7%. For the application of moxibustion and acupoints sticking only, the above obvious improvement was 34.4%, 46.7% and 69.9% for within in a year, two years and three years of duration,

夹杂型较差，经统计学处理后 $P < 0.05$，亦有显著性差异。敷灸后食欲增加，体力增加，感冒次减少，还能减少或停用平喘药，但对长期服用激素者疗效较差。

预防胃肠病

胃肠病泛指发生于胃肠道的多种疾病，如胃炎、十二指肠溃疡、肠炎、痢疾、胃肠道肿瘤等，针灸不仅可以治疗胃肠疾病，而且还有预防和保健作用。

中医认为，各种胃肠病均属于"脾胃病"的范畴，脾胃病的发生与脾胃虚弱关系最为密切。因此，对于素体脾胃虚弱的人积极采取一些健运脾胃的预防保健措施，不仅可以预防脾胃病的发生，针对各种

respectively. The improvement increases with the years of treatment, and the best results are being demonstrated for three consecutive years of treatment. The statistics show that P<0.005 demonstrates the most obvious differences, and the treatment is most effective for symptoms caused by Cold factor, and then for symptoms caused by Heat factors, and the least to the symptoms caused by combination of Cold and Heat factors. The statistics show that P<0.05 demonstrates the obvious differences. The application of moxibustion and acupoints sticking has positive effects. It increases one's appetite and stamina, reduces the frequency of catching cold. It also reduced the intake amount of anti-asthmatics medicine or even makes one have no reliance on such medicine. However, it is less effective for patient who has been taking long term hormone therapy.

Prevention of Gastro-intestinal Diseases

Gastro-intestinal diseases include a range of diseases such as gastritis, enteritis, diarrhea and gastrointestinal tumor, etc. Acupuncture can cure gastro-intestinal disease and at the same time prevent and improve health conditions.

Traditional Chinese Medicine generally regards gastro-intestinal disease as the range of "spleen and stomach disease". The spleen and stomach disease is closely linked with disfunction of spleen and stomach. Therefore, it is useful for those with relatively weak spleen and stomach to actively take enhancement and prevention methods to prevent the reoccurrence of symptoms and

慢性脾胃病的患者,还可以防止疾病的传变,促进其早日康复。

一、预防方法

(一)电热针疗法或毫针疗法

处方 足三里(ST36)、三阴交(SP6)、脾俞(BL20)、胃俞(BL21)、中脘(CV12)、天枢(ST25)。

方义 足三里是足阳明胃经合穴,可和胃、健脾、润肠,是培补后天之本及强壮全身之要穴;三阴交与足太阴脾经穴,又是肝、脾、肾三经交会穴可健脾、益肾、调肝,同样也是全身保健要穴;脾俞、胃俞是脾胃之气输注于背部之穴,具有健运脾胃,输转中焦,生化气血之功效;中脘、天枢为胃与大肠腑之气汇集于腹部的募穴,可和胃润肠,促进运化。诸穴相伍,对脾胃病起到预防和保健作用。

方法 电热针对一般人采用40mA(平补平泻法),对脾

prevent the exacerbation of the existing chronical symptoms.

I. Prevention methods

(I) Electrothermal needle acupuncture and filiform needle acupuncture

Prescription: Zusanli(ST36), Sanyinjiao(SP6), Pishu(BL20), Weishu(BL21), Zhongwan(CV12), Tianshu(ST25).

Mechanism of prescription: Zusanli is the He acupoint of Yang-Ming Stomach Meridian of Foot, and it is important for enhancing stomach, spleen and intestines. Sanyinjiao is on the Tai-Yin Spleen Meridian of Foot. It is also the confluent acupoint of Liver Meridian, Spleen Meridian and Kidney Meridian, whose function includes invigorating spleen, enhancing kidney and smoothing liver. At the same time, it is also useful for improving the overall health conditions. Pishu and Weishu is where the Qi of spleen and stomach and transfers to the acupoints of one's back. It is useful to boost the function of spleen and stomach, transfer in MiddleJiao, enhance the flow of blood and Qi. Zhongwan and Tianshu is the Mu acupoint which converge the Qi of stomach and intestine and useful for smoothing intestine. The co-effect and harmony among the acupoints demonstrate relatively positive effects for the prevention of gastro-intestinal diseases.

Methods: Electrothermal needle acupuncture can apply 40mA (mild reinforcing-attenuating method) for

胃虚弱者宜采用60mA（补法）。选定穴位皮肤常规消毒，足三里直刺0.8～1.0寸，三阴交直刺0.5～0.7寸，脾俞、肾俞向脊柱方向斜刺0.6～0.8寸，中脘、天枢直刺0.6～0.8寸，一般预防保健时，每次选2～4个穴位，轮流交替使用。

疗程 每日或隔日1次，7次为1个疗程，疗程间休息5天。

（二）耳针疗法

处方 神门、脾、肾、大肠、小肠、交感。

方法 采取埋耳针或压王不留行籽法，两耳交替应用，先取一侧耳穴，保留3～5天。取下后再换另一侧耳穴，每次选2～3穴，7次1疗程，疗程间休息5天。

（三）灸疗法

处方 足三里（ST36）、中脘（CV12）、天枢（ST25）。

方法 采用艾条灸法，将艾条一端点燃对准穴位，距离皮肤3cm左右，当患者感到穴位局部温热舒适就固定不动，

people in normal condition. For patients with relatively week spleen and stomach, 60mA can be applied (enhancing method). Select acupoints and conduct conventional skin disinfection. Apply vertical needling insertion towards Zusanli for 0.8-1.0" and Sanyinjiao for 0.5-0.7". For Pishu and Shenshu, apply oblique insertion towards spinc for 0.6-0.8". Apply vertical insertion towards Zhongwan and Tianshu for 0.6-0.8". For general prevention and health improvement purpose, it is recommended to select 2-4 acupoints each time and use alternatively.

Therapeutic course: Once a day or once every other day, 7 times as a course of treatment and can take 5 days off during the interval time.

(Ⅱ) Auriculotherapy

Prescription: Shenmen, spleen, kidney, large intestine, small intestine and Jiaogan.

Methods: Use ear needle embedding or ear bean and interchange between the two ears. Apply the chosen method to one ear and retain for 3-5 days and switch to the other ear. Locate 2-3 acupoints, 7 times for one course of treatment and can rest for 5 days during the interval time.

(Ⅲ) Moxibustion

Prescription: Zusanli(ST36), Zhongwan(CV12), Tianshu (ST25).

Methods: Apply moxa roll, ignite one side of the roll and locate it to the acupoints, and 3cm of distance from the skin. When patient feels the acupoints get warm, then fix the position. Leave the moxa roll for 10-

每穴灸至皮肤红润为度，约10～15分钟，对腹部穴位也可以用温灸器施灸。

二、注意事项

1. 针灸对胃肠病的预防保健效果可靠，但要坚持治疗至脾胃恢复强壮或康复为止。

2. 必要时还可以配合其他保健措施，如中药、按摩。

预防高血压

高血压是以动脉血压高，特别是舒张压持续升高为主要临床表现的慢性全身性血管性疾病。早期有头晕、头痛、心悸、失眠、耳鸣、心烦、乏力、记忆力减退、颜面潮红或肢体麻木等，晚期可发生脑、心、肾等器官的病变，本病40～50岁以上者较为多见。

中医认为，本病属"眩晕""头痛""肝阳""肝风"等病症范畴，并与"中风"有直接联系，多由情志抑郁，精神过度紧张或饮酒过度，嗜食肥甘厚味等，导致肝阳偏亢，痰湿壅阻，肝肾阴虚，阴阳两虚而发。针灸预防本病，首先是未病先防，特别对35～40岁

15 minutes until the skin of each acupoint turns to reddish. A warming moxibustion apparatus can be applied to acupoints at abdomen.

II. Cautions

Acupuncture has positive effect for prevention of gastro-intestinal disease, and it is important to maintain the treatment until the spleen and stomach recover their functions.

When needed, it can also be combined with other methods such as Chinese Herb Medicine and massage.

Prevention of High Blood Pressure

High blood pressure is caused by high blood pressure at artery, due to continuously increases of diastolic pressure, and it is a typical chronical blood vessel disease. The early symptom includes dizziness, headache, palpitate, insomnia, tinnitus, be vexed, feeble, decrease of memory, reddish face and numbness of limb. At the late stage, it is possible to cause pathological changes to brain, heart and kidney. High blood pressure is often observed at the age group of above 40-50 years old.

Traditional Chinese Medicine regards high blood pressure as the range of "dizziness", "headache", "liver Yang", and "liver Wind", having direct linkage with apoplexy. It is caused by many factors including depression, overstress and alcohol, intake of fat and heavy taste food, etc. Acupuncture can prevent high blood pressure, and it is particularly applicable to the potential patients aged between 35-40, who have accumulated stress with fluctuating emotions, and those with family history of high

左右具有潜在致病因素的人群，如长期精神紧张而缺乏体力劳动者，平时性情急躁易发怒者，有高血压家族史、体重、饮食中食盐含量多和大量吸烟者，都可以采取针灸预防高血压的发生；其次是对已患有Ⅰ期高血压患者，通过针灸保健可以防止其传变。

一、预防方法

（一）电热针疗法或毫针疗法

处方 曲池（LI11）、足三里（ST36）、三阴交（SP6）。

方义 曲池为手阳明经穴，足三里为足阳明经穴，两穴均为中老年保健要穴，具有降逆潜阳、调和气血功能；三阴交为足三阴交合穴，具有健脾、益肾、调肝的功效。诸穴合用，能有效预防高血压的发生。

配穴 长期精神过度紧张者，加神门、百会；平素性情急躁者，加肝俞、太冲；体质肥胖伴有脘痞恶心、头晕、头

blood pressure, heavy weights, the habit of smoking and too much intake of salt. Acupuncture can also prevent the deterioration of high blood pressure symptom, particular to the first phase patient. Therefore, acupuncture is useful for the prevention and early phase of treatment of high blood pressure.

I. Prevention methods

(I) Electrothermal needle acupuncture or filiform needle acupuncture

Prescription: Quchi(LI11), Zusanli(ST36), Sanyinjiao(SP6).

Mechanism of prescription: Quchi is one of the acupoints of Yang-Ming Meridian of Hand. Zusanli is one of the acupoints of Yang-Ming Meridian of Foot. Both of the acupoints are important for enhancing the health condition of middle aged and elder people. These can submerse exuberance Yang, adjust and smooth the function of blood and Qi. Sanyinjiao is the He acupoint of the confluence of the three Yin Meridians of Foot, which can boost the function of spleen, kidney and adjust the function of liver. The co-effects can effectively prevent the symptoms of high blood pressure.

Matching acupoint: Add Shenmen and Baihui for patient who is under long-term stress. Add Ganshu and Taichong for patient who is impetuous. Obese type of people may feel dizziness, bloating, nauseous or heavi-

重，脉滑，苔腻者，加内关、中脘、丰隆、公孙；平素房劳过度易出现神疲腰酸，耳鸣如蝉，头晕眼花，舌红，脉细数者，加肾俞、太溪。

方法 电热针40mA（毫针平补平泻），选定穴位，皮肤常规消毒，电热针直刺0.6～0.8寸，足三里直刺0.7～1.0寸，三阴交直刺0.5～0.7寸，神门直刺0.3～0.5寸，百会沿皮刺0.3～0.5寸，内关直刺0.5～0.7寸，公孙直刺0.3～0.5寸，肾俞直刺0.6～0.8寸，太溪直刺0.5寸，得气后接通电热针仪，分别给予电流50mA，以出现胀而舒适或温热为度，留针30分钟。

疗程 每日1次，10次为1个疗程，疗程间休息5天。

（二）耳穴疗法

处方 神门、心、内分泌。
配穴 肝、肾、肾上腺。
方法 采用耳穴埋针，耳穴压王不留行籽。先埋一侧保留3～5天，取下后再换另一侧耳穴，左右交替应用。

ness in the brain, for whom with greasy tongue fur and slippery pulse, add Neiguan, Zhongwan, Fenglong and Gongsun. For patient who easily feel fatigue after excessive intercourse and experiencing soreness in waist, ear ringing, dizzy spell, red tongue and thready rapid pulse, it will be useful to add Shenshu and Taixi.

Methods: Electrothermal needle acupuncture 40mA (filiform needle reinforcing-attenuating method), select acupoints and conduct conventional skin disinfection. Apply perpendicular insertion with electrothermal needle for 0.6-0.8", perpendicular insertion at Zusanli for 0.7-1.0", Sanyinjiao for 0.5-0.7", Shenmen for 0.3-0.5", shallow insertion at Baihui for 0.3-0.5", perpendicular insertion at Neiguan for 0.5-0.7", perpendicular insertion at Gongsun for 0.3-0.5", perpendicular insertion at Shenshu for 0.6-0.8" and perpendicular insertion at Taixi for 0.5". After obtainment of Qi, turn on the electrothermal equipment, apply 50mA of electric current and retain the needles for 30 minutes with comfortable warmth.

Therapeutic course: Once a day, ten times as one course, can take 5 days off during the interval.

(Ⅱ) Ear acupoint therapy

Prescription: Shenmen, heart and internal secretion.
Matching acupoint: Liver, kidney and adrenal gland.
Methods: Use ear needle or ear bean embedding for one side of ear first and retain for 3-5 days and then switch to the other side, and use alternatively.

（三）艾条灸疗法

处方 足三里（ST36）、曲池（LI11）。

方法 采用艾条分别于每穴灸10～15分钟，每日1次，每月灸10次，每年春夏之交、秋冬之交各灸1次，已有高血压症状者可连续灸数次以进行保健。

（四）穴位贴敷疗法

处方 气海（CV6）、关元（CV4）。

方法 取附子、马兰子、蛇床子、木香、肉桂、吴茱萸各等分，共研细末，混合均匀，密瓶备用，应用时取药末用姜汁调如膏状，分别贴至穴位上，外盖油纸，胶布固定，每日或隔日1次，每次保留12小时左右。

二、注意事项

1. 针灸预防疾病，重在调节脏腑气血功能，需坚持治疗才能取得满意疗效。

2. 耳穴埋耳针，夏季时间不宜过久，1～3天即可，以防汗出造成感染。

(Ⅲ) Moxa roll therapy

Prescription: Zusanli (ST36), Qushi(LI11).

Methods: Use moxa roll therapy for each acupoint for 10-15 minutes, once a day, 10 times a month. Once for the changing season between spring and summer, and fall and winter. For those experiencing high blood pressure, the moxa roll therapy can be continued for several courses.

(Ⅳ) Acupoints sticking

Prescription: Qihai (CV6), Guanyuan (CV4).

Methods: Take aconm lateralis radix praeparaia, Malanzi, cnidii fructus, aucklandiae radix, cinnamomi cortex, euodiae fructus, mill them into powder, mix them and store them in a bin. Take the powder, mix it with ginger juice and to be pasted to the acupoint. Then put oil paper on top of it and stick it with rubberized fabric. Once a day or every other day. Retain for 12 hours each time.

Ⅱ. Cautions

1. Acupuncture prevent one from having the disease and the important point is to adjust the Qi and blood of the organs. Continuous treatment can lead to improvement.

2. Ear acupoint therapy with ear needles embedding during the summer season should not be too long and normally 1-3 days will be enough to avoid infection.

三、现代临床研究

中医认为,老年高血压发病本质在于本虚标实,气血失和,兼夹有风、痰、瘀,病位主要在肝、脾、肾。辨证施治当治标在肝,治本在肾,调理脾胃贯穿始终。据此,近年来临床上对百会、足三里与风池、三阴交,两组穴位交替应用,探讨对老年高血压的治疗,取得了较满意的疗效,现介绍如下。

临床资料 246例老年高血压患者纳入标准:年龄66岁以上,收缩压＜21kpa(160mmHg)或舒张压＞13kpa(95mmHg),非同日2次测定,并伴有头晕、目眩、心悸、失眠、耳鸣、烦躁、腰酸腿软。246例中,病程1年以内有16例,1～5年有154例,6～10年有28例,10年以上有18例;属高血压Ⅰ期86例,Ⅱ期65例,Ⅲ期95例;合并脑动脉硬化12例,冠心病44例,中风后遗症15例,糖尿病6例。

III. Modern clinical research

Traditional Chinese Medicine considers that high blood pressure is caused by asthenia in origin and asthenia in superficiality, loss of harmony between Qi and blood accompanied by Wind, phlegm and stagnation. The origin of the problem comes from liver, spleen and kidney, so it is essential to adjust these organs. Through the alternative usage of two pairs of acupoints, namely Baihui together with Zusanli and Fengchi with Sanyinjiao, we have achieved the following positive results in dealing with high blood pressure of the elders.

Clinical findings: 246 elders with the following standard symptoms: aged 66 and above—systolic pressure ＜ 21kpa (160mmHg), or diastolic pressure ＞ 13kpa(95mmHg), and this was measured twice at two different days. These people at the same time experienced dizziness, palpitation, insomnia, irritation, ear ringing, soreness on waist and legs and are being regarded as high blood pressure symptom for those elderly people. Among the 246 cases, those who had symptom within a year accounted for 16 cases, within 1-5 years accounted for 154 cases, within 6-10 years accounted for 28 cases, and more than 10 years accounted for 18 cases. Phase I high blood pressure accounted for 86 cases, phrase II accounted for 65 cases. The phase III in combination with cerebral arteriosclerosis accounted for 12 cases, with coronary heart disease accounted for 44 cases, with sequela of apoplexy accounted for 15 cases and with diabetes accounted for 6 cases.

治疗选穴 百会,别名三阳五会,出自《针灸甲乙经》,位于前顶后一寸五分,现代取穴采用正坐位,后发际正中直上七寸,当头部的中线与两耳尖连线交点处。此穴位为高血压反应点,高血压患者按之必痛。《针灸甲乙经》记载风池穴位置为"颞颥后发际陷中"。现代取法采用俯卧位,在项后枕骨下两侧,当斜方肌上端与胸锁乳突肌之间凹陷中,寻找压痛明显处。足三里、三阴交常规取穴。

治疗方法 上述穴位,毫针与电热针交替使用。先针头部穴位,后针下肢穴位,留针30～40分钟。亦可教患者自行灸治,方法是先灸头部穴位,后灸下肢穴位,操作时艾条从远处缓慢向穴位靠近,艾条点燃一端与皮肤表面距离以患者感到温热舒适为度,每次灸10～15分钟,每日1次,30次为1疗程。疗程间休息7天,定期测血压。

246例患者治疗期间均停

Locating the acupoints: Baihui, another name is Sanyangwuhui. *Jia Yi Jing* indicates that Baihui is 1.5" behind the top of the head. Sit straight when locating the acupoint. Identify the acupoint from the rear concave along the hairline for 6-7" and the convergence point between the middle line of the head and the line of the top edge of the two ears. This acupoint is the reflection point of high blood pressure, and high blood pressure patient may feel pain when pressed with this acupoint. With regard to Fengchi, the *Jia Yi Jing* indicates that it is in the concave along the hairline behind the Nao Kong acupoint. Lying on one's stomach, Fegnchi acupoint is located behind the occipital bone, in a concave between the upper part of trapezius and sternocleidomastoid. Once being pressed, one may feel the pain. In combination with Fengchi, take the acupoints of Zusanli and Sanyinjiao.

Treatment methods: The above mentioned two pairs of acupoints can be adjusted between the applications of electrothermal acupuncture and filiform needle acupuncture. Start with acupoints at the heads, and then towards the legs and retention is about 30-40 minutes for each needle. One can also teach the patient to conduct self-moxibustion. Similarly, starting with the head towards the legs, from approaching the moxa rolls in far distance towards closer distance until feeling comfortable with temperature. Each moxibustion is about 10-15 minutes, once a day, 30 times for one course and can take 7 days off during the interval. Monitor blood pressure regularly.

Among the 246 patients, the medicine for con-

用降压药，电热针治疗后大多数有不同程度的降压效果，针前收缩压平均值为169.5mmHg，针后为144.4mmHg，降低25.1mmHg；针前舒张压平均值为100.2mmHg，针后为95.2mmHg，降低14mmHg。

疗效评定 在1个疗程中，舒张压较治疗前降低10mmHg以上并到达正常水平范围，或舒张压未降至正常，但已下降20mmHg以上，伴随症状消失为显效，共186例，占75.6%；舒张压较治疗前下降10～19mmHg，但未达到正常范围，收缩压较治疗前下降30mmHg为以上，伴随症状减轻，为有效，共46例，占18.7%；未达到以上标准者为无效，共15例，占6.1%。

结论 百会、风池穴有平肝息风、升清降浊、醒脑开窍等功效。足三里为强身要穴，可健脾和胃、调理气血。三阴交可调补肝肾、通经活络。研究表明，针刺上述穴位对血压、心率、血流动力学和动脉血氧均有双向调节作用。

trolling high blood pressure was stopped during the treatment. The electrothermal acupuncture has positive effects for lowering the blood pressure. Before the treatment, the average systolic pressure was 169.5mmHg. After treatment, it reached 144.4mmHg, reduced by 25.1mmHg. Before the treatment, the average diastolic pressure was 100.2mmHg. After the treatment, it reached 95.2mmHg, reduced by 14mmHg.

Assessment: Through one course of treatment, diastolic pressure was reduced by 10mmHg, reaching normal range or systolic pressure was not lowered to normal range yet, however, the later was reduced by more than 20mmHg and with obvious improvement. About 186 cases, 75.6% demonstrated that diastolic pressure reduced by 10-19mmHg compared with pre-treatment, but still had not reached normal range. Systolic pressure was reduced by more than 30mmHg compared with pretreatment, and the high blood pressure symptoms had lessened, and these accounted for 46 cases, 18.7%. About 15 cases, 6.1%, did not reach the above standards or had no effects.

Conclusion: Baihui and Fengchi, the two acupoints can calm the liver Wind, ascending the clear and descending the turbid. Zusanli is an important acupoint for strengthen the body, improve the function of stomach and adjust Qi and blood. Sanyinjiao can adjust and enhance the function of liver, kidney, clearing and activating the channels and collaterals. Through the research findings, it is observed that acupuncture at the above mentioned acupoints can have positive effects on blood pressure, heart beats, dynamic movement of blood and oxygen

预防冠心病

冠心病全称冠状动脉粥样硬化性心脏病，是由冠状动脉发生粥样硬化导致心肌缺血性的心脏病。临床主要表现为胸闷，气短，心前区疼痛，心悸，汗出肢冷、脉微细等。严重者可致死亡，是中老年血管疾病中最常见的一种，并有逐年增多的趋势。因此，预防应放在首位，尤其是对40岁以上的中老年人应该加强对此病预防。

中医认为，本病属"真心痛""胸痹"等病症范畴。其发病主要由气滞血瘀所致，与心、肝、脾、肾诸脏功能失调有关。针灸对未病的预防和保健有较好的效果，主要体现在两方面：一是通过针灸预防本病的发生；二是对冠心病患者可通过针灸进行保健以改善症状，预防或减少心绞痛和心肌梗死（塞）的发作次数，促进康复。

supply to artery.

Prevention of Coronary Heart Disease

Coronary heart disease is caused by atherosclerosis at coronary artery, which would cause ischemia myocardiosis. The clinical symptoms include breathing difficulty, short of breath, precordial pain, palpitation, sweating, weak and small pulse, etc. Serious sumptom may also lead to death. It is one of the common disease among middle aged and elder people and it has been an increasing trend. Therefore, prevention task is important, particular for people aged 40 and above.

Traditional Chinese Medicine regards this disease as in the range of "angina pectoris" and "chest apoplexy". It is caused by stagnation of Qi and blood and lose of proper function of heart, liver, spleen, kidney, etc. Acupuncture has preventional effects and can also improve the conditions. Meanwhile, it can reduce the frequency of angina pectoris and myocardial infarction and improve one's health conditions.

一、预防方法

（一）电热针疗法或毫针疗法

处方 内关（PC6）、膻中（CV17）、心俞（BL15）、厥阴俞（BL14）。

方义 内关为手厥阴心包经络穴，是调理上焦气机、活血通络的要穴之一；膻中隶属于任脉，位于胸部正中，又为气会，可宽胸理气；心俞、厥阴俞分别是心、心包络的背俞穴，是强心宁神、调节心脏功能的要穴。诸穴合用，可收强心宽胸、行气活血、通络止痛的功效，是冠心病预防与保健的常用方法。

方法 选定穴位，常规消毒，电热针直刺0.6～0.8寸，膻中向下平刺0.6～0.7寸，得气即可，不要求传导，均留针30～40分钟。心俞、厥阴俞向脊柱方向斜刺0.6～0.8寸，得气后，接通电热针仪，分别给予50mA，留针30～40分钟。

疗程 每日或隔日1次，

I. Prevention methods

(Ⅰ) Electric thermal acupuncture and acupuncture

Prescription: Neiguan (PC6), Danzhong(CV17), Xinshu(BL15), Jueyinshu(BL14).

Mechanism of prescription: Neiguan is one of the acupoint at Jue-Yin Pericardium Meridian of Hand. Danzhong belongs to Ren Channel and is at the center of the chest, is also the confluence point of Qi. It can adjust and smooth Qi. Xinshu and Jueyinshu are the Back-Shu acupoint of Heart and Pericardium Meridian and can enhance heart and calm down spirit. It is an important acupoint for adjusting the function of heart. The co-effects of the acupoints can enhance heart, broaden mind, smooth the flow of Qi and circulation of blood and meridian. It can also ease pain and therefore has good preventional and health effects to coronary heart disease.

Methods: Select acupoints, conduct conventional disinfection, apply perpendicular insertion of electrothermal needle for 0.6-0.8", apply horizontal insertion towards the bottom of Danzhong for 0.6-0.7", obtainment of Qi is good enough and no need to wait for transfer, and then retain for average 30-40 minutes. Apply oblique insertion at Xinshu, Jueyinshu towards the backbone for 0.6-0.8", after obtainment of Qi, turn on the electrothermal equipment, apply current of 50mA and retain the needle for 30-40 minutes.

Therapeutic course: Everyday or every other day,

10次为1个疗程，每月1个疗程即可。

（二）耳针疗法

处方 心、神门（HT7）、皮质下、交感。

方法 针刺（毫针或皮内针）用平补平泻法，留针20～30分钟，还可以埋耳针或压王不留行籽，保留3～4天（夏季2天），左右两耳交替应用。

（三）灸疗法

处方 膻中（CV17）。

方法 艾条雀啄灸，将燃着的一端对准穴位，像麻雀啄米一样，距穴位皮肤2～3cm处，对准穴位上下移动施灸，患者感到温热感，即固定不动，以穴位部有温热舒适感为度。

（四）穴位贴敷疗法

处方 膻中（CV17）、内关（PC6）。

方法 取川芎3g，冰片1g，硝酸甘油1片，共研细末，制成黄豆粒大丸剂，备用。应用时，取药丸分别贴敷于膻中、内关穴处，用胶布固

10 times for a course, one course for a month.

(Ⅱ) Ear acupoint therapy

Prescription: Heart, Shenmen(HT7), Pizhixia. Jiaogan.

Methods: Needle insertion (filiform needle or intradermal needle) can use mild reinforcing-attenuating method, retain needle for 20-30 minutes. Alternatively, it can also use ear needle embedding or ear bean, retain for 3-4 days (2 days at most during summer), and interchange between left and right side.

(Ⅲ) Moxibustion

Prescription: Danzhong (CV17).

Methods: Moxa rolls moxibustion like sparrow peaks, locate the ignited side towards the acupoint, like sparrow peaking, move up and down and to be detached from the skin of acupoint at 2-3cm until the patient feels warm at the surface of the acupoint and then fix the position.

(Ⅳ) Acupoints sticking

Prescription: Danzhong (CV17), Neiguan (PC6).

Methods: Take chuanxiong rhizoma 3g, borneolum syntheticum 1g, nitroglycerin tablets 1 piece, mill them into powder and make them into soybean sized bolus for usage. Take one bolus each time and attach to Danzhong and Neiguan, and fix it with bandage. Once a day and 7

定即可，每日1次，7次为1个疗程。

二、注意事项

电热针或毫针对冠心病的预防与保健，简便经济，见效快，又无药物的毒副反应。但需长期坚持，方能取得远期疗效。除此之外，还要配合饮食调理，注意劳逸结合，保持心情舒畅，忌烟酒和浓茶。

三、现代临床研究

本病以气虚为主（本），治疗以养心益气为主，助阳通窍、活络宣痹为辅。取穴以心包经和背俞穴为主，心绞痛发作时，速取内关配通里、膻中，选定穴位后，常规消毒，电热针直刺内关0.5～0.7寸，直刺通里0.5～0.8寸，向下斜刺膻中0.6～0.8寸，接通电热针仪，分别给予60mA，得气后即可留针30～40分钟；或以毫针针刺亦可，待至心绞痛减缓。其次，还可以用毫针透刺膻中穴，用长针沿皮刺入鸠尾穴。对心绞痛严重者，可用0.5%普鲁卡因10mL，分别注入心俞、内关、膻中穴，每

times as one course of treatment.

II. Cautions

Electrothermal acupuncture and filiform needle acupuncture have health benefits and prevention effects to coronary heart disease. It is economical, convenient and fast acting without side effects caused by medicine. It is important to continue with the treatment to achieve long-term improvement. In addition, it is important to eat healthy with regular exercise to keep a relaxed mind. It is prohibited to drink alcohol or strong tea.

III. Modern clinical research

Prevention and treatment of coronary heart disease by electrothermal acupuncture and filiform needle acupuncture: The disease is mainly caused by deficiency of vital energy (Ben), treatment is mainly based on nourishing heart and Qi. Secondly it is based on reinforcing Yang and dredging the meridian, and activating collaterals and reducing the numbs. The acupoints mainly include Pericardium Meridian and Back-Shu acupoint. When there is angina pectoris, it is recommended to immediately take the acupoint of Neiguan together with Tongli and Danzhong. Conduct regular disinfection, apply electrothermal needle in a perpendicular manner towards Neiguan for 0.5-0.7" and the same to Tongli for 0.5-0.8". Apply the electrothermal needle in an oblique manner towards the bottom of Danzhong for 0.6-0.8", apply electric current separately for 60mA (obtainment of Qi is good enough for needle retainment), retain for

次 2mL 以治其标；待心绞痛缓解后，再治其本，取内关、大陵、巨阙、膻中、心俞等穴，行电热针疗法，轮流交替施以补法，每日 1 次。气滞血瘀者，加太冲、期门、血海、膈俞；胸阳阻痹者，加丰隆、脾俞；心脾两虚者，加足三里、三阴交；心肾阳虚者，加关元、肾俞、足三里；阳气欲脱者，加百会、关元、气海。若以上诸证中出现心动过速者加间使，过缓者加通里；惊恐者加神门，气喘者加太渊、尺泽。

30-40 minutes. Alternatively, it can apply only filiform needle until the pain of angina pectoris ceases. Secondly, it can also use filiform needle to point through the acupoint of Danzhong and use a long needle to insert into the acupoint of Jiuwei alongside of the skin. Thirdly, for a patient with severe pain of angina pectoris, it can apply 10mL of 0.5% procaine and inject into Xinshu, Neiguan, Danzhong acupoints separately, each time with 2mL (treat the superficial symptoms), and wait until the pain cases. After the pain ceases, then treat the root of the symptom. Take acupoints of Neiguan, Daling, Juque, Danzhong and Xinshu (electrothermal therapy) and rotate the above mentioned acupoints. It is an reinforcing method and can practice once a day. If the patient experiences stagnation of Qi and blood, it is recommended to add Taichong, Qimen, Xuehai and Geshu. For those with chest Yang obstruction, add Fenglong and Pishu. For those with heart and spleen deficiency, add Zusanli and Sanyinjiao. For those with heart-kidney Yang deficiency, add Guanyuan and Shenshu and Zusanli. For those who are going to releasing process of Yang Qi, add Baihui, Guanyuan and Qihai. For those experience tachycardia, it is recommended to add Jianshi. For those experience bradycardia, add Tongli. For those who easily feel alarmed or panicky, add Shenmen. For those who are short of breath, add Taiyuan and Chize.

预防中风

中风是以突然口眼㖞斜，言语謇涩不利，肌肤麻木不仁，或部分肢体运动障碍，半

Stroke Prevention

Stroke is a kind of disease whose clinical manifestations are sudden facial distortion, dysphasia, skin numbness or part of limbs dyskinesia, hemiplegia, and

身不遂，甚至突然昏倒，不省人事为特征的一类疾病。本病包括现代医学的脑出血、脑血栓形成，脑血管痉挛，蛛网膜下腔出血等脑血管病，多发于中老年人，且有高血压和动脉硬化病史患者发病率较高。本文主要介绍脑血栓形成、脑出血、脑血管痉挛的电热针预防方法。

中医认为，本病多因平素气血虚衰，心、肝、肾三脏阴阳失调，情志郁结，起居失常，导致肝肾之阴不足，心火肝火偏旺；或因饮酒暴食，生痰化热而生内风所致。电热针可通过调整脏腑气血功能，使之恢复正常状态，防患于未然。

一、预防方法

（一）电热针疗法或毫针疗法

处方 曲池（LI11）、合谷（LI4）、足三里（ST36）、太冲（LR3）、三阴交（SP6）。

方义 曲池、三阴交两穴具有降逆明目、调和气血的作

even sudden faint without consciousness. This syndrome includes series of cerebrovascular diseases defined in modern medicine such as cerebral hemorrhage, cerebral thrombosis, cerebral embolism, cerebral vasospasm, subarachnoid hemorrhage and so on. It's mostly seen in middle-aged and old people, and high morbidity generally with medical histories of high blood pressure and arteriosclerosis. This article mainly introduces the cerebral thrombosis development and electrothermal acupuncture prevention methods for cerebral hemorrhage and cerebral vasospasm.

Traditional Chinese Medicine believes that this disease mostly is caused by Qi and blood deficiency, emotion stagnation, lifestyle disorder, leading to Yin deficiency of liver and kidney and exuberance of heart Fire and liver Fire in the context of Yin-Yang imbalance in heart, liver, and kidney; or caused by drinking and gluttony, phlegm generation, Heat-transmission leading to endogenous Wind. Electrothermal acupuncture may regulate Qi, blood of viscera to recover the functions to prevent stroke consequently.

Ⅰ. Prevention Methods

（Ⅰ）Electrothermal acupuncture therapy or filiform needle therapy

Prescription: Quchi(LI11), Hegu(LI4), Zusanli(ST36), Taichong(LR3), Sanyinjiao(SP6).

Mechanism of prescription: The acupoints Quchi and Sanyinjiao can increase eyesight, lower adverse Qi,

用；太冲为平肝息风的要穴；三阴交为肝、脾、肾三经的合穴，具有健脾益肾、平肝养肝的作用。诸穴配伍，可调气和血，降逆息风，祛邪扶正而达预防目的。

配穴 平时痰湿重者，加丰隆、中脘；心火亢盛者，加中冲；肾阴虚甚肝阳亢盛者，加太溪、足临泣。

方法 电热针疗法，可酌情交替使用，曲池直刺0.6～0.7寸，合谷直刺0.5～0.7寸，足三里直刺0.6～0.8寸，太冲直刺0.5～0.6寸，三阴交直刺0.5～0.7寸，丰隆直刺0.6～0.8寸，中脘直刺0.5～0.7寸，太溪直刺0.4～0.5寸，足临泣直刺0.3～0.5寸，留针30～40分钟。

疗程 每日1次，10次为1个疗程，疗程间可休息5天。

（二）耳穴疗法

处方 降压沟、心、肾、肾上腺、肝。

配穴 血压过高者，加耳尖、皮质下。

regulate Qi-blood. Taichong is an important acupoint for calming liver and checking endogenous Wind. Sanyinjiao, which is a He acupoint from meridians of Liver, Spleen and Kidney, can invigorate spleen, replenish kidney, calming liver and nourish liver. Applying treatment on all acupoints may regulate Qi-blood, lower adverse Qi, check endogenous Wind, strengthen vital Qi and eliminate pathogenic factors to prevent stroke.

Matching acupoints: For phlegm-Damp, add Fenglong, Zhongwan. For flaring heart-Fire, add Zhongchong. For deficiency of kidney Yin and hyperactivity of liver Yang add Taixi, Zulinqi.

Method: Electrothermal acupuncture therapy, use alternately if it's appropriate. Perpendicular insertion into Quchi for 0.6~0.7", perpendicular insertion into Hegu for 0.5-0.7", perpendicular insertion into Zusanli 0.6-0.8for", perpendicular insertion into Taichong for 0.5-0.6", perpendicular insertion into Sanyinjiao for 0.5-0.7", perpendicular insertion into Fenglong for 0.6-0.8", perpendicular insertion into Zhongwan for 0.5-0.7", perpendicular insertion into Taixi for 0.4-0.5", perpendicular insertion into Zulinqi for 0.3~0.5", leaving the needles for 30-40 minutes.

Therapeutic course: Once a day, 10 times for a course, a break of 5 days between courses.

(II) Auricular-plaster therapy

Prescription: Groove of posterior surface, heart, kidney, paranephros, liver.

Matching acupoints: For high blood pressure, add ear apex, subcortex.

方法 采用毫针刺入，以快速捻针的治法，留针30分钟，每日1次，10次为1个疗程，亦可埋耳针。皮质下采用压耳籽法，两侧交替，每3天更换1次，7次为1个疗程，疗程间休息3天。其次，血压过高还可以在降压沟、耳尖采用三棱针放血（点刺），每日1次，至血压平稳为止，适用于高血压患者以预防中风。

（三）灸疗法

处方 足三里（ST36）。

配穴 患者有高血压配曲池，已出现中风先兆，即突然眩晕、头痛、一过性半身麻木失用、足踝酸沉者配悬钟。

方法 采用艾条温和灸法，将艾条点燃的一端距穴位皮肤3cm处施灸，待局部有温热舒适感后固定不动，每次约10～15分钟，灸至面部稍红润为度，隔日灸1次，每月灸10次。对已出现中风先兆者，或已患高血压且平素血压过高者，可采用艾炷瘢痕灸法，用黄豆或蚕豆大小的艾炷，两侧穴位各灸5～6壮，7天左右穴位处会化脓，脓液呈白色，约45天左右施灸穴位处愈合；

Method: Using the filiform needles, twisting needles rapidly, leave needles in for 30 minutes. Once a day, 10 times for a course, auricular needle-embedding therapy if necessary. Auricular Point Sticking for subcortex, two ears in turn, renew once for every 3 days, 7 times for a course, a break of 3 days between courses. For hypertensive, bloodletting (swift pricking) on ear apex and groove of posterior surface by three-edged needles once a day till blood pressure recovery to prevent stroke.

(Ⅲ) Moxibustion therapy

Prescription: Zusanli (ST36).

Matching acupoints: For high blood pressure, match Quchi, for aura of apoplexy (sudden dizziness, headache, transient hemianesthesia, apraxia, soreness of ankle), match Xuanzhong.

Method: Mild moxa-roll moxibustion, put burning point of moxa roll about 3 centimeters away from the skin to warm and fumigate the acupoint. The suitable position of the moxa roll is that the patient feels partial warm and comfortable. 10 to 15 minutes each time, and the limit is that the patient's complexion turns red, once every two days, 10 times each month. For aura of apoplexy or too high blood pressure, perform moxa-stick scarring-moxibustion, places a small cone of moxa soybean or broad bean shaped on the skin at an acupoint and burns it, 5-6 cones of moxa for each acupoint. Aseptic suppuration with white pus will be generated after 7 days and about 45 days later recovered. After the crust of scar

结痂脱落后再灸，待血压平稳，或中风先兆症状消失后，可于每年春夏、夏秋之交定期施灸。

falling, perform moxibustion again. When the patient's blood pressure is recovered to normal level or apoplectic prodrome disappeared, perform moxibustion regularly during the turns of spring and summer or summer and autumn each year.

（四）穴位贴敷疗法

处方 涌泉（KI1）。

方法 取生附子切片如五分硬币大小，放于盐水中浸泡备用，于每晚临睡前取咸附子2片，分别贴在双侧涌泉穴上，用胶布固定，翌日起床时取下，每日或隔日贴敷1次，7次为1个疗程，疗程间休息3天。此法适用于高血压患者的中风预防。

（Ⅳ）Acupoint Stiking Therapy

Prescription: Yongquan (LI1).

Method: Steep 5 cent coin sized slices of unprocessed aconite root in brine. Plaster two slices of salty aconite root to bilateral Yongquan acupoints respectively and fix it by tape before bedtime every night, withdraw it next morning. Once every day or two days, 7 times a course, a break of 3 days between courses. This method is applicable for hypertensive to prevent stroke.

二、注意事项

1. 应用电热针对预防中风有效果，因此必须听从医生指导。特别是灸法效果较好，灸法和穴位贴敷法，操作简单易于掌握，医生可以指导患者进行家庭自灸。

2. 采用艾炷瘢痕灸时，因烧灼疼痛较重，应让患者仰卧，观察患者耐受程度，防止晕灸，产生灸疮后应注意保护疮面，以防细菌感染；对出现

Ⅱ. Precautions:

1.The application of electrothermal acupuncture to prevent stroke must follow the guidance of doctors to guarantee efficacy. Even though moxibustion is particularly efficacious and easy to operate, patients must adhere to long-term treatment. Due to easy operation for moxibustion and acupoints stiking, doctors can guide the patients to do self-healing.

2.Let the patient lie at supine position due to severe "burning" pains when perform moxa-stick scarring-moxibustion. Check whether the patient can bear the pain and prevent fainting during moxibustion. Protect the post-moxibustion sore to prevent infections. Infected pa-

细菌感染者（脓液由白色变为黄绿色）可按外科感染处理，对灸后不化脓者，可于原处续灸，并嘱患者多食用含蛋白质的食物。

3. 应注意饮食、起居、情志的影响，合理调节，以巩固针灸预防中风的效果。

三、现代研究

1. 辨证施灸治疗原发性高血压及预防中风的临床研究。

据文献报道，临床观察原发性高血压患者105例，采用随机分组的方法，分为观察组与对照组。两组辨证分型情况近似，观察组63例分为4型，阴虚阳亢型取穴足三里、蠡沟，阴阳两虚型取穴足三里、三阴交，痰湿型取足三里、丰隆，肝热型取足三里、太冲，每日灸1次，共灸3个月；对照组43例，继服中西药物，耳穴压丸22例，对照组观察3个月。结果显示：①灸治后，收缩压、舒张压均有下降，与对照组比较有显著差异，且对高血压有双向调节作用，使血压保持相对稳定，提示有预防

tients (The pus changes from white to yellow-green.) can be treated by surgical infection. For patients without suppuration, repeat scarring-moxibustion at original point and ask patients to have more rich protein food.

3.The patients should pay attention to regulation of diet, daily life, work and leisure balance to enhance efficacy of acupuncture on stroke prevention.

Ⅲ. Modern research

1.Apply acupuncture for primary high blood pressure based on the principles of Traditional Chinese Medicine "syndrome differentiation", clinical research on stroke prevention.

According to the descriptions in literatures, 105 primary high blood pressure patients were divided randomly into two groups: control group and observation group. Two groups have nearly the same differentiation of syndrome. 63 patients in observation group can be classified into 4 types. For Yin deficiency and Yang hyperactivity, use acupoints Zusanli, Ligou. For Yin and Yang deficiency, use Zusanli, Sanyinjiao. For phlegm Damp, use Zusanli, Fenglong. For liver Heat, use Zusanli, Taichong. Moxibustion once a day for 3 months. Patients in control group took traditional Chinese Herb Medicine and Western Medicine with 22 cases by auricular acupoint seed-pressing therapy. After 3 months observation, the results show: ① Patients' both systolic pressure and diastolic blood pressure decreased after moxibustion. Compared with the control group, there were significant differences, and there was a bidirectional regulation ef-

中风的作用和价值。②灸治后，纤维蛋白原明显下降，与对照组比较有显著差异。FDP高值者下降，低值者上升，两者变化保持血凝和纤维蛋白系统的平衡，有效预防了中风的发生。③灸治后，血液黏稠度中，全血比黏度与对照组比较有明显下降，对改善血液循环起了一定作用。④灸治后，部分病例眼底有一定变化，推测脑血管会有相应地改善，为预防中风提供了依据。

2. 艾灸足三里对血浆蛋白原及纤维蛋白降解产物的影响观察。

选择47例诊断为Ⅲ期高血压合并脑血栓形成恢复期的患者。取双侧足三里用艾条施灸，每次灸20分钟，每灸2～3次，10次为1个疗程。艾灸后足三里处起泡者共33例（相当于Ⅰ度烧伤），灸疮在直径1cm以上者26例，0.5cm以下者11例。结果显示：16例血浆蛋白原高于正常值者，灸后明显下降（$P<0.05$）；34例纤维蛋白降解产物高于正常值者，治疗后下降（$P<0.05$）。提示

fect on high blood pressure, which kept the blood pressure relatively stable, proving efficacy on preventing stroke. ② After moxibustion treatment, the fibrinogen was significantly decreased, which was significantly different from that of the control group. FDP high value decreases, low value increases; both changes maintain the balance of blood coagulation and fibrin system, which effectively prevent the occurrence of stroke. ③ The total blood ratio in blood viscosity after moxibustion treatment was significantly decreased compared with that of the control group, which took certain effect on improving blood circulation. ④ After the moxibustion therapy, there is a certain change in the eye base of some patients, and it is speculated that the cerebral blood vessels can be improved, providing proofs for preventing stroke.

2.Effect observation of moxibustion over acupoint Zusanli regarding plasma protein and fibrin degradation products.

Selected 47 patients in recovery phase diagnosed as Ⅲ period high blood pressure with cerebral thrombosis. Perform moxibustion on bilateral acupoints Zusanli, 20 minutes each time, 2 or 3 times each moxibustion, 10 times a course. 33 cases with blisters on Zusanli after moxibustion (equivalent to a first degree burn). There are 26 cases with post-moxibustion sore whose diameter is more than 1 centimeter, 11 cases with the sore whose diameter is less than 0.5 centimeter. The results show 16 patients whose plasma protein was higher than normal at the beginning got significantly decreased value ($P<0.05$) after moxibustion; 34 patients whose fibrin degradation products level was higher than normal got decreased val-

对已患中风恢复期的患者有预防复发的作用。

ue after treatment ($P < 0.05$). It indicates that moxibustion have efficacy of preventing recurrence of stroke for apoplexy patients in recovery phase.

预防感冒

感冒是因风寒邪病毒侵袭人体后而引发，以头痛、鼻塞流涕或恶寒、发热等为主要症状的外感疾病。本病一年四季均可发生，尤其是在春冬两季，更为多见，而且不分男女老幼。感受外邪是本病的主要发病因素，但机体抗病能力的下降，也是导致本病不可忽视的内在因素。老年人、婴幼儿和素体虚弱者比常人更易患感冒，不但症状重，且有转变为其他疾病的可能，因此对易感人群采取积极的预防措施，有着重要的意义。

Cold Prevention

Cold is caused by invasion of external Wind-Cold pathogen. It's an exogenous disease with symptoms of headache, stuffy nose, aversion to cold and pyrexia. This disease can occur all the year round especially in spring and winter regardless of male, female, young and old. Invasion of external pathogen is the main cause, but the immunity is the non-negligible internal factor. Infants, older people, young children and the weak are more likely to catch a cold than others, who have not only severe symptoms but also possibility of transformation to other diseases. Therefore it's significantly important to take active prevention measures before the disease occurrence.

一、预防方法

（一）电热针疗法或毫针疗法

处方 大椎（GV14）、风门（BL13）、足三里（ST36）。

方义 大椎为督脉穴，并为诸阳之会，有振奋阳气、通阳解表的作用，是预防感冒的经验要穴；风门隶属于足太阳

Ⅰ. Prevention Methods

（Ⅰ）Electrothermal acupuncture therapy or filiform needle therapy

Prescription: Dazhui(GV14), Fengmen(BL13), Zusanli(ST36).

Mechanism of prescription: Dazhui is the acupoint of Du Collateral and the confluent acupoint of all Yangs. It can invigorate Yang Qi, clear Heat and relieve exterior syndrome. Dazhui is the important acupoint to prevent

膀胱经，膀胱主一身之表，针刺风门可卫外固表，抵御外邪侵入；足三里为全身强壮要穴，可增强机体抗病祛邪能力。诸穴合用，有宣行卫气、固表强身的功效。

方法 大椎向下斜刺0.5～0.7寸，风门向脊柱方向斜刺0.5寸，足三里直刺0.6～0.8寸，以上诸穴一般情况下电热针50mA（毫针平补平泻手法）；体虚易汗出者用补法，电热针60mA（毫针提插补法）每针30～40分钟。

（二）灸疗法

1. 艾条灸

处方 身柱（GV12）。

方法 制成烟卷大小的艾条，用火点燃一端，对准穴位，距皮肤3cm左右固定不动，灸至皮肤红晕为度，约5～10分钟，在春冬易患感冒季节，每日1次，每月灸5～7次即可，此法适用于婴幼儿。

2. 隔姜灸

处方 风门（BL12）、肺俞（BL13）。

cold. Fengmen belongs to the meridian acupoint of Tai-Yang Bladder Meridian of Foot, and bladder masters the exterior syndrome of the whole body. Acupuncture of Fengmen can guard the surface of the body against exopathogen. Zusanli is an important tonifying acupoint and can eliminate pathogenic factors. The use of combination of these acupoints can invigorate Wei Qi and guard the surface of the body.

Method: Obliquely puncture downward into Dazhui for 0.5-0.7", obliquely puncture into Fengmen towards spine for 0.5", perpendicular insertion into Zusanli for 0.6-0.8", apply a current of 50mA (mild tonifying and attenuating for filiform needle). For patients of deficiency and easily sweaty, apply the method of tonifying, electrothermal acupuncture with 60mA(lifting and thrusting tonifying method for filiform needle), leaving the needles in for 30-40 minutes.

(II) Moxibustion therapy

1. Moxibustion with moxa roll

Prescription: Shenzhu (GV12).

Method: Make moxa into a cigar-shaped stick, put burning point of moxa stick about 3 centimeters away from the surface of the skin to warm and fumigate the acupoint until the skin is flushed, about 5-10 minutes. Once a day during spring and winter when it is easy to catch cold, 5-7 times each month. This method is applicable for infants.

2. Ginger-separated moxibustion

Prescription: Fengmen (BL12), Feishu(BL13).

方法　取新鲜生姜一块，切成厚约0.3cm的薄片，用针在姜片中心穿刺数孔，放在穴位皮肤上，其上放置黄豆大小艾炷，用火点燃施灸，每次可灸10～15壮，以灸至局部温热舒适、皮肤潮红为度。每日1次，连续灸5～7天即可。适用于体虚易感冒者，常于感冒流行时在人群中普遍推广使用。

(三) 梅花针疗法

处方　颈部前后、鼻窦部、前额部、颞部。

方法　取梅花针，在以上部位每侧3～4行，每行隔1cm，前额及颞部轻度扣刺，额部前后重度扣刺，鼻翼部中度扣刺。

二、注意事项

1. 针灸预防感冒，有经济简便、效果可靠的优点。

2. 针刺胸部腧穴时，要严格掌握针刺深度，不要过深，避免发生气胸；采用灸法时，应避免造成皮肤烫伤。

3. 体质虚弱之人应加强身体锻炼，劳逸结合，寒温调适，配以针灸预防。

Method: Cut fresh ginger into pieces of 0.3cm thick, puncture into the center of ginger slice for several holes and put it on the acupoint, put the soybean sized moxa cone on ginger slice and burn it. 10-15 cones of moxa for each moxibustion. The limit is that patient feels warm and comfortable, and the skin turns red. Once a day, 5-7 days a course. It's applicable for the deficiency patients who are easier to catch cold or widely used in flu season.

(Ⅲ) Plum-blossom needle therapy

Prescription: Back and front of neck, paranasal sinus, forehead, tempus

Method: Puncture into positions mentioned above, 3-4 rows each side, line space is 1 centimeter, mild manipulation on forehead and tempus, forceful manipulation on frontal part, moderate manipulation on nose-wing.

Ⅱ. Precautions

1. Acupuncture and moxibustion are economic efficacious and convenient methods to prevent cold.

2. When applying acupuncture over acupoints on the chest, the angle and depth of application is strictly regulated. Excessive perpendicular insertion is prohibited to avoid pneumothorax. Avoid scald during moxibustion.

3. People with weak physique should strengthen the physical exercise, balance work and rest, apply acupuncture to prevent cold.

三、现代临床研究

1. 针刺预防流行性感冒1090例。

某校园于某年5月29日开始流行本病,至同年7月2日达高峰,在1449人中,发病率为23.4%,预防措施从7月2日开始,7月8日流行停止,针刺预防共1090例,取穴足三里(双侧)行弱刺激手法,每针30分钟,针刺感应达足趾部,每人仅针1次,针后发病者39例,发病率为3.6%。

2. 梅花针预防流行性感冒60例。

选在感冒流行地区居住的60例小学生,进行分组。第一组35人,每人治疗1次;第二组10人,每天1次连续治疗2天;第三组15人,每天1次,连续治疗3天;另有240人做对照组。具体操作方法为:①刺激部位,取颈前后及鼻翼部,配合前额及颞部,采用双侧刺法,每侧3～4行,每行隔1cm;②刺激强度,额前部及颞部用轻刺激,颈部前后用重刺激,鼻翼部用中度刺激,刺激时要分清部位界线;③对针具及刺激部位的皮肤进行严

III. Modern clinical study

1. 1090 cases of influenza prevention by acupuncture.

On May 29 X year, influenza occurred in some campus, reaches to a peak on July 2. The incidence was 23.4% among 1449 persons. The preventive measures were taken from July 2, and the epidemic of flu was stopped on July 8. 1090 prevention cases received acupuncture. Mild puncture into acupoint Zusanli on both sides, 30 minutes per puncture. The needling sensation should reach toe site. Only one puncture for each person, 39 cases of reoccurrence after puncture, the incidence was 3.6%.

2. 60 cases of influenza prevention by Plum-blossom needle therapy.

60 patients are primary school students living in epidemic area of flu. Method: 35 patients in Group 1, 1 time treatment per person; 10 patients in Group 2, once a day for two days; 15 patients in Group 3, once a day for 3 days; there were 240 patients in control group. Operation: ① Acupuncture positions: Puncture on back and front of neck, nose wing, along with forehead and tempus. Bilateral puncture with 3 ~4 lines on each side, 1 centimeter line space. ② Manipulation intensity: Mild manipulation on forehead and tempus, forceful manipulation on neck, moderate manipulation on nose-wing. Distinguish the boundary of each side during puncture. ③ Perform strict disinfection for skin and needles. Result: 60 cases in prevention group, 3 influenza cases after half month observation, the incidence is only 5%

格消毒。结果显示：预防组60例，通过半个月观察，发病者3例，发病率仅为5%，其中发病轻微者，1～2日自愈。未行梅花针者240例，在同一时间的发病率达30%以上。

(slight symptoms and self-healing after 1 or 2 days). The incidence is more than 30% in 240 cases without Plum-blossom needle treatment.

预防流行性腮腺炎

流行性腮腺炎是腮腺病毒引起的一种急性传染病，以耳下腺部非化脓性肿胀疼痛为主要特征。多流行于冬春两季，儿童多见，成人亦可发生，但病情较儿童为重，也有伴发睾丸炎和脑膜炎者。

中医学成本病为"痄腮"，俗称"虾蟆瘟""含腮疮"等，多由感受时邪与胃火上攻，壅滞于少阳、阳明经而成，在流行季节和地区，对未患本病的儿童采用针灸预防措施，可预防本病的发生。

Mumps Prevention

Mumps is an acute infectious disease caused by parotid gland virus, whose main symptom is nonsuppurative swelling and pain in parotid gland. It's usually epidemic in winter and spring, mostly seen in children, some in adult as well. But the syndrome in children is more severe, sometimes along with comorbid orchitis and meningitis.

In Traditional Chinese Medicine this disease is called "mumps", common known as "Ha Ma Pestilence", "Cheek Boil of Newbor", etc. All the factors, affecting of seasonal pathogenic factors, blazing up of stomach Fire, stagnation in Shao-Yang and Yang-Ming Meridians, may cause mumps. Acupuncture therapy as prevention measures for children not infected by mumps may prevent this disease.

一、预防方法

（一）毫针疗法

处方 合谷（LI4）。

方义 合谷是手阳明经原穴，具有疏通手足阳明经络，清热泻火的功效，又为防治头

Ⅰ. Prevention Methods

（Ⅰ）Filiform needle therapy

Prescription: Hegu (LI4).

Mechanism of prescription: Hegu is the Yuan acupoint from Yang-Ming Meridian of Hand, which is a key acupoint preventing and curing diseases in face and

面疾患的要穴，故针刺合谷可以预防本病的发生。

方法 常规消毒，选双侧合谷直刺 0.5～0.7 寸，得气后留针 30 分钟，间歇行针 3～4 次。如幼儿不配合可不留针，进针 3 分钟，提插 1 分钟即可出针，每日 1 次。

（二）灸疗法

处方 角孙（TE20）、翳风（TE17）。

方法 艾条灸防治流行性腮腺炎，取艾条一支点燃一端，在距穴位皮肤 3cm 处施灸，使局部达到温热而舒适为度，灸 15 分钟，每日灸 1 次，两个穴交替应用。

二、现代临床研究

某幼儿园有幼儿 183 人，1977 年 5 月发生第 1 例流行性腮腺炎，之后病例逐月上升，至同年 7 月上旬已有 70 人患本病，占总数的 38.2%。7 月 9 日对在园的 95 例未发病的幼儿用艾条灸双侧角孙穴各 1 次，疫情迅速下降，92 例幼儿未发本病；另 3 例在施灸后在 15 天

head. Hegu can soothe Yang-Ming Meridians of Hand and Foot, clear Heat and purge Fire. Therefore, applying acupuncture therapy to Hegu can prevent mumps.

Method: Perform routine disinfection, select bilateral Hegu acupoints and perpendicular insertion for 0.5-0.7", leave the needles in for 30 minutes after Qi acquisition, intermittent manipulating needles for 3-4 times. No need to retain needles if children cannot cooperate for treatment, insert for 3 minutes and lifting-thrusting for 1 minute then withdraw needles. Once a day.

(Ⅱ) Moxibustion therapy

Prescription: Jiaosun (TE20), Yifeng (TE17).

Method: Moxibustion with moxa roll to prevent mumps. Burn moxa roll and put the burning point towards acupoints 3 centimeters over the skin. Comfortably warm and fumigate the acupoints for 15 minutes. Once a day, apply on two acupoints in turn.

II. Modern clinical study

In May 1977 the first mumps case occurred in one kindergarten where there were 183 children. Later the number of cases increased month by month. There were 70 children infected in the first third of July, account for 38.2% of total. After moxibustion was applied on bilateral acupoints Jiaosun for one time for 95 children not infected by mumps on July 9th, the outbreak of mumps went down. 92 children were not attacked by the disease and 3 children got slight symptom including slight

内先后出现轻微症状,如腮轻痛、微肿,但不发热,吃饭玩耍如前,经艾灸耳根翳风穴1次后痊愈,艾条灸防治腮腺炎的复发率为3.2%;另有18例幼儿,在本病流行期间,先后接回家中未做预防性施灸,其中有3例在7月中下旬分别患本病,高热达39℃以上,发病率为16.6%,说明本法可作为防治腮腺炎之法。

防治痢疾

痢疾是夏秋季节流行的肠道疾病之一,临床以腹痛、里急后重、便脓血为主要特征,严重者会出现昏迷、休克,甚至危及生命,食入或饮入被痢疾杆菌污染的食物或饮料为主要发病因素。防止病从口入,注意饮食卫生,是预防痢疾的重要措施。电热针从提高机体抗病能力角度出发,作为在痢疾流行地区和季节对曾与痢疾患者密切接触的人群而采取的一种有效的预防措施,经济简便,效果可靠,常优于药物治疗,值得推广应用。

swelling and pain in cheek but no fever within 15 days after moxibustion; they could eat and play as usual. These 3 infected children were cured by moxibustion for one time on acupoint Yifeng. The reoccurrence rate is 3.2% on mumps prevention and treatment by moxibustion. Besides, there were 18 children back home and no moxibustion treatment at home. 3 of them were attacked by mumps respectively with fever of 39 degrees in the third and second third of July. The incidence was 16.6%, which proved moxibustion could be used for mumps prevention.

Dysentery Prevention

Dysentery is one of the epidemic bowel diseases in summer and autumn. The main clinical symptoms are abdominal pain, tenesmus, stool containing pus and blood. Coma and shock may occur for severe infected patients, which would be life threatening. Food or drinks infected by dysentery bacillus are the main risky factors. Preventing illness finding the way in by mouth and paying attention to dietary health, are key prevention measures. Electrothermal acupuncture which can reinforce immunity is an efficacious prevention measure for people who have close contact with dysenteric patients in epidemic areas or seasons. The operation of electrothermal acupuncture is simple and continent, and the efficacy is reliable, better than that of drug therapy. This therapy is worth being promoted.

一、预防方法

(一) 电热针疗法或毫针疗法

处方 足三里（ST36）、上巨虚（ST37）、合谷（LI4）。

方义 足三里是足阳明胃经合穴，是调理胃肠、防止胃肠疾病的有效穴之一；上巨虚为胃经穴，又是大肠下合穴，具有通滞清肠、健脾益气的作用；合谷是手阳明大肠经原穴，除调理大肠外还可通条全身气机。诸穴合用，可通调肠胃、健身御邪。

方法 选定穴位，皮肤常规消毒，针直刺足三里0.5～0.8寸，上巨虚直刺0.5～0.8寸，合谷直刺0.3～0.5寸，接通电热针仪，分别给予每个穴60mA电流，使患者感到穴位处有舒适温热感为度，留针30～40分钟，每日1次。毫针给予中度刺激，平补平泻手法，留针30分钟。

I. Prevention Method

(I) Electrothermal acupuncture therapy or filiform needle therapy

Prescription: Zusanli (ST36), Shangjuxu (ST37), Hegu (LI4).

Mechanism of prescription: Zusanli is a He acupoint of Stomach Meridian and Yang-Ming Meridian of Foot, a key tonifying acupoint. It's one of the effective acupoints to tonify stomach and intestine and prevent gastrointestinal diseases. Shangjuxu is the acupoint of Stomach Meridian and He acupoint of Large Intestine, which can soothe stagnation, clean intestine, invigorate spleen and tonify Qi. Hegu is a Yuan acupoint from Large Intestine Meridian, which can nourish Qi of the whole body and regulate large intestine. The use of combination of these acupoints can soothe the stomach and intestine, improve bodyhealth, and remove pathogenic factors.

Method: Selecting the relevant acupoints, perform routine skin disinfection. Using electrothermal acupuncture needles, perpendicular insertion into Zusanli for 0.5-0.8", perpendicular insertion into Shangjuxu for 0.5-0.8", perpendicular insertion into Hegu for 0.3-0.5", turn on the electrothermal acupuncture equipment, apply a current of 60-70mA to each acupoint, the limit is that the patient feels warm and comfortable. Leave the needles for in 30-40 minutes. Once a day. Moderate stimulation for filiform needle acupuncture (use the method of mild reinforcing and attenuating). Leave the needles for 30 minutes.

（二）灸疗法

处方 天枢（ST25）、关元（CV4）、足三里（ST36）。

方法 选艾条灸，将艾条一端点燃，在距穴位上皮肤3cm左右处施灸，使患者感到有温热舒适为度，灸5～10分钟左右，每日1次，连续治疗3～5天即可。

（三）隔盐灸

处方 神阙（CV8）。

方法 将纯细盐末纳入脐中，将脐窝填平，上面置放黄豆大小的艾炷，用火点燃，燃尽换另1柱，连灸10～15壮，每日1次，连灸7天即可。

二、注意事项

1. 电热针或毫针预防痢疾，多在痢疾流行季节或密切接触了痢疾患者后应用。

2. 对多年反复发作的慢性菌痢患者，在发作前采用上述针法及灸法均有预防作用。

3. 采用灸法时，应注意避免烫伤皮肤，或烧坏衣服等。

(Ⅱ) Moxibustion therapy

Prescription: Tianshu(ST25), Guanyuan (CV4), Zusanli(ST36).

Method: Burn moxa roll and put the burning point towards acupoints 3 centimeters over the skin. Comfortably warm and fumigate the acupoints for 5 to 10 minutes. Once a day, 3 to 5 days consecutive treatment.

(Ⅲ) Salt suspension-moxibustion

Prescription: Shenque(CV 8).

Method: Place fine salt dust on navel and fill it in. Put soybean sized moxa cone on navel, burn it and renew one after burnout, 10 to 15 cones per moxibustion. Once a day, 7 days consecutive moxibustion treatment.

Ⅱ. Precautions:

1. Electrothermal acupuncture treatment or filiform needle treatment is frequently used for people who have close contact with dysenteric patients or in epidemic seasons.

2. Acupuncture methods mentioned above can prevent the disease for long years of repeated onset of chronic bacillary dysentery before its onset.

3. Avoid skin and clothes burns during moxibustion.

减肥

肥胖症是指人体脂肪积聚过多而造成体重超重的疾病。引起肥胖症的原因很多，概括起来有三个方面，一是外源性肥胖，由过量饮食引起，又称"营养性肥胖"；二是内源性肥胖，多由体内代谢或内分泌紊乱造成，如垂体性肥胖、肾上腺皮质机能亢进性肥胖、甲状腺机能减退性肥胖、性腺机能不足性肥胖、多源性肥胖等；三是内外源混合性肥胖。

肥胖的临床表现，一般可分为单纯性肥胖和继发性肥胖两类。前者脂肪分布较均匀，男性表现为多血型肥胖，即体质发育好，肌肉强壮，血色素正常或略高，耳唇常充血，颈粗厚，腹膨隆，很少有其他营养不良的症状；女性多表现贫血型肥胖，脂肪组织松弛，脉搏细小，贫血貌，体力弱，易于心慌气短，食欲差，不愿吃肉食，常伴有蛋白质缺乏、缺铁性等营养不良的症状。由于肥胖程度不同，临床表现各异，轻者可无任何症状，肥胖显著者因体重超重而耗氧量较正常者常增加30%～40%，故

Antiobesity

Obesity is a disease caused by accumulation of excess body fat that results in overweight. Several factors would cause obesity, summarized in three aspects: First is exogenous obesity caused by overeating, also called "nutritional obesity"; second is endogenous obesity mostly caused by disorder of metabolism or endocrine, such as pituitary obesity, adrenocortical hypertrophy obesity, hypothyroidism obesity, hypogonadism obesity, multiple sources obesity, etc.; third is hybrid internal and external source obesity.

The clinical manifestations of obesity can be divided into two types: simple obesity and secondary obesity. The fat is equally distributed in simple obesity. The disease for male is multi-blood type obesity: well developed physique, strong muscles, normal or slightly high the blood pigment level, hyperaemia in ear and lip, thick neck, bulged abdomen, rarely malnutrition syndrome. The disease for women is anemia obesity: flabby adipose tissue, small pulse, anemia, weak physical strength, easily flustered and short of breath, poor appetite, unwilling to have meat, often along with adverse syndrome such as lack of protein, iron-deficiency malnutrition. Clinical symptoms are quite different due to varying degrees of obesity. In mild case it may have no symptom. In serious case due to overweight the patients' oxygen consumption is often increased by 30% - 40%, therefore they often fear heat, sweat, easy fatigue, unable to take physical

常畏热、多汗、易疲乏、不能承受体力劳动，并有头痛、头晕、心慌、气短、腹胀、下肢浮肿等症。检查有端坐呼吸、血压升高、皮肤痤疮、平足等。继发性肥胖，脂肪分布不匀，如肾上腺皮质机能亢进时，为向心性肥胖，表现为躯干胖、四肢细。男性机能不全性肥胖则出现臀部、大腿脂肪积聚多，乳房大，伴有各类代谢内分泌紊乱的表现。由于肥胖症患者较正常体重者抵抗力低，常易患动脉硬化、高血压、心血管病、胆结石、糖尿病、肝硬化、关节退行性病变等疾病，且预后较差。通过人群死亡统计，肥胖者患心、脑、肾、血管疾病的死亡率明显高于体重正常和偏瘦的人群。

随着社会的进步以及预防、保健医学的发展，人们对肥胖影响形体美及危害人体健康的认识日益加深，多种多样的减肥方法应运而生。针灸减肥是20多年前兴起的一种新的减肥方法，经过临床验证效果较好。尤其近10年来，采用电热针疗法减肥取得了较好的疗效，且方法简便，无副作用，值得提倡推广。

work, along with headache, dizziness, palpitations, shortness of breath, abdominal distension, swollen limbs; examination shows orthopnea, elevation of blood pressure, acne, flat foot. Fat distribution is not equal in secondary obesity. When adrenocortical hormone is hyperfunctional, it's centripetal obesity with symptoms of fat truncus, thin limbs. The symptoms of male insufficiency functions obesity includes fat accumulating in thigh and buttocks, big breast, along with some symptoms of metabolic endocrine disorder. Obesity patients' immunity are poorer than healthy people, along with some complications such as arteriosclerosis, high blood pressure, cardiovascular disease, gallstones, diabetes, cirrhosis of the liver, joints degenerative diseases, etc. The prognosis of obesity patients is not good. From people death statistics, the death rate of obesity patients who suffer from heart, brain, kidney, vascular disease is obviously higher than that of the normal physique and the thinner.

With development of society, prevention and health medicine, people have increasingly known that obesity would affect physical beauty and harm to health. A variety of methods to reduce weight arises. Acupuncture to lose weight created nearly 20 years ago, is a new kind of method for reducing weight, proven good efficacy by clinical application. Especially in the past 10 years electro thermal acupuncture therapy has got better efficacy without side effect. Its operation is simple and worth being promoted.

中医认为，肥胖与患者恣食肥甘有密切联系，而胃火亢盛、脾虚湿滞、肾虚是本病发病的内在因素。

一、辨证要点

1. 胃中蕴热证。饮食较多，大便干结，口渴溲黄，口臭难闻，颈粗厚，腹膨隆，肌肉组织结实，血压有时偏高，舌红苔黄厚，脉数有力。

2. 脾虚湿滞证。饮食不多，倦怠嗜睡，动则气短，口不渴或渴不欲饮，小便少，大便溏薄，脂肪组织多而松弛，肌肉组织少而虚弱，舌淡而胖，边有齿痕，脉濡缓而无力。

3. 肾虚证。饮食一般，大便尚好或不成形，小便频数，腰酸膝软，女子月经不调，经量少或闭经，男子阳痿早泄，腹部、臀部胖而松弛，乳房肥大，舌淡而胖，脉沉细或濡细。

二、治疗方法

（一）电热针疗法或毫针疗法

1. 胃中蕴热证

处方　内庭（ST44）、曲

Traditional Chinese Medicine believes that obesity is highly related with patients' diet. Some internal factors such as exuberance of stomach Fire, spleen deficiency and Damp stagnation, and kidney deficiency are related factors for the disease attacks.

I. Key Points for Syndrome differentiation

Syndrome of Heat within stomach: Eat and drink too much, dry and hard stool, thirsty, yellowish urine, ozostomia, thick neck, bulged belly, strong muscle, high blood pressure sometimes, red tongue with thick and yellow fur, powerful pulse.

Syndrome of spleen deficiency and Damp stagnation: Eat less, tired and sleepy, shortness of breath when move, not thirsty or thirsty but unwilling to drink, less urine, sloppy and thin stool, rich adipose tissue but flabby, less muscle and weak, light tougue with teeth marks, weak and slow pulse.

Kidney deficiency syndrome: Simple diet, shapeless stool, frequent urination, aching lumbus and limp knees, menoxenia, scanty period or amenorrhea, asynodia, premature ejaculation, fat and flabby belly and hip, breast hypertrophy, light and fat tongue, soft and thin pulse.

II. Therapeutic Methods

(I) Electrothermal acupuncture therapy or filiform needle therapy

1. Syndrome of Heat within stomach

Prescription: Neiting(ST44), Quchi(LI11), Zhigou

池（LI11）、支沟（TE6）、大横（SP15）。(TE6), Daheng (SP15).

方义 内庭是胃经荥穴，可清泄胃火；曲池是大肠经合穴，泄热通腑；支沟是三焦经经穴，可泄三焦相火而通便，是治肠燥便秘之要穴；大横隶属于脾经位于腹部，可助大肠传导以通便。诸穴配伍，胃热得清而饮食减少，肠中积热得消而泻胃火，共奏减肥之功效。

Mechanism of prescription: Neiting is a Xing acupoint of the stomach meridian, clear stomach and disperse Heat; Quchi is a He acupoint from Large Intestine Meridian, clean Heat and soothe internal organs; Zhigou is the acupoint of San-Jiao Meridian and can disper Sanjiao Heat to promote defecation, which is a key acupoint for treatment of intestinal Dryness with constipation; Daheng belongs to spleen channel located in belly, support large intestine transmission to promote defecation. All the combination of these acupoints can be used together. Stomach Heat is cleared so as to reduce diet, intestine Heat and stomach Fire are cleared, and therefore it can reduce weight.

操作 内庭向上斜刺0.5寸，曲池直刺0.7～0.8寸，支沟斜刺0.4～0.6寸，大横直刺0.5～0.7寸，得气后接通电热针仪，分别每个穴位给予30～40mA电流（毫针给予泻法），留针30～40分钟，以患者感到胀而舒适为度。

Operations: Obliquely puncture upward into Neiting for 0.5", perpendicular insertion into Quchi for 0.7-0.8", obliquely puncture into Zhigou for 0.4-0.6", perpendicular insertion into Daheng for 0.5-0.7", after Qi acquired, turn on the electrothermal acupuncture equipment, apply a current of 30-40mA to each acupoint(reducing method for filiform needle), leave needles in for 30-40 minutes, the limit is the patient feels swell and comfortable.

疗程 每日或隔日1次，10次为1个疗程，疗程间可休息3天。

Therapeutic course: Once a day or two days, 10 times a course, a break of 3 days between courses.

2. 脾虚湿滞证

处方 脾俞（BL20）、章门（LR13）、阴陵泉（SP9）、水分（CV9）、天枢（ST25）。

2. Syndrome of spleen deficiency and Damp stagnation

Prescriptions: Pishu(BL20), Zhangmen(LR13), Yinlingquan(SP9), Shuifen(CV9), Tianshu(ST25).

方义 脾俞、章门分别为脾之背俞穴与腹募穴，二穴为俞募配穴，是健脾益气常用穴；阴陵泉为脾经合穴，可健脾化湿、通利三焦；水分是任脉穴，助小肠泌别清浊，利水道以通小便；天枢为募穴，刺之可调大肠传导而实大便。诸穴合用健脾气以助水湿运化，利小便而使其有出路，水湿得清则浮肿肥胖自消。

配穴 动则气短者加内关，自幼肥胖者加肾俞、三阴交。

方法 脾俞向脊柱方向斜刺 0.6～0.8 寸，章门刺 0.6～0.8 寸，得气后接通电热针仪分别给予电流 50～60mA，以患者感到温热或胀或舒适为度；阴陵泉直刺 0.4～0.6 寸，水分直刺 0.5～0.8 寸，天枢直刺 0.5～0.8 寸，得气后给予接通电热针仪，分别给予电流 20～30mA，以感觉胀而舒适为度；肾俞直刺 0.6～0.8 寸，三阴交直刺 0.5～0.8 寸，得气后给予接通电热针仪，分别给

Mechanism of prescription: Pishu, Zhangmen are respectively the Back-Shu acupoint of the Spleen and the Mu acupoint, both of them are the method of Shu-Mu acupoints combination as well as the commonly-used acupoints invigorating spleen and replenishing Qi; Yinlingquan acupoint is the He point of Spleen Meridian, can invigorate the spleen for eliminating Damp, and unchoke three Jiaos. Shuifen is the acupoint of Ren Channel, helps small intestine separate the useful from the waste and alleviate urine retention; Tianshu is Mu acupoint, can be punctured to adjust large intestine's function and to cure diarrhea. Joint using of these acupoints can help strengthen Qi of the spleen to transport and transform Water-Damp, induce diuresis, and the edema and the obesity would be cured.

Matching acupoints: Additionally select Neiguan for ones breathing short for movement, select Shenshu and Sanyinjiao for ones being obese from a child.

Methods: Obliquely puncture Pishu for 0.6-0.8" toward the patient's spine, Zhangmen for 0.6-0.8". After arrival of Qi, turn on the electrothermal acupuncture apparatus and apply the electric current 50-60mA respectively to the extent that patients feel warm or swelling or comfortable; perpendicularly puncture Yinlingquan for 0.4-0.6", Shuifen for 0.5-0.8", Tianshu for 0.5-0.8". After arrival of Qi, turn on electrothermal acupuncture apparatus and apply the current 20-30mA respectively to the extent that patients feel swelling and comfort; perpendicularly puncture Shenshu for 0.6-0.8", perpendicularly puncture Sanyinjiao for 0.5-0.8". After arrival of Qi, turn on the electrothermal acupuncture apparatus and apply the current 60mA (for Shenshu) or 30mA (for Sanyinjiao) respectively to the extent that patients feel swelling and comfortable, then apply electrothermal needle for 30-40 minutes.

Therapeutic course: 1 time every day, 10 times per course of treatment, 3 days interval between courses

3. Kidney deficiency syndrome

Prescription: Shenshu(BL23), Mingmen(GV4), Guanyuan(CV 4), Sanyinjiao(SP6).

Mechanism of prescription: Shenshu is the acupoint where the Qi of kidney is infused into the back. Mingmen is attached to the Du Channel between two Shenshus and is the gate of life. Guanyuan attaching to the Ren Channel is a key acupoint for the strong body. Sanyinjiao attaching to the Spleen Channel is the intersection acupoint of liver, spleen and kidney. The joint application of these acupoints may tonify kidney and strengthen Yang, reinforce vital essence and foundation, and replenish vitality, nurse Chong Channel and Ren Channel to lose weight.

Matching acupoints: Additionally select Shimen and Ququan for postpartum obesity.

Methods: Perpendicularly puncture Shenshu for 0.5-0.8", perpendicularly puncture Mingmen for 0.4-0.6", perpendicularly puncture Guanyuan for 0.5-0.8", perpendicularly puncture Sanyinjiao for 0.5-0.7", perpendicularly puncture Shimen for 0.5-0.8", perpendicularly puncture Ququan for 0.5- 0.8". After arrival of Qi, turn on the electrothermal acupuncture instrument and apply the current 60-70mA respectively to the extent that

电针 30～40 分钟。

疗程 每日 1 次，10 次为 1 个疗程，疗程间休息 3 天，（毫针施补法）。

（二）耳针疗法

处方 口、脾、肾、胃、内分泌、脑点、丘脑、肾上腺。

配穴 交感、卵巢、皮质下。

方法 每次选 3～4 个穴（亦可用耳针探测仪选敏感点进行治疗），耳穴埋针法、耳穴压籽法、耳穴毫针治法，采用针刺泻法，毫针 30 分钟，两侧耳交替，每日 1 次，10 次为 1 疗程，疗程间休息 5 天；耳穴埋针法和耳穴压籽法，先选一侧耳穴，压 3～5 天，每日令患者自行按压数次，每穴按压 1 分钟，待取下耳穴的针或籽后，换另侧耳穴，左右耳穴交替，10 次为 1 个疗程，疗程间休息 1 周，一般需坚持 1～2 个疗程。对严重肥胖者，要坚持 3～4 个疗程。

patients feel swelling and comfortable, then keep electrothermal acupuncture for 30-40 minutes.

Therapeutic course: 1 time every day, 10 times per course of treatment, 3 days interval between courses, (apply the reinforcing method with filiform needles).

(Ⅱ) Auriculotherapy

Prescription: Mouth, spleen, kidney, stomach, endocrine acupoint, Central Rim (Brain), thalamus, adrenal gland.

Matching acupoints: Sympathetic, ovary, subcortex.

Methods: Select 3-4 acupoints each time (acupuncture may also be applied at sensitive points with an auriculo-acupuncture detector), apply auricular embedding acupuncture, sticking and pressing auricular acupoint, auricular filiform-needle acupuncture therapy, take twirling reducing manipulation with filiform needle acupuncture for 30 minutes, conduct rotation surgery alternately over two ears, once each day, 10 times for a course of treatment, an interval of 5 days during a course; as for auricular embedding acupuncture method and sticking and pressing auricular acupoint method, select one side auricular point firstly, keep the point pressed for 3-5 days, advise patients to press the point several times by themselves each day, 1 minute for pressing each auricular point per time. After the auricular needle or seeds removed, proceed another side auricular point, left and right sides auricular acupoints applied alternately, 10 times for a course of treatment, with an interval of 1 week between courses, generally 1-2 courses shall be required. For serious obesity, at least 3-4 courses are required.

(Ⅲ) Moxibustion therapy

Prescription: Yangchi(TE 4), Sanjiaoshu(BL22).

Matching acupoints: Diji, Mingmen, Dazhui.

Methods: Select 1 main acupoint and 1 matching acupoint each time, apply moxibustion with moxa-roll, ignite one end of the moxa-roll, fix revolving moxibustion 3cm away from the acupoints, apply moxibustion for 10-15 minutes to each acupoint, 1 time each day or 1 time every other day, 1 month for a course of treatment.

Ⅲ. Precautions

1. The needling depth of acupoints for treating obesity is deeper than that of common people, the overweight ones should be punctured deeper or to the extent the arrival of Qi being achieved, otherwise ineffective.

2. Application of auriculotherapy shall be strictly sterilized in case of infection.

3. Advise patients to correct irrational diet habits in combination with acupuncture and moxibustion, and prevent relapse of disease.

4. Patients with secondary obesity should also be actively treated for primary disease.

Ⅳ. Modern clinical study

1. Observation on the curative effect of 350 cases of auricular needle-embedding therapy for losing weight.

Select 3 acupoints each time among auricular

分泌、神门、皮质下，每次3穴，埋揿针后用胶布固定，每3天（最多5天）更换1次，7次为1个疗程。观察结果：体重下降3～5公斤者115例，下降6～7公斤者78例，下降11～16公斤者26例，下降16公斤者14例，无效者117例，有效率66.6%[《中国针灸》1984，4（6）：17]。

2. 针灸减肥300例疗效分析。

一般资料：参与疗效评价者年龄在20岁以下有22例，20～30岁有265例，50岁以上有13例；其中男性43例，女性257例；体重最重者为116公斤，最轻者为65公斤；腹围最大者为127cm，最小者为80cm；肥胖史两年以上者35例，2～5年的215例，5年以上的41例，自幼肥胖者9例。治疗选穴：气虚湿滞、脾失健运型，取内关、水分、天枢、关元、丰隆平补平泻手法（电热针疗法40mA电流），三阴交、列缺施补法（电热针疗法给60mA）；胃强脾弱、湿热内蕴型，取曲池、支沟、四满、三阴交（平补平泻手法、电热针疗法给予电流40mA），内庭、腹

acupoints, including lung, spleen, stomach, endocrine, Shenmen and subcortex, embed needles and fix them with rubberized fabric, the needles shall be replaced once every 3 days (the maximum 5 days), 7 times for a course of treatment, the clinic results show that 115 cases of the weight lost by 3-5kg, 78 cases lost by 6-7kg, 26 cases lost by 11-16kg, 14 cases lost by 16kg, 117 cases ineffective, the effective rate accounts for 66.6% [*Chinese Acupuncture and Moxibustion*, 1984.4 (6):17].

2. Analysis on curative effect of 300 cases acupuncture for weight loss.

General information: 22 cases under 20 years of age, 265 cases of 20-30 years of age, 13 cases of above 50 years of age, among them, 43 cases for male and 257 cases for female, the largest weight was 116kg, the lightest 65kg, the longest abdominal circumference was 127cm, the shortest 80cm, 35 cases with an obesity history for more than two years, 215 cases for 2-5 years, 41 cases for more than 5 years, and 9 cases of obesity from children. For treatment of deficiency of Qi and Damp stagnation and dysfunction of spleen in transport type, apply even reinforcing-reducing method (electrothermal acupuncture therapy, at 40mA electrical current) at Neiguan, Shuifen, Tianshu, Guanyuan and Fenglong points; reinforcing method (electrothermal acupuncture therapy, at 60mA current) at Sanyinjiao and Leique points; for sthenia of stomach and asthenia of spleen and Damp-Heat syndrome, apply reinforcing-reducing method (electrothermal acupuncture therapy, at 40mA current) at Quchi, Zhigou, Siman, Sanyinjiao points, apply

结（泻法、电流 30mA）；冲任失调、带脉不和型，取支沟、中注（平补平泻手法、电流 40mA），关元、带脉、血海、三阴交、太溪（均补法、电流 60mA），每隔日治疗 1 次，每次电针 30～40 分钟，20 次为 1 个疗程。结果显示：显效 75 例（经 1 个疗程，体重下降 4 公斤以上者或腹围减少 10 厘米以上）占 25%，有效 192 例（经 1 个疗程，体重下降 2～4 公斤者或腹围减少 5～10 厘米）占 64%，无效 33 例（经 1 个疗程，体重下降不到 2 公斤者或腹围减少不足 5 厘米）占 11%，总有效 89%[《上海针灸》1988，7（3）：8]。

3. 耳穴压籽疗法减肥 540 例。

主穴：饥点、口、肺、脾。配穴：内分泌、直肠下端、肾。方法：将白芥子或王不留行籽，压在穴位上，按压 2 分钟之后用胶布固定，每 5 天换 1 次，7 次为 1 个疗程，休息 3 周再进行第 2 个疗程。结果：体重减轻 3 公斤以上者 81 例，减轻 0.5～2.5 公斤者 292 例，

reducing method (electrothermal acupuncture therapy, at 30mA current) at Neiting and Fujie points; for incoordination between the Chong and Ren Channels syndrome, apply even reinforcing-reducing method (electrothermal acupuncture therapy, at 40mA current) at Zhigou and Zhongzhu points; apply reinforcing method (electrothermal acupuncture therapy, at 60mA current) at Guanyuan, Daimai, Xuehai, Sanyinjiao and Taixi points. electrothermal acupuncture for 30-40 minutes once every other day, 20 times for a course of treatment. Clinical results: 75 cases with significant effect (the weight lost by 4kg or abdominal circumference reduced by over 10cm after a course of treatment) accounted for 25%; 192 cases effective (weight lost by 2-4kg or abdominal circumference reduced by 5-10cm after a course of treatment) accounted for 64%, 33 ineffective cases (weight lost by 2kg or abdominal circumference reduced by less than 5cm after 1 course of treatment) accounted for 11%, the total effective rate was 89% [*Shanghai Journal of Acupuncture and Moxibustion*, 1988.7 (3):8].

3. 540 cases of weight loss by auricular acupoint seed-pressing therapy.

Main acupoints: Jidian, mouth, lung, spleen. Matching acupoints: Endocrine, rectum, kidney. Method: Press semen brassicae or cowherb seed on the auricular acupoint for 2 minutes, then fix them with rubberized fabric, and replace them once every 5 days, 7 times for a course of treatment, 3 weeks interval for the second course of treatment. Clinic results: 81 cases of the weight lost by over 3kg, 292 cases of the weight lost by 0.5-2.5kg, 167 cases ineffective [*Shaanxi Journal of Traditional Chi-*

无效者167例［《陕西中医》1983，4（3）：23］。

nese Medicine, 1983.4(3):23］.

美容

面部特别是颜面部是最受人们注目的部位，当颜面部出现瘢痕、畸形、皮肤病（如痤疮、湿疹、疱疹）等，以及随着年龄增长出现皱纹、褐色斑，或皮肤松弛、眼睑下垂等一些生理老化现象时，容易影响美观。随着社会物质生活水平的不断提高，人们越来越重视自己的容颜。因此，各种各样的美容技术也应运而生。针灸美容主要是通过治疗面部的痤疮、扁平疣、色素斑、色素痣、血管瘤、酒渣鼻、斑秃等疾病，以及延缓或消除面部生理性衰老现象以达到美容的作用。本文重点讨论祛斑、除痣、消皱的美容方法。

一、美容方法

（一）毫针疗法

处方 斑纹部位、局部络穴。如额前部选阳白（GB14）、印堂（EX-HN3）、头维（ST8）；颧颊部选四白（ST2）、下关（ST7）、颊车（ST6）、大迎（ST5），

Cosmetology

The face, especially facial appearance, is the most conspicuous part, so when facial scars, deformities, skin diseases, such as acne, eczema, herpes, etc., are found in the face, and with aging, facial wrinkles, brown spots, skin laxity, eyelid drooping and other physiological aging phenomenon occur, it is most likely to affect the beauty of appearance. With the increasing improvement of the living level in China, people pay more and more attention to their facial appearance. So, a variety of cosmetology develops in the context, the acupuncture application to cosmetology is mainly by treating acne, flattened verruca, pigmented spots, pigmented nevus, hemangioma, rosacea, alopecia and other dermatoses, to delay or eliminate the physiological senescence of the face, for achieving cosmetic effect. This section focuses on the cosmetic method of removing spot and nevus, and eliminating wrinkles.

Ⅰ. Cosmetic method

(Ⅰ) Therapy of filiform needles

Prescription: Fleck location, part of Collateral points, e.g. select Yangbai (GB14), Yintang (EX-HN3), Touwei (ST8) in the anterior frontal part; select Sibai (ST2), Xiaguang(ST7), Jiache (ST6), Daying (ST5) at cheek; select Taiyang (EX-HN5), Sizhukong(TE23),

颞及眼角部选太阳（EX-HN5）、丝竹空（TE23）、瞳子髎（GB1），鼻部选迎香（LI20），下颌部选承浆（CV24）、合谷（LI4）、足三里（ST36）、三阴交（SP6）。

方义 针刺斑皱部位及附近络穴可疏通经络、行气活血，促进血液循环，改善皮肤组织营养状况。合谷、足三里、三阴交是调整全身脏腑功能的要穴，针刺有健脾和胃、调肝补肾、益气养血，使全身代谢功能旺盛或恢复正常的生理作用。诸穴合用，一是从局部着眼，二是从整体出发，共收祛斑除皱之功。

方法 皱纹部位及附近络穴宜浅刺或平刺，采用轻刺激或提插手法。合谷直刺0.5～0.7寸，足三里直刺0.6～0.8寸，三阴交直刺0.5～0.7寸，宜用中度刺激量（即平补平泻手法）针刺，每针20分钟。

疗程 每日1次或隔日1次，5次1个疗程，疗程间休息2天。

Tongziliao(GB1)between the ear and the eye on each side of the head; choose Yingxiang(LI20) at partes nasalis; select Chengjiang (CV（RN）24), Hegu (LI4), Zusanli (ST36), Sanyinjiao (SP6) at mandibular part.

Mechanism of prescription: Needling flecks location and nearby Collateral points can dredge the meridians, promote Qi to activate blood, improve blood circulation, improve the nutrition of skin. Hegu, Zusanli and Sanyinjiao are the key acupoints adjusting the internal organs of human body, the needling of which can strengthen spleen and stomach, tonify liver and invigorate kidney, replenish Qi, nourish and activate blood, make the entire body metabolism vigorous or recover to the normal. Jointedly using the acupoints, based on not only local but also entirety, can achieve the function of eliminating flecks and wrinkles.

Method: Shallow puncturing or horizontally puncturing are recommended to apply to parts with wrinkle and their nearby Collateral points, take slight-stimulation or lifting and thrusting manipulation. Perpendicularly puncture Hegu for 0.5-0.7", Zusanli for 0.6-0.8", Sanyinjiao for 0.5-0.7", it is advisable to use a moderate degree acupuncture, such as manipulation of even reinforcing and reducing movement, and the retention time of needling is 20 minutes.

Therapeutic course: 1 time each day or 1 time every other day, 5 times for a course of treatment, two days interval between courses.

（二）电火针疗法

处方 色素痣、血管瘤、瘢痕、色素斑局部。

方法 采用电火针治疗色素痣时，先在其周围点刺，然后在病灶中央点刺 1 针，使其整个病灶炭化；色素斑施术时，先在整个病灶上点刺，使其炭化；血管瘤施术时先在瘤中央（即病灶中央）刺入 1 针，然后沿病灶周围进行围刺。以上刺法宜浅刺，切忌深刺。其炭化组织多在治疗后 3～7 天之内自行脱落，局部皮色在 1 至 1 个半月恢复正常。一般 1 次即可结束治疗，若 1 年未愈可酌情增加治疗 1 次。

（三）耳针疗法

处方 肺、脾、肾、肝、内分泌。

方法 用 5 分长的毫针快速刺入耳穴，中度刺激，每针 30 分钟，每隔 10 分钟加强刺激 1 次。亦可压王不留行籽或耳针，3～5 天换 1 次。

疗程 10 次为 1 个疗程，

(II) Electric pyropuncture therapy

Prescription: Pigmented nevus, hemangioma, cicatrix, pigment spot.

Method: Select electric pyropuncture and make it aim at pigmented nevus and use pricking method at its periphery, then prick a needle at the center of lesions, make the lesions carbonization; when puncture at plain speckle of blood, first prick a needle at the entire lesions, make the lesions carbonization; when puncture at hemangioma, first prick a needle at the center of hemangioma (i.e. central tumor lesions of the central), then apply the method of encircling needling at the periphery of lesions. The aforesaid acupuncture should be the shallow puncturing, avoid deep puncturing by all means. The carbonized tissue mostly get off itself 3-7 days after the treatment, local skin color may turn normal in 1 month to 1 and half a month. Generally, it can be cured for one time, if it is not cured in one year, it may be given an additional treatment based on patient's conditions.

(III) Auriculotherapy

Prescription: Lung, spleen, kidney, liver, endocrine acupoint.

Method: Apply 5cm-long filiform needle and insert into auricular point at medium level of stimulation, 30 minutes retaining time per needling, and conduct strong stimulation one time with 10 minutes interval. Also press the seed of cowherb on the auricular acupoint, or change the auricular needle one time with 3-5 days interval.

Therapeutic course: 10 times for a course of treat-

每日1次或隔日1次，疗程期间休息3天。

（四）水针疗法

处方 肺俞（BL13）、脾俞（BL20）、肾俞（BL23）、病灶局部。

方法 此法适用于面部肌肉萎缩。根据辨证，血虚者用当归注射液，血瘀者用川芎注射液，肝郁兼血瘀者用丹参注射液，体虚者用胎盘注射液、维生素B12注射液。每次2个穴位，每个穴注0.5mL，隔日1次。

疗程 10次为1个疗程。

（五）耳穴刺血疗法

处方 耳前（热穴）、耳后（疖肿穴）、皮质下、内分泌，根据全身状况辨证，配脾穴、胃穴等。

方法 患者端坐，选定穴位常规消毒，用眼科15号小手术刀片，划破穴位表皮0.1cm，出血后以75%酒精棉球3个，连续拭净血迹，再用消毒干棉球压盖刺孔，防止感染。

ment, 1 time every day or 1 time every other day, 3 days interval between courses.

(Ⅳ) Hydro-acupuncture therapy

Prescription: Feishu(BL13), Pishu(BL20), Shenshu(BL23), local lesion.

Method: Suitable for facial muscle atrophy, in accordance with dialectics, blood deficiency patient is injected with angelica parenteral solution, patient with blood stasis is applied with chuanxiong injection, patients with stagnation of liver and blood stasis applied with Danshen injection. For patients with deficiency, placental histosolution and vitamin B12 injections are applied. Select 2 acupoints each time, and administrate 1 dose of 0.5ml injection for each acupoint, one time every other day.

Therapeutic course: 10 times for a course of treatment

(Ⅴ) Blood-pricking therapy of auricular acupoint

Prescription: Pre-auricula (hot acupoint), retroauricular (furuncle acupoint), subcortex acupoints, endocrine acupoint, and match spleen acupoint and stomach acupoint in term of the syndrome differentiation.

Method: Patient sits up straight; selecting the relevant acupoints and make routine disinfection, cut the epidermis of acupoint in the depth of 0.1cm with 15# small surgical blade of ophthalmology, continuously wipe off blood with three 75%-ethanol cotton balls after bleeding, then apply and squeeze the sterilized dry cotton ball to

疗程　根据病情选穴，隔日刺血1次，穴位交替使用，每次只刺1穴，15次为1个疗程，疗程间休息7～10天。

二、注意事项

1. 针对清除面部色斑及皱纹，若采用一种针刺方法效果不佳时，可采用多种方法综合治疗，可提高疗效。

2. 采用火针疗法时，治疗前要用麻沸散于病灶局部进行麻醉，以减少或清除火针点刺时的疼痛感。

3. 采用水针疗法时，一定要对所用器具及皮肤严格消毒，以防感染。

4. 施术前，对患者血常规及凝血时间进行检测，避免刺血后出血不止。

5. 向患者说明治疗方法，取得患者信任，减少患者的恐惧。

6. 体位的选择，对精神紧张的患者尤其重要，可防止晕针现象的发生。

7. 用75%酒精棉球擦拭耳部穴位出血时，要轻轻活动耳郭，避免用力挤捏。

cover the puncture hole in case of infection.

Therapeutic course: Selecting the relevant acupoints based on the condition of patients, one time blood-pricking every two day, alternate apply acupoints, prick one acupoint each time, 15 times for a course of treatment, and 7-10 days interval between courses.

II. Precautions:

1. In order to eliminate the facial stains and wrinkles, if the effect of a kind of acupuncture is not obvious, a variety of acupuncture methods can be comprehensively applied to improve the curative effects.

2. Using fire needle therapy, make Mafeisan soaked in local lesions for anesthesia before treatment, it can reduce or eliminate the pain-feeling of burning when fire needle prick.

3. When apply hydro acupuncture therapy, appliance and skin must be sterilized in case of infection.

4. Prior to needle insertion, give patients a blood routine examination and clotting time test, avoid bleeding post-blood-pricking.

5. Explain the treatment method to the patient, get the patient to cooperate with and not be afraid of the treatment.

6. It is particularly important for patients with mental stress to choose a right body position for avoiding fainting during his/her acupuncture treatments.

7. Wipe blood off ear with 75%-ethanol cotton ball, gently exercise helix to avoid vigorously squeezing and pinching.

8. 刺孔敷盖干棉球并固定，嘱患者保持棉球24小时不脱落，避免感染及着水；如遇耳部针孔愈合欠佳者，避免重复在原处刺血，防止感染或延误愈合。

三、现代临床研究

1. 电火针美容。

100例患者中，黄褐斑13例，色素痣47例，血管瘤2例，疣38例。先对病灶处消毒，将电火针对准病灶速刺疾出，根据病种不同，针刺方法略有差异。黄褐斑在整个病灶处，轻轻点刺，使其炭化；色素痣先在痣的周边刺，后在痣的中央刺1针，使整个病灶炭化；血管瘤先在病灶中央刺1针，然后沿病灶周边围刺，以上刺法切勿刺入皮下组织；针刺疣时，须围刺范围略大于病灶，稍深入皮下，以免复发。术后一般无须包扎，其炭化组织多在3～7天内自行脱落，局部肤色一个半月左右便可恢复正常。一般1次即可治愈。若1次未愈，可于5天后再行电火针1次［《中国针灸》1990，（4）］。

8. The puncture is covered with a dry cotton ball, patient is advised to keep the ball 24 hours for avoiding infection and water; in case of poor healing of hole in ears, avoid duplication of pricking blood in one location to prevent infection or delayed healing.

III. Modern clinical study

1. Electric pyropuncture for cosmetology.

Among 100 cases, 13 cases of chloasma, 47 cases of pigmented nevus, 2 cases of hemangioma, 38 cases of warts, firstly disinfect lesion, and then apply electric pyropuncture quickly and exactly at focal lesion. The acupuncture method varies slightly depending on the disease. Chloasma is located on the entire lesion, gently prick at the lesion and carbonize it; for pigmented nevus, puncture around the nevus firstly, and then apply one acupuncture in the center of the nevus to carbonize the entire lesion; for hemangioma, one acupuncture in the center of the lesion, and then conduct encircling needling around the lesion. Be sure not to puncture into the subcutaneous during applying the above-mentioned acupuncture manipulations. When warts are punctured, the scope of encircling needling shall be slightly larger than the lesion, slightly deeper into the subcutaneous to avoid recurrence. Generally, postoperative bandaging is not required. Most of carbonized tissues were off on their own within 3-7 days, local skin color came back to normal about 1 and a half months. Generally, it can be cured by 1 time acupuncture. If it wasn't cured for 1 time, the electric pyropuncture might be applied in 5 days for one

2.耳穴刺血疗法治疗黄褐斑283例临床观察。

临床资料：患者283例，均来源于门诊，其中男性54例，女性229例；最小年龄17岁，最大年龄44岁；大多为青年工人和学生。患者发斑部位多在面颊、鼻柱、眉或口唇上方，斑块小如硬币、或大如鹅卵，边界明显，或模糊不清；斑形多呈蝶翼状占全部病例的83.2%，呈褐色素沉着者占35%。病例病程：1～3年者131例，4～6年者62例，7～10年者57例，11～13年者33例，多数病例病程在1～6年。在治疗前曾经外治和内饮中药治疗者85%，未经过治疗者仅占15%。治疗方法及穴位选择：以耳前（热穴），耳后（疖肿穴），皮质下穴为主；再根据患者全身状况配用内分泌或脾穴、胃穴。操作方法：患者端坐，选定穴位常规消毒后，用眼科15号小手术刀片，划破穴位表皮0.1cm，出血后以75%酒精棉球3个，连续拭净血迹，再用消毒干棉球压盖刺孔，防止感染。疗程：根据病情选穴，

additional treatment [*Chinese Acupuncture and Moxibustion*, 1990. (4)].

2. Clinical observation of 283 cases of blood-pricking in auricular acupoint for chloasma treatment.

Clinical data: There were 283 cases in this group, all from outpatient services, 54 males and 229 females, of which, the youngest was aged 17, the oldest 44, who were mostly young workers and students. The patients in this group suffered from spots mostly on the cheeks, bridge of the nose, eyebrows or the upper lip. The plaques were as small as coin at size, or as large as the goose egg, with clear or vague edges. Spots were mostly shaped as butterfly wings, which accounted for 83.2% of all cases, 35% of patients with brown pigmentation. As for the patients' course of disease in this group, 131 cases for 1-3 years, 62 cases for 4-6 years, 57 cases for 7-10 years, 33 cases for 11-13 years, as you can see, the majority of cases were for 1-6 years. Before this treatment, 85% patients in the group had received external treatment and intake of Chinese Herd Medicine treatment, while only 15% untreated. For treatment method and acupoints selection, pre-auricula (hot acupoint) or retro-auricular (furuncle acupoint), subcortex acupoints take the leading role, and endocrine acupoint or spleen acupoint and stomach acupoint are matched for use in term of the general conditions of patients. Operation method: Patients sit up straight, the selected acupoints go through routine disinfection, and the epidermis of the disinfected acupoints are cut into 0.1cm with an ophthalmic No. 15 small scalpel blade. After bleeding, continuously wiped off blood with 3 cotton balls of 75%- ethanol, and then

隔日刺血1次，穴位交替使用，每次只刺1穴，15次为1个疗程，疗程后进行复查，如不愈者可继续2～3个疗程，疗程间可休息7～10天。治疗结果：痊愈165例，占58.3%；显效52例，占18.3%；好转24例，占8.4%；无效42例，占15%[《中国针灸》1983，（3）]。

3. 针刺和药物穴位注射治疗黛黑斑100例。

毫针主穴取大椎、曲池、血海、足三里、三阴交、风岩（耳垂下端与后发际中央连线的中点微前0.5寸处），每日或隔日1次，10次为1个疗程。不留针，多为平补平泻手法。耳穴取神门、交感、肾上腺、内分泌、皮质下、肺、肝、肾，每日每侧取2穴，每半小时按压针柄1次，以增强刺激，每针4小时后取针；穴位注射取肺俞、心俞、肝俞、肾俞，血虚者用当归注射液，血瘀者用川芎注射液，肝郁兼血瘀者用丹参注射液，体虚者用胎盘和

covered acupuncture holes with disinfected dry cotton ball to prevent infection. Course of treatment: Select acupoints according to the patient's condition, conduct blood-pricking once every other day, acupoints are alternately applied, one acupoint pricked each time, 15 times for a course of treatment, reviewing is conducted after a course of treatment, the uncured may continue to get 2-3 courses of treatment, and rest for 7-10 days between courses. Treatment results: 165 cases were cured, accounting for 58.3%, 52 cases were markedly effective, accounting for 18.3%, 24 cases were improved, accounting for 8.4%, and 42 cases were ineffective, accounting for 15% [(*Chinese Acupuncture and Moxibustion*, 1983. (3)].

3. 100 cases of curing black spots through acupuncture and injection of medicine into acupoints.

The main acupoints for filiform needle are Dazhui, Quchi, Xuehai, Zusanli, Sanyinjiao, Fengyan(0.5" in the middle of the middle point of the central line of the lower end of the earlobe and the back of the hairline), 1 time daily or once every other day, 10 times as a course of treatment. Do not leave the needle in the body. The method of mild reinforcing and attenuating are mostly applied. Among ear acupoints, choose Shenmen, point sympathetic, point adrenal gland, point endocrine, point subcortex, point lung, point liver, point kidney for acupuncture, and take 2 points per side per day for 4 needles, press needle once every half hour to enhance stimulating, withdraw needle in four hours for per needle; Choose Feishu, Xinshu, Ganshu, Shenshu for acupoint injection, blood deficiency patient is injected with angelica paren-

维生素 B12 注射液，每次选 2 穴，均取双侧，注射 1～2 支，每日或隔日 1 次，10 次为 1 个疗程；皮肤瘙痒者，每次用维丁胶性钙 2 支分别注于大椎、曲池、血海。针刺和穴位注射同时进行，每疗程间休息 2～3 天，5～6 个疗程休息半个月，一般需 20～25 个疗程。结果：治愈 16 例，显效 39 例，好转 40 例，无效 5 例。2 年后随访其中 44 例，疗效巩固和继续好转者共 38 例，轻度复发 5 例，复发 1 例［《中国针灸》1990，(4)：46］。

teral solution, patient with blood stasis is applied with chuanxiong rhizoma injection, patients with stagnation of liver and blood stasis applied with Danshen injection. For patients with deficiency, placental histosolution and vitamin B12 are applied. Take 2 acupoints each time, and administrate 1 dose or 2 doses of injection for each side, one time a day or two days, 10 times for a course of treatment. For cutaneous pruritus, for a dose, 2 vials of calcium colloidal et vit D are respectively injected into points, i.e. Dazhui, Quchi, Xuehai. Acupuncture and injection into acupoints are conducted simultaneously, 2-3 days interval following a course of treatment, half month interval follows 5-6 courses of treatment, generally 20-25 courses of treatment are needed. Result: 16 cases were cured, 39 cases were markedly effective, 40 cases were improved, 5 cases were ineffective. 44 cases were site-visited after 2 years, 38 cases were in stable curative effect and continued improvement, 5 cases of minor recurrence and 1 cases of recurrence [*Chinese Acupuncture and Moxibustion,* 1990. (4): 46].